ADVANCED
Assessment and Treatment of
Trauma

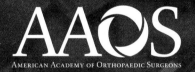

AMERICAN ACADEMY OF ORTHOPAEDIC SURGEONS

Michael D. Panté, NREMT-P, FP-C
Editor

Andrew N. Pollak, MD, FAAOS
Medical Editor

JONES AND BARTLETT PUBLISHERS
Sudbury, Massachusetts
BOSTON   TORONTO   LONDON   SINGAPORE

AAOS

AMERICAN ACADEMY OF ORTHOPAEDIC SURGEONS

World Headquarters

Jones and Bartlett Publishers
40 Tall Pine Drive
Sudbury, MA 01776
978-443-5000
info@jbpub.com
www.jbpub.com

Jones and Bartlett Publishers Canada
6339 Ormindale Way
Mississauga, Ontario L5V 1J2
Canada

Jones and Bartlett Publishers
  International
Barb House, Barb Mews
London W6 7PA
United Kingdom

Jones and Bartlett's books and products are available through most bookstores and online booksellers. To contact Jones and Bartlett Publishers directly, call 800-832-0034, fax 978-443-8000, or visit our website, www.jbpub.com.

Substantial discounts on bulk quantities of Jones and Bartlett's publications are available to corporations, professional associations, and other qualified organizations. For details and specific discount information, contact the special sales department at Jones and Bartlett via the above contact information or send an email to specialsales@jbpub.com.

Production Credits

Chief Executive Officer: Clayton Jones
Chief Operating Officer: Don W. Jones, Jr.
President, Higher Education and Professional Publishing:
  Robert W. Holland, Jr.
Sr. V.P., Sales and Marketing: James Homer
V.P., Design and Production: Anne Spencer
V.P., Manufacturing and Inventory Control: Therese Connell
Publisher: Kimberly Brophy
Acquisitions Editor—EMS: Christine Emerton
Associate Editor: Amanda Brandt
Production Manager: Jenny L. Corriveau

Senior Production Editor: Susan Schultz
Director of Sales: Matthew Maniscalco
Director of Marketing: Alisha Weisman
Marketing Associate: Meagan Norlund
Cover Design: Anne Spencer
Photo Research Manager and Photographer: Kimberly Potvin
Associate Photo Researcher: Jessica Elias
Compositor: Shepherd, Inc.
Cover Image: © Bob Keyes/*Jackson Citizen Patriot*/AP Photos
Printing and Binding: Courier Kendallville
Cover Printing: Courier Kendallville

The procedures and protocols in this book are based on the most current recommendations of responsible medical sources. The American Academy of Orthopaedic Surgeons and the publisher, however, make no guarantee as to, and assume no responsibility for, the correctness, sufficiency, or completeness of such information or recommendations. Other or additional safety measures may be required under particular circumstances.

This textbook is intended solely as a guide to the appropriate procedures to be employed when rendering emergency care to the sick and injured. It is not intended as a statement of the standards of care required in any particular situation, because circumstances and the patient's physical condition can vary widely from one emergency to another. Nor is it intended that this textbook shall in any way advise emergency personnel concerning legal authority to perform the activities or procedures discussed. Such local determination should be made only with the aid of legal counsel.

The patients and providers described in the case studies throughout this textbook are fictitious.

Library of Congress Cataloging-in-Publication Data

Advanced assessment and treatment of trauma/American Academy of Orthopaedic Surgeons;   Michael Pante.
  p. ; cm.
Includes bibliographical references and index.
ISBN-13: 978-0-7637-5131-9
ISBN-10: 0-7637-5131-6
1. Traumatology. 2. Wounds and injuries. 3. Emergency medical technicians. I. Panté, Michael D. II. American Academy of Orthopaedic Surgeons.
[DNLM: 1. Wounds and Injuries—diagnosis. 2. Wounds and Injuries—therapy. 3. Emergency Medical Services—methods. 4. Emergency Medical Technicians. WO 700 A846 2010]
RD93.A855 2010
617.1—dc22

2009000289

6048
Printed in the United States of America
16 15 14 13 12   10 9 8 7 6 5 4 3

Brief Contents

Contents

Resource Preview

Advanced Assessment and Treatment of Trauma (ATT) represents the state-of-the-art in prehospital trauma assessment and management. Based on the most current medical information and best practices, this concise and highly interactive continuing education course covers the critical knowledge and skills necessary to rapidly evaluate, stabilize, and transport the trauma patient.

This textbook is the core of the ATT Course with features that will reinforce and expand on the essential information. These features include:

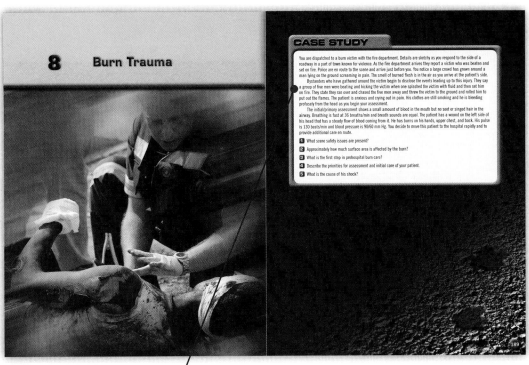

Case Study: A pictorial case study takes readers immediately to the scene of the emergency. Found in each chapter, these compelling case studies grab the reader's attention and promote their critical thinking skills. Questions posed in the case study are discussed in the Chapter Resources section at the end of the chapter.

Tip: Tips are featured throughout the chapters to reinforce the most critical concepts.

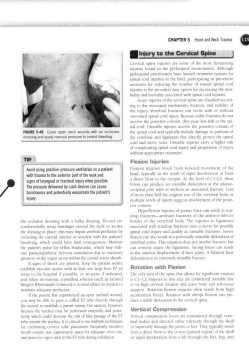

Sample page — Chapter 3

PRO/CON

Digital intubation is a technique using just the provider's fingers to guide the endotracheal tube past the epiglottis and into the trachea. The provider places the first two fingers on one hand in the patient's mouth, locates the tip of the epiglottis with the middle finger, and slides the ETT down the groove between the two fingers, helped over the epiglottis by the middle finger.

Digital intubation may be a useful tool with patients who have a mandibular fracture or open facial trauma requiring immediate intubation to secure an airway. This technique has several negatives, however, including patients with an intact gag reflex, the chance for the provider to be bitten, and the provider's hand being too short to reach the epiglottis. A blind technique also increases the chance for a misplaced ETT.

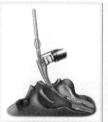

FIGURE 3-18 The gum elastic stylet can assist with an intubation when direct visualization of the airway cannot be accomplished.

Nasotracheal Intubation

Nasotracheal (nasal) intubation is an alternative to orotracheal intubation but with limited applications in the trauma patient **PROCEDURE 10**. The primary indication for nasal intubation is the patient who is expected to have a difficult airway but has spontaneous ventilations.

Nasotracheal intubation requires the patient to be placed into the sniffing position. Suspected cervical spine injury will limit the ability to position the patient to receive the nasal intubation. Contraindications to nasotracheal intubation include:

- Mid-face trauma or suspected basilar skull fracture
- Apnea

Relative contraindications include:

- Combativeness
- Increased intracranial pressure (ICP)
- Suspected hypertension
- Coagulopathy

Nasotracheal intubation should also be avoided in patients who have low oxygen or ventilatory reserves, because the procedure will take more time than the previously discussed procedures.

After lubricating the tube, it is advanced through one of the nares into the hypopharynx. When breath sounds (or whistling through the tube) are heard, the tube should be advanced quickly during inhalation. When the tube enters the trachea the patient will cough. Placement must be confirmed. If no breath sounds are heard, the tube does

not advance, or gastric sounds are present, the tube must be repositioned and the procedure attempted again.

An alternative to the standard endotracheal tube is the Endotrol tube. It is more flexible and has an attached line to help the provider curve the end up to enter the trachea when advanced.

Retrograde Endotracheal Intubation

Another technique used to guide a tracheal tube into the trachea is retrograde endotracheal intubation (REI). The technique requires advanced skill and additional time, making it a rarely used technique in the hospital setting and even less frequently used technique in the prehospital setting. REI requires a catheter to be placed through the cricothyroid membrane and a flexible wire inserted through the catheter, then advanced upward into the mouth. The tracheal tube is then placed over the wire and advanced into the trachea. The wire and catheter are then removed and the tracheal tube advanced slightly into position. There are commercial kits available for the procedure. Given the infrequent use and potential complications, REI should be reserved for when conventional intubation techniques have failed to ventilate the patient and only if local protocols allow.

Pharmacologically Assisted Intubation

Rapid sequence intubations (RSIs) are the standard for intubations in the trauma center. Prehospital systems have begun to investigate this technique and some have developed protocols for usage. Drug-facilitated intubations commonly use a sedative and paralytic agent. Not all patients will require RSI, because many can be intubated with a sedative or an induction agent alone.

Premedication Agents

Several medications may be helpful before intubating a patient. These are referred to as premedication agents The mnemonic LOAD is often used to remember these agents **TABLE 3-2**.

Pro/Con: Pros and cons are a concise discussion of various controversies in prehospital trauma assessment and treatment.

Key Terms: Key terms noting essential terminology are identified throughout the chapters. A comprehensive glossary of key terms is found at the end of the textbook.

Sample page — Glossary

Glossary

abandonment The termination of the provider-patient relationship without preventing for the appropriate continuation of care.

acceleration (a) The rate of change of velocity that an object is subjected to, whether speeding up or slowing down.

Achilles tendon The strong, fibrous cord that attaches the muscles in the back of the leg to the heel.

acidosis An excess of hydrogen ions in the body, which causes the pH to drop below 7.35.

acidosis Increased acid in the blood plasma.

acromioclavicular joint The shoulder.

active external rewarming Applying heat directly to the skin to rewarm the body.

active internal rewarming Directing the heat into the core and essentially warming the body from the inside.

adventitious Abnormal.

afterdrop Situation in which cold blood sequestered in the peripheral areas of the body is moved into the core.

afterload The pressure against which the heart must pump.

agnosia The inability to comprehend auditory, visual, or sensational stimuli, even though the eyes, ears, and other sensory organs are intact.

air embolism A process caused by sudden expansion of dissolved gas in the bloodstream. This results in embolization and occlusion of blood flow to a vital organ such as the brain, heart, or lungs.

alkalosis A decrease in the number of hydrogen ions in the body, causing the pH to increase above 7.45.

alveoli Small air sacs in the lungs.

amputation The complete separation or loss of a body part, usually a finger, toe, arm, or leg.

angiotensin II Hormone that helps reduce urine production.

anterior-posterior compression fracture (straddle fracture) Fracture associated with a slight widening of the pubic symphysis along with a fracture at the sacroiliac joint, whereby the pelvis is separated both front and back.

anterograde (posttraumatic) amnesia A loss of memory relating to events that occurred after an injury.

antidiuretic hormone (ADH) Hormone released from the pituitary gland to stimulate the kidneys to retain water and sodium, also called vasopressin.

aorta The large blood vessel near the heart.

aortic balloon pump A mechanical device used to decrease oxygen demand while increasing cardiac output. The device uses a balloon inserted in the aorta to inflate and deflate timed with the cardiac cycle.

aphasia The inability to communicate through speech, writing, or signs because of brain dysfunction.

apraxia The inability to perform purposeful movements when the motor and sensory organs are not directly impaired.

aqueous humor Clear watery fluid that fills the anterior chamber of the globe of the eye.

arachnoid mater The second meningeal layer, a delicate, transparent membrane.

arterial pressure points Locations on extremities where large arteries from the trunk of the body pass near bones as they enter the extremity.

arteriosclerosis The stiffening of vessel walls.

ataxia Lack of muscular coordination.

autonomic nervous system System that controls the cardiovascular system and is composed of two competing subsystems.

avulsion A three-sided cut that leaves a flap of skin and soft tissue attached to the body on the fourth side.

avulsion fracture An injury to the bone where a tendon or ligament attaches to the bone.

axon A long, slender extension of a neuron that conducts electrical impulses away from the neuronal soma in the brain.

bariatrics The branch of medicine that deals with obesity and related health issues.

barometric energy Energy resulting from sudden and radical changes in pressure, often during diving or flying.

basal metabolic rate (BMR) The number of kilocalories created by the body per hour.

Bennett's fracture Fracture of the base of the thumb.

biomechanics The study of the physiology and mechanics of a living organism using the tools of mechanical engineering.

blast front The leading edge of a shock wave.

blunt trauma Injuries in which the tissues are not penetrated by an external object.

boxer's fracture Metacarpal neck fracture of the little finger.

Boyle's law A gas law that states that pressure and volume of gas are directly proportional. Important because the volume of air will increase if the patient is moved to a higher altitude, as occurs during flight transfers.

bradypnea Slow respiratory rate.

brain stem Structure located at the base of the brain that connects the spinal cord to the remainder of the brain. It houses many structures that are critical to the maintenance of vital functions.

breach of duty When the provider deviates from what would be considered good and accepted practice.

bronchi The two main branches of the trachea.

bronchiole Small tube that branches from the bronchi to the alveoli in the lungs.

bronchorrhea Excessive mucus production by the bronchial mucus membrane.

burn Diffuse soft tissue injury created by destructive energy transfer via radiation, thermal energy, or electrical energy.

burn shock Shock that occurs because of fluid loss across the damaged skin and because of a series of volume shifts within the body itself.

bursa A synovial-like membrane around the joint to protect it and to decrease the friction of rubbing tendons over their boney prominences.

calcaneus The bone in the back of the foot, commonly referred to as the heel.

383

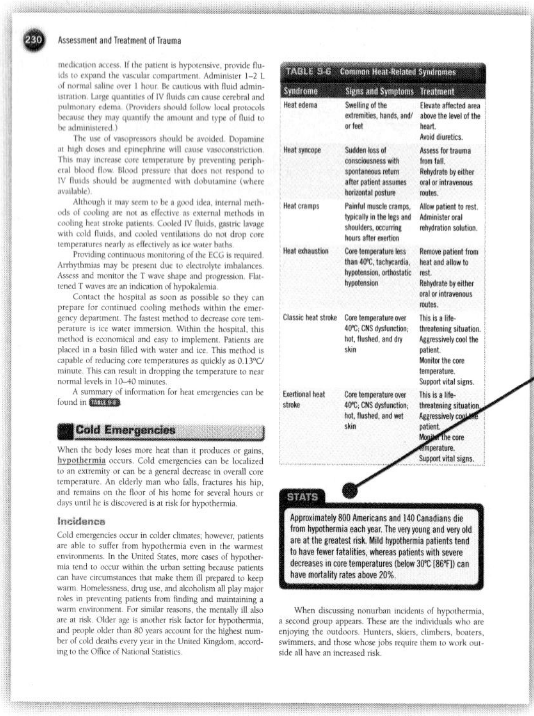

Sample page — Assessment and Treatment of Trauma

230 Assessment and Treatment of Trauma

medication access. If the patient is hypotensive, provide fluids to expand the vascular compartment. Administer 1–2 L of normal saline over 1 hour. Be cautious with fluid administration. Large quantities of IV fluids can cause cerebral and pulmonary edema. (Providers should follow local protocols because they may quantify the amount and type of fluid to be administered.)

The use of vasopressors should be avoided. Dopamine at high doses and epinephrine will cause vasoconstriction. This may increase core temperature by preventing peripheral blood flow. Blood pressure that does not respond to IV fluids should be augmented with dobutamine (where available).

Although it may seem to be a good idea, internal methods of cooling are not as effective as external methods in cooling heat stroke patients. Cooled IV fluids, gastric lavage with cold fluids, and cooled ventilations do not drop core temperatures nearly as effectively as ice water baths.

Providing continuous monitoring of the ECG is required. Arrhythmia may be present due to electrolyte imbalances. Assess and monitor the T wave shape and progression. Flattened T waves are an indication of hypokalemia.

Contact the hospital as soon as possible so they can prepare for continued cooling methods within the emergency department. The fastest method to decrease core temperature is ice water immersion. Within the hospital, this method is economical and easy to implement. Patients are placed in a basin filled with water and ice. This method is capable of reducing core temperatures as quickly as 0.13°C/minute. This can result in dropping the temperature to near normal levels in 10–40 minutes.

A summary of information for heat emergencies can be found in **TABLE 9-6**.

Cold Emergencies

When the body loses more heat than it produces or gains, hypothermia occurs. Cold emergencies can be localized to an extremity or can be a general decrease in overall core temperature. An elderly man who falls, fractures his hip, and remains on the floor of his home for several hours or days until he is discovered is at risk for hypothermia.

Incidence

Cold emergencies occur in colder climates; however, patients are able to suffer from hypothermia even in the warmest environments. In the United States, more cases of hypothermia tend to occur within the urban setting because patients can have circumstances that make them ill prepared to keep warm. Homelessness, drug use, and alcoholism all play major roles in preventing patients from finding and maintaining a warm environment. For similar reasons, the mentally ill also are at risk. Older age is another risk factor for hypothermia, and people older than 80 years account for the highest number of cold deaths every year in the United Kingdom, according to the Office of National Statistics.

TABLE 9-6	Common Heat-Related Syndromes	
Syndrome	Signs and Symptoms	Treatment
Heat edema	Swelling of the extremities, hands, and/or feet	Elevate affected area above the level of the heart. Avoid diuretics.
Heat syncope	Sudden loss of consciousness with spontaneous return after patient assumes horizontal posture	Assess for trauma from fall. Rehydrate by either oral or intravenous routes.
Heat cramps	Painful muscle cramps, typically in the legs and shoulders, occurring hours after exertion	Allow patient to rest. Administer oral rehydration solution.
Heat exhaustion	Core temperature less than 40°C, tachycardia, hypotension, orthostatic hypotension	Remove patient from heat and allow to rest. Rehydrate by either oral or intravenous routes.
Classic heat stroke	Core temperature over 40°C, CNS dysfunction; hot, flushed, and dry skin	This is a life-threatening situation. Aggressively cool the patient. Monitor the core temperature. Support vital signs.
Exertional heat stroke	Core temperature over 40°C, CNS dysfunction; hot, flushed, and wet skin	This is a life-threatening situation. Aggressively cool the patient. Monitor the core temperature. Support vital signs.

STATS

Approximately 800 Americans and 140 Canadians die from hypothermia each year. The very young and very old are at the greatest risk. Mild hypothermia patients tend to have fewer fatalities, whereas patients with severe decreases in core temperatures (below 30°C (86°F)) can have mortality rates above 20%.

When discussing nonurban incidents of hypothermia, a second group appears. These are the individuals who are enjoying the outdoors. Hunters, skiers, climbers, boaters, swimmers, and those whose jobs require them to work outside all have an increased risk.

Stats: Statistics are highlighted throughout the textbook to offer perspective on the occurrence of particular trauma situations.

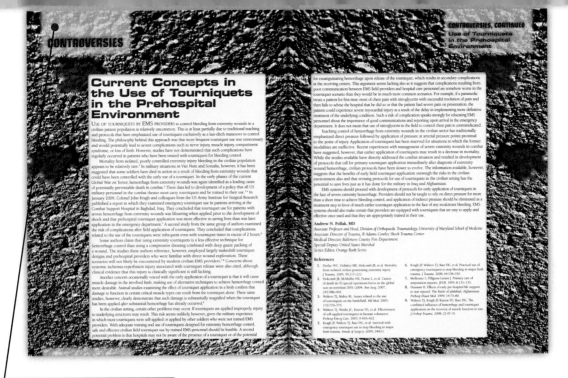

Controversies: Leading physicians weigh in on current controversies in trauma treatment and management, including controversies brought on by changing technology or very recent changes in treatment modalities.

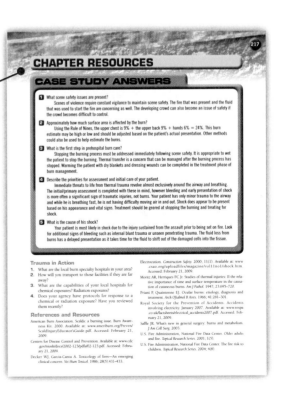

Chapter Resources: This section provides answers to the questions posed in the case study, suggests additional resources that may supplement the chapter content, and presents additional discussion questions.

PROCEDURE 3
Glasgow Coma Scale Assessment and Grading

Introduction

It is important to determine the level of consciousness for trauma patients. From levels of disorientation to the severity of a trauma patient's head injury, the ability to qualify and quantify the level can be difficult for the provider to do on-scene. The Glasgow Coma Scale (GCS) provides a simple and relatively reproducible assessment of the level of consciousness. Based on an evaluation of the patient's eye opening and verbal and motor responses, the on-scene provider can determine the general severity of the head injury and effectively communicate this to the receiving facility.

Indications, Contraindications, and Equipment

Indications	Altered levels of consciousness Head trauma
Contraindications	None
Equipment	Exam gloves and goggles

Rationale

Patients who have experienced an injury often present with a decreased or decreasing level of consciousness or coma. Prehospital providers must be able to assess the level of responsiveness both to determine the need for treatment and to present a baseline medical exam to the receiving facility to further the patient's care. The GCS is an easily repeated exam tool that enables providers to obtain and relay this information to others quickly and in a useful format.

Possible Complications

Mistaking patient responses while assessing the GCS can lead to incorrect prioritization and/or treatment both prehospitally and during the initial phase of in-hospital care.

Procedure

1 Assess eye opening.
  a. If the patient's eyes are open, the score is 4.
  b. If the eyes are closed, say the patient's name or ask them to open their eyes. If they open, the score is 3.

  c. If the eyes remain closed, apply a painful stimulus such as pressure over a fingernail. If the eyes open, the score is 2.
  d. If the eyes do not open, the score is 1.
  e. Note: If the eyes are swollen and cannot open, the score is omitted for the section and a "C" (for closed) placed in the comments.

2 Assess motor response.
  a. Ask the patient to complete a task ("Lift your arm"). If the patient completes the task with no prompting, the score is 6. Note: Do not ask the patient to squeeze your fingers because this response can be confused with a grasp reflex.
  b. If the patient does not complete the task, apply a painful stimulus to one side of the body. This can be done by putting pressure on a fingernail of one hand, squeezing the trapezius muscle, or applying supraorbital pressure to the rim above the eye. If the patient reaches across the midline in response to the pain (as to push you away), the patient is said to localize pain and the score is 5. Do not use a sternal rub because the result may be confusing to interpret so close to the center.
  c. If the patient responds to the pain by withdrawing from the pain, the score is 4. The trapezius pinch may be better suited to a centralized response and will produce a shrug of the shoulder.

  d. If the patient responds to pain by abnormal flexion of the extremity, as seen by wrist flexion, upper arm adduction, or flexion of the fingers over the thumb, the patient is said to be decorticate posturing and receives a score of 3. Also common to the upper arm movements are extension of the head and neck and extension of the lower extremities.

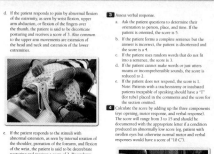

  e. If the patient responds to the stimuli with abnormal extension, as seen by internal rotation of the shoulder, pronation of the forearm, and flexion of the wrist, the patient is said to decerebrate posturing and receives a score of 2. Decerebrate posturing also has extension of the head and neck with extension of the lower extremities. Posturing is a primitive response by the brain to attempt to remove the painful stimuli.

  f. If there is no response the score is 1. Note: If the patient is chemically paralyzed or sedated, a "P" or "S" should be inserted into the comments, respectively, and the score omitted for the section.

3 Assess verbal response.
  a. Ask the patient questions to determine their orientation to person, place, and time. If the patient is oriented, the score is 5.
  b. If the patient forms a complete sentence but the answer is incorrect, the patient is disoriented and the score is 4.
  c. If the patient uses random words that do not fit into a sentence, the score is 3.
  d. If the patient cannot make words or just utters moans or incomprehensible sounds, the score is reduced to 2.
  e. If the patient does not respond, the score is 1. Note: Patients with a tracheostomy or intubated patients incapable of speaking should have a "T" (for tube) placed in the comments and the score for the section omitted.

4 Calculate the score by adding up the three components (eye opening, motor response, and verbal response). The score will range from 3 to 15 and should be documented with the appropriate letter if a condition produced an abnormally low score (eg, patient with swollen eyes but otherwise normal motor and verbal responses would have a score of "10 C").

5 Repeat the assessment every 15 minutes to trend changes to the baseline or anytime a significant change is noted.

Procedures: The 36 procedures provide a step-by-step guide to the most critical ALS-level trauma skills. Each procedure includes:
- Introduction
- Indications
- Contraindications
- Equipment
- Rationale
- Possible Complications
- Step-by-step pictorial walk-through

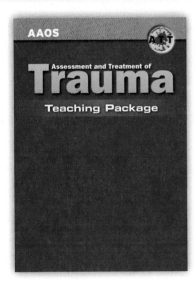

Teaching Package

ISBN: 978-0-7637-7380-9

The ATT program is supported by a comprehensive Teaching Package that includes all the components you need to teach the course. This package can be used to teach either the Basic or Advanced ATT Course. Included in the package are:

ToolKit CD-ROM

This invaluable resource includes:
- Helpful tips and guidelines for teaching an ATT Course
- Administrative information for the Course Coordinator's convenience
- Compelling PowerPoint presentations and lecture notes
- Detailed scenarios for small-group discussions
- Skills station strategies and activities

DVD

Containing real-life footage from the field, this DVD will engage participants' interest and show them the skills that are central to the assessment and treatment of trauma patients.

www.ATTrauma.com

Make full use of today's teaching and learning technology with www.ATTrauma.com, a community of ATT users and providers. This site has been specifically designed to complement ATT and is updated regularly.

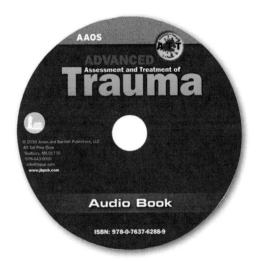

Included in each copy of *Advanced Assessment and Treatment of Trauma* are:

Advanced Assessment and Treatment of Trauma Audio Book

This CD-ROM contains an audio version of the ATT textbook so that you can prepare for class while sitting in your car or office. The files are provided in .mp3 format.

Precourse Online Module Access Code

An access code to the 2-hour Precourse Online Module is packaged in each textbook. This module is designed to guide the participant through much of the cognitive material associated with the Advanced ATT Course. The module provides an opportunity to refresh knowledge of basic trauma concepts using cutting-edge technology to create a colorful, dynamic, and interesting learning environment that maximizes retention. At the end of the module, participants take a final exam and print a certificate of completion.

Acknowledgments

The American Academy of Orthopaedic Surgeons and Jones and Bartlett Publishers would like to thank the many authors, contributors, and reviewers who enhanced this textbook and course with their knowledge and their dedication to trauma education.

Authors

Lead Author
Michael D. Panté, NREMT-P, FP-C
BMA Education
Flemington, New Jersey

Chapter 1
Michael D. Panté, NREMT-P, FP-C
BMA Education
Flemington, New Jersey

Chapter 2
Michael D. Panté, NREMT-P, FP-C
BMA Education
Flemington, New Jersey

Chapter 3
Michael D. Panté, NREMT-P, FP-C
BMA Education
Flemington, New Jersey

Chapter 4
Bruce Butterfras, MS-Ed, LP
The University of Texas Health Science Center at San Antonio
San Antonio, Texas

Chapter 5
Alan Heckman, BS, NREMT-P, NCEE
Program Coordinator
Lehigh Valley Health Network
GEM-Emergency Medicine Institute
Allentown, Pennsylvania

Stephen J. Rahm, NREMT-P
EMS Professions Educator
Bulverde-Spring Branch EMS
Spring Branch, Texas

Chapter 6
Michael D. Smith, NREMT-P, CCEMT-P, EMSI
City of Grandview Heights Division of Fire, Paramedic/
 Fire Fighter
Coordinator, Ohio University–Lancaster EMS Education
Grant LifeLink, Outreach Educator
Flight Paramedic, MedFlight
Columbus, Ohio

Chapter 7
David J. Filtranti, PA-C
Orthopaedic Surgery Physician Assistant
Hunterdon Orthopedic Institute, PA
Flemington, New Jersey

Randy A. Smith, NREMT-P
Evangelical Community Hospital
Paramedic Coordinator
Pre-Hospital Services
Lewisburg, Pennsylvania

Chapter 8
Charles Bortle, MEd, NREMT-P, RRT
Director EMS Education
Albert Einstein Medical Center
Philadelphia, Pennsylvania

Chapter 9
Charles W. Sowerbrower, MEd, NREMT-P, NCEE
Sinclair Community College
Dayton, Ohio

Chapter 10
Samuel A. Getz, Jr, BS, NREMT-P, EMSI
President and CEO, EMS/QA Systems Consulting Service
EMS Coordinator, Western Reserve Joint Fire District
Paramedic/Fire Fighter, Newton Falls Joint Fire District
Austintown, Ohio

Christopher B. Haber, NREMT-P
EMS Educator
Owner, MEDPRO EMS Education
Hulmeville, Pennsylvania

Chapter 11
Alan J. Azzara, Esq, EMT-P
EMS Attorney and Consultant
Former Vice President and Legal Counsel
North East Mobile Health Services
Scarborough, Maine

Chapter 12
Scott C. Donohue, BS, NREMT-P
Somerset Medical Center
Somerville, New Jersey

Chapter 13
Sophia Hazel, DO
Endocrinologist, Sacramento County Department of Health
    and Human Services
Assistant Clinical Professor, Division of Endocrinology,
Clinical Nutrition, and Vascular Medicine
University of California Davis Medical Center
Sacramento, California

C. Nathan Hox, BS, LVN, NREMT-B
University of California Davis Medical Center
Sacramento, California
Core Cadre Instructor
349th Medical Group, USAFR
Travis Air Force Base, California

Matthew J. Sena, MD, NREMT-P
Assistant Professor, Division of Trauma and Emergency
    Surgery
University of California Davis Medical Center
Sacramento, California
Medical Director, EMT Basic and Pre-Hospital Trauma Life
    Support Program
349th Medical Group, USAFR
Travis Air Force Base, California

Procedures
Brian D. Bricker, EMT CFC
REACH Air Medical
Santa Rosa, California

Senior Contributor

Mark Woolcock BSc(Hons), PG Dip, Cert Ed, MPara, MiFL
Emergency Care Practitioner
College of Paramedics
Truro, United Kingdom

Contributors

Jonathan Borak, MD, DABT
Clinical Professor of Epidemiology and Medicine
Yale School of Medicine
New Haven, Connecticut

Raymond L. Fowler, MD, FACEP
Professor of Emergency Medicine, Surgery
Associate Professor of Allied Health Professions
Chief of EMS Operations
Co-Chief in the Section on EMS, Disaster Medicine,
    and Homeland Security
University of Texas Southwestern Medical Center
Attending Faculty, Parkland Memorial Hospital Emergency
    Department
Dallas, Texas

Marianne Gausche-Hill, MD
Department of Emergency Medicine
Harbor–UCLA Medical Center
Torrance, California

Henry Guly, MD, FCEM, FRCP
Consultant in Emergency Medicine
Derriford Hospital
Plymouth, United Kingdom

Timothy Horeczko, MD
Department of Emergency Medicine
Harbor–UCLA Medical Center
Torrance, California

Russell D. MacDonald, MD, MPH, FCPC, FRCPC
Medical Director, Research Program, Ornge Transport
    Medicine
Assistant Professor, Division of Emergency Medicine
Faculty of Medicine, University of Toronto
Toronto, Ontario, Canada

Evadne Marcolini, MD
Assistant Professor
Division of Surgical Critical Care and Emergency Medicine
R Adams Cowley Shock Trauma Center
University of Maryland Medical Center
Baltimore, Maryland

Donald L. Parsons, PA-C, MPAS
Department of Combat Medic Training
Fort Sam Houston, Texas

Andrew N. Pollak, MD
Associate Professor and Head, Division of Orthopaedic
    Traumatology, University of Maryland School of Medicine
Associate Director of Trauma, R Adams Cowley Shock
    Trauma Center
Medical Director, Baltimore County Fire Department
Special Deputy United States Marshal
Series Editor, Orange Book Series
Baltimore, Maryland

Dave Spear, MD, FACEP
Clinical Assistant Professor
Emergency Ultrasound Programs
Parkland Hospital
Dallas Children's Medical Center
Dallas, Texas

Henry E. Wang, MD, MS
University of Alabama at Birmingham
Birmingham, Alabama

Joseph P. Wood, MD, JD
Consultant and Vice-Chair
Department of Emergency Medicine
Mayo Clinic in Arizona
Phoenix, Arizona

Reviewers

George P. Abraham, MD, FACS, FRCS (Edin)
Troy Community Hospital
Troy, Pennsylvania

Lewis Andrews, Paramedic
USAR Paramedic Instructor
East of England Ambulance Service NHS Trust
Bedfordshire, United Kingdom

Leaugeay C. Barnes, BS, CCEMT-P, NREMT-P
Oklahoma City Community College
Oklahoma City, Oklahoma

Helga Bell
Retired
Sao Paulo, Brasil

Robert Bernini, EMT-P
Harrisburg Area Community College
Shumaker Public Safety Center
Harrisburg, Pennsylvania

T. J. Bishop, AAS, NREMT-P
Clinical Division Chief
North Country EMS
Yacolt, Washington

Susan Boardman, Paramedic, PG Dip, FHEA, MIFL
Course Leader in Paramedic Practice
Faculty of Health and Wellbeing
Sheffield Hallam University
Sheffield, United Kingdom

Lea Ann Bobbitt
National College of Technical Instruction (NCTI)
Mesquite, Texas

Alfie Bondoc
USAF
California State University Sacramento
University of Saint Eustatius School of Medicine
Sacramento, California

David Bradley
Senior Lecturer
Liverpool John Moores University
Liverpool, United Kingdom

John Bray, BS, NREMT-P, CCEMT-P
Saint Vincent's Hospital–Manhattan
Institute of Emergency Care
New York, New York

Justin Carding, HEMS Paramedic
Helicopter Emergency
Surrey Sussex Medical Services
Surrey, England

Graham Chalk, Bsc (Hons), Paramedic
Paramedic Training Department
London Ambulance Service NHS Trust
London, United Kingdom

Vince Clarke, BSc (Hons), Paramedic, PGCE
Paramedic Tutor
London Ambulance Service NHS Trust
London, England

Glen William Clegg
Administration Chief
Zephyrhills Fire Rescue
Zephyrhills, Florida

Heidi P. Cordi, MD, MPH, MS, EMT-P, FACEP
Associate Medical Director
Emergency Medical Services
The New York Presbyterian Hospital
New York, New York

Ray Crooks, PGCEd, Paramedic
London Ambulance Service NHS Trust
London, England

Mark Cutler, Paramedic, QTS, MIFL
Senior Lecturer in Pre-Hospital Medicine
Faculty of Health and Wellbeing
Sheffield Hallam University
Sheffield, United Kingdom

Dr Paul de Jong
Honorary Medical Director, PHTLS Australia
District Director Emergency Medicine
Fraser Coast Health, Hervey Bay Hospital
Hervey Bay, Australia

Clyde Deschamp, PhD, NREMT-P
University of Mississippi Medical Center
Jackson, Mississippi

Paul Down, BSc (Hons), Paramedic, Cert Ed (PCET)
Emergency Care Practitioner
South Western Ambulance Service NHS Trust
Barnstable, United Kingdom

Martha Driscoll, EMT-P, NREMT
Assistant Professor
Daytona Beach College
Daytona Beach, Florida

Christopher Ebright, BEd, NREMT-P
EMS Education Program Director
MedCorp, Inc. Training and Education Center
Toledo, Ohio

Bob Elling, MPA, REMT-P
Clinical Instructor
Albany Medical Center
HVCC Paramedic Program
Troy, New York

Ricky Ellis, H Dip EMT
Advanced Paramedic, Clinical Tutor
Dublin Fire Brigade/Royal College of Surgeons
Dublin, Ireland

Jonathan L. Epstein, MEMS, NREMT-P
Executive Director
NorthEast Emergency Medical Services, Inc.
Wakefield, Massachusetts

Leif Erickson, CCEMT-P
Flight Paramedic/Education Coordinator
EMS Instructor/Coordinator
Madison Area Technical College
Flight For Life—Milwaukee/Waukesha
Madison, Wisconsin

John Bastian Etti
EMS Education Coordinator
TUV Rheinland Akademie GmbH EMS School
Associate National Coordinator, PHTLS Germany
Neuwied, Germany

Bob Fellows, BSc, Paramedic, PGCE
University of Hertfordshire
Hatfield, United Kingdom

Graham Fisher, CPO, SRP
West Midlands Ambulance Service NHS Trust
West Midlands, United Kingdom

Nichola Fothergill, Paramedic
Organisational Learning Department
Midlands Ambulance Service
Lincolnshire, England

Steven K. Frye, BS, NREMT-P
Faculty, University of Maryland
Maryland Fire and Rescue Institute
College Park, Maryland

Scott Garrett, NREMT-P
Fire Chief
Westview-Fairforest Fire & EMS Department
Spartanburg, South Carolina

Jennifer M. K. Glass, CRT, USAF, CCATT
United States Air Force
USAFA, Colorado

Steve Greisch, CRNA
National Coordinator, PHTLS Luxembourg
CFPC Widong
Centre Hospitalier Emile Mayrisch Esch/Alzette
Esch-sur-Alzette, Luxembourg

Wiro J. G. G. Gruijters, RN
National Coordinator, PHTLS The Netherlands
Programmemanager Ambulancezorg Nederland
Zwolle, Netherlands

Henry Guly, MD, FCEM, FRCP
Consultant in Emergency Medicine
Derriford Hospital
Plymouth, United Kingdom

Carol Gupton, BS (EMS), NREMT-P
EMS Education Coordinator
Omaha Fire Department
Omaha, Nebraska

Kathy Haack, RN, CEN
Avera Heart Hospital of South Dakota
South Dakota

David Halliwell, MSc, Paramedic
Head of Education
South Western Ambulance NHS Trust
Bournemouth, United Kingdom

Glyn Harding, Paramedic/ECP
Clinical Tutor
South Western Ambulance Service NHS Trust
Exeter, United Kingdom

Sharon Hardwick, BSc (Hons), Paramedic
Course Leader/Senior Lecturer Paramedic Foundation
    Degrees
University of Worcester Institute of Health and Society
Worcester, United Kingdom

Christopher E. Harris, BSHA, MICT, I/C
Sedgwick County Emergency Medical Service
Wichita, Kansas

Graham Harris, BSc, PGCE, MSc, Paramedic
Training Officer
Higher Education Programme Team
Department of Education and Training
London Ambulance Service NHS Trust
Bromley, England

Robert Hawkes, MS, PA, NREMT-P
Southern Maine Community College
South Portland, Maine

Thomas Herron, EMT-P
Cape Fear Community College
Castle Hayne, North Carolina

Lizi Hickson
Senior Lecturer in Paramedic Science
University of Central Lancashire
Lancashire, England

Rick Hilinski, BA, EMT-P
CCAC Public Safety Institute
Pittsburgh, Pennsylvania

Graham A. F. Hill
Military Medic (Reserves)
Fenton Pharmaceuticals
London, United Kingdom

David Hiltbrunn, NREMT-P, MICP
EMS Coordinator
St. Mary Corwin Regional Medical Center
EMS Institute of Prehospital Care
Pueblo, Colorado

Rob Holborn, EdD, Paramedic
Reedy Creek Emergency Services
Orlando, Florida

Conni Holder, NREMT-P
Instructor/QI Coordinator
CGH Medical Center
Sterling, Illinois

Dr Anil Hormis, MBChB, FCARCSI
Sheffield Teaching Hospitals NHS Trust
Sheffield, United Kingdom

Roxane Horowitz, NREMT, EMT-B(I)
Education Manager/EMS Program Coordinator
MONOC
Wall, New Jersey

C. Nathan Hox, BS, LVN, NREMT-B
University of California Davis Medical Center
Sacramento, California

Annie Jenkin, MSc, PGDE, BSc (Hons), RGN
Senior Lecturer in Emergency Care
School of Nursing and Community Studies
Faculty of Health and Social Work
University of Plymouth
Plymouth, United Kingdom

Sandra Jones, RN, BSN, EMT-P, CEN
Vanderbilt Medical Center
Nashville, Tennessee

Daniel Kane, MEd, BSN, RN, CEN, CCRN, CFRN, EMT-P
Clinical Assistant Professor, School of Nursing
MGH Institute of Health Professions
Boston, Massachusetts

Paul Kattenhorn, Paramedic, PGCE, DMS
Clinical Operations General Manager
East of England Ambulance Trust
Bedford, United Kingdom

William R. Kerney, MA, EMT-P (ret.)
Professor of Emergency Medicine
College of Southern Nevada
Las Vegas, Nevada

Dave Kerr, BSc (Hons), CertEd, Paramedic
Higher Education Programme Team
London Ambulance Service NHS Trust
London, England

Lieutenant Timothy M. Kimble, NREMT-P
Fauquier County Department of Fire, Rescue,
   and Emergency Services
Warrenton, Virginia

Gerard King, BSc (Hons)
Emergency Care Practitioner
South Western Ambulance Service NHS Trust
Penzance, United Kingdom

Robert W. Knappage, EMT-P
EMS Lieutenant
Sachse Fire Rescue
Sachse, Texas

Lieutenant Rob Kuhl, APA-C, MPAS
Aeromedical Physician Assistant
US Coast Guard
Air Station Barbers Point, Hawaii

Mark Langley, HEMS Paramedic
Devon Air Ambulance/SWAST
North Devon Air Ambulance
Exeter, United Kingdom

John Lewis, MEd, CCEMT-P, NREMT-P
Paramedic Program Director
Brigham Young University–Idaho
Rexburg, Idaho

Tony Little, BSc, Dip Mgmnt, Paramedic, PGCEd
PHTLS Coordinator, London
Clinical Tutor
London Ambulance Service NHS Trust
London, England

Larry Macy, NREMT-P
Safety Specialist, Instructor/Coordinator
Western Wyoming Community College
Rock Springs, Wyoming

Scott A. Matin
Vice President
MONOC Mobile Health Services
Wall, New Jersey

William M. Mehbod, BS, EMT-P
Cincinnati State Technical and Community College
Cincinnati, Ohio

Antoinette Melton-Tharrett, NREMT-P, CCEMT-P, KYEMT-P
Instructor
Air-Evac Lifeteam
Albany, Kentucky

Dominador O. Mendoza, Jr, RN, MANc
Emergency Medicine Institute
Riyadh, Kingdom of Saudi Arabia

Dr Ognyan Milev
General Surgeon
PHTLS International Instructor
St. Petka County Hospital
Vidin, Bulgaria

Steve Monsam, NREMT-P, BS
Tappan, New York

Tracy Nicholls, PGC (TLHE), FHEA
East of England Ambulance Service NHS Trust
Bedfordshire, United Kingdom

Fernando da Costa Ferreira Novo, MD
Hospital das Clinicas, University of Sao Paulo School
    of Medicine
Sao Paulo, Brasil

Michael Page, BSc (Hons) Pre Hospital Care, PGC Spr. Practice,
Paramedic, Cert Ed. AASI
Great Western Ambulance Service NHS Trust
Chippenham, United Kingdom

Guy Peifer, BS, NREMT-P, CIC, RF/PC
Paramedic Program Coordinator, Borough of Manhattan
    Community College
EMS Education Coordinator, Yonkers Fire Department
New York, New York

Richard Pilbery, BMedSci (Hons), PGCert
Paramedic Team Educator
Yorkshire Ambulance Service
Sheffield, United Kingdom

Dr Neil Pryde, MBChB, MRCGP
General Practitioner, Howe of Fife Medical Practice
Chief Medical Officer, Knockhill Racing Circuit
Fife, United Kingdom

Wright N. Randolph, Jr, CEP
EMS Program Director
Pima Community College
Tucson, Arizona

John Reed, MPH, BSN, RN, EMT-P
Education Coordinator
Birmingham Regional Emergency Medical Services System
Birmingham, Alabama

Gina Riggs, BS, CCEMT-P
Kiamichi Technology Center, EMS Training Program
Poteau, Oklahoma

Roberto Rivera-Rosario, RN, BSN, EMT-B
Trauma-Flight Nurse
MCPR/ITLS Puerto Rico Chapter Coordinator
San Juan, Puerto Rico

Dr Katharine Robinson, MBBS, BSc, MRCS, FCEM
Consultant Emergency Physician
Emergency Department
Torbay Hospital
Torquay, United Kingdom

Eric Sacht, NREMT-P
EMS Director, Sacramento City Unified School District
Sacramento, California

Scott P. Sherry, MS, NREMT-P, PA-C
Oregon Health and Sciences University
Division of Trauma/Surgical Critical Care
Portland, Oregon

Terry G. Skidmore, Jr, NREMT-P
Training Coordinator
Georgetown County Emergency Services
Georgetown, South Carolina

Captain Katharine R. Smith, AS, NREMT-P
Professional Standards and Training Officer
Florence County EMS
Florence, South Carolina

Captain Scott Smith, MBE, RAMC, Paramedic
HM Forces Paramedic Tutor
United Kingdom

Nicky Smy, Paramedic
PHTLS, AMLS, GEMS Instructor
West Midlands Ambulance Service NHS Trust
Stafford, United Kingdom

João Manuel da Silva Sousa
Crupo Trauma e Emergência Portugal
Caldas da Rainha, Portugal

Kent R. Spitler, MSEd, RN, NREMT-P, CPP
Gaston College Department for EMS Education
Dallas, North Carolina

Michelle Starbuck, RN, CCRN, CFRN
California Shock Trauma Air Rescue (CALSTAR)
Concord, California

Dr Carrie Stevenson, Paramedic, BMBS
South Western Ambulance Service NHS Trust
Royal Devon and Exeter Hospital Trust
Redruth, United Kingdom

Bill Sugiyama, MA, RN, NREMT-P
Prehospital Care Coordinator
Alameda County Emergency Medical Services
San Leandro, California

Richard Taffler, MSc, BSc (Hons), BEng, FASI, Paramedic
South Western Ambulance Service NHS Trust
Exeter, United Kingdom

Pete Thorpe, Paramedic, Dip IMC RCS (ed)
Aid Training and Operations Ltd
Warminster, United Kingdom

Gustavo Jorge Tisminetzky, MD, MAAC, FACS
Jefe Unidad Urgencia Hospital J A Fernandez
Coordinador Comisión de Trauma Asociación Argentina de Cirugía
Chairman of COT ATLS, Capítulo Argentino American College of Surgeons
Ex Presidente Sociedad Argentina de Medicina y Cirugía del Trauma
Buenos Aires, Argentina

John Todaro, BA, REMT-P, RN, TNS, NCEE
Director/Chief Operating Officer
Emergency Medicine Learning and Resource Center
Orlando, Florida

Rachel Toft, Paramedic
South Western Ambulance Service NHS Trust
Ilfracombe, United Kingdom

Mike Tonkay, AS, EMT-P
Harrisburg Area Community College
Harrisburg, Pennsylvania

Stephen Traynor
Training Officer, Education and Development
London Ambulance Service NHS Trust
Bromley, England

Vanni Vincenzo, NREMT, WEMT, EMT-T
Instructor AHA, ITLS, AMLS
Course Coordinator, TC APT
Air Rescue
Pavia, Italy

Wilma Vinton, MICP, NREMT-P
Interior Region EMS Council, Inc.
University of Alaska, Fairbanks Tanana Valley Campus Paramedic Academy
Fairbanks, Alaska

Sandy Waggoner, BA, EMT-P, EMSI
President
Resource Solutions Associates, LLC
Milan, Ohio

Jimmy Walker
Midlands EMS
West Columbia, South Carolina

Adam Watts, Paramedic, Dip IMC RCS Ed
South Western Ambulance NHS Trust
Bournemouth, United Kingdom

Brad D. Weilbrenner
NH Fire Standards and Training and EMS
Concord, New Hampshire

Bob Willis
Program Lead Paramedic Science
The University of Northampton
Northampton, United Kingdom

Dennie Wulterkens, RN, EMT-P, RMA-P
Training Institute for Emergency Medicine
Dutch Association of Physicians
Houten, Netherlands

Doug York, NREMT-P, PS
EMSLRC, University of Iowa Hospitals and Clinics
Iowa City, Iowa

Jodi Kae Zufelt, Paramedic
Kuna Rural Fire District
Kuna, Idaho

Matt Zukosky, MA, NREMT-P
Emergency Medical Care Program Coordinator
Suffolk County Community College
Selden, New York

A Tribute to Chris Haber

After completing the work on his chapter but before he was able to see it in print, Chris Haber lost his battle with cancer. Chris was passionate about EMS and he touched the lives of many providers as a paramedic, fire fighter, instructor, and author. Thank you, Chris, for your enduring commitment and desire to make EMS a better place. The EMS world has lost and will truly mourn "one of the good ones."

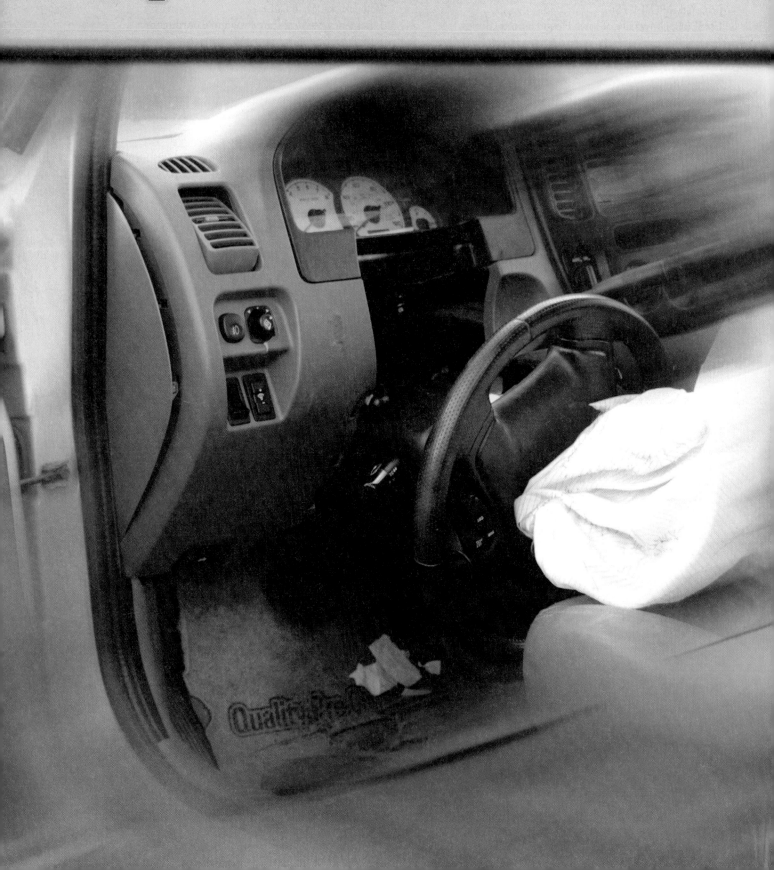

You have been dispatched to a motor vehicle collision on a high speed roadway. Dispatch notifies you that there is a 60-year-old man complaining of chest pain. Via the radio you learn that a disabled vehicle was parked on the side of the roadway and another vehicle struck it at highway speed. When you arrive on scene, you find a sport utility vehicle with moderate front end damage with a patient still seated in the driver's seat. There is a compact car pushed off the roadway with significant rear end damage.

Your patient is a 60-year-old man who complains of chest pain when he breathes. He states that he dropped his coffee and that when he looked back up at the road the other car was right in front of him. He states that he was not wearing his seatbelt and he denies loss of consciousness. As you assess your patient, you note that the air bag has deployed. The steering wheel is bent and the steering column has broken from its mounting position.

Your assessment reveals the patient has tenderness to the anterior chest wall when you palpate it and he complains that each breath hurts worse than the last. He has no facial injury but complains of neck pain. There are abrasions and bruising across the lower chest and abdomen. His pelvis has no injury and the lower extremities appear to have no injury.

1 What is the effect of speed on energy? How can energy be a predictor of injury?

2 Describe the three impacts seen in this collision as the energy of speed is dissipated through the car and patient.

3 What are some of the clues available from the vehicle that can help predict the body areas that may have sustained injury? How would the injury pattern differ if the patient had worn his seatbelt? What if there were no seatbelt or air bags?

4 What injuries would you suspect with this patient based on the available information?

5 Using the process of predicting injury based on the review of trauma, what types of clues could help predict the injury if the mechanism was a fall? A gunshot wound? A knife wound?

Introduction

Globally, young people between the ages of 15 and 44 years account for nearly 50% of the world's injury-related deaths. In addition to the considerable number of deaths, millions more are wounded or suffer other nonfatal health consequences due to injuries.

The Eastern European States have the highest overall injury mortality rates, whereas North America, Western Europe, Australia, and New Zealand have the lowest. Indeed, the World Health Organization (WHO) reports that 7 of the 15 leading causes of deaths for people 5 to 29 years old are injury-related: motor vehicle–related injuries, suicide, homicide, war, drowning, poisoning, and burns. The patterns of injury deaths differ by region. Whereas death rates from road traffic, burns, and drowning are particularly high in Africa and Asia, death rates due to falls are highest in Western Europe.

Important lessons have been learned about injuries during the past few decades. Among them is that injuries are not inevitable; they are preventable. Many injury prevention strategies have already been shown to be effective. Using seatbelts in cars and helmets when riding motorcycles, calming traffic to protect pedestrians, enforcing policies against drunk driving and speeding, training parents and conducting home visitations to stop abuse, wearing protective equipment at work or when playing sports, storing firearms and ammunition in separate and locked places, using flame-resistant material for children's clothes, and using special packaging to prevent poisoning are among the measures that have contributed to decreasing the burden of injuries.

Basic concepts of the mechanics and biomechanics of trauma will help the provider to analyze and manage a patient's injuries. Analyzing a trauma scene is a vital skill because you are the eyes and ears of the emergency department physicians. The patient care report is what physicians and surgeons use to understand the events and mechanisms that led to the trauma patient's injury. Scene information is critical as a foundation when attempting to visualize and search for injuries that may not be apparent on initial physical examination.

STATS

The top five causes of trauma death worldwide are motor vehicle collisions, falls, poisonings, burns, and drowning.

Trauma, Energy, Biomechanics, and Kinematics

Trauma is the acute physiologic and structural change (injury) that occurs in a patient's body when an external source of energy dissipates faster than the body's ability to sustain and dissipate it.

If a person falls while working on scaffolding 20′ (6 m) in the air, the energy delivered by gravity is released when the movement is stopped by the ground. If the energy is not absorbed in other ways, the patient's body absorbs it, often breaking bones and rupturing internal organs—traumatic injuries.

Different forms of energy produce different kinds of trauma. These external energy sources can be mechanical, chemical, thermal, electrical, and barometric.

Mechanical energy is energy from motion (**kinetic energy**) or energy stored in an object (**potential energy**). Kinetic energy can be found in two moving vehicles just before they collide. Potential energy would be present in a person standing at the top of a ladder. If he were to fall, then gravity would be the source of *potential* energy that can cause the object to fall. **Chemical energy** can be found in an explosive or an acid, or even from a reaction to an ingested or medically delivered agent or drug. **Thermal energy** comes from the energy stored in objects and is seen as a change in temperature, like the friction in braking on a car or burning of materials. Trauma from **electrical energy** can be seen in the form of a high-voltage electrocution or a lightning strike. **Barometric energy** can result from sudden and radical changes in pressure, often occurring during explosions, diving, or flying.

Biomechanics is the study of the physiology and mechanics of a living organism using the tools of mechanical engineering. Biomechanics provides a way of analyzing the mechanisms and results of trauma sustained by the human body. **Kinetics** studies the relationships among speed, mass, direction of force, and, for emergency medical providers, the physical injury caused by speed, mass, and force. Knowledge of kinetics and biomechanics can help you predict injury patterns found in a patient.

The Physics of Injury

Although drivers of motor vehicles might not obey traffic laws, they must—whether they want to or not—obey the laws of physics that govern all objects on our planet. A little familiarity with these laws will help you understand more about the mechanisms of trauma.

Velocity (V) is the distance an object travels per unit of time. The difference between velocity and speed is that velocity is also defined by movement in a specific direction. **Acceleration (a)** of an object is the rate of change in velocity that an object is subjected to, whether speeding up or slowing down. **Gravity (g)** is the downward acceleration that is imparted to any object on earth by the effect of the earth's mass. During each second of a fall, the velocity or speed of the falling object increases by 9.8 m/sec^2.

The kinetic energy (KE) of an object is the energy associated with that object in motion. It reflects the relationship between the weight (mass) of the object and the velocity at which it is traveling, and is expressed mathematically as:

$$\text{Kinetic energy} = \frac{\text{Mass} \times \text{Velocity}^2}{2}$$

or

$$KE = (M \times V^2)/2$$

Thus, **velocity** has a much greater effect on KE than weight.

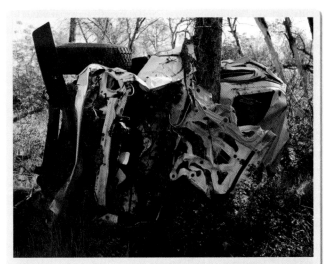

FIGURE 1-1 The kinetic energy of a speeding car is converted into the work of stopping the car, usually by crushing the car's exterior.

In other words, an object increases its kinetic energy more by increasing its velocity than by increasing its mass. The kinetic energy of an object involved in a collision must be dissipated as the object comes to rest. The kinetic energy of a car in motion that stops suddenly must go somewhere. In a car, kinetic energy can be dissipated by braking, transforming it to heat or thermal energy. If all the energy is not transformed into heat, however, the KE that is left at the time of the collision is transformed into deformed metal (mechanical energy), which results in damage to the car and its occupants **FIGURE 1-1**. The mechanics of dissipation can result in injury. For example, a car traveling at 35 mph (56 km/h) hits a wall, which stops the car, but the driver is still traveling at 35 mph (56 km/h) until stopped by the seatbelt or the air bag, or, if not wearing a seatbelt, the steering wheel, dashboard, or windshield.

Speed kills exponentially: look what happens to the KE when velocity increases incrementally versus when the weight of a person increases:

- Mass (in kg) × Velocity (in meters/sec)² divided by 2 = KE (in Joules)
- 154-lb (70-kg) person at 50 mph (22.352 m/sec) = 17,486 Joules
- Increased velocity: 154-lb (70-kg) person at 60 mph (26.8224 m/sec) = 25,180 Joules
- Increased weight: 164-lb (74.5-kg) person at 50 mph (22.352 m/sec) = 18,610 Joules

Note that when weight increases by 10 lb (4.5 kg) but velocity remains the same, the change in kinetic energy is only 1,124 J. However, when the velocity increases from 50 to 60 mph (80 to 96 km/h), a difference of only 10 mph (16 km/h), the KE (energy in motion) increases by 7,694 J, an almost seven-fold increase.

Remember the laws of physics that no driver can break? Here is a quick review of physics. The **law of conservation of energy** states that energy can be neither created nor destroyed; it can only change form. Energy generated from a sudden stop or start must be transformed into one of the following energy forms: thermal, electrical, chemical, radiant, barometric, or mechanical.

Energy dissipation is the process by which KE is transformed into one of these forms of energy. When a car stops slowly, its KE is converted to thermal energy—heat—by the friction of the braking action. If the car crashes, KE is also dissipated into mechanical energy as the car body crumples in a collision. Mechanical energy is further dissipated in the form of injury as the occupants sustain fractures or other bodily harm.

Protective devices such as seatbelts, air bags, and helmets are designed to manipulate the way in which energy is dissipated into injury **FIGURE 1-2**. For example, a seatbelt converts the kinetic energy of the occupant into a seatbelt-to-body pressure force rather than into a steering wheel deformation against the torso or a windshield shattering against the head.

Newton's first law of motion states that a body at rest will remain at rest unless acted on by an outside force. Similarly, a body in motion tends to remain in motion at a constant velocity, traveling in a straight line, unless acted on by an outside force. Most bodies in motion tend to stop eventually, owing to the action of forces of friction, wind resistance, gravity, or another force resulting in deceleration.

Newton's second law of motion states that the force an object can exert is the product of its mass times its acceleration:

$$\text{Force} = \text{Mass (Weight)} \times \text{Acceleration (or deceleration)}$$

The higher an object's mass and acceleration, the higher the force that needs to be applied to make a change of course or to stop the object. Force equals mass multiplied by acceleration or deceleration. Rapid deceleration, as may occur in a collision, dissipates tremendous forces, which may cause major injuries. This leads to **Newton's third law of motion**, which states that for every action there is an equal and opposite reaction. When a patient falls to the ground, his weight (mass) multiplied by the speed that now suddenly stops (deceleration) equals the force applied to the body.

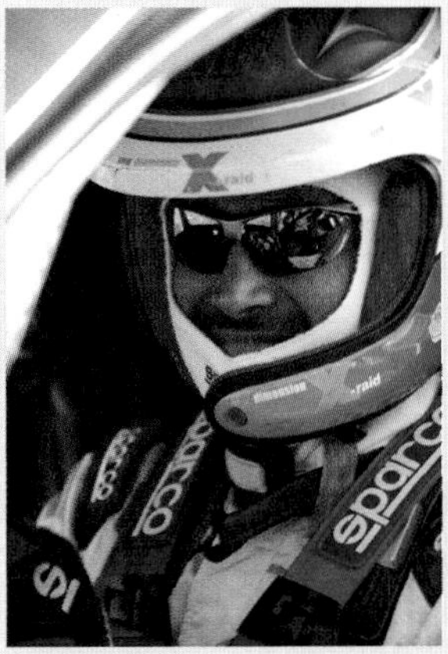

It is important to understand these laws of physics because they help define the types and patterns of trauma you will see in the field. You are the most important witness the hospital trauma team has. The information you gain from observing and understanding physics will affect your patient's outcome.

FIGURE 1-2 Protective devices are used to dissipate the energy involved in a collision.

Factors Affecting Types of Injury

The kind of injury resulting after trauma is sustained is determined by the ability of the patient's body to disperse the energy delivered by the traumatic event. Some patients' bodies can stretch and bend to absorb the energy of the traumatic event, whereas another patient's bone and tissue cannot absorb the energy. For example, a healthy football player can absorb a hit on the playing field better than an older man with diminished bone mass can.

External factors that determine types of injury include the amount of force and energy delivered. The amount of injury your patient sustains varies with the:

- Size (or mass) of the objects delivering the force and energy
- Change in velocity (how fast your patient is traveling)
- Acceleration or deceleration (how much the object or your patient speeds up or slows down)
- Body area where the force is applied

Duration and direction of the force of application are also important. Injuries from vehicle collisions follow directional patterns related to the vehicular damage seen in front-end, side, and rear-end collisions **FIGURE 1-3** . The larger the area of force dissipation, the more the pressure is reduced to a specific spot on the body, often without making a visible cut. Bullet impact is less if the energy in the bullet is dissipated over the ceramic plate inside a bulletproof vest than if all the force of the bullet is applied at a small location on the skin. In trauma medicine, this spreading of impact where tissues are not penetrated is described as **blunt trauma**.

The position of the trauma victim—how he or she is standing or sitting—at the time of the event is an external factor. Seatbelts have done a great deal to reduce lethal car collision injuries by keeping occupants in positions least likely to cause fatal injuries.

The impact resistance of body parts also will have a bearing on types of tissue disruption. Impact resistance is often determined by what is inside your patient's organs: gas, liquid, or solid. Biomechanical engineers measure the densities of tissues that are traumatized. Organs that have gas inside, such as in the lungs and intestinal tract, will disperse energy more than liquid or solid organs. This means that the organ containing the gas will be easily compressed, so look for lung and intestinal trauma first. Water-bearing organs include the vascular system, liver, spleen, and muscle. Water-bearing tissues are less compressible than gas-containing tissues. Solid density impact occurs mostly in bones such as in the cranium, spine, and long bones.

Because many injuries are not obvious on first presentation, understanding the effects of forces and energy transfer patterns will help in the assessment of the mechanism of injury (MOI), which in turn can help predict the most likely types of injuries you will see when you are in the field.

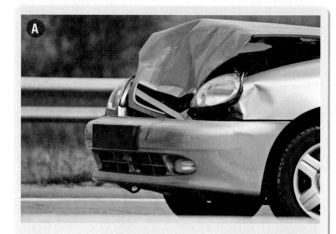

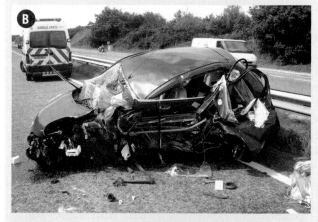

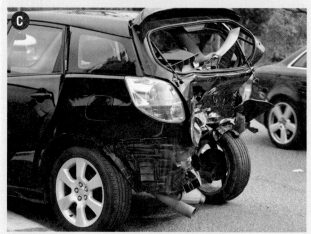

FIGURE 1-3 In a motor vehicle collision, the direction from which a vehicle is hit or strikes another vehicle or object can affect the injuries of the drivers and passengers. **A.** Front impact. **B.** Side impact. **C.** Rear impact.

TIP

Index of Suspicion

Suspect a spinal injury when you see a cracked windshield, steering wheel or dashboard intrusion into a vehicle, or head injuries after a fall. It will make a difference in how you handle the ABCs.

Types of Trauma

Injuries are generally described as the consequence of blunt or penetrating trauma **FIGURE 1-4**. Blunt trauma refers to injuries in which the tissues are not penetrated by an external object. Blunt trauma typically occurs in motor vehicle collisions, in pedestrians hit by a vehicle, in motorcycle crashes, in falls from heights, assaults, in serious sports injuries, and in blasts when no shrapnel is involved and the pressure wave is the primary cause of the injuries.

Penetrating trauma results when tissues are penetrated by single or multiple objects. Penetrating trauma results from gunshot wounds caused by a single or multiple projectiles, stab wounds, and blasts with shrapnel or secondary projectiles. Penetrating trauma may also occur in combination with blunt injuries such as in impalement injuries during a motor vehicle collision or a fall out of a tree and onto a fence.

Injuries Caused by Deceleration

Abrupt deceleration injuries are produced by a sudden stop of a body's forward motion. Whether from a fall, shaking a baby, or a high-speed vehicle collision, decelerating forces can induce shearing, avulsing, or rupturing of organs and their restraining fascia, vasculature, nerves, and other soft tissues. These injuries are often invisible during examination, so every provider needs to understand how such injuries are sustained.

The head is particularly vulnerable to deceleration injuries. The brain is a fairly heavy organ surrounded by fluid inside the skull. Any trauma that will jerk the patient's head can cause the brain to hit the inside of the skull, causing bleeding, bruising, tearing, and crushing injuries **FIGURE 1-5**. All of these injuries are extremely dangerous and might not show up on a cursory examination.

The aorta is vulnerable to injury with chest trauma. The aorta, the largest blood vessel exiting the heart, is the most common site of deceleration injury in the chest. The aorta is often torn away from its points of fixation in the body when the weight of the heart pulls against it. Shearing or tearing of the aorta can result in rapid loss of all the body's blood and immediate death.

Abdominal blunt trauma results as the forward motion of the body stops but internal organs continue their forward motion, resulting in tearing at their points of attachment, or shearing injuries, and compression against abdominal walls or crushing injuries. Organs that can be affected include the liver, kidneys, small intestine, large intestine, pancreas, and spleen.

Kidneys are injured as forward motion produces tears to the organ at the points that attach with the abdominal aorta to the renal arteries **FIGURE 1-6**. Also, as forward motion is restrained by the large bowel, the small bowel can tear and result in free air in the abdomen. Trauma can also damage without tearing but by causing an insufficient supply of blood to the bowel through bruising. The spleen and the liver can also be torn or split, sometimes resulting in life-threatening internal bleeding.

Injuries Caused by External Forces

Crush and compression injuries are the result of forces applied to the body by things external to the body at the time of impact. Crush and compression injuries occur *at the* time of impact, unlike deceleration injuries, which occur

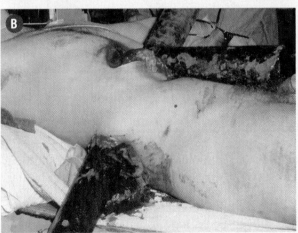

FIGURE 1-4 There are two main types of trauma the provider will treat. **A.** Blunt trauma. **B.** Penetrating trauma.

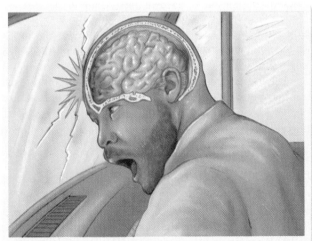

FIGURE 1-5 In a sudden deceleration, the brain continues to move and strikes the inside of the skull, causing bruising, bleeding, and changes in level of consciousness.

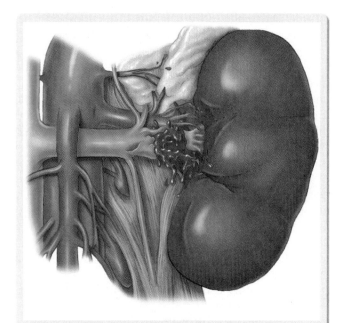

FIGURE 1-6 Kidneys and the other organs of the abdomen continue to decelerate when the body has come to a stop; they are at risk of tearing away from their blood supply.

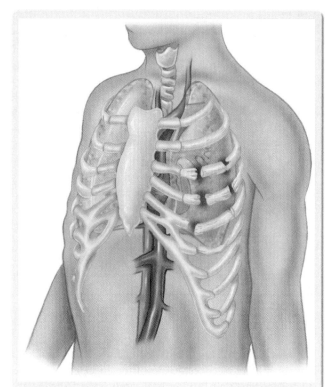

FIGURE 1-7 Compression of the chest wall may cause rib fractures and internal injury.

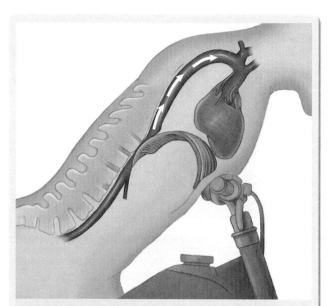

FIGURE 1-8 A compression injury to the abdomen can cause a rush of blood to return to the heart causing valve damage.

after impact. Crush and compression injuries are often caused by dashboards, windshields, the floor, and heavy objects falling on the body.

Compression injuries of the chest may produce fractured ribs, which can lead to internal injuries of the lungs and heart **FIGURE 1-7**. If the lungs are compressed, large pulmonary contusions can require positive-pressure ventilations to maintain your patient's breathing. Blunt cardiac injury can compress the heart between bones in the chest, causing arrhythmias and direct injury to the heart muscle.

Almost all abdominal organs can be affected by hitting an external object. The organs most often injured are the liver, spleen, pancreas, and, occasionally, kidneys. Compression against the seatbelt may result in bowel rupture, bladder rupture, tearing of the diaphragm, and spinal injuries. The aorta continues from the chest into the abdomen. A large blow to the abdomen may push blood flow backward up the aorta and create a rupture or inversion of the cardiac valves **FIGURE 1-8**.

Pelvic fractures also result from external compressive trauma, potentially injuring the bladder, vagina, rectum, lumbar plexus, and pelvic floor and leading to severe bleeding in the large arteries in the pelvis.

Motor Vehicle Collisions

When a motor vehicle collides with another object, trauma in the collision is composed of five phases tied to the effects of progressive deceleration. The first phase, *deceleration of the vehicle,* occurs when the vehicle strikes another object and is brought to an abrupt stop. The forward motion of the car continues until its KE is dissipated in the form of mechanical deformation and damage to the vehicle and occupant or until the restraining force of the object is removed (eg, sheared-off pole or tree) and the vehicle motion continues until its KE is gently dissipated by drag or continued braking.

The second phase is *deceleration of the occupant,* which starts during sudden braking and continues during impact and collision. This results in deceleration, compression, and shear trauma to the occupants. The effects on vehicle occupants will vary depending on the mass of each occupant,

STATS

- According to 2006 National Highway Transportation Safety Administration (NHTSA) statistics, the overall US traffic fatality rate dropped to a record low of 1.41 fatalities per 100 million vehicle miles traveled in 2006.
  - This still represents a total of 5.973 million collisions across the United States.
- In 2006 alone, 42,642 people were killed; 32,092 were vehicle occupants, 4,810 were motorcycle riders, and 5,740 were nonmotorists.
  - There were 2,575,000 injured.
  - Of the 42,642 killed, 41% involved alcohol-related collisions.
  - Of drivers killed, males accounted for 70% of traffic fatalities, 69% of pedestrian fatalities, and 88% of pedacyclist fatalities.
  - Of passengers killed, 55% were not wearing seatbelts.
- The age group with the most fatalities was 16- to 24-year-olds, accounting for 24% of fatalities.
- The fatality rate of all drivers over the age of 55 was also 24%.

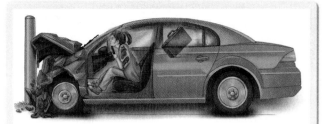

FIGURE 1-9 Five phases of trauma in motor vehicle collisions are deceleration of the vehicle, deceleration of the occupant, deceleration of internal organs, secondary collisions, and additional impacts.

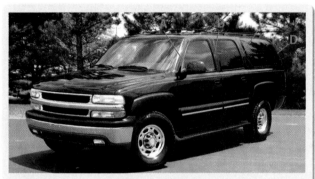

FIGURE 1-10 When looking at a motor vehicle it is important to be able to describe the damaged area. Areas of concern are the front end, rear end, and lateral or side impacts, which can be subdivided by which pillar the damage is near.

protective mechanisms in the vehicle such as restraints and air bags, body parts involved, and points of impact.

The third phase, *deceleration of internal organs*, involves the body's supporting structures (skull, sternum, ribs, spine, and pelvis) and movable organs (brain, heart, liver, spleen, and intestines) that continue their forward momentum until stopped by anatomic restraints. Energy is dissipated by internal organs as they are injured. Movement of fixed and nonfixed parts may result in tears and shearing injuries.

The fourth phase is the result of *secondary collisions*, which occur when a vehicle occupant is hit by objects moving within the vehicle such as packages, animals, or other passengers. These objects may continue to travel at the vehicle's initial speed and then hit a passenger who has come to rest. These types of collisions have been known to cause severe spine and head trauma and even death of the front seat passengers by unrestrained rear seat passengers.

The final phase is the result of *additional impacts* that the vehicle may receive, for example when it is hit and deflected into another vehicle, a tree, or another object. This may increase the seriousness of original injuries or cause further injury. For example, a frontal collision may cause a posterior hip dislocation and an acetabular fracture via an impact with the dashboard and a subsequent side impact from another vehicle may add a lateral compression pelvic ring injury, resulting in complex pelvic and acetabular trauma **FIGURE 1-9**.

Modern cars are designed to have crumple zones to maximize the amount of energy dissipated by deformation before the passenger compartment is involved **FIGURE 1-10**. Damage to the exterior of the automobile is often an indicator to how fast the car was going. The amount of damage can provide information to help in your decision about transferring your patient to a trauma center.

In addition to the velocity at which the car (and its passengers) are traveling, the vehicle's angle of impact (front collision versus side impact) will provide clues to the mechanism of injury the patient may have sustained. Additional clues include:

- How your patient was positioned inside the automobile
- The differences in the sizes of the two vehicles
- The restraint status and protective gear the occupants used will affect the amount of energy dissipation that affects your patient

TABLE 1-1 shows the structural clues, body clues, and resulting injuries for different types of collisions.

TIP

Don't forget that the collision of internal organs striking against the body can result in severe damage, though this damage may not always be obvious.

TABLE 1-1	Motor Vehicle Collision: MOI	
Structural Clues	**Body Clues**	**Look for These Injuries**
Head-on collision		
Deformed front end, cracked windshield	Bruised head	• Brain injury • Scalp, facial cuts • Cervical spine injury • Tracheal injury
Deformed steering column	Bruised neck Bruised chest	• Sternal or rib fracture • Flail chest • Myocardial contusion • Cardiac tamponade • Pneumothorax or hemothorax • Exsanguination from aortic tear
Deformed dashboard	Bruised abdomen Bruised knee	• Ruptured spleen, liver, bowel, or diaphragm • Fractured patella • Dislocated knee • Femoral fracture • Dislocated hip
Lateral collision		
Deformed side of car	Bruised shoulder	• Clavicular fracture • Fractured humerus • Multiple rib fractures
Door smashed in	Bruised pelvis	• Fractured hip • Fractured iliac wing
B pillar deformed	Bruised temple	• Brain injury • Cervical spine fracture
Broken door or window handles	Bruised arms	• Contusions
Broken window glass	Dicing lacerations	• Multiple square or angulated injuries
Rear-end collision		
Posterior deformity of the vehicle Headrest not adjusted Check for secondary anterior deformity	Neck pain	• "Whiplash" injuries • Deceleration injuries of a head-on collision

Predicting Types of Injury

Important clues to predict injury types can be obtained by paying attention to the history of the collision and by examining the scene. Using your knowledge of the physics of trauma, you can make a good estimate of how injured your patients might be by looking at the amount of damage around the scene. How dented and deformed the vehicle looks is a clear indication of the forces involved and of the degree of deceleration sustained by your patient. Dents and deformities on the inside of the vehicle will show you the point of impact on the patient. Quickly check for injury types visible on your patient: head injury or seatbelt marks show what parts of the body may have been involved in energy absorption. Tire skid marks at the scene indicate whether significant energy was dissipated by braking before collision. Debris along the course of the crash may indicate multiple collisions and different force vectors acting on the victim along the course of the collision.

There are primarily five types of impact patterns: frontal or head-on, lateral or side impact, rear impact, rotational, and rollover.

Frontal (Head-on) Impact

In frontal (head-on) collisions, the front end of the car distorts as it dissipates kinetic energy and decelerates its forward motion **FIGURE 1-11**. Passengers decelerate at the same rate as the vehicle. At a 30-mph (48-km/h) collision, the front end of an average car will crush 2′ (0.6 m) at the rough estimate of 1″ (2.5 cm) of deformity for each 1 mph (1.6 km/h). The forces applied to the driver will differ based on car design, materials, and safety features of the vehicle. The interior will also suggest possible injuries by the damage your patient's body has done to the dash, windshield, or steering wheel **FIGURE 1-12**.

The occupant's position at the precise time of impact is very important in determining an occupant's movements

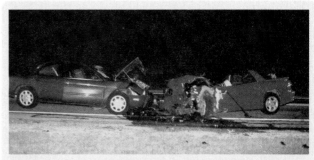

FIGURE 1-11 Front-end collisions impart a large amount of energy to the occupants.

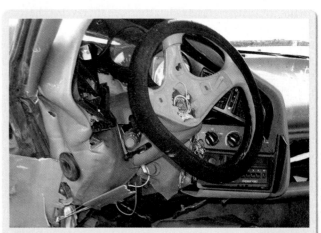

FIGURE 1-12 Damage to a vehicle's interior may indicate potential injuries to the driver and passengers.

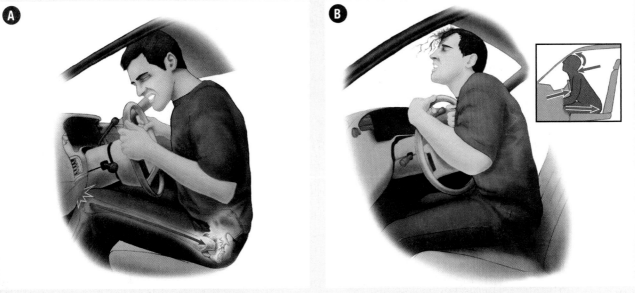

FIGURE 1-13 An unrestrained vehicle occupant will likely follow **A.** the down-and-under trajectory or **B.** the up-and-over trajectory.

and injuries during a collision. Unrestrained occupants usually follow one of two trajectories, a *down-and-under pathway* or an *up-and-over pathway* **FIGURE 1-13** .

The down-and-under pathway is traveled by an occupant pushed under the steering column. As the vehicle is decelerating, the occupant continues to travel downward and forward into the dashboard or steering column, led by the knees. The knees hit the dashboard, transmitting the energy of the deceleration up the femur to the pelvis. With knees locked in the dash and hips in the seat, force vectors go down the tibia and along the femur. If the feet are not locked by folding floorboards or foot pedals, energy along the tibia will be transferred to the lower leg with no immediate injury. If the feet are locked in place, midshaft femur fracture can occur. In some cases, the heads of the femurs will dislocate. If the occupant's knees hit the dashboard, look for a fracture-dislocation of the knee or other injuries. Look also for hip and pelvic fractures or hip dislocation. Your patient's torso can twist in such a way that his or her head hits the steering column. Always look for spinal injuries.

The upper torso continues forward until it impacts the car, be it the steering wheel or the seatbelt and air bag protection system. Look for rib fractures or pulmonary or cardiac injuries caused by internal organs being struck or compressed.

In the up-and-over pathway, the lead point is the head. In this sequence, rotation occurs around the ankles with the torso moving in an upward and forward direction. The head takes a higher trajectory, impacting the windshield, roof, mirror, or dashboard, causing compression and deceleration injuries in your patient that can include significant head and cervical spine trauma. The anterior part of the neck may strike the steering wheel, causing laryngeal fracture, serious lacerations, and other soft-tissue injury. The chest is particularly at risk. As it crosses over the steering wheel, it may impact, causing fractured ribs and internal trauma.

Ejection is possible if the windshield does not stop the head from projecting through it. This leads to a second set of impact injuries when the body contacts the ground or objects outside of the car. These injuries can be as severe as initial-impact injuries, and they increase the likelihood of great vessel damage and death. The spine absorbs energy as it is compressed between the stationary head and the moving torso, which leads to injury.

A dangerous lung injury may occur because your patient can reflexively take a deep breath just before impact, hyperinflating the lungs and closing the glottis. The impact of the steering wheel can injure the lungs via generation of pressures beyond the capabilities of lung tissue, like a paper bag being exploded (60% to 70% of pneumothoraces may occur this way) **FIGURE 1-14** .

The abdomen, pelvis, or upper thigh contacts the lower aspect of the steering wheel or dash, and lower leg fractures could be present.

Lateral (Side) Impact Collisions

Lateral impact, T-bone, and side collisions impart energy to the near-side occupant almost directly to the pelvis, chest, and extremities on the side of the impact. Unrestrained occupants remain almost motionless, literally having the car pushed out from under them. Seatbelts do little to protect passengers in these collisions because they are designed to

TIP

When there is damage to the steering assembly, there is critical injury to the driver until proved otherwise.

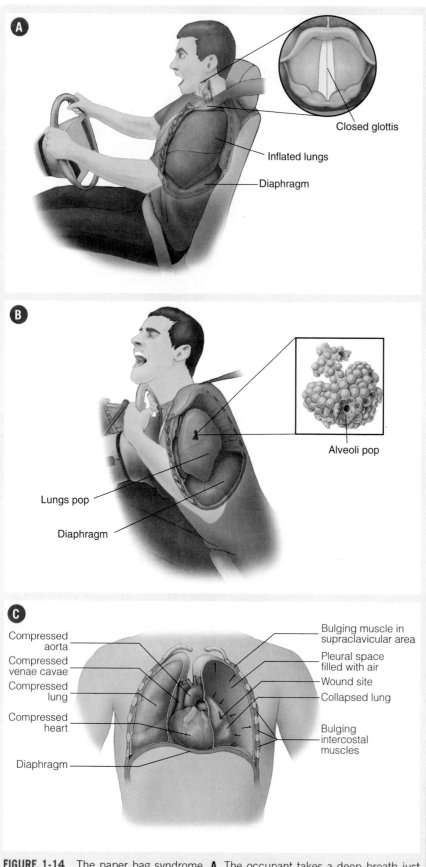

FIGURE 1-14   The paper bag syndrome. **A.** The occupant takes a deep breath just before crashing, closing the glottis and filling the lungs with air. **B.** The occupant's chest hits the steering wheel, popping the alveoli in the lungs. **C.** A tension pneumothorax results.

limit forward hinging injuries, not side impacts. As one vehicle makes contact with the side of the other vehicle, the occupant nearest the impact is hit by the door of the car as the passenger compartment begins to deform and collapse. The head can strike the inside of the vehicle as well as the hood of the impacting vehicle or object. Injury results from direct trauma to the affected side and to tension developed on the far side.

Upper extremity trauma depends on the spatial orientation of the arm at impact. The shoulder frequently rotates externally and posteriorly, exposing the chest and ribs to injury. Forces transmitted to the chest cause rib fractures, lateral flail chest, and lung contusions. If the humerus remains between the door and chest, the clavicle may absorb side motion and fracture. As the body of the occupant is pushed in one direction the head moves toward the impacting object, creating a line of tension along the cervical spine **FIGURE 1-15**. This may result in ligamentous disruption and dislocation of the spine on the opposite side of the impact. The far-side occupant, if properly restrained, has the advantage of "riding down" with the car, thereby receiving considerably less force. If unrestrained, he or she may move in a direction parallel but opposite to the impact. This passenger receives forces similar to any unrestrained occupant. Furthermore, because both passengers travel in a direction parallel to impact but in opposite directions, they collide with each other, causing additional injury.

In a lateral collision, the greater trochanter of the femur is impacted and transmits forces to the pelvis, sometimes being driven through the acetabulum into the pelvis. If the force reaches the ilium, the pelvis may also fracture. The typical pattern of pelvic injury that occurs in this scenario is a lateral compression injury that trauma surgeons call pelvic ring disruption. Lateral compression injuries are less serious than anterior compression injuries. Death in lateral collisions is usually the result of associated torso or head injuries.

Rear Impact Collisions

Rear-impact collisions have the most survivors if the driver and passengers are properly restrained. If the vehicle coming from the rear is traveling at excessive speed, however, morbidity increases. Most often in this kind of collision, a stationary (or slower moving) vehicle is struck from behind and the impact energy is transmitted as a sudden forward accelerating force. The neck hyperextends as the body moves forward relative to the head. The head does not move forward with the body unless a headrest is in the proper position; if the headrest is not in proper position, the head is snapped backward and then forward. Because most seats have some degree of elasticity after the sudden forward acceleration has ended, the stored potential energy in the seat is converted to an energy of forward motion, which can aggravate the hyperextension trauma to the neck and then follow with some rebound forward flexion of the head on the chest, resulting in hyperflexion. A third episode of extension may occur as the chest moves forward. This is the so-called **whiplash injury**.

In a rear-impact collision, energy is imparted to the front vehicle, which accelerates rapidly, while frontal impact energy to the rear driver is reduced because energy is being transferred to the front car. One concern with rear-impact collisions is the frequency with which seat backs collapse, causing unrestrained occupants to be propelled into the back seat. Head restraints developed to prevent the head and torso from moving separately are not always adjusted correctly. Many are placed too low and act as a fulcrum that may actually facilitate the extension injury. They need to be adjusted so they are behind the head and not just behind the neck **FIGURE 1-16**.

Rotational Impact

A rotational or corner impact occurs when the collision is off center. In this case, rotation occurs as part of the car continues to move and part of the car comes to a stop. The vehicle stops at the point of impact, but the opposite side continues in rotational motion around the impact point. The point of greatest speed loss of the vehicle is the site where the greatest damage to the occupant will occur. Occupants tend to receive a combination of frontal and lateral injuries. Because rigid objects may be in line with vector forces, head injuries may result **FIGURE 1-17**. Three-point belts are effective in preventing injury in angled collisions of up to 45°.

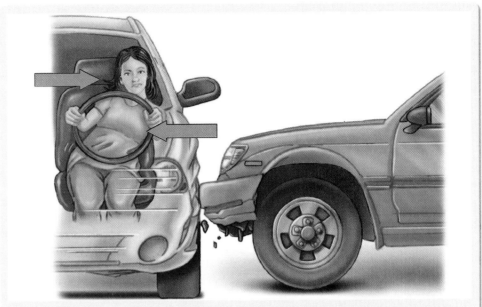

FIGURE 1-15 A lateral impact causes the body of the occupant closest to the impact to be pushed away from the impact while the head moves toward the impact.

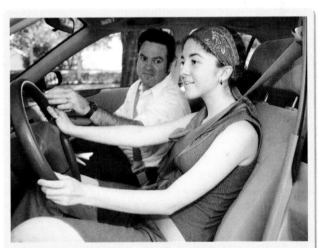

FIGURE 1-16 A properly adjusted headrest can protect the occupant's neck from hyperextension.

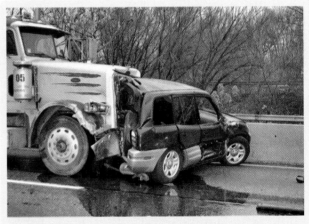

FIGURE 1-17 A rotational impact usually results in the occupants receiving both frontal and lateral injuries.

Rollover

Rollover scenarios have the greatest potential to cause lethal injuries. Injuries will be serious even if seatbelts are worn. However, if your patients did not wear seatbelts, they probably will be ejected, and they will have been struck hard with each change in direction the car makes with the rollover. Even a restrained occupant's head and neck will change direction with each change in the vehicle's position.

Ejection of the victim from the vehicle increases the chance of death by 25 times **FIGURE 1-18**. One of three ejected victims will sustain a cervical spine fracture. A partial ejection can result in an arm or leg injured by being caught between the vehicle and the ground.

Restrained Versus Unrestrained Occupants

Seatbelts are highly effective because they stop the motion of any automobile occupant who will otherwise travel at the same speed as the vehicle until stopped. The seatbelt, although capable of delivering some injury at high speeds, will prevent the serious-to-fatal injuries of being unrestrained in the car and being ejected from the car. One of every 13 victims of ejection sustains major and permanent cervical spine damage. Restrained victims "ride down" the deceleration with belt elasticity and crush time of the car, with a nearly 45% reduction in fatalities. Restraints limit the contact of the occupants with the interior of the vehicle, prevent ejection, distribute deceleration energy over a greater surface, and prevent the occupants from violently contacting each other. As a result, all types of injuries are decreased, including head, facial, spine, thoracic, intra-abdominal, pelvic, and lower extremities, and ejection is also limited.

All arguments against seatbelt use are unfounded. Every unrestrained passenger poses a hazard to themselves and to other occupants in the vehicle, especially for front seat passengers who are at double risk for injury in a front-end collision if the back seat occupants are unrestrained.

Specific injuries associated with seatbelt use include cervical fractures due to flexion stresses and neck sprains due to deceleration and hyperextension. Most serious injuries occur because the patient did not use the seatbelt correctly. If the occupant does not use the lap strap, severe upper body injuries, including spinal injuries and decapitation, can occur. If the seatbelt is placed above the pelvic bone, abdominal injuries and lumbar spine injuries result.

Air bags are another great step up for patient safety. In the United States, it is estimated that air bags have reduced deaths in direct frontal collisions by about 30%. Front air bags will not activate in side impact collisions or impacts to the front quarter panel, and without the use of a seatbelt, they are insufficient to prevent ejection. They are self-deflating and function only for a first impact, not the secondary ones. The rapidly inflating bag can also result in secondary injuries from direct contact with the air bag or from the chemicals used to inflate it. Common injuries include abrasions and burns to the face, chest, and arms; minor corrosive toxic effects; chemical keratitis; conjunctivitis or corneal abrasion; and inhalation injuries **FIGURE 1-19**.

Small children can be severely injured or killed if air bags inflate while they are in the front seat. That is why all EMS providers are encouraged to participate in teaching parents how to use children's car seats correctly.

Unique Patient Populations

Increased morbidity and mortality, especially chest trauma, is more common in elderly patients. This is particularly the case for rib and sternal fractures. Fatalities also increase if child restraint devices are improperly installed or used. Children who have outgrown a car seat but are too small to be restrained by belts designed for adults are at risk for hyperflexion and abdominal injury.

Pregnant women in general wear seatbelts less frequently than do nonpregnant women owing to the unproven concern that the seatbelt may increase damage to the unborn child in the case of a collision. However, no study has reported that seatbelts increase fetal mortality. If lap belts are worn alone and too high, they allow enough forward flexion and subsequent compression to rupture the uterus because deceleration forces are transmitted directly to

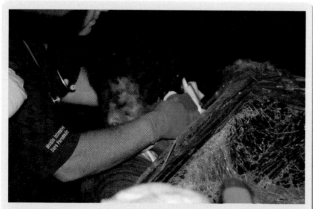

FIGURE 1-18 Occupants who have been ejected or partially ejected may have struck the interior of the car many times before ejection.

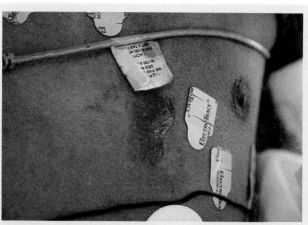

FIGURE 1-19 Air bags can cause abrasions to the face, chest, and arms.

the uterus. Lap belts with shoulder harnesses are essential to provide equal distribution of forces and to prevent forward flexion of the mother. Without the shoulder harness, the protuberant uterus will also receive the impact of the steering wheel or dashboard. Steering wheel or dashboard injuries sustained because seatbelts were not worn or were worn improperly are associated with a 50% fetal death rate.

Motorcycle Collisions

In a motorcycle collision, any structural protection afforded to the victims is not derived from a steel cage, as is the case in an automobile, but from protective devices worn by the rider—that is, helmet, leather or abrasion-resistant clothing, and boots. Although helmets are designed to protect against impact forces to the head, they transmit any impact into the cervical spine, and as such do not protect against severe cervical injury. Leather and synthetic gear worn over the body was initially designed to protect professional riders in competition, where falls tend to be controlled and result in long sliding mechanisms on hard surfaces rather than multiple collisions against road objects and other vehicles. Leather clothing will protect mostly against road abrasion but offers little or no protection against blunt trauma from secondary impacts. In a street crash, collisions usually occur against other larger vehicles or stationary objects.

When assessing the scene of a motorcycle collision, attention should be given to the deformity of the motorcycle, the side of most damage, the distance of skid marks in the road, the deformity of stationary objects or other vehicles, the distance between the rider and the bike following the collision, and the extent and location of deformity in the helmet **FIGURE 1-20**. These findings can be helpful in estimating the extent of trauma in a patient.

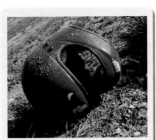

FIGURE 1-20 After a motorcycle collision, check the patient's helmet for damage.

There are four types of motorcycle impacts: head-on, angular, ejection, and laying the motorcycle down **FIGURE 1-21**.

Head-on Collision

In a head-on collision, the motorcycle strikes another object and stops its forward motion while the rider and any parts

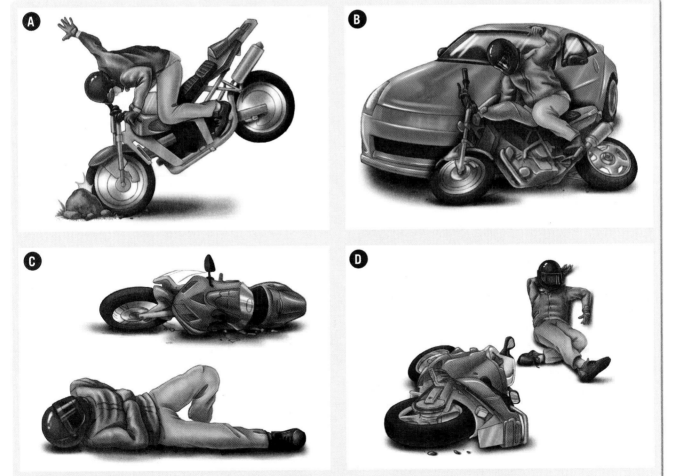

FIGURE 1-21 There are four types of motorcycle collisions. **A.** Head-on collision. **B.** Angular collision. **C.** Ejection. **D.** Laying the motorcycle down.

of the motorcycle that are broken off continue their forward motion until stopped by an outside force, such as drag from the road or from a secondary collision. Because the motorcycle's center of gravity is above the front axle, there is a forward and upward motion at the point of the collision, causing the rider to go over the handlebars. If the rider's feet remain on the pegs or pedals, the forward and upward motion of the upper torso is restrained by the lower extremities, producing bilateral femur or tibia fractures and severe foot injuries.

For motorcycles with a low riding seat below the level of the gas tank, such as Japanese racing bikes or Italian transalpine-style motorcycles, the tank can act as a wedge on the pelvis during the initial phase of the collision, resulting in severe anterior-posterior compression (APC) injuries to the pelvis, which in turn often result in severe neurovascular compromise **FIGURE 1-22**. Open pelvic fractures are also common, resulting in severe perineal injuries with loss of the pelvic floor. Mortality associated with open pelvic fractures approaches 50%.

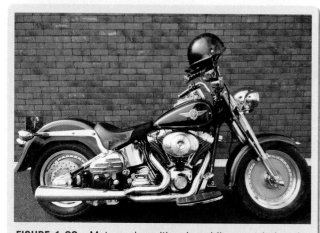

FIGURE 1-22 Motorcycles with a low riding seat below the level of the gas tank, such as racing bikes or transalpine-style motorcycles, can pose additional dangers to the rider. The tank can act as a wedge on the pelvis during the initial phase of the collision, often resulting in severe neurovascular compromise.

Angular Collision

In an angular collision, the motorcycle strikes an object or another vehicle at an angle so that the rider sustains direct crushing injuries to the lower extremity between the object and the motorcycle. This usually results in severe open and comminuted lower extremity injuries with severe neurovascular compromise, often requiring surgical amputation. Often the rider is propelled over the front of the colliding vehicle. Because the collision is at an angle, severe thoracoabdominal torsion and lateral bending spine injuries can result, in addition to head injury and pelvic trauma.

Ejection

An ejected rider will travel at high speed until stopped by a stationary object, another vehicle, or road drag. Severe abrasion injuries down to bone can occur with drag. An unpredictable combination of blunt injuries can occur from secondary collisions.

Laying the Motorcycle Down

A technique used to separate the rider from the body of the motorcycle and the object to be hit is referred to as *laying the motorcycle down*. It was developed by motorcycle racers and adapted by street bikers as a means of achieving a controlled crash. As a collision approaches, the motorcycle is turned flat and tipped sideways at 90° to the direction of travel so that one leg is dropped to the grass or asphalt. This slows the occupant faster than the motorcycle, allowing for the rider to become separated from the motorcycle. If properly protected with leather or synthetic abrasion-resistant gear, injuries should be limited to those sustained by rolling over the pavement and any secondary collision that may occur. When executed properly, this maneuver prevents the rider from being trapped between the bike and the object. However, a rider unable to clear the bike will continue into the collision, often with devastating results.

To immobilize the spine and secure the airway, the motorcycle helmet will need to be removed from the patient. Dents and abrasions seen on the exterior of the helmet must be assumed to have caused cervical spine fractures until proven otherwise by radiographs. Precautions should be taken to remove the helmet, which should be cut if it cannot be removed without introducing further deformation to the neck **PROCEDURE 21**.

Pedestrian Injuries

Pedestrians, skaters, cyclists, and skateboarders are at greater risk for injury than vehicle occupants and usually bear the greatest burden of injury. This is especially true in low-income and middle-income countries, because of the greater variety and intensity of traffic mix and the lack of separation from other road users. Of particular concern is the mix between the slow-moving and vulnerable nonmotorized road users, as well as motorcycles, and fast-moving, motorized vehicles.

There are some 800 million bicycles in the world, which is twice the number of cars. In Asia alone, bicycles carry more people than do all the world's cars. Nonetheless, in many countries, bicycle injuries are not given proper recognition as a road safety problem and attract little research.

Recent studies have shown that pedestrians and motorcyclists have the highest rates of injury in Asia. Injured pedestrians and passengers in mass transportation are the main issue in Africa. In Latin America and the Caribbean, injuries to pedestrians are the greatest problem. By contrast, in Western Europe, car occupants represent more than 60% of all traffic-related fatalities, a reflection of the greater number of motor vehicles in use. Although there are fewer motorcyclist, cyclist, and pedestrian casualties, these groups of road users bear higher fatality rates.

Older pedestrians in particular are associated with a very high rate of road injury and death. This is mainly due to the increased physical frailty of the elderly. Given the same type of impact, an older person is more likely to be injured or killed than a younger one.

More than 85% of pedestrians are struck by the vehicle's front end, sustaining a predictable pattern of injuries starting with those caused by direct impact with the bumper. Adult injuries are generally lateral and posterior because adults tend to turn to the side or away from impact, whereas children will face forward into oncoming traffic FIGURE 1-23.

Pediatric patterns of pedestrian injury are different from patterns in adults. Small children are shorter, so the car bumper is more likely to strike them in the pelvis or torso, causing severe injuries from direct impact. Although they are less likely than adults to fly over the front of the car, they are more likely to be run over by the vehicle as they are propelled to the ground by the impact.

Falls from Heights

High falls most commonly involve children younger than 5 years old who are left unsupervised near a high window (more than 10' [3 m]) or on a porch higher than 10' (3 m) with inadequate railings. Adult falls from heights usually occur in the context of criminal activity, attempted suicide, or intoxication such as in alcohol, narcotic, or hallucinogen use, including PCP or LSD.

Remember that a fall produces acceleration downward at 9.8 m/sec^2. On contact with the floor or ground, an instantaneous deceleration occurs forcing the victim from whatever velocity had been achieved at the end of the fall to zero velocity. If a person falls for 2 seconds, the speed at impact will be nearly 20 m/sec^2 (or about 45 mph).

The severity of injuries you can expect to find in your patient will depend on a number of factors, all of which will be important in your patient assessment FIGURE 1-24.

Height

The height from which the victim has fallen will determine the velocity of the fall. Height plus stopping distance predicts the magnitude of deceleration forces. A fall greater than

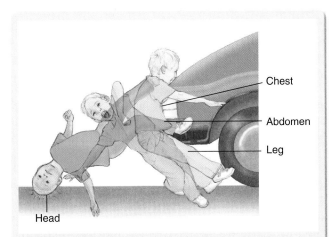

FIGURE 1-23 Waddell's triad refers to the pattern of automobile pedestrian injuries that can be predicted in children. First, the bumper hits the pelvis and femur, instead of the knees and tibias; second, the chest and abdomen hit the grill or low on the hood of the car (sternal and rib fractures); third, the head strikes the ground (skull and facial fractures, facial abrasions, and closed head injury).

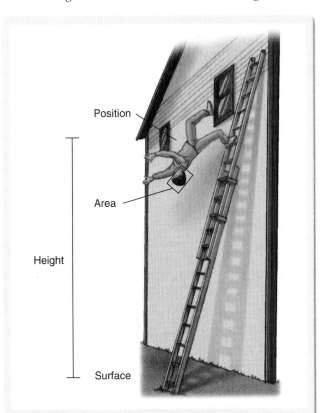

FIGURE 1-24 The five factors of falls are height, position, area, surface, and physical condition.

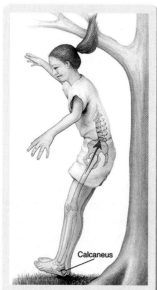

FIGURE 1-25 When an adult falls and lands on his or her feet, the energy is transmitted to the spine, sometimes producing a spinal injury in addition to injuries to the legs and pelvis.

15′ (4.6 m) or 2.5 to 3 times the height of the patient will have a greater incidence of morbidity and mortality, although it is usually assumed that a fall from four stories may be survivable. At five stories, survival is questionable; at six stories, survival is unlikely; and a fall from seven stories or higher is rarely survivable.

Position

The position or orientation of the body at the moment of impact will also be a determinant in the types of injuries sustained and their survivability. Children tend to fall headfirst, owing to the relatively greater mass of a child's head, so head injuries are common in children, as are injuries to the wrists and upper extremities when the child attempts to break his or her fall with outstretched arms. Adults, on the other hand, usually try, when not intoxicated, to land on their feet, thus controlling their fall. However, they often tilt backward, landing on their buttocks and outstretched hands. The group of potential injuries from a vertical fall to a standing position is commonly referred to as the *Don Juan syndrome* or *lover's leap* pattern of injuries **FIGURE 1-25**. Injuries include foot and lower extremity fractures, along with hip, acetabular, and pelvic ring and sacral fractures. Lumbar spine axial loading also results in vertebral compression and burst fractures, particularly of T12-L1 and L2. Vertical deceleration forces tend to injure organs (liver, spleen, and aorta). Fractures of the forearm and wrist (Colles fracture) are also common.

Area

This refers to the area over which the impact is distributed. The larger the area of contact at the time of impact, the greater the dissipation of the force and the lower the peak pressures generated. Landing on the buttocks and legs will spread the energy over a larger surface than just landing on the feet.

Surface

The surface onto which the person has fallen and the degree to which that surface can deform (degree of plasticity) under the force of the falling body can help dissipate the forces of sudden deceleration. Deep snow, for example, has a relatively large capacity to deform, whereas concrete has scarcely any plasticity. Also, contrary to what may be expected, water also has very little plasticity at high-speed impacts. The surface of contact may also present hazards in the form of irregularities or protruding structures; it is far more dangerous to fall onto a wrought-iron fence, for example, than onto the grass beside it. If the surface does not conform, the unprotected body will.

Physical Condition

The physical condition of the victim in the form of preexisting medical conditions may also influence the injuries sustained. Most notably is the case of older patients with osteoporosis, a condition that predisposes them to fractures even with minimal falls. Patients with hematologic conditions resulting in an enlarged spleen may also be more prone to a ruptured spleen in a fall. Children younger than 3 years old have fewer injuries from falls than do older children and adults, most likely because of the more elastic nature of their tissues and less ossification.

Penetrating Trauma

Unlike blunt trauma, which can involve a large surface area, penetrating trauma involves a disruption of the skin and underlying tissues in a small, focused area. Although a variety of objects may cause penetrating injuries in a variety of settings, penetrating trauma is usually interpreted as being more specific to injuries caused by knives, firearms, and other devices used as a means to cause intentional or accidental harm.

Stab Wounds

The damage a stabbing can create is limited to what the weapon can reach when it is in place. Wounds are classified as low energy because the speed of the weapon is limited to human force. Stab wounds are often caused by a knife but ice picks, screwdrivers, and pencils have all been used to cause bodily injury. Damage from low energy weapons is limited to the path that the weapon takes within the body.

The severity of a stab wound depends on the anatomic area involved, depth of penetration, blade length, and angle of penetration. When possible, the provider should try to identify the type of weapon used, including the length and cutting edge. Knowing the gender of the attacker can also help determine the path of the wound track. Men tend to grasp the knife with the blade in the thumb side of the hand and strike forward or upward, while women grasp the knife with the blade at the pinky finger side and strike in a downward motion. If the wound is in a hand, the injury may create permanent disability but is rarely life threatening. If it is in the abdomen, the possibility of life threats expands if the location is over an organ and the weapon was long enough to reach the organ.

A stab wound may also involve a cutting or hacking type force such as in machete wounds, which not only can result in laceration, but also can cause fractures,

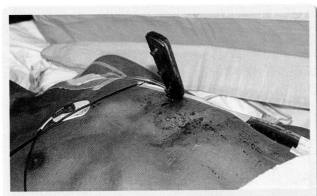

FIGURE 1-26 The severity of a stab wound depends on the anatomic area involved, depth of penetration, blade length, and angle of penetration.

blunt injury to underlying soft tissues and bone, and amputation. Wounds can also look smaller on the external surface but have more tissue damage on the inside when the attacker moves the blade while the blade is inserted in the body.

Neck wounds can involve critical anatomic structures such as the carotid arteries, subclavian vessels, apices of the lung, upper mediastinum, trachea, esophagus, and thoracic duct. Deep neck wounds of sufficient energy can result in spinal cord involvement and cervical fracture.

Lower chest or upper abdominal wounds have the potential of involving the thoracic and abdominal cavities, depending on the location of the diaphragm at the time of injury, that is, whether the person was inhaling or exhaling **FIGURE 1-26**.

The pattern of stab wounds closely relates to the mechanism involved and should be documented in detail because your records may be needed in criminal proceedings. Be sure to record the directions of the stab wounds.

STATS

In the United States, the most common sources of penetrating injuries are firearms. According to the US Department of Justice, 29,573 people died by gunfire in the United States in 2001. Although a staggering number, this actually represented a 25% decline in firearm-associated deaths from a peak in 1993 of 39,595 deaths. Of the gun-related deaths in 2001, 57% were suicides, 39% were homicides (including justified shootings by law enforcement personnel and gun owners), 3% were unintentional, and 1% were unclassified.

Gunshot Wounds

Firearms are the primary mechanism resulting in penetrating trauma. The amount of damage a firearm can cause will depend on a number of factors, including the type of firearm, the velocity of the projectile, the physical design of the projectile, the distance to the target from the muzzle of the firearm, and the type of tissue struck. There are hundreds if not thousands of firearm models and designs; however, they can be classified primarily into three types: shotguns, rifles, and handguns.

Shotguns fire round pellets (referred to as "shot") from about half a dozen to several dozen at a time depending on the type of load used. The load denominated 00 or 000, "buckshot," is a larger pellet; smaller shot such as No. 7 is a common fowl hunting shot or "birdshot." At short range, even the smaller shot can cause devastating injuries. Shotgun shells can also be loaded with a single large and heavy projectile called a sabot, which can cause even worse harm. A shotgun typically has a smooth bore, and its numerous projectiles are not stabilized in flight by spin, as is the single projectile fired from a rifle barrel. The pellets, therefore, leave the barrel and immediately start dispersing so that the shot density (that is, the separation between any two pellets) at the time of impact on a target will be determined by the distance traveled.

At very close range (less than 10′ [3 m]), a shotgun can induce destructive injuries. Entrance and exit wounds can be very large, with shotgun wadding, bits of clothing, skin, and hair driven into the wound that can cause massive contamination, leading to increased infection potential should the patient survive the initial trauma.

Rifles are firearms firing a single projectile at very high velocity through a grooved barrel that imparts a spin to the projectile that stabilizes the projectile's flight for accuracy.

Handguns are of two types: revolvers and pistols. Revolvers have a cylinder holding from 6 to 10 rounds of ammunition, and pistols have a separate magazine holding as many as 17 rounds of ammunition in some models. Handguns also have rifled barrels to impart spin to a bullet, but their accuracy is more limited than a rifle's because their barrels (and sight radius) are shorter. The ammunition handguns fire is also, in general, less powerful than ammunition fired from rifles, and handguns fire at much lower velocities.

The most important factor for the seriousness of a gunshot wound is the type of tissue through which the projectile passes. Tissue of high elasticity (eg, muscle) is better able to tolerate stretch (temporary cavitation [cavity formation]) than tissue of low elasticity, like the liver. A high-velocity bullet fired through a fleshy part of the leg may do much less damage than a relatively low-velocity bullet that punctures the aorta or the liver.

An entry wound is characterized by the effects of initial contact and implosion. Skin and subcutaneous tissues are pushed in, cut, or abraded externally as missile fragments pass and heat is transferred to the tissues. At close range,

TIP

It is often difficult, if not impossible, to determine entrance wounds from exit wounds in the field. Report the number of wounds and, if known, the number of shots fired, to the trauma team.

of cavitation at the point of exit. Exit wounds usually have irregular edges and may be larger than the entry wound **FIGURE 1-29** . There may be multiple exit wounds in the case of fragmentation. The number of exit wounds and the extent of tissue damage encountered must be assessed and carefully documented.

tattoo marks from powder burns can occur **FIGURE 1-27** . At extremely close ranges, burns can occur from the muzzle blast. Heavy wound contamination results from negative pressure generated behind the traveling projectile, which sucks surrounding elements such as clothing into the wound, greatly increasing infection potential.

Deformation and tissue destruction sustained in soft tissues and bone is based on a combination of factors, including density, compressibility, missile velocity, and missile fragmentation. The initial path of tissue destruction is caused by the projectile crushing the tissue during penetration. This creates a permanent cavity that may be a straight line or an irregular pathway as the bullet is deflected into a number of angles after initial penetration. Pathway expansion refers to the tissue displacement that occurs as the result of low-displacement shock waves (sonic pressure waves) that travel at the speed of sound in tissue (four times the speed of sound in air). These shock waves push tissues in front of and lateral to the projectile and may not necessarily increase the wound size or cause permanent injury, but they result in cavitation **FIGURE 1-28** . Tissue is compressed and accelerated away, causing injury. The waves of tissue are similar to throwing a rock into a pond. The rock creates a hole in the pond that quickly refills while waves emanate from the penetrating "wound," or hole in the pond.

Bowel, muscle, and lung are relatively elastic, resulting in fewer permanent effects of temporary cavitation. Liver, spleen, and brain are relatively inelastic, and the temporary cavity may become a permanent defect. Missile fragmentation is a major cause of tissue damage as the projectile may break apart and send off fragments that create their own separate paths through tissues. Secondary missiles can also be generated by pieces of bone, teeth, buttons, or other objects encountered in the projectile's path as it enters the body. Exit wounds occur when the projectile has sufficient energy that is not entirely dissipated along its trajectory through the body. The projectile then exits the victim and can injure other bystanders as well.

The size of the exit wound depends on the energy dissipated and the degree

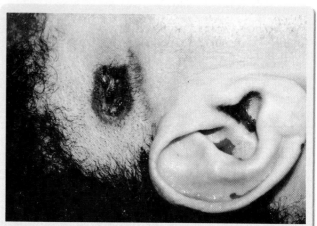

FIGURE 1-27 Tattoo marks can result from powder burns when a victim is shot at close range.

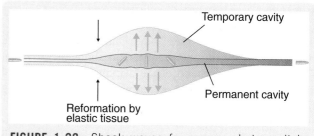

FIGURE 1-28 Shock waves from a gunshot result in cavitation.

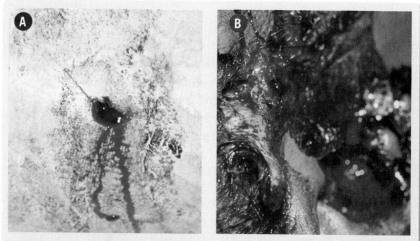

FIGURE 1-29 **A.** Entrance wound from a gunshot. **B.** Exit wound from a gunshot.

To give the trauma team at the hospital as much information as possible, try to obtain the following information:

- *What kind of weapon* was used (handgun, rifle, or shotgun; type and caliber if known)?
- At *what range* was it fired?
- *What kind of bullet* was used? (Ideally, see if you can find an unfired cartridge.)

What to look for:

- Powder residue around the wound
- Entrance and exit wounds (the exit wound is usually larger and more ragged)

In the real world, the assailant is usually gone, along with the weapon, and patient care is the first goal of providers, a far more pressing matter than obtaining answers to the previous questions.

Blast Injuries

Although most commonly associated with military conflict, blast injuries are also seen in civilian practice in mines, shipyards, chemical plants, and, increasingly, in association with terrorist activities. People who are injured in explosions may be injured by any of four different mechanisms **FIGURE 1-30**:

- **Primary blast injuries:** These are due entirely to the blast itself, that is, damage to the body caused by the pressure wave generated by the explosion.
- **Secondary blast injuries:** Damage results from being struck by flying debris, such as shrapnel from the device or from glass or splinters that have been set in motion by the explosion. Objects are propelled by the force of the blast and strike the victim, causing injury.
- **Tertiary blast injuries:** These occur when the victim is hurled by the force of the explosion against a stationary object. A "blast wind" also causes the victim's body to be hurled or thrown, causing further injury.
- **Miscellaneous blast injuries:** These include burns from hot gases or fires started by the blast, respiratory injury from inhaling toxic gases, and crush injury from the collapse of buildings, among others.

The vast majority of patients who survive an explosion will have some combination of the four types of injury mentioned. We will confine our discussion here to primary blast injuries because they are the most easily overlooked.

The Physics of an Explosion

When a substance is detonated, a solid or liquid is chemically converted into large volumes of gas under pressure with resultant energy release. This generates a pressure pulse in the shape of a spherical blast wave that expands in all directions from the point of explosion. Flying debris and high winds commonly cause conventional blunt and penetrating trauma.

Components of a Blast Shock Wave

The leading edge of the shock wave is called the blast front. A positive wave pulse refers to the phase of the explosion in which there is a pressure front higher than atmospheric pressure. The peak magnitude of the wave experienced by a victim becomes lessened the farther the person is from the center of the explosion. Tissue damage is dependent on the magnitude of the pressure spike and the duration of force application. The negative wave pulse refers to the phase in which pressure is less than atmospheric; it may last 10 times as long as the positive wave pulse. It occurs as air displaced by the positive wave pulse returns to fill the space of the explosion. It can lead to massive movements of air, resulting in high-velocity winds **FIGURE 1-31**.

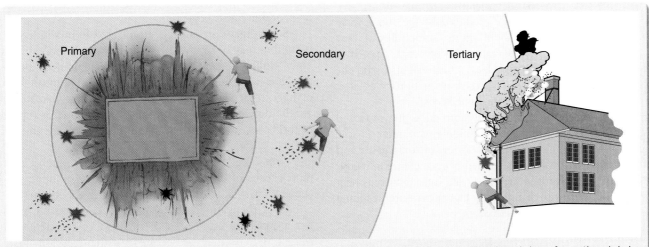

FIGURE 1-30 Blast injuries come in several phases: primary injury from the blast; secondary injury from the debris; injury from being thrown into other objects; miscellaneous injuries from crushing, burning, or secondary collapse.

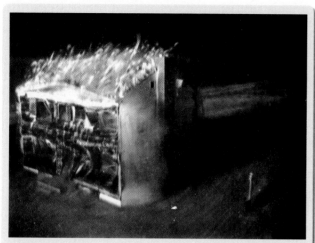

FIGURE 1-31 Blast waves produce a positive and negative pressure change that affect the air-containing organs of the body.

The speed, duration, and pressure of the shock wave are affected by the following:

- **The size of the explosive charge:** The larger the explosion, the faster the shock waves and the longer they will last.
- **The nature of the surrounding medium:** Pressure waves travel much more rapidly in water, for example, and are effective at greater distances in water.
- **The distance from the explosion:** The farther one is from the explosion, the slower the shock wave velocity and the longer its duration.
- **The presence or absence of reflecting surfaces:** If the pressure wave is reflected off a solid object, its pressure may be multiplied several times. For example, a shock wave that might cause minimal injury in the open can cause devastating trauma if the victim is standing beside a wall or similar solid object.

The changes in pressure produced by the shock wave are accompanied by transient winds, sometimes of very high velocity, that can accelerate small objects to speeds of hundreds of feet per second. Blast winds can also send the human body flying against larger, more stationary objects, or as mentioned previously, amputate limbs.

An explosion is significantly more damaging in closed spaces because of a limited dissipation environment for the forces involved and for the generation of toxic gases and smoke. The blast wave is magnified when it comes into contact with a solid surface such as a wall, causing victims near a wall to be hit with significantly higher pressure, resulting in increased risk of injury and death.

Tissues at Risk

Air-containing organs such as the middle ear, lung, and gastrointestinal tract are most susceptible to pressure changes. Junctions between tissues of different densities and exposed tissues such as the head and neck are prone to injury as well. The ear is the organ system most sensitive to blast injuries. The tympanic membrane evolved to detect minor changes in pressure and will rupture at pressures of 5 to 7 pounds per square inch (psi) above atmospheric pressure. Thus, the tympanic membranes are a sensitive indicator of the possible presence of other blast injuries. The patient may complain of ringing in the ears, pain in the ears, or some loss of hearing, and blood may be visible in the ear canal. Dislocation of structural components of the ear, such as the ossicles conforming the inner ear, may occur. Permanent hearing loss is possible.

Primary pulmonary blast injuries occur as contusions and hemorrhages. When the explosion occurs in an open space, the side facing the explosion is usually injured, but the injury can be bilateral when the victim is located in a confined space. The patient may complain of tightness or pain in the chest and may cough up blood and develop tachypnea or other signs of respiratory distress. Subcutaneous emphysema (crackling under the skin) over the chest can be palpated, indicating air in the skin. Pneumothorax is common and may require emergency decompression in the field for your patient to survive **PROCEDURE 13**. Pulmonary edema may ensue rapidly. If there is *any* reason to suspect lung injury in a blast victim (even just the presence of a ruptured eardrum), administer oxygen. Avoid giving oxygen under positive pressure, however (ie, by bag mask or demand valve), because that may simply increase the damage to the lung. Be cautious as well with intravenous fluids, which may be poorly tolerated in patients with this lung injury and result in pulmonary edema.

One of the most concerning pulmonary blast injuries is arterial air embolism, which occurs on alveolar disruption with subsequent air embolization into the pulmonary vasculature **FIGURE 1-32**. Even small air bubbles can enter a coronary artery and cause myocardial injury. Air emboli that enter the cerebrovascular system can produce disturbances in vision, changes in behavior, changes in state of consciousness, or other neurologic signs.

Solid organs are relatively protected from shock wave injury but may be injured by secondary missiles or a hurled body. Hollow organs, however, may be injured by similar mechanisms as lung tissue is. **Petechiae**, or pinpoint hemorrhages that show up on the skin, to large hematomas are the dominant form of pathology. Perforation or rupture of the bowel and colon is a risk because they are air-filled organs.

Neurologic injuries and *head trauma* are the most common causes of death from blast injuries. **Subarachnoid** (beneath the arachnoid layer covering the brain) and **subdural** (beneath the outermost covering of the brain) hematomas are often seen. Permanent or transient neurologic deficits may be secondary to concussion, intracerebral bleeding, or air embolism. Instant but transient unconsciousness, with or without retrograde amnesia, may be initiated not only by head trauma, but also by

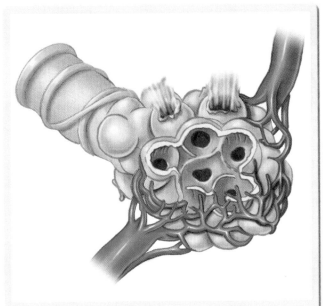

FIGURE 1-32 Damage to the lung may cause air to leak from the alveoli into the bloodstream, causing an air embolism that may enter the heart, lung, or brain.

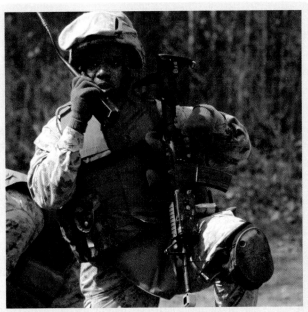

FIGURE 1-33 Improvements to military body armor have decreased the number of fatal injuries to the torso.

cardiovascular problems. Bradycardia and hypotension are common after an intense pressure wave from an explosion. This is a vagal nerve–mediated form of cardiogenic shock without compensatory vasoconstriction (eg, vasovagal syncope).

Extremity injuries, including traumatic amputations, are common. Other injuries are often associated with tertiary blasts. Patients with traumatic amputation by postblast wind are likely to sustain fatal injuries secondary to the blast. In present combat, improved body armor has increased the number of survivors of blast injuries from shrapnel wounds to the torso **FIGURE 1-33**. The number of severe orthopaedic and extremity injuries, however, has increased. In addition, although body armor may limit or prevent shrapnel from entering the body, it also "catches" more energy from the blast wave, possibly resulting in the victim being thrown backward, thus increasing potential spine and spinal cord injury.

CHAPTER RESOURCES

CASE STUDY ANSWERS

1 What is the effect of speed on energy? How can energy be a predictor of injury?

Speed or velocity plays a much bigger role in the amount of energy an object has than does its weight or mass. The more energy an object has to dissipate, the more the body will have to absorb, causing injury.

2 Describe the three impacts seen in this collision as the energy of speed is dissipated through the car and patient.

The first impact that begins to exchange energy is the vehicle striking the other vehicle. As the vehicle suddenly slows down, the occupant has not yet changed speed and crashes into the steering wheel. In this case, the air bag deployed in an attempt to slow the occupant's speed. The third impact is the major internal organs of the body suddenly decelerating and stopping when they strike the chest and abdominal wall. The amount of energy decreases with each impact; however, the more energy there is initially, the more energy the body has to withstand.

3 What are some of the clues available from the vehicle that can help predict the body areas that may have sustained injury? How would the injury pattern differ if the patient had worn his seatbelt? What if there were no seatbelt or air bags?

From the history of the scene we can deduce that the vehicle was traveling at highway speeds when it struck a parked vehicle. By the patient's account, he had no opportunity to brake and decrease the amount of speed. The SUV has moderate damage directed in the center of the front end and no damage to any other part of the vehicle. The second vehicle was pushed off the roadway, taking some of the energy with it. Internally, the vehicle has deployed air bags and a broken steering wheel. This patient appears to have slid forward and impacted the steering wheel.

Had the patient worn his seatbelt, the energy would have been spread more evenly over his skeletal frame. A seatbelt should fit snugly across the pelvis and then over the chest, crossing the midclavicle to distribute the energy from a sudden stop more evenly over the whole body. In motor vehicle collisions, passengers protected by air bags alone have been shown to have similar rates of abdominal injury that require surgery as compared to those who were wearing seatbelts and whose vehicle had no air bag deployment.

An unrestrained patient in a vehicle involved in a frontal impact has a tendency to travel forward and then either up and over the steering wheel (with injury to the head, neck, and chest) or down and under the steering wheel, impacting the lower dashboard (with injury to the knees, legs, pelvis, and abdomen).

4 What injuries would you suspect with this patient based on the available information?

This patient sustained several rib fractures, bilateral pulmonary contusions, and a laceration to the liver. Other injuries that could have been possible include: C-spine injury, sternal fracture, additional lung injury, cardiac injury, and additional abdominal trauma.

5 Using the process of predicting injury based on the review of trauma, what types of clues could help predict the injury if the mechanism was a fall? A gunshot wound? A knife wound?

Injury and the extent of injury from a fall can be predicted by looking at the height of the fall (falls over 20′ (6 m) are significant trauma producers), the surface on which the patient fell (concrete is worse than a soft surface), and the body part on which the patient landed (energy will travel through the body from the feet up or the head down).

Factors that affect the amount of energy a patient will sustain from a gunshot wound include the speed of the bullet (high power weapons have more speed than handguns), the type of bullet (some bullets are designed to fragment or mushroom to create more injury when they hit the body), the area on the body that was struck (bullets go through different tissue with different injury patterns), the number of bullets or projectiles (shotguns cause more damage because they have more projectiles), and any safety gear that can slow the speed of the bullet (bulletproof vests or even standing behind something that will slow the bullet will decrease the amount of injury).

The amount of damage a knife wound can produce is based on several factors: The length of the knife (the longer the knife, the further it can reach), the depth it was inserted (when the weapon can be located, the depth can sometimes be determined by examining the blade), the direction the stab wound follows (women often stab downward while men tend to stab horizontally forward), the number of wounds (more wounds equals more injury), the location of wounds on the body (knife wounds are limited to the areas that the knife can reach), and whether the knife was twisted when it was in the body (injury can be worsened if the wound track is expanded by twisting the knife).

Trauma in Motion

1. What types of injury would you expect to see if a patient were hit in the chest with a bat? Would the injury be different if they were hit on the right or left side?
2. If a person dove into shallow water head first, what types of injuries would you suspect? Would they be different if a heavy object fell on top of their head?
3. What unique mechanisms of injury do you see in your agency and what types of injury are associated with them?
4. If your ambulance were in a collision, what would you expect to see for injury patterns for the caregiver in the back?
5. What are the three most important safety devices used to reduce injury and why?

References and Resources

American Academy of Orthopaedic Surgeons. *Emergency Care of the Sick and Injured.* 9th ed. Sudbury, MA: Jones and Bartlett; 2005.

American Academy of Orthopaedic Surgeons. *Nancy Caroline's Emergency Care in the Streets.* 6th ed. Sudbury, MA: Jones and Bartlett; 2007.

Findlay G, Smith N, Martin IC, et al. *Trauma: Who Cares? A Report of the National Confidential Enquiry into Patient Outcome and Death (NCEPOD).* London, UK: 2007.

Mock C, Lormand JD, Goosen J, et al. *Guidelines for Essential Trauma Care.* Geneva: World Health Organization; 2004.

National Highway Traffic Safety Administration, Center for Statistics and Analysis. Traffic safety facts 2006 data, DOT HS 810 809. Available at: http://www.nhtsa.gov. Accessed Mar. 20, 2007.

Peden M, Scurfield R, Sleet D, et al. *World Report on Road Traffic Injury Prevention.* Geneva: World Health Organization; 2004.

Royal College of Surgeons of England and the British Orthopaedic Association. *Better Care for the Severely Injured.* London, UK: July 2000.

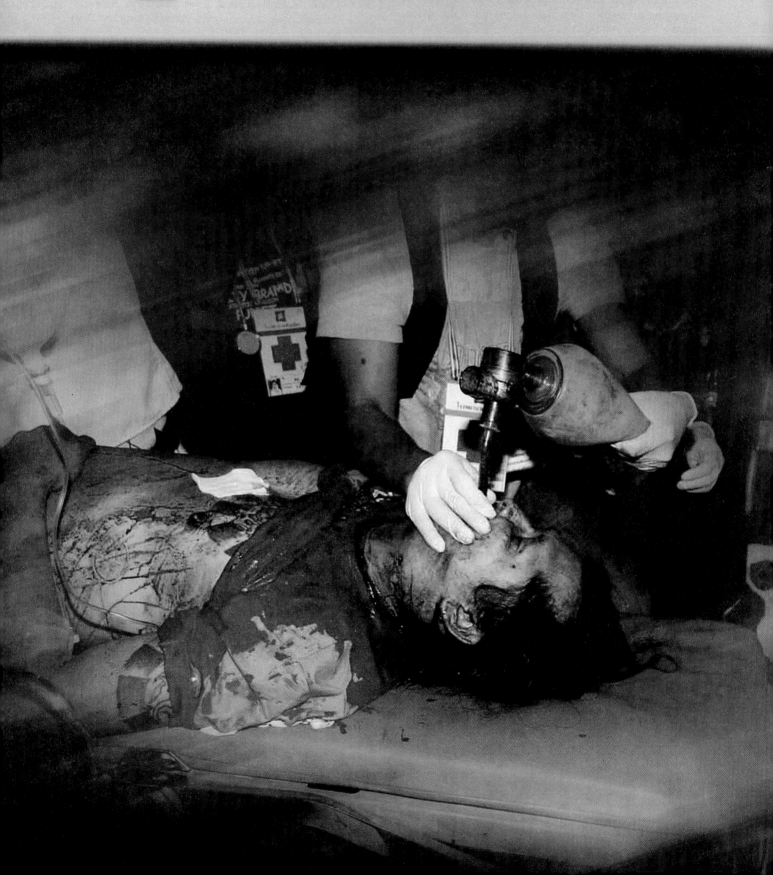

CASE STUDY

You are dispatched for a shooting at a local market. While monitoring the radio en route to the call, you learn that a fight has broken out following the shooting. Police report there is a male patient who was shot once in the chest and the person who shot him was attacked by the crowd and is now in police custody. Police report the patient is unresponsive at the scene with difficulty breathing.

Upon your arrival you are quickly ushered through a loud crowd into a café where you see a middle-aged man covered in blood lying on the ground. He is lying on his side breathing erratically and with difficulty. As you continue to scan the scene you see that more police have shown up for crowd control and that they have cleared an area for you to work.

As you log roll the patient to begin care, you find the patient struggling to breathe. The patient has snoring respirations and abnormal chest movement with breaths. You open the airway and the breathing becomes easier with less snoring. Turning your attention to his breathing you notice erratic breathing at 8 to 10 breaths/min with increased accessory muscle use. Quickly exposing his chest you note a single wound in the mid sternum that has bubbling air and a small amount of blood coming from the wound. You cover the wound with a gloved hand but notice no change in breathing. The patient has no distal pulses but has a weak carotid pulse that is very rapid. No additional wounds are located following a rapid trauma/secondary assessment of the head, neck, and torso (including the back). Lung sounds are absent on the right side and the patient has jugular venous distension.

1 What are the issues related to scene safety at this scene?

2 Describe the conditions found in the initial/primary assessment and the management required to support life.

3 How does the additional information from the rapid trauma/secondary assessment help to define the priorities for patient care?

4 Does this patient require rapid transport to a trauma center?

5 Why are frequent reassessments required for this priority patient?

Introduction

Patient assessment is the single most important skill a provider brings to a patient. Several elements make up the skill of patient assessment: information gathered from the caller, the patient, and the patient's family and friends; the emergency scene itself; and eyewitnesses to the emergency event. That information is then added to the data you obtain from your diagnostic tools and tests (such as physical assessment, vital signs, cardiac monitor, glucometer, pulse oximetry, and capnography).

Patient assessment, however, does not start with the patient; it starts with an assessment of the scene. Due to the nature of trauma scenes, the prehospital provider must consider his or her own safety. Crash and rescue scenes often include multiple risks, such as unstable vehicles, moving traffic, jagged metal and broken glass, fire or explosion hazards, downed power lines, and possibly hazardous materials. There is also the potential for violence at scenes from bystanders or assailants. Just because the scene is safe when you arrive does not mean it will stay safe. Always be aware of your surroundings before and during a call.

Scene Size-up and Evaluation

The process of scene size-up is conducted in a very short time and involves processing the dispatch information, evaluating the overall scene and safety, determining the mechanism of injury (MOI), and requesting additional help **FIGURE 2-1**.

Body Substance Isolation and Standard Precautions

The first step of the patient assessment process is the scene size-up. Your first and foremost concern on any call is ensuring your own safety and the safety of the other prehospital providers. Blood and fluids are prevalent on the trauma call. These fluids may contain the ability to transfer bloodborne pathogens such as hepatitis or human immunodeficiency virus (HIV). You should wear properly sized gloves on every call. If blood or other fluids could potentially splash or spray, wear eye protection **FIGURE 2-2**. Even covering up exposed skin with clothing can provide an initial barrier to fluid contact. When inhaled particles are a risk factor, wear a properly sized mask. In many trauma calls a gown or outer covering is also indicated.

Scene Safety

In the assessment and evaluation of the emergency scene, the main focus is to ensure the safety and well-being of the EMS team and any other emergency responders **FIGURE 2-3**. Roadways have many hazards including moving traffic, damaged electric wires, fluids from damaged vehicles, and glass or sharp metal on the vehicle itself. Construction sites that have excavating equipment or debris or

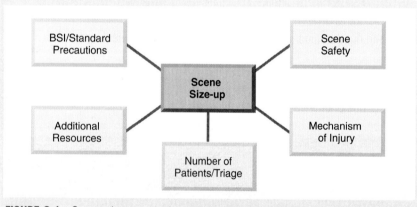

FIGURE 2-1   Scene size-up requires the provider to multitask to gain the required information.

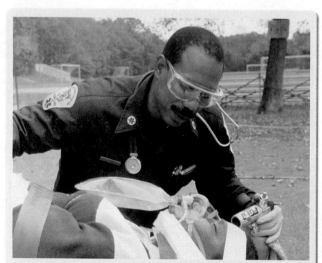

FIGURE 2-2 Providers must take precautions on every trauma call to avoid body fluids.

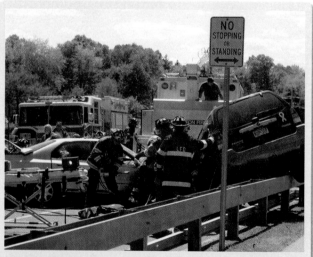

FIGURE 2-3   Your assessment begins with looking at the scene for potential hazards.

involve ladders to access patients have a set of hazards unique to the situation FIGURE 2-4 . Technical rescues often require specially trained personnel to access the patient. If you are injured while accessing or caring for the patient, you will do them no good. Extra resources will be needed to resume care for the patient and to provide care for you.

STATS

> The most common injuries experienced by providers are exposure to bloodborne pathogens from needlesticks, injuries from lifting and moving patients, various wounds inflicted by violent patients, and injuries caused by traffic accidents involving ambulances.

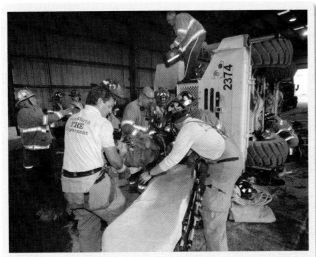

FIGURE 2-4 Equipment at construction sites presents unique hazards.

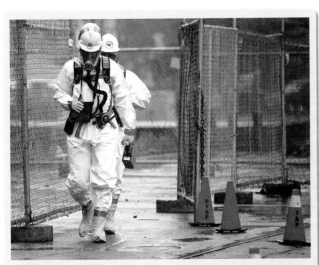

FIGURE 2-5 Hazardous material scenes present the prehospital provider with unique challenges.

Toxic substances are found at many scenes. From the lawn and garden chemicals found in almost every home to the countless chemicals used in industry and manufacturing, you should always be alert for the presence of toxic substances FIGURE 2-5 . If multiple victims are present and have similar symptoms or complaints, consider carbon monoxide poisoning or exposure to some other noxious agent as prime candidates. You should also be wary of working in toxic environments, for example confined spaces, fire scenes, or hazardous material scenes, which are all high risk. Smoke is the by-product of incomplete combustion and can contain many toxins, pathogens, and carcinogens. In these cases, having proper body and respiratory protection is a must before entering the scene and initiating patient care.

Don't just think of crime scenes in the past tense because there is always the possibility that more violence may occur FIGURE 2-6 . Under ideal circumstances, when dispatched to a potential crime scene, law enforcement personnel should enter and secure the scene first. All too frequently, the medical team arrives first and unknowingly enters a crime scene. For example, dispatch might receive a call for an "unconscious person." On arrival, the prehospital providers might discover that the patient has been stabbed in the chest. Law enforcement personnel should be requested immediately in such cases because it is nearly impossible for you and your partner to control the scene and care for the patient at the same time; the perpetrator could return with more weapons.

When faced with an unstable scene or a scene that begins deteriorating, such as a scene where bystanders become progressively louder or more unruly or make aggressive gestures or threats, consider retreating to a safe location until the scene is secured and deemed safe. If you believe that you can do so safely, remove the patient from the scene with you. Making such an attempt is clearly a judgment call on your part. Proper planning and situational awareness are important in keeping yourself and other rescuers safe.

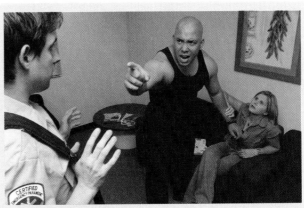

FIGURE 2-6 Emergency calls may be made in response to violence, or violence may develop during the call.

Remember that unsafe environments are everyday occurrences in the field. In some areas, snow- or ice-covered surfaces can persist for 3 or 4 months out of the year or more **FIGURE 2-7**. In other areas, it may rain for several months. Working on unstable surfaces is an inevitable part of prehospital medicine. Many areas have terrain issues ranging from minor hills to mountains to sandy beaches. Take the time to make all of your patient lifts and moves as safe and controlled as possible. Also, if footwear is not provided as part of your uniform, consider investing in a good pair of boots that will serve to keep your feet comfortable and to provide good traction to avoid slips.

Although protecting the emergency response team is clearly a priority, so is protecting the patient and bystanders. Establishing a perimeter around an emergency scene may prevent bystanders from entering a dangerous scene and potentially becoming patients themselves. Environmental issues can also influence scene safety and the patient care process. A patient involved in a motorcycle accident, lying on the roadway, exposed to wind and rain, may potentially develop hypothermia. Leaving a patient lying on a hot asphalt roadway as the midday sun beats down poses risks of burns or heat exposure. When the environment is unfriendly, perform the initial assessment, address life threats, and get the patient into a controlled environment (eg, an ambulance) as quickly as possible.

Mechanism of Injury

The **mechanism of injury (MOI)** is the way in which traumatic injuries occur—the forces that act on the body to cause damage (as seen in Chapter 1). Assessing and evaluating the MOI can help you predict the likelihood of certain injuries having occurred and estimate their severity.

At this point, if there is more than one patient or the patient requires rescue, helicopter transportation, or advanced care (eg, specialty teams) you should call for addi-

tional resources. The presence of multiple patients requires that they be triaged appropriately to determine which additional resources you need and how you will allocate the resources. When you have multiple patients at a trauma scene you must triage all patients (see Chapter 12).

Initial Assessment (Primary Assessment)

The initial assessment (or primary assessment) is the most intensive portion of the trauma assessment because it focuses on the identification and management of life-threatening problems **PROCEDURE 1**. The goal is to provide a rapid survey of the patient for life threats. In the first 60 to 90 seconds, as you observe, speak with, and assess the patient, you should be able to identify threats to the ABCs. More often than not, you will form a general impression of your patient based almost solely on the initial presentation and chief complaint.

Whether the emergency is medical or trauma, the first question is a qualification and the second is quantification. "Is my patient sick?" has a yes or no answer, whereas "How sick is my patient?" attempts to rate the event's severity. With time and experience, you should be able to answer both questions in that 60- to 90-second window, forming your general impression. Once these questions are answered, you can move forward with determining your priorities of care, developing a care plan, and putting the care plan into action.

The information gleaned from the initial assessment is crucial to the overall outcome for your patient. Treat life threats as you find them, but also decide what additional care is needed, what should be done on scene versus en route, when to initiate transport, and which facility is most appropriate given your patient's needs.

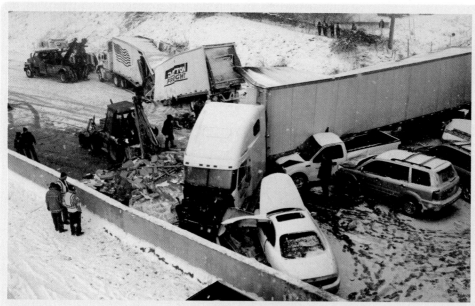

FIGURE 2-7 Weather can have an effect on the safety of a trauma scene.

Assess the Patient's Airway Status

For air to be drawn into the lungs, the airway has to be properly positioned and not obstructed (that is, open from an anatomic perspective). If you hear sonorous (snoring) respirations, think "position problem"—the sounds you are hearing are most likely from the tongue partially obstructing the airway **TABLE 2-1**. If you hear gurgling or bubbling sounds, think "suction"—there are most likely fluids such as blood, mucus, or vomit in

TIP

Immediate trauma care is geared toward finding and treating life threats. This approach follows the ABCs, but two issues have to be addressed first: c-spine control and catastrophic bleeding control. C-spine control will change how the provider opens the airway. Catastrophic hemorrhage control is needed to stop red blood cell loss, allowing all the remaining care to make an impact.

the mouth or posterior pharynx. Whistling, wheezing, or other noises coming from the upper airway are a sign of an obstruction from a foreign body (teeth, food, or another object) or may be from damage to the airways from direct trauma to the larynx or trachea. More aggressive airway management may be needed to handle this patient.

Assessment of a patient's airway is completed in the same way regardless of the patient's age. In responsive patients of any age, talking or crying will give clues about the adequacy of the airway. For all unresponsive patients, you must look, listen, and feel for breathing. If breathing is ineffective or absent, you must open the airway with a jaw thrust maneuver in the trauma patient with suspected spinal injury.

If you determine that the patient cannot maintain his or her airway and you cannot maintain it with manual maneuvers, you will need to use a more invasive technique. If mechanical means are required to keep the airway open and patent, you must choose an airway adjunct (see Chapter 3). If you opt to place an oropharyngeal or nasopharyngeal airway, choose the appropriate device and the right size for the patient. Endotracheal intubation involves several pieces of equipment, including (but not limited to) a laryngoscope handle, a laryngoscope blade, a properly sized endotracheal tube, a syringe, a stylet, an oropharyngeal airway (OPA), an end-tidal carbon dioxide ($ETCO_2$) detector, a bag-mask device, and a method to secure the tube once it is placed. Obviously, gathering the equipment, preparing the patient, and performing the intubation procedure are time consuming; quicker airway maneuvers should be used first.

Two additional components that must be considered as you begin your hands-on assessment and management of a trauma patient are cervical spine (c-spine) control and excessive hemorrhage control. The need for c-spine control must be determined based on the mechanism of injury and

patient status PROCEDURE 15. The unconscious patient following a traumatic event must have c-spine control and stabilization during the initial steps of airway control FIGURE 2-8. The second component is control of exsanguinating hemorrhage. Continual loss of large amounts of blood must be controlled quickly in trauma care. Extreme external bleeding that goes uncontrolled will leave your patient with fewer red blood cells to transport oxygen throughout the body. Without these cells, time spent managing airway and breathing issues may be unrewarded.

Assess the Patient's Breathing

Breathing is proportional and related to airway adequacy. The assessment of breathing focuses on two questions:

1. Is the patient breathing? If not, then you have to provide ventilatory support for the patient.
2. If the patient is breathing, is breathing adequate?

It is easy to answer the first question, but the second requires more thought. Adequate breathing requires the body to move enough air into and out of the lungs for the body to extract the oxygen it needs and eliminate carbon dioxide. But what is the correct amount? This question can be best answered by looking at how much air is moved over time rather than with each breath.

The respiratory rate multiplied by the amount inspired (tidal volume) with each breath equals the minute volume. Normal minute volume for an adult is between 5 and 8 liters. For example, a patient breathing slowly and deeply at 10 breaths/min with a tidal volume of 500 mL/breath, has a minute volume of 5,000 mL. By comparison, a patient breathing faster and shallower at a rate of 25 breaths/min and 200 mL/breath would also have a minute volume of 5,000 mL TABLE 2-2. On a per-minute basis, the volumes of the two patients are virtually identical, even though the second patient is breathing more than twice as fast as the first patient. The difference in the patients involves how much air is moved through the alveoli each time. Air that sits in the space of the airway that remains open is referred

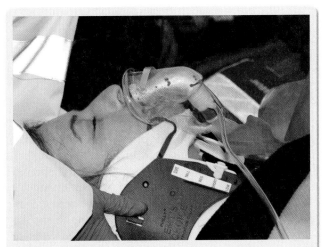

FIGURE 2-8 Cervical spine stabilization must be provided during the initial care of the airway.

TABLE 2-1	Assessment of Airway Sounds	
Sound	**Problem**	**Solution**
Snoring	Tongue and soft tissue	Position
Gurgling	Fluids	Suction
Stridor	Obstruction	Airway adjunct

CONTROVERSIES

Advanced Monitoring

EMERGENCY MEDICAL SERVICES (EMS) HAS deep historical roots and has adapted over time to meet the needs of the population as well as to improve its services according to current research and technology. Today, many health care administrators and legislators ask whether EMS has gone too far with its technologic advances and whether it should scale back to the basics of retrieval and transport.

In the United States it seems to be part of our makeup, our human nature, to want the latest and greatest. How many of you have purchased a new cell phone or handheld device when your old one worked just fine? And, how many of us know how to use all our personal gadgets to the full capacity for which they were intended?

In today's world of advanced technology and highly skilled care providers, it is important to ensure that the activities of EMS are consistent with its mission. The fundamental six stages of high-quality prehospital care are represented by the six arms of the "star of life" emblem of EMS: early detection, early reporting, early response, good on-scene care, care in transit, and transfer to definitive care. Within these parameters, we will consider whether new technologic advances support or detract from these goals.

I know from my work as a paramedic that when a new device was added to our ambulances, we all tried to come up with a good reason to use the device. And I also know from experience that when we had a protocol change that changed a medication from online medical control to a standing order, the medication use increased, at least in the short term.

The automated external defibrillator (AED), introduced in 1979, is now placed not only in ambulances but also in community and public gathering places. The treatment for ventricular fibrillation or ventricular tachycardic arrest is defibrillation, and the time it takes to defibrillate a patient correlates to outcome. In the hands of first responders and emergency medical technicians (EMTs), this technology has started many patients on their return from cardiac arrest to their prior quality of life. With respect to the goal of good on-scene care, this tool has clearly brought advancement to the field. The limitation of automated external defibrillation centers on delay in transport. Taking time at the scene to monitor a patient who does not need defibrillation can delay transport to a site that can provide definitive care. The key to proper use of the AED is to quickly assess and treat a patient and to simultaneously deliver the patient to the appropriate medical facility.

The ability to obtain a 12-lead electrocardiogram (ECG) is available on many ground and air ambulances. Diagnostic readouts from 12-lead monitoring can be transmitted to a hospital physician and allow resources to be mobilized for primary cardiac intervention. Some services use this technology to enable paramedics to initiate preparation of the catheterization lab from the field. This practice has dramatically decreased the times from door to catheterization lab and from door to thrombolytic administration.[1,2] Some ambulance services have diversion protocols that allow transport of patients with documented myocardial infarction to dedicated cardiac centers. The pitfalls of the use of 12-lead technology in the field are delay in transport and misdiagnosis. The cornerstone of effective use of this technology is paramedic education in ECG interpretation, timely acquisition of ECG tracings, and avoiding delay in transport. A well-structured protocol focuses on communication of the results of patient assessment, transmission of an ECG strip, and activation of the proper therapeutic intervention, whether it is cardiac catheterization and angioplasty or thrombolytics.

Reliance on technology can enable us to become less fluid with assessment skills. Consider the seasoned paramedic team that picked up a patient in cardiac arrest. Utilizing a brand new monitor with pacing capabilities, they placed the pads, adjusted the gain until they noted capture on the screen, and transported the patient. Unfortunately, a pulse check was neglected, and they walked into the emergency department with a patient in electrical-mechanical dissociation. It is human nature to use the technology at hand, and care must be taken not to become out of practice with our physical exam skills.

Carbon dioxide capnography allows EMTs to confirm and monitor the position of an endotracheal tube and, as an indirect measurement of cardiac output, can indicate the effectiveness of chest compressions. In the care of patients with head trauma, CO_2 levels can guide the use of hyperventilation, which, if not used judiciously, can be deleterious to neurologic outcome.[3] The two most important parameters for care of the brain-injured patient are hypoxia and hypotension. With capnography, progress toward end-tidal CO_2 goals can guide the ventilation of these patients and thus improve outcome.

Pulse oximetry can be a very useful tool in the prehospital environment; however, actions based on the incorrect interpretation of pulse oximetry readings heighten the risk of inducing harm. SaO_2 levels can be influenced by mild hypothermia, poor baseline perfusion, and even nail polish. In a patient with severe asthma, intubation is the decision of last resort, because the risk of morbidity and mortality associated with the intubation of a severe asthmatic is very high. Overdependence on pulse oximetry can lead to early intubation, aggressive ventilation, increased PEEP, hypotension, and cardiorespiratory arrest. The best indicator of when to intubate a patient with status asthmaticus is non-response to treatment or patient fatigue resulting from respiratory effort. Lack of knowledge of the pitfalls of pulse oximetry may lead to misdiagnosis of carbon monoxide poisoning or cyanide poisoning. Proper use of pulse oximetry can help the EMT determine and treat poor oxygenation levels, such as in the hypovolemic trauma patient who needs supplemental oxygen because of a lack of circulating red blood cells. The key to any medical tool is to know its uses and, more importantly, its limitations.

One of the problems with use of the technology is that it can cause delays in patient care, including transport. It is not only a prehospital phenomenon, there are several studies that point toward delays of patients being transferred to a tertiary care center as smaller community hospitals use all their technology to assess a patient, diagnose a problem, but then don't have the resources to treat the diagnosed problems. Consider the trauma patient brought to a small community hospital that has access to CT scan, but no surgeon on call. The trauma patient in hypovolemic shock needs to be moved expeditiously toward a facility with a surgeon, not wasting valuable time in diagnosing a liver laceration in the CT scan.

The repeating theme of this topic is that technology can indeed improve patient care and long-term outcome but, as with all therapeutic measures in medicine, each technologic tool has benefits as well as limitations. The key to proper utilization of technology and excellent patient care lies with the person using the technology. Each of us must be aware of the limitations of each tool and use it within those limitations. In the end, the most important tool is an excellent history and physical exam, followed by appropriate response to available information. Over-reliance on tools does not improve patient care, but a well-prepared EMT can make a difference in someone's life.

Evadne Marcolini, MD
Assistant Professor
Division of Surgical Critical Care and Emergency Medicine
R Adams Cowley Shock Trauma Center
University of Maryland Medical Center
Baltimore, Maryland

References

1. Sejersten M, Sillesen M, Hansen PR, et al. Effect on treatment delay of prehospital teletransmission of 12-lead electrocardiogram to a cardiologist for immediate triage and direct referral of patients with ST-segment elevation acute myocardial infarction to primary percutaneous coronary intervention. *Am J Cardiol.* 2008 Apr 1; 101(7):941–6. Epub 2008 Jan 25.

2. Garvey JL, MacLeod BA, Sopko G, Hand MM. Pre-hospital 12-Lead electrocardiography programs: a call for implementation by emergency medical services systems providing advanced life support. National Heart Attack Alert Program (NHAAP) Coordinating Committee, National Heart, Lung, and Blood Institute (NHLBI), National Institutes of Health. *J Am Coll Cardiol.* 2006; 47:485–491.

3. Lal D, Weiland S, Newton M, et al. Prehospital hyperventilation after brain injury: a prospective analysis of prehospital and early hospital hyperventilation of the brain-injured patient. *Prehosp Disast Med.* 2003; 18(1):20–23.

TABLE 2-2	Air Usage Affected by Ventilatory Rates		
Pt A	10 breaths/min ×	500 mL/breath =	5,000 mL minute volume
Pt B	25 breaths/min ×	200 mL/breath =	5,000 mL minute volume
Pt A	150 mL dead space ×	10 breaths/min =	1,500 mL unused air/min
Pt B	150 mL dead space ×	25 breaths/min =	3,750 mL unused air/min
Pt A	5,000 mL minute volume −	1,500 mL unused air/min =	3,500 mL air available for exchange in the alveoli
Pt B	5,000 mL minute volume −	3,750 mL unused air/min =	1,250 mL air available for exchange in the alveoli

to as *dead space*. In an average-sized adult, dead space is approximately 150 mL. When a patient breathes shallowly, the amount of new air that enters the lung is decreased due to this space. Adequate breath depth should be assessed by looking for chest expansion. Always keep in mind that the amount of air actually moved into and out of the lungs each minute is the best measure of breathing adequacy. Compare the two patients in Table 2-2. They have an equal minute volume, but faster ventilatory rates can affect the air available for exchange in the alveoli if breaths are shallow.

Besides the assessment of tidal volume and breathing rate, note the **work of breathing**, breath sounds, skin color, and level of consciousness or mental status as part of the breathing assessment. Because the brain is very sensitive to oxygen, an early indication of hypoxia is restlessness or anxiety. This restless state is often confused with intoxication from drugs or alcohol or sometimes just the emotions at a highly charged scene. While anxiety is a dangerous sign to watch for, an even more ominous sign in the level of consciousness is somnolence. As the body moves through states of hypoperfusion, acidosis builds up increasing the levels of CO_2 in the bloodstream. Hypercarbia presents with a tired appearance and can be seen in the patient that responds to verbal stimuli but fades back to sleep without stimulation.

Work of breathing is the effort a person uses to breathe. Signs of increased work of breathing include retractions or recession of the skin in between the ribs or around the sternum, excessive use of accessory muscles to breathe, nasal flaring, and using the tripod position when breathing. When the body begins to compensate for hypoperfusion, it attempts to move more air in and out of the lungs. Effortless tachypnea is often a sign seen in shock. The respiratory rate increases and the rate alone is enough to bring in the oxygen that the body requires. If rate alone will not satisfy the need for oxygen, the body enlists additional muscles in the chest to force a deeper breath. The pectoral, trapezius, scalene, and sternocleidomastoid muscles all work to pull the upper chest upward and outward while the abdominal muscles pull the lower rib cage downward, increasing the functional size of the chest. Often this forced expansion of the chest wall creates such negative pressure inside the chest that the skin between the ribs or just above the sternum or clavicles will be pulled inward. The body also attempts to make air movement easier to reduce the amount of energy needed to breathe. Flaring of the nares opens the airway to

TABLE 2-3	Breathing Assessment
Look	Chest movement and symmetry
Listen	Breathing sounds
Feel	Air movement

allow more air to pass with less resistance while moving the upper body into the tripod position straightens the airway and produces more movement of the diaphragm.

When evaluating the patient's breathing, the more signs of increased work of breathing that are seen, the worse the patient is. Increased respiratory rates indicate the patient's need for oxygen while an increase in the work of breathing is a sign that the patient requires oxygen and possible additional airway or ventilatory care. A patient who has been breathing hard will begin to tire and the signs of increased work of breathing may decrease as the accessory muscles tire and stop working. This is a sign of impending failure of the respiratory system and should be assessed during frequent patient reassessments. Children have less developed chest muscles and will often present with increased work of breathing earlier than an adult but will tire earlier as well (see Chapter 10).

The techniques used to assess a patient's breathing status are not new: Look, listen, and feel **TABLE 2-3**. Look for chest rise and fall, noting symmetry of the chest wall and depth of respirations. Observe the chest wall looking for abnormal movement or lack of movement of the rib cage. Rib fractures or flail segments often present with the surrounding muscles splinting the injury and decreased movement in the area (see Chapter 6). Listen for breath sounds by using your sense of hearing and by auscultation with a stethoscope. Lung sounds should be evaluated for equality and depth of air movement. Listen over the apices and the middle chest and at the bases of each lung. Note **adventitious** (abnormal) lung sounds, and treat the patient accordingly. If the patient is in spinal immobilization, use the anterior chest and mid axillary positions. If the posterior surface is available, lung sounds can be assessed both anteriorly and posteriorly. Finally, when in doubt, feel for chest movement by placing your cheek or the palms of your hand around the chest wall. Continue by palpating the chest wall for continuity of the rib cage. Palpate for crepitus, subcutaneous emphysema, or deformity which may indicate internal injury.

Patients breathing slower than 12 breaths/min or faster than 20 breaths/min, or who have a significant mechanism of injury, should have high-flow oxygen applied as early as possible. For patients with breathing rates of less than 9 breaths/min or greater than 28 breaths/min, consider the need for artificial ventilations with a bag mask. If the patient requires ventilations, begin them immediately. When in doubt, ventilate. Continue with the rest of the assessment after ventilations have been managed.

Several other life-threatening conditions should be managed if they are noted during the breathing assessment. For example, if a tension pneumothorax is present or highly suspected, a needle thoracentesis is indicated immediately **PROCEDURE 13** (see Chapter 6). If, during the visual assessment of the chest, an open chest wound is found, the wound should be covered by a gloved hand immediately and then an occlusive dressing applied. Paradoxical motion of the chest wall should be stabilized, as soon as it is noted, by holding pressure. The patient should then be evaluated to see if ventilation is required. (See Chapter 6 for more on chest injuries.)

Assess the Patient's Circulation

Assessing the pulse gives a rapid check of the patient's cardiovascular status and provides information about the rate, strength, and regularity of the heartbeat. The pulse is best palpated over the radial or carotid artery by using the tips of your index and middle fingers. In infants the pulse is better checked proximally at the brachial or femoral arteries. The presence of the pulse may help determine the ability of the body to provide blood to the vital organs. For example, the presence of a femoral pulse indicates that blood has moved along the aorta, past the major abdominal organs, to the legs.

First measure the pulse rate by counting the number of beats during 15 seconds, then multiply by 4. As you count the pulse rate, note the force of the pulse. A normal pulse feels "full," as if a strong wave has passed beneath your fingertips. When there is severe vasoconstriction or in the case of hypotension with a fast pulse (as in a shock state), the pulse may feel weak or "thready." By comparison, a patient who is hypertensive may produce a pulse that is more forceful than usual—a "bounding" pulse (as might be found in patients with a closed head injury).

Finally, note the rhythm of the pulse. A normal rhythm is regular, like the ticking of a clock. If some beats come early or late or are skipped, the pulse is irregular. Although many cardiac arrhythmias are not life threatening, in the case of heart blocks or ventricular ectopy, an irregular pulse can indicate a serious condition. Therefore, you should consider patients with an irregular pulse at risk until an ECG can be monitored and evaluated.

While checking a pulse, assess the patient's skin for color, temperature, and condition. Remember to compare extremities to the body's core. Collectively, these criteria provide insight into the patient's overall perfusion. Use the back of your hand to assess the warmth and condition of the patient's skin because it tends to be more sensitive than your palm.

When the blood vessels supplying the skin are fully dilated, the skin becomes warm and pink or flushed. When the blood vessels supplying the skin constrict or the cardiac output drops, the skin becomes pale or mottled and cool **FIGURE 2-9**. The color of the skin, especially in light-skinned patients, reflects the status of the circulation immediately underlying the skin, including the oxygen saturation of the blood. In dark-skinned patients, changes may not be readily evident in the skin but may be assessed by examining the mucous membranes (such as the lips or conjunctivae). If the patient is not receiving enough oxygen, the blood will desaturate as the oxygen level drops; the skin will turn a dusky gray or blue (**cyanosis**). Pallor occurs if arterial blood flow decreases to part of the body, as in the case of a blood clot or massive bleeding. Hypothermia will also result in pallor as the body shunts blood to the core and away from the extremities and the skin.

Normal skin is moderately warm and dry. The dryness or moistness of the skin is largely determined by the sympathetic nervous system. Stimulation of the sympathetic nervous system, as in shock or any other severe stress, causes sweating. The most common skin condition that providers will see in trauma patients will be cool, clammy skin. Depression of the sympathetic nervous system, as in an injury to the thoracic or lumbar spine, can cause the skin in the affected area to become abnormally dry and warm. Skin temperature rises as peripheral blood vessels dilate; it falls as blood vessels constrict. Fever and high environmental temperatures usually stimulate vasodilation, whereas shock elicits vasoconstriction.

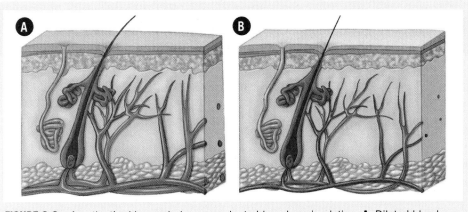

FIGURE 2-9 A patient's skin can help you evaluate his or her circulation. **A.** Dilated blood vessels make the skin pink and dry. **B.** Constricted blood vessels make the skin pale and moist.

Any visible active bleeding must be controlled at this point. Begin with bulky bandages and direct pressure. Pulsatile bleeding is usually arterial; if direct pressure does not control the bleeding, placing pressure on a proximal pulse point can slow the flow, allowing better control. Tourniquets are also an option if used early in patient care to control catastrophic hemorrhage (see Chapter 7). A steady flow of blood is more often from a vein. Venous bleeding is under less pressure, and if it continues through the first bandage additional bandages should be added. Clots need to form in the opening of the vein, and removing the initial bandaging may tear the clot loose allowing more bleeding. Clotting agents have become more available to control bleeding but still have not become accepted globally for use (see Chapter 4).

While assessing for bleeding, several internal sites should be examined if the patient presents with shock but little external bleeding. Internal bleeding cannot be managed in the field, and rapid transport is indicated. Areas of greatest concern are the chest, abdomen, pelvis, and femur fractures. A **hemothorax** (blood collecting between the lung and chest wall) may present with only mild respiratory distress although a large amount of blood may be present in the chest cavity. Abdominal bleeding can be assessed by palpating the abdomen looking for tenderness, distension, or firmness. Pelvic fractures can lose large amounts of blood that can pool in the **retroperitoneal space** (the space behind the abdomen). Long bone fractures are also of concern when evaluating blood loss. Quickly check the femurs, because multiple long bone fractures can lead to shock (see Chapter 7). IV fluid therapy should be initiated en route to the hospital.

Assess the Patient's Mental Status and Neurologic Function

The patient's mental status is often one of the prime indicators of how sick the patient really is. Changes in the state of consciousness may provide the first clue to an alteration in the patient's condition, so it is important to establish a baseline as soon as you encounter the patient. At the same time you are assessing mental status, if trauma is involved, you need to decide whether you will need to implement spinal immobilization procedures.

The quickest and simplest way to assess the patient's mental status or level of consciousness (LOC) is to use the AVPU mnemonic:

A *Awake* and alert
V Responsive to *verbal* stimuli
P Responsive to *pain*
U *Unresponsive*

You can further assess mental status by considering whether the patient is alert and oriented (A × O) in four areas: person, place, day, and the event itself. Assessing whether the patient can recall his or her name and the day tests long-term memory, whereas assessing whether the patient knows where he or she is and what happened tests short-term memory.

The most reliable and consistent method of assessing mental status and neurologic function is the **Glasgow Coma Scale (GCS)** TABLE 2-4, which assigns a point value (score) for eye opening, verbal response, and motor response; these values are added for a total score PROCEDURE 3. Although it may take slightly longer to perform than the AVPU and A × O, the GCS provides much greater insight into the patient's overall neurologic function. For more on the GCS and further assessment of level of consciousness, see Chapter 5.

Any trauma patient who is unresponsive or has altered mentation should be considered a high-risk priority patient and requires immediate transport to a trauma center. An unconscious, unresponsive patient may have experienced a traumatic brain injury, stroke, hypoglycemia, or alcohol or drug intoxication. All are bad—even potentially lethal—events, with some (such as traumatic brain injury) being devastating injuries.

Injuries to the spine should also be evaluated by quickly assessing movement and sensation in the distal extremities. Have the patient wiggle their toes to assess whether the motor nerves of the spinal cord are intact and touch each foot to determine the sensory abilities. The same should be done for the upper extremities.

TABLE 2-4 Glasgow Coma Scale for Adults					
Eye Opening		**Best Verbal Response**		**Best Motor Response**	
Spontaneous	4	Oriented and converses	5	Follows commands	6
To verbal command	3	Disoriented conversation	4	Localizes pain	5
To pain	2	Speaking but nonsensical	3	Withdraws from pain	4
No response	1	Moans or makes unintelligible sounds	2	Decorticate flexion	3
		No response	1	Decerebrate extension	2
				No response	1

Scores:
14–15: Mild dysfunction
11–13: Moderate to severe dysfunction
10 or less: Severe dysfunction (The lowest possible score is 3.)

Exposure, Examination, and Environment

To evaluate injuries effectively, the provider must be able to view them. Clothing must be removed or cut away to assess the underlying tissue. This may be an awkward part of the exam due to the invasion of personal space and patient modesty, but missing an important injury can have life-altering implications. Try to respect modesty by moving the patient to a less public area or at least covering the patient with sheets or blankets. The environment will also play a big part in how well you will be able to assess your patient. Cold environments can make the patient hypothermic if clothing is removed to assess them. Keep the patient covered as much as possible and use warm IV fluids and warmed blankets if possible to prevent hypothermia and coagulopathies (blood clotting disorders).

Identifying Priority Patients

Early in the assessment process, you need to identify priority patients who will benefit from limited time at the scene and rapid transport, as in the case of a hypotensive patient with suspected internal bleeding from trauma. Such a patient needs to reach definitive care, preferably a trauma center where a surgeon is readily available to control internal bleeding and replace the lost blood, neither of which can be accomplished in the field setting.

When you have a priority patient, it is important that you expedite transport and minimize scene time. You should do only what is absolutely necessary at the scene and handle everything else en route, including the appropriate focused history and physical examination. Determining a priority patient requires that you think through a variety of possibilities:

- **Poor general impression:** The patient is in obvious distress and does not "look well."
- **Unresponsive patients:** Unresponsiveness is never a good sign and typically points to a patient in serious or critical condition.
- **Responsive but doesn't or can't follow commands:** Altered mentation is another indication of the seriousness of the injury.
- **Difficulty breathing:** Breathing problems are one of the most common chief complaints in prehospital care. Patients who have difficulty breathing are in trouble; those who are "working to breathe" are at high risk for deterioration.
- **Hypoperfusion or shock:** This is an obvious sign of a high-risk patient. Weak or absent peripheral pulse, sustained tachycardia, and pale, cool, wet skin are critical indications of serious injury.
- **Uncontrolled bleeding:** Whether internal or external, such bleeding is a serious life threat.
- **Severe pain:** Any person with severe pain, especially pain that is unexplained by outward visible injury, should be considered a priority patient.
- **Multiple injuries:** A patient may have multiple minor injuries that, when taken together, can add up to one big problem.

Patients who present with a problem in the initial/primary assessment should receive necessary life-sustaining care and should be transported to the appropriate hospital as soon as possible. A failure to pass the initial/primary assessment means the patient is unstable; additional assessment may not be able to be completed if the provider is supplying care.

Rapid Trauma/Secondary Assessment

The rapid trauma assessment is a specialized assessment tool that comes between the initial assessment and the detailed physical exam of a trauma patient. This assessment is usually performed on patients with any significant mechanism of injury.

The rapid trauma/secondary assessment is performed after the initial assessment and after all life threats to airway, breathing, and circulation have been identified and addressed. If the patient is responsive, identify the chief complaint(s) and symptoms; then use this information to guide and direct your assessment. Keep in mind that the most visible injury you may be looking at (the scalp laceration) or the most painful injury the patient complains about (the fractured and dislocated ankle) may not be nearly as serious as the most lethal injury the patient has (the ruptured spleen).

If you decide the patient needs immediate transport, you should perform the rapid trauma assessment either while the patient is being immobilized and prepared for transport or as you are en route to the hospital. The rapid trauma exam consists of quickly examining the patient systematically from the head to the toes **PROCEDURE 2**.

After you complete the rapid trauma assessment, obtain a set of baseline vital signs **FIGURE 2-10**. If you have the resources, have another provider take the vital signs while you do your secondary assessment; it is efficient, saves time, and is a good practice. Baseline vital signs are an integral part of any focused history and physical exam. Clues provided will help you determine the seriousness of the patient's condition and the functioning of internal organs. Remember that shock is seen in different stages. Changes in a patient's blood pressure are often a late finding, as the patient deteriorates and shock progresses. Keep in mind that blood pressure must be sufficient to maintain adequate end-organ perfusion.

The rapid trauma assessment will help you find any other potential life threats you may have missed in the primary assessment, but it needs to be done quickly. Although it generally follows the pattern of a detailed physical exam, the rapid trauma assessment is done much quicker. With practice, you can perform a rapid trauma assessment in 2 or 3 minutes.

At the completion of the rapid trauma/secondary assessment, the patient who is in need of rapid transportation to the trauma center can be secured to a long backboard. The board can be used to splint the body globally and minimize the chance of further injury to isolated fractures. Even patients secured to backboards must be evaluated frequently to maintain a clear airway. Additional assessment and treatment can be conducted en route to the hospital.

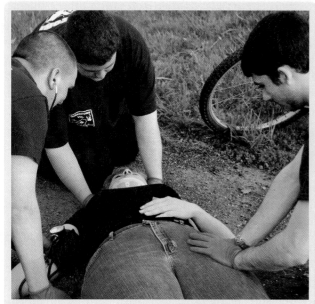

FIGURE 2-10 If a second provider is available, vital signs can be obtained while the assessment is going on, speeding up the process.

Focused History and Detailed Physical Examination

Patients With Minor Injuries or No Significant Mechanism of Injury

Most trauma calls involve patients with a single, isolated injury or, on occasion, several minor injuries. In almost all of these cases, the lack of serious or critical injuries is consistent with the lack of a significant mechanism of injury: A collision on the basketball court results in a sprained ankle; a skater crashes and ends up with a Colles fracture; a loose piece of metal spins off a lathe in the machine shop, lacerating the machinist's forearm. These types of patients should not show any signs of systemic involvement (hypotension). If they do, suspect more than an isolated injury. You need to continue your assessment with the goal of finding the more serious problem.

Additional History and Exam

Trauma patients may be classified into two major groups: patients with an isolated injury and patients with multisystem trauma **FIGURE 2-11**. The biggest difference from an assessment perspective is that an isolated injury allows you to focus on the main problem immediately. In contrast, with multisystem trauma you must first find all (or as many as you can reasonably find) of the various problems—for example, a hematoma on the forehead, a fractured arm, and neck or lower back pain. Then you need to prioritize

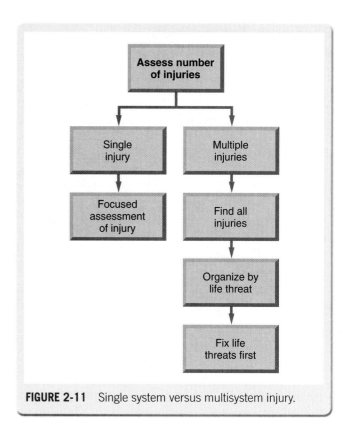

FIGURE 2-11 Single system versus multisystem injury.

the injuries by severity and the order in which you plan to address them. During the assessment, you must continually think about how each injury or condition relates to the others. For example, the survival rate for a patient with a serious traumatic brain injury who has a single episode of hypotension decreases by approximately 50%. In such a case, not recognizing and addressing the hypotension and the lack of adequate perfusion pressure has a huge impact—in some cases a fatal impact.

Another important consideration is the high visibility factor of many injuries, which sometimes creates a visual distraction. A compound fracture of the lower leg and ankle, with the foot twisted sideways and jammed under the brake pedal in a car, is not a pretty sight—but it is not a life-threatening injury. Because of the visual distraction, you might focus on the grossly deformed ankle and miss the early signs and symptoms of shock caused by the internal injuries and bleeding that you can't see.

A number of mechanisms have the potential to produce life-threatening injuries:

- Ejection from *any* vehicle (car, motorcycle, or all-terrain vehicle [ATV])
- Death of another patient in the same passenger compartment
- Falls from more than 20′ (6 m) (or three times the patient's height)
- Vehicle rollover (unrestrained occupant)
- High-speed motor vehicle crash
- Vehicle–pedestrian collision
- Motorcycle crash
- Penetrating wounds to the head, chest, or abdomen

If the patient is an infant or a child, mechanisms of injury that would indicate a high-priority patient include falls from more than 10′ (3 m) (or 3 times the child's height), a bicycle collision, or being a passenger in a vehicle in a medium-speed collision.

During the assessment of patients who have the ability to converse with the provider, a SAMPLE (signs and symptoms, allergies, medications, pertinent medical history, last oral intake, and event) history should be completed. It is often the initial provider who is able to gain valuable information about a patient. Medications the patient may take can alter the body's ability to compensate for injury (eg, beta-blockers and blood thinners). Knowing about allergies may prevent a patient from receiving a lethal medication, and the knowledge of a patient's previous medical conditions may alter the patient's treatment (eg, congestive heart failure [CHF] or previous cerebrovascular accident [CVA]).

The detailed physical exam continues the assessment begun in the rapid trauma assessment. In many cases, you won't need to do this assessment (such as for a finger laceration) or won't have time (such as when you have a patient in serious or critical condition). The detailed physical exam can take 15 minutes or more to gather a more detailed and comprehensive history and perform a detailed and thorough physical examination (such as checking range of motion [ROM] and distal pulses, motor function, and sensory function [PMS]). See Chapters 5, 6, and 7 for more information on detailed examinations.

In the majority of cases when you perform a detailed physical exam, it will be done on a trauma patient en route when you have extended transport time (usually more than 15 minutes). Frequently, you will find yourself modifying the exam based on the patient's chief complaint. Use this tool as you see fit—or not at all, if you are providing lifesaving care.

Motor Vehicle Collisions

In many cases, multiple mechanisms of injury have come into play—for example, a T-bone collision that leaves the patient with a crushed upper arm and pelvic girdle and also penetrating trauma from the piece of door trim impaled in his chest. A patient with any of the previously mentioned mechanisms should immediately raise your index of suspicion. Two or more mechanisms of injury markedly increase the chance of a patient sustaining a serious or fatal injury PROCEDURE 22 .

Several other mechanisms of injury are also worth considering. Seatbelts, even when properly positioned, can cause injuries as the car and its occupants decelerate in a crash FIGURE 2-12 . Check the clavicles where the shoulder strap crosses. The clavicles are small bones, and the subclavian vein and arteries run directly underneath them. In shorter patients, the shoulder strap mounted on the B post in a car can ride up across the neck, increasing the risk of soft-tissue and cervical spine injury. Examine the area where the lap belt crosses the pelvic girdle. If the belt is not across the iliac crests but has ridden up over the lower abdomen, the patient has an increased risk of organ damage and thoracic or lumbar spine injury. Passengers who tuck the shoulder harness under their arms for comfort and are then

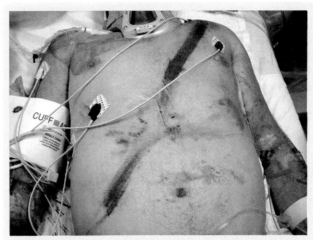

FIGURE 2-12 Bruises from seatbelts are a clue to internal injury.

involved in rollover accidents are at high risk of death from liver injuries caused by the improperly positioned belt.

Air bags have saved countless lives, but many people don't realize that an air bag is a secondary restraint system, designed to work with seatbelts to reduce injuries. When the seatbelt is not used and a crash occurs, the air bag deploys, momentarily catching the patient. As the air bag deflates, it releases the driver or passenger, who continues moving forward and may go down-and-under (into the dashboard) or up-and-over (into the steering wheel and/or windshield). When working any crash with air bag deployment, lift the bag and look underneath for a bent steering wheel—another potential source of life-threatening internal injuries. Remember that air bag deployment in vehicles during patient extrication can injure rescuers.

Child safety seats also have saved countless lives FIGURE 2-13 . If they are improperly installed or positioned in

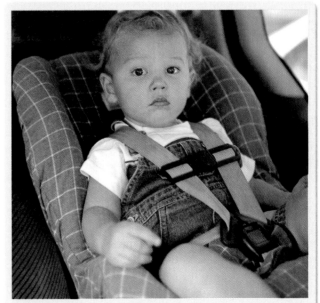

FIGURE 2-13 Child safety seats work best when correctly installed according to their instructions.

the vehicle, however, they can be rendered useless as a safety device. If the car seat comes loose during a crash, the risk of face, head, neck, and spine trauma to the child increases markedly. Similarly, if the child is too large or too small for the seat, the seat will not provide the intended level of protection.

Penetrating Trauma

When evaluating a patient with penetrating injury, several factors can assist in the overall care of the patient. The type and size of weapon used can help the surgeons determine the extent of injury and the need for immediate surgery. With projectile weapons such as firearms, the caliber and distance from the weapon when it was fired can determine the amount of internal injury.

Reassessment

After the initial/primary assessment, the reassessment may be the single most important assessment process you will perform. It represents a continuous, yet cyclical, process that you perform throughout transport, right up to the time you turn patient care over to the emergency department staff. For patients in stable condition, you should do a reassessment every 15 minutes. For patients in unstable condition, you need to make a concerted effort to repeat the reassessment every 5 minutes.

Reassessment of Mental Status and the ABCs

The reassessment combines repetition of the initial/primary assessment, reassessment of vital signs and breath sounds, and repetition of the secondary assessment. During the reassessment, continue to evaluate and reevaluate the patient's status and any treatments already administered. Trends in the patient's current condition may give clues about the effectiveness of treatments: Have they improved the patient's condition? Are identified problems better or worse? This information indicates which changes have occurred and which critical conditions have been addressed and corrected.

First, compare the patient's LOC with your baseline assessment. Is the LOC changing? The Glasgow Coma Scale is a useful tool. If the level of consciousness is decreasing, can the patient still protect the airway? If you have doubts, consider inserting an advanced airway (see Chapter 3).

Second, review the patient's airway. Is it patent? Swelling, bleeding, or just a change of position can obstruct the airway in the blink of an eye, so make certain that the airway is properly positioned and dry. Always be prepared to suction, and don't delay if you hear gurgling in the upper airway. It's far better to prevent aspiration than to treat it later. If the airway needs to be secured, *do it immediately*, and place an airway in the patient (see Chapter 3). Once the airway is secured, recheck lung sounds and assess oximetry and capnography to confirm that the airway is properly placed.

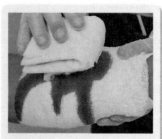

FIGURE 2-14 Reassess bleeding for additional intervention.

Third, reassess breathing. Is the patient breathing adequately? If not, figure out why and fix the problem. For hypoventilation, assist breathing with oxygen and a bag-mask device. Correct hypoxia with high-concentration oxygen therapy. For patients with diminished or absent breath sounds, jugular venous distension (JVD), and progressive dyspnea (signs of pneumothorax), decompress the chest PROCEDURE 13.

Stay alert for signs that the patient is experiencing ventilatory fatigue (eg, decreasing pulse oximetry reading or the patient looks increasingly tired). Be especially alert for this possibility in children because it is a classic sign that precedes disaster for the patient. Patients of any age who are going into ventilatory fatigue need to have their airway managed for them.

Finally, reassess the patient's circulation. Assess overall skin color as an initial measure of cardiovascular function and hemodynamic status. With pale, cool, wet skin, think shock; with cyanosis, think oxygen desaturation; with mottling, think late-stage shock (see Chapter 4).

Make certain that all bleeding is controlled FIGURE 2-14. If you find blood-soaked dressings, add more fresh dressings to the stack and rebandage in place. Reassess the blood pressure, watching closely for signs that the patient is beginning to decompensate.

Reassess the pulse, including its rate, strength, and regularity. Progressive tachycardia may indicate that the patient is still bleeding, is hypoxic, or is developing cardiogenic shock (see Chapter 4). In contrast, sustained or progressively worsening bradycardia may reflect rising intracranial pressure (from trauma or a stroke) or end-stage shock.

Reassessment of Patient Care and Transport Priorities

After repeating the initial assessment as part of your reassessments, think about your present care plan. Have you addressed all life threats? Based on what you now know, do you need to revise your priority list? If so, make the change and get on with patient care. In contrast, if your plan is working well and you've addressed most or all of the patient's complaints, there is no need to revise the care plan.

While you are reevaluating your patient care priorities, you should reassess the transport plan as well. Should routine transport be stepped up to priority? Is the patient's condition worsening to the point that you need to consider diverting to a closer facility? Do you need to set up a rendezvous with an air ambulance and fly the patient to a trauma center? If your patient's condition has improved and stabilized (eg, extreme pain controlled with analgesia), you should step down from priority and transport the patient as a routine case, the clearly safer choice.

CHAPTER RESOURCES

CASE STUDY ANSWERS

1 What are the issues related to scene safety at this scene?

Just because the police have declared the scene safe for you to move into does not make the scene safe. Trauma scenes with victims of violence often become unstable as passions reignite and the fight continues or when your patient was the target of the violence and you are now seen as stopping the process. You and your crew may become involved in the situation only because you happen to be in the wrong place at the wrong time. At the scene where violence has erupted, you and your partner may decide to take separate roles; one as the caregiver and one as a safety monitor who is alert for signs that more trouble may develop.

2 Describe the conditions found in the initial/primary assessment and the management required to support life.

The initial or primary assessment looks at immediate threats to life. Your patient has an airway obstruction, breathing difficulty, and decreased circulation. As these problems are found you should try to provide care to fix them. The airway obstruction was helped immediately by opening the airway and the open hole in the chest wall was covered to fix part of the breathing difficulty. BVM ventilations will help provide continued care and the decrease noted in the circulation exam reveals signs of shock and blood loss. External bleeding is minimal at this point, so rapid transportation to a facility capable of surgery is indicated.

3 How does the additional information from the rapid trauma/secondary assessment help to define the priorities for patient care?

While the crowd reported only one shot was heard, the chaos that occurs at the time of these events does not always lead to correct information. The patient should be checked for additional wounds that may have been inflicted or additional injury when he fell to the ground. The rapid trauma or secondary assessment has indicated a pneumothorax on your patient that must be evaluated and additional priority care may be needed.

4 Does this patient require rapid transport to a trauma center?

Yes. This patient requires immediate surgery and the supportive care offered at a center that specializes in trauma.

5 Why are frequent reassessments required for this priority patient?

Your patient is unstable and may require additional resuscitation or a change in care several times before you are able to complete your transport. He may require additional airway support, treatment for a tension pneumothorax, or volume replacement for blood losses to maintain perfusion.

Trauma in Motion

1. Does your agency have a policy regarding responses to violent scenes to ensure provider safety? Is there a policy for incidents on roadways? Hazardous material incidents?
2. What gear does your agency supply for protection from bloodborne pathogens?
3. Our eyes provide us with the ability to assess most injuries. How could you alter your assessment if you had no light to work under?
4. How does technology help make assessments easier? Harder?
5. During your response to a bombing, how could you prepare for the incident?

References and Resources

American Academy of Orthopaedic Surgeons. *Emergency Care and Transportation of the Sick and Injured.* 9th ed. Sudbury, MA: Jones and Bartlett; 2005.

American Academy of Orthopaedic Surgeons. *Nancy Caroline's Emergency Care in the Streets.* 6th ed. Sudbury, MA: Jones and Bartlett; 2007.

American College of Surgeons Committee on Trauma. *Advanced Trauma Life Support for Doctors.* 7th ed. Chicago, IL: American College of Surgeons; 2004.

Deakin CD, Low JL. Accuracy of the advanced trauma life support guidelines for predicting systolic blood pressure using carotid, femoral, and radial pulses: observational study. *BMJ.* 2000; 321:673–674.

Feliciano DV, Mattox KL, Moore EE. *Trauma.* 6th ed. New York, NY: McGraw-Hill Medical; 2008.

Norwood SH, McAuley CE, Berne JD, et al. A prehospital Glasgow Coma Scale score ≤14 accurately predicts the need for full trauma team activation and patient hospitalization after motor vehicle collisions. *J Trauma Injury Infect Crit Care.* 2002; 53(3):503–507.

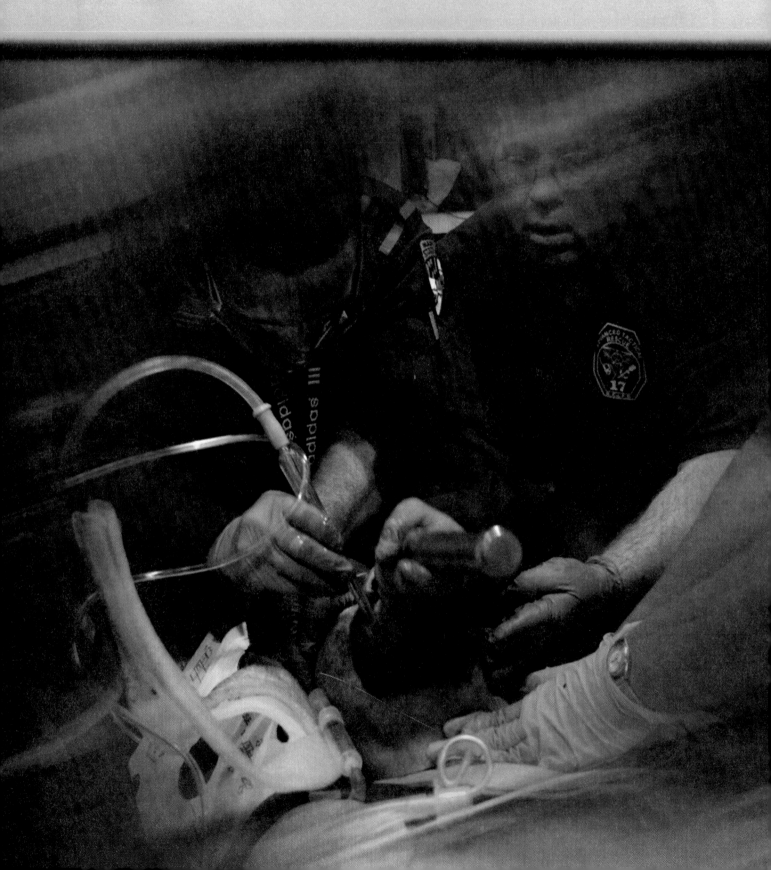

You are dispatched for a construction worker who fell from scaffolding. Dispatch tells you that the patient is reported to be unconscious following a 32′ (11 m) fall. You arrive on scene to be guided into a large warehouse where a patient is on the concrete floor next to a motorized lift. Workers state the patient was working at the top of the fully extended lift when he fell to the floor.

Your patient is a 32-year-old man who has irregular snoring respirations. His coworkers have kept him from moving and state he has not been conscious since the fall. You immediately move the patient into a neutral in-line position and open the airway with a trauma jaw thrust maneuver.

The patient has irregular respirations at a rate of 12 breaths/min, a pulse of 136 beats/min, blood pressure of 100/64 mm Hg, and Spo_2 of 84% on room air. High-flow oxygen by nonrebreathing mask is applied and the Spo_2 increased to 92%. The patient has blood coming from an unseen wound in his mouth. While your partner prepares to suction the patient's airway, your rapid trauma/secondary assessment reveals injury to the left side of the head, sluggish pupil response, and a flail segment located on the left chest. Lung sounds are shallow, especially on the left but present throughout, crepitus is noted with every breath, and an open fracture of the left forearm is noted. After immobilizing the patient in a cervical collar and securely placing him on a long backboard, the patient is moved to the ambulance.

1 What are the priorities for this patient?

2 Are his ventilations adequate?

3 Why does a chest injury affect how you will manage his airway?

4 What steps should be taken to manage this patient's airway?

5 What steps should be taken to monitor his airway following placement of an airway adjunct?

Introduction

The provider can make very few interventions that will so profoundly and broadly affect the trauma patient as managing an airway and providing necessary ventilations. Primary hypoxia, secondary hypoxia, and prolonged hypoxic events are all stepping stones toward the patient's death. The provider has many tools in his or her proverbial toolbox, with the strongest being the ability to evaluate the patient's status during the assessment and follow-up care.

Many conditions can affect the airway. Direct injury of the airway can result from blunt or penetrating trauma to the face, neck, or chest. Burns can cause the airway to swell and/or constrict movement. Blood or vomitus can continue to obstruct an airway, whereas teeth or foreign objects can be removed. Lack of control of the muscles due to head trauma can cause the airway to relax, leading to difficulty ventilating; lack of muscle control from a c-spine injury may halt the body's ability to ventilate at all.

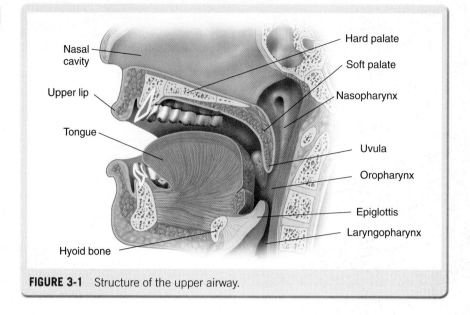

FIGURE 3-1 Structure of the upper airway.

Anatomy and Physiology

The physical structure of the airway provides a passage for air movement from outside the body to the alveoli. Because of the differences of the structures it is easiest to divide the airway into upper and lower segments for review. The alveoli allow gasses to pass between the inspired air and the blood and vice versa to form a mixture to be expired. The muscles of ventilation are required to move the air physically and affect the patient's ability to respire as dramatically as an open airway. To work properly, the system requires regulation to allow the body to stimulate ventilation when needed.

Upper Airway

The upper airway consists of all anatomic structures above the level of the vocal cords, including the nasopharynx, the oropharynx, and the hypopharynx or laryngopharynx **FIGURE 3-1**. The nasopharynx is divided into two passages by the nasal septum. Three turbinates protrude from the wall of the nasopharynx parallel to the floor of the nasal cavity. The oropharynx forms the larger opening to the airway but is not the usual pathway used for breathing. The oropharynx meets up with the nasopharynx where the soft tissue of the tongue and the soft palate allow air to pass when they are kept separated.

The upper airway ends at the larynx, a structure made up of independent cartilaginous elements **FIGURE 3-2**. Palpable from the outside of the body, the thyroid cartilage is made of two plates that form a V-shape. The cricoid carti-

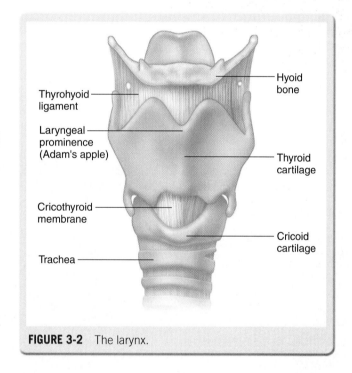

FIGURE 3-2 The larynx.

lage (or cricoid ring) is the first ring of the trachea and the only one to encircle the trachea completely. Separating the thyroid and cricoid cartilages is the cricothyroid membrane. This thin membrane is the site where the internal airway passes closest to the external surface of the body. The glottis (or glottic opening) is the space in between the vocal cords. Airway patency is very dependant on adequate muscle tone to keep this passage open.

Lower Airway

The lower airways consist of air passages that divide into smaller passages until they end at the alveoli **FIGURE 3-3**. The trachea begins at the cricoid cartilage and descends until the first of many branches occur at the left and right mainstem bronchi. This branching occurs at approximately the fifth or sixth thoracic vertebra. The right mainstem bronchus is shorter and straighter than the left, allowing easier passage for a misplaced endotracheal tube. Upon entering the lungs, the mainstem bronchi branch into increasingly smaller bronchioles.

The bronchioles pass into alveolar ducts, then into the alveoli. These balloon-like structures are surrounded by capillaries and are the functional site for respiration. The exchange of oxygen and carbon dioxide occurs by simple diffusion between the thin wall of the alveoli and the pulmonary capillaries.

Ventilation

Ventilation is the process of moving air into and out of the lungs FIGURE 3-4. It consists of two phases: inhalation and exhalation. Inhalation is an active process initiated by the contraction of the respiratory muscles. The diaphragm flattens, pulling the lungs downward while the intercostal muscles contract to pull the chest wall upward and outward. The lungs, which are highly elastic and held to the chest wall by visceral and parietal pleura, increase in volume following the chest cavity. The relative pressure within the chest decreases and air rushes in to fill the void (a process known as negative pressure ventilation).

In contrast, exhalation is a passive process that occurs from the relaxation of the muscles of ventilation and the related decrease in size of the chest cavity.

Respiration

Every living cell in the body requires oxygen to carry out its metabolic process. During aerobic metabolism, the cells use oxygen and produce carbon dioxide as a waste product. This waste must be

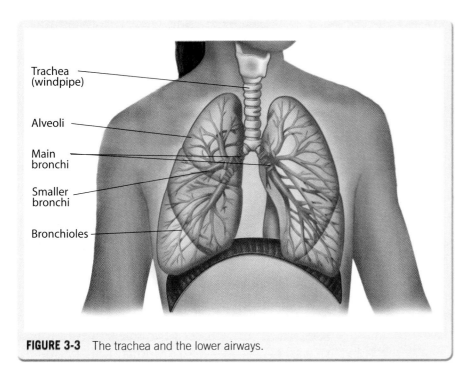

FIGURE 3-3 The trachea and the lower airways.

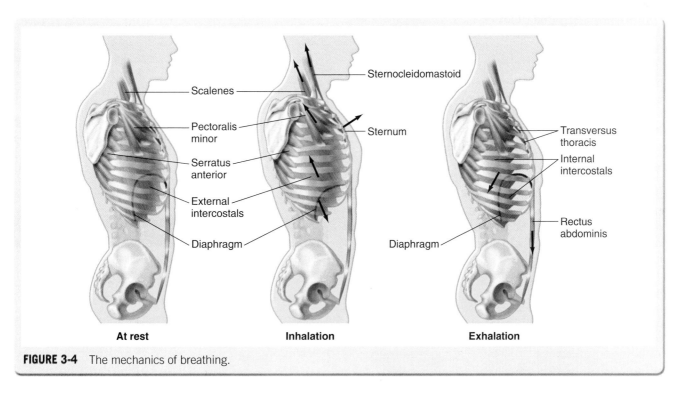

FIGURE 3-4 The mechanics of breathing.

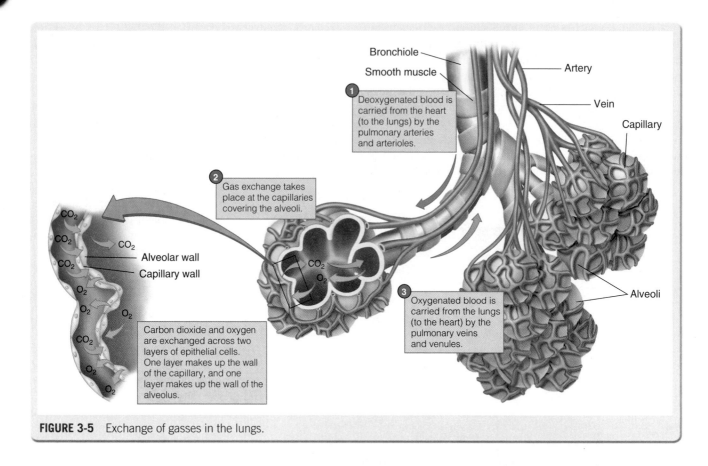

FIGURE 3-5   Exchange of gasses in the lungs.

carried away or it may accumulate to toxic levels. The body uses the process of respiration to both supply oxygen and remove carbon dioxide through the blood.

Gas exchange in the body occurs by **diffusion**, a process in which a gas moves from an area of higher concentration to an area of lower concentration **FIGURE 3-5**. Both oxygen and carbon dioxide pass through the alveolar membrane by diffusion. Dissolved oxygen passes through the pulmonary capillary membrane and binds to the hemoglobin molecule of the red blood cells. The majority of carbon dioxide is transported back to the lungs in the form of bicarbonate ions. As oxygen passes into the blood, carbon dioxide diffuses from the blood and passes into the lungs.

The brain controls respiration through the respiratory center in the medulla oblongata. Receptors in the medulla sense changes in the pH of the cerebrospinal fluid while chemoreceptors in the aortic arch detect changes in the oxygen and carbon dioxide levels. Chemoreceptors in the carotid bodies combine with the aortic receptors and the medulla to stimulate ventilations. The main respiratory stimulus is accumulation of carbon dioxide in the blood; low oxygen levels have a much lesser effect. It is for this reason that all patients who have the potential for decreased levels of oxygen to be delivered to the cells should have high concentrations of oxygen applied.

Assessment of the Trauma Airway

Most of the conditions that affect the ability to keep the airway open can be found using the simple look, listen, and feel technique. As you begin your approach, look at the patient to determine the work of breathing. Look for trauma to the face, neck, or chest that may indicate injury to the airway. Asking a patient a question like, "What's your name?," "What hurts?," or "What happened?" can provide useful information. The answer can provide some history, but how the patient answers can tell you about the airway.

Listen carefully for abnormal airway sounds **TABLE 3-1**. Most will be audible, but using a stethoscope may help determine more subtle sounds. Gurgling indicates fluid and the need for suctioning. A hoarse voice may indicate swell-

TABLE 3-1	Airway Sounds
Gurgling	Fluid (blood or vomitus)
Hoarseness	Swelling around the vocal cords
Stridor	Upper airway obstruction
Snoring	Intermittent obstruction from the tongue and soft tissue

ing near the vocal cords or direct trauma to the airway. Stridor is an indication of obstruction or swelling in the upper airway. Snoring indicates a patient who has a decreased level of consciousness, allowing the muscles of the airway to relax and causing the tongue and soft tissues to obstruct the airway intermittently.

If you find that during your initial assessment of the airway the airway is not completely open, provide a jaw thrust or other appropriate manual maneuver to open it. If fluid or blood is noted in the oropharynx, suction it out before moving to evaluate or provide ventilations. If objects such as teeth, food, or other foreign bodies are noted in the airway, remove them immediately before they move deeper into the airway and/or cause further obstruction.

Finally, when abnormalities are noted, palpate the external structure to look for **crepitus** (crunching of the bone or cartilage) or **subcutaneous air** (crackling of air under the skin) along the anterior neck. Fractures of the lower jaw can make the structure supporting the tongue fail, leading to obstruction of the airway. An airway adjunct will most likely be needed to support this patient.

Airway obstructions from a foreign object should be managed immediately. Begin by looking into the mouth to see if the object can be removed. If the object cannot be seen, determine the level of severity of the obstruction. Partial airway obstructions may cause stridor but allow some air to pass, whereas a complete obstruction will not allow stridor or air. Partial airway obstructions should be managed as soon as time and equipment permit. Direct visualization by laryngoscopy may be required to remove the object safely.

Assessment of Ventilation

Many injuries can affect the body's ability to move enough air into and out of the lungs to sustain life. Ventilation must be assessed by how much air is moved over a period of time. Adults exchange 5 to 8 liters of air each minute. This is based on an average breath of 500 mL with a respiratory rate of 10 to 16 breaths/min. A breath of 500 mL will produce visual chest movement.

TV (Tidal Volume) × RR (Respiratory Rate) = MV (Minute Volume)

500 mL × 12 breaths/min = 6,000 mL/min

Rates above 29 breaths/min or below 10 breaths/min are concerning. Conditions such as shock will compensate for the loss of tissue perfusion by increasing the ventilation rate. Anxiety, pain, or fear can also increase ventilations. Therapy should be geared to normalizing the minute volume. High-flow oxygen may help the body sense the increasing oxygen and decrease the body's need to continue hyperventilating. However, care should be taken to reassess the patient with high or low ventilatory rates.

Injuries to the chest wall can affect how well a patient can move air into and out of the lungs. Fractured or bruised ribs often create enough pain to make a patient hypoventilate by reducing the depth of breath in an attempt to reduce the pain. Pulmonary contusions under the external injury decrease the lung's ability to use that part of the lung effectively. This requires the patient to breathe more to compensate. Injury to the nervous system may also affect how well the muscles in the chest can do their job. This can be seen when chest injuries are combined with spinal injuries.

Injuries to the lungs may cause a pneumothorax (see Chapter 6). Lung sounds should be auscultated to determine any adventitious sounds and determine the equality of air entry into the chest. Absence of lung sounds most often indicates a collapsed lung and requires further evaluation. If a tension pneumothorax exists, immediate decompression should be done **PROCEDURE 13**.

Management of the Trauma Airway

Care of the airway should begin with the simplest maneuvers and progress rapidly until effective ventilation is achieved, at which point you should continue your assessment to determine the need for a more definitive airway. If an airway can be achieved with the use of manual maneuvers, do not progress to the use of other adjuncts until you have finished your initial/primary assessment and addressed other immediate life threats. After the life threats have been addressed, reevaluate the effectiveness of your airway control and determine if an additional step will be required to control the airway for transport. A prehospital provider must think ahead to determine where the best place for intervention may be. Many adjuncts are available to help providers. Each has its pros and cons for the management of different traumatic conditions.

Manual Maneuvers

The trauma jaw thrust and the trauma chin lift are two maneuvers that can be used to help lift the tongue from the soft tissue at the back of the pharynx. These maneuvers both limit the flexion of the neck to protect against additional injury to the c-spine. Neither maneuver allows for complete opening of the airway.

The trauma jaw thrust can be completed with the patient's cervical spine in neutral position **PROCEDURE 6**. Place two or three fingers under the patient's mandible while the thumbs of each hand are placed on the zygomatic arches. Squeeze the fingers toward the thumbs, moving the jaw forward. The mouth can be opened or a mask applied to the face with the fingers.

The trauma chin lift should be done only on an unresponsive patient who will not bite down on the provider's fingers **PROCEDURE 7**. Open the patient's mouth and pinch the lower teeth and the chin between the thumb and fingers. Pull the jaw forward to move the tongue from the posterior airway.

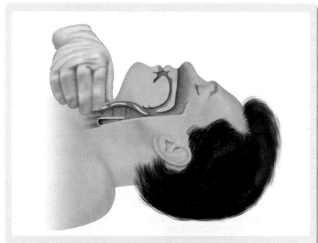

FIGURE 3-6 Cricoid pressure can be used to help guard against regurgitation in the airway.

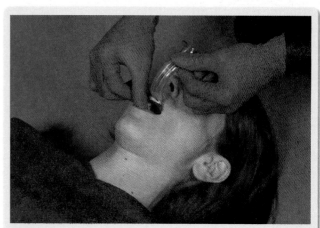

FIGURE 3-7 Oral airways provide a means to keep the airway open but do not guard against bleeding or fluid entering the lower airways.

If the patient is immobilized on a backboard and begins to vomit or secretions build up before suctioning is readily available, turn the patient and board to one side to allow the obstruction to drain from the mouth. Solid materials such as food, teeth, or vomitus should be swept from the mouth with a gloved hand.

Manual maneuvers have limited ability to manage bleeding within the airway or to protect the airway in the case of vomiting. A combination of the jaw thrust and chin lift can effectively clear the tongue from the hypopharynx. Another tool the provider has is cricoid pressure, which can be used to prevent gastric regurgitation into the airway FIGURE 3-6 .

Airway Adjuncts

An airway adjunct should be considered for any trauma patient who:

- Is not able to ventilate or oxygenate
- Cannot maintain their own airway
- Has an injury that makes it hard to maintain ventilation, oxygenation, or an open airway

In general, patients with any of the following presentations will require an airway adjunct to assist in keeping the airway open.

- Acute airway obstruction
- Decreased effective ventilations (< 10 or > 29)
- Severe hypoxia despite high-flow oxygen
- Glasgow Coma Scale (GCS) score < 9
- Severe hemorrhagic shock and hypotension
- Cardiac arrest

Basic Airways

Oropharyngeal airways (OPA) are a simple adjunct to help the provider keep the tongue forward, away from the soft tissue of the oropharynx. The oral airway can help even when the mandible has been deformed. Limiting its use-

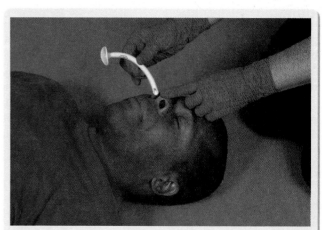

FIGURE 3-8 Nasal airways are better tolerated in patients with a gag reflex. Caution should be used when the patient has mid-face trauma.

fulness is the need for the patient to be unconscious and without a gag reflex. It also has no ability to manage blood or vomit FIGURE 3-7 . Oral airways are foreign objects in the airway and must be continually monitored to make sure they do not change position.

Nasopharyngeal airways have the flexibility to be used with patients who require assistance but still maintain some level of consciousness. The nasopharyngeal airway (NPA) (sometimes called a nasal trumpet because of its shape) provides an opening through the nose to the pharynx to allow air to pass. Because of its flexibility, it does not provide as much support to the tongue where it meets the soft tissue FIGURE 3-8 . The nasal airway should *not* be used on patients with mid-face injury because of the possibility of basilar skull fracture. These fractures may provide access for any object (eg, suction catheter, nasogastric tube, or airway) placed in the nose to enter the skull cavity.

Suction is another skill available to all providers and its importance should not be overlooked when dealing with the trauma airway. Blood, secretions, and vomitus are all problems facing the provider when attempting to keep the airway clear. Reassess the airway frequently for the need to suction.

Intermediate Airways

Several airway adjuncts are available to providers, and in recent years some have begun to provide better control of the airway. Dual-lumen airways (Combitube or PtL), esophageal intubation devices (esophageal obturator airway [EOA] or esophageal gastric tube airway [EGTA]), supraglottic airways such as the laryngeal mask airway (LMA) or the i-gel airway, laryngeal tube airways (LTAs; King LT-D and LTS-D), and the perilaryngeal airway (Cobra perilaryngeal airway [CobraPLA]) all enter the airway in a blind technique. These airways all pass through the oropharynx to introduce air into the airway, usually above the level of the glottis. These devices all use a standard 15-mm adapter to fit a ventilation device. Because these airways are not intended to intubate the trachea, bleeding or fluids in the upper airway may not be prevented from entering the trachea. Also, because the placement of these devices is blind, trauma in the upper airway can prevent proper placement of the devices. It is important to remember that although several airways are discussed here, they may not all be accepted in your organization. Always follow local protocols.

Dual-Lumen Airways

Dual-lumen airways use a connected pair of tubes at differing lengths to pass through the upper airway and enter either the trachea or the esophagus. When the tube is inserted to the correct depth, a pair of cuffs is inflated near the end of the distal tube and just above the proximal opening for the shorter tube. If the airway has passed into the esophagus, as it is designed to do, air will enter into tube number 1 and pass between the cuffs from the pharynx into the trachea. If the airway passes into the trachea (which is

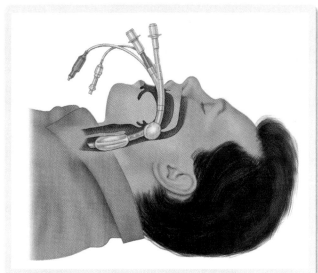

FIGURE 3-9 The dual-lumen airway has two openings for air depending on where the device is placed.

less likely), the provider will not hear lung sounds or be able to provide ventilation through tube number 1 and must switch to tube number 2 to ventilate through the distal end of the airway **FIGURE 3-9**.

Because this dual-lumen airway is placed with a blind technique it requires far less skill than intubation, making it available to a wider number of providers. It can be used as a backup to a failed intubation, when a patient is entrapped and intubation cannot be performed, or when an endotracheal intubation is unavailable. Contraindications to dual-lumen airways include the following:

- Patients younger than 16 years old
- Patients shorter than 5' (1.5 m) tall
- Patients with an intact gag reflex
- Patients who have ingested caustic substances

Another relative contraindication is a patient who will require continuous tracheal suctioning, because these devices will not allow for the passage of a catheter. Providers should use caution with patients suspected of having tracheal injury, because the dual-lumen airway uses positive pressure from a bag-mask device to inflate the lungs, and bleeding below the level of the airway can be pushed into the lungs.

Supraglottic Airway Devices (SAD)

The **laryngeal mask airway (LMA)** is available in several different styles that allow for different patient conditions **FIGURE 3-10**. The LMA consists of a tube connected to a pointed oval-shaped inflatable cuff with an opening in the center. The LMA is placed blindly through the oropharynx and over the larynx. The large mask-like cuff is then inflated, sealing the airway and allowing air to pass through to the trachea **FIGURE 3-11**. In its newer versions, the Proseal LMA has a port placed into the distal end allowing for esophageal suctioning, and the LMA Fastrach and Intubating LMA (ILMA) have become useful tools in the management of trauma situations. The sizes of LMAs range from

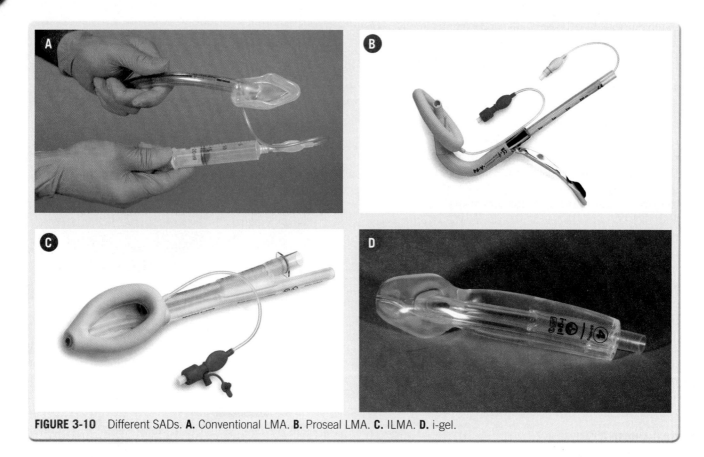

FIGURE 3-10   Different SADs. **A.** Conventional LMA. **B.** Proseal LMA. **C.** ILMA. **D.** i-gel.

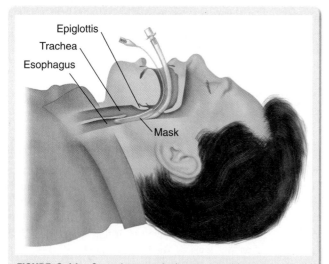

Epiglottis
Trachea
Esophagus
Mask

FIGURE 3-11   Supralaryngeal airways provide an anatomically shaped mask that is inflated above the glottis.

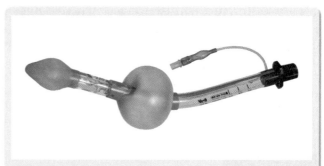

FIGURE 3-12   The King LT-D and LTS-D have been incorporated into many local protocols/guidelines.

neonate to large adult. Similar in its airway position is the i-gel supraglottic airway. It is inserted blindly but does not have a cuff to inflate. Little investigation of this airway has been completed in the trauma patient.

There are contraindications to the use of an LMA:

- Patients with an intact gag reflex
- Patients with severe facial or pharyngeal trauma (because it may worsen the trauma)
- Patients who require high ventilatory pressures due to chest trauma (because it may increase the risk for aspiration)

Because the SAD does not occlude the esophagus, the risk for aspiration following vomiting is present. If the patient vomits, immediately evaluate the airway to determine whether vomitus has entered under the airway mask and toward the trachea before continuing positive pressure ventilations. Trauma to the pharynx, hematomas affecting the airway, or swelling in the pharynx or glottic opening may affect the ability to place the device.

The **laryngeal tube airway (LTA)** is an airway with similar form and function to the dual-lumen airways, though it is reported to have less resistance on insertion. It was designed as an emergency airway device with a single tube for ventilation **FIGURE 3-12**. The tube has inflatable cuffs at the distal end and a larger one midway up the tube. The design of the airway is for insertion into the esophagus. After the cuffs are inflated, ventilations are passed down through the tube into the pharynx and through

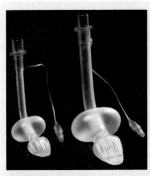

FIGURE 3-13 The Cobra-PLA is another airway adjunct available to some users.

the larynx with a bag-mask device. With the distal cuff inflated in the esophagus, the risk for aspiration is lower. The LTA allows for higher airway pressures to be used for ventilation if required. LTAs are available in sizes from pediatric to large adult. Contraindications include:

- Patients with an intact gag reflex
- Patients who have ingested caustic substances

One other device that deserves mentioning is the Cobra perilaryngeal airway (CobraPLA) **FIGURE 3-13**. This supraglottic airway has been used in the anesthesia setting in scenarios where intubation and ventilation are difficult. The airway consists of a ventilation tube (with variable sizes) and a large inflatable cuff surrounding it. The end is designed with a gentle curve to fit into the hypopharynx, directing the air toward the larynx. When the cuff is inflated, the upper airway is sealed off and the tongue and soft tissues are held apart for better air movement.

The device does not guard against regurgitation. Gastric distension due to overpressure of the airway can occur with aggressive ventilations. This device has limited prehospital research to support it as more than a rescue airway.

Advanced Airways

Intubation of the trachea is considered the gold standard for definitive airway control for the acutely ill trauma patient. Intubation can be achieved via an oral or nasal route of insertion. It allows the provider to bypass the structures of the upper airway and secure the airway through to the larynx. Intubation is in the skill set of most ALS providers but can become more difficult under traumatic circumstances. Patients with suspected cervical spine trauma will require special handling, including a second provider to maintain stabilization during the intubation **PROCEDURE 8**.

Successful intubation requires a thorough knowledge of anatomy and the skills required to intubate the trachea. Emergency providers will be required to control an airway for a patient trapped in a vehicle, in a confined space such as in a helicopter, or in other positions that are less than optimal. Positioning for a patient with no cervical compromise requires the patient to be placed into extension; however, most patients requiring airway control following a traumatic event will require manual c-spine stabilization during intubation **FIGURE 3-14**.

Choice of blade style—either straight (Miller) or curved (Macintosh)—is a matter of personal preference and comfort level and, to some extent, prior experience. Careful preparation must be completed prior to an attempt at intubation. Once the blade is placed into the mouth and advanced into

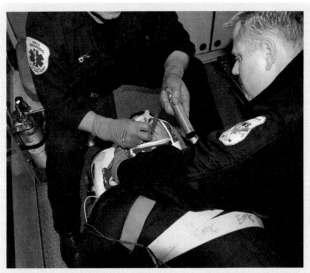

FIGURE 3-14 Cervical spine stabilization may be required during intubation attempts.

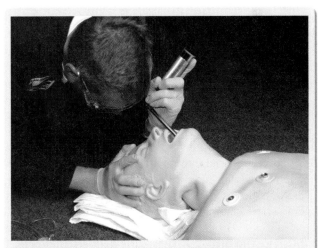

FIGURE 3-15 A rocking motion of the laryngoscope can cause dangerous extension of the c-spine.

the oropharynx, the provider should use a forward motion along the angle of the laryngoscope **FIGURE 3-15**. Rocking the laryngoscope can place dangerous extension on the cervical spine and may break teeth.

Confirmation of tube placement following intubation is critical. The first step in confirming tube placement is to view the tube passing through the vocal cords. Confirmation by auscultation of breath sounds requires that the provider know the condition of the lungs prior to intubation. Unequal lung sounds can be the product of a misplaced endotracheal tube in either mainstem bronchus, pneumothorax, lung contusion, or uneven muscular ability in the ribcage. Esophageal intubation may occur because of distortion of the airway due to trauma or because of blind intubation, where the provider cannot see the vocal cords. Recognizing the misplaced endotracheal tube as early as possible is the key to good airway care. Visualization of rise

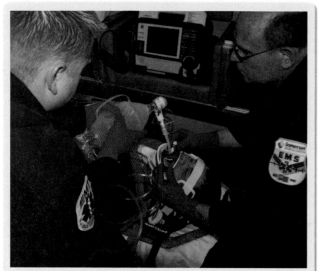

FIGURE 3-16 Capnometry is vital, along with other assessments, when trying to monitor the placement of an ETT.

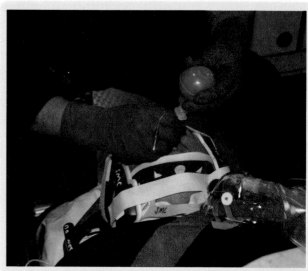

FIGURE 3-17 An esophageal detection device is a good way to confirm ETT placement.

and fall of the chest and misting of the endotracheal tube are also indications of proper placement.

Carbon dioxide monitoring is considered one of the best methods of confirming correct endotracheal tube (ETT) placement **FIGURE 3-16**. Typically, end-tidal carbon dioxide ($ETCO_2$) detecting has been used to confirm placement of an endotracheal tube. Disposable detectors indicate the presence of CO_2 in the expired breath by a change of color. The presence of CO_2 in the expired air strongly suggests that the tube has been placed into the trachea in perfusing patients. Capnometers (with wave form display) or colormetric $ETCO_2$ detectors should be used regularly to establish correct endotracheal placement. Electronic capnometers measure exhaled CO_2 over time. This curved shape can be viewed on a monitor. End-tidal CO_2 levels have been used to predict outcome from resuscitation. False positive detection may occur after ingestion of carbonated beverages and the like, but the effect is transient. Six breaths should clear any residual CO_2 and color change on the device will stop. Detection of carbon dioxide may be difficult in severe hypoperfusion states or during cardiac arrest. The use of these monitors should be secondary to visualizing the tube entering the cords, the visual rise of the chest, and listening to the breath sounds with your stethoscope.

In the absence of $ETCO_2$ detection for ETT placement, an esophageal (bulb or syringe) detection device can be used **FIGURE 3-17**. The esophageal detector may be more accurate in cardiac arrest or low perfusion states than the $ETCO_2$ detector. Squeeze the bulb to remove the air and place it on the ETT immediately following intubation. Because the trachea and mainstem bronchus contain a column of air supported by cartilaginous rings, a collapsed bulb attached to the end of an ETT should inflate rapidly. The syringe style is placed on top of the ETT and the plunger pulled back to confirm air movement in the tube. Use caution when a patient has been ventilated aggressively prior to intubation, as gastric

distension may give a false positive result. Caution should also be given if a ruptured esophagus is suspected.

An adjunct to difficult intubation is the gum elastic bougie (GEB) or Eschmann stylet. When good visualization of the vocal cords is not available during intubation, the GEB is advanced to the level of the epiglottis with the angled end pointing anteriorly. When advanced further, the stylet may enter the trachea, where it will create a washboard or ripple effect as it passes over the tracheal rings. If that is not felt, pull the stylet back and make another attempt. After the stylet is placed in the trachea, the ETT can be passed over the GEB and advanced into place **FIGURE 3-18**. Two providers are often required to advance the tube into place. The GEB is then removed and the patient ventilated. Because the bougie stylet is passed blindly beyond the provider's view, it should be used with caution when airway trauma is suspected.

Several other tools are available to assist the provider with an intubation attempt. The GlideScope and the Bullard laryngoscope are two fiberoptic devices that facilitate the provider's view of the vocal cords. The GlideScope uses a small external LCD screen whereas the Bullard laryngoscope uses an eyepiece. Both have been shown to increase the number of successful intubation attempts in difficult situations. Unfortunately, unfamiliarity and cost limit their use in the prehospital setting.

The use of fiberoptic bronchoscopy may facilitate the placement of an endotracheal tube in difficult airway situations, but it is rarely available to the street-level provider of trauma care. Intubation by fiberoptic visualization is required for all patients suspected of airway tear or rupture. Positive pressure ventilations above the level of the tear can cause additional injury. If a patient is in need of direct airway visualization by bronchoscopy, notify the receiving facility and determine the next best means to oxygenate and ventilate the patient during rapid transport.

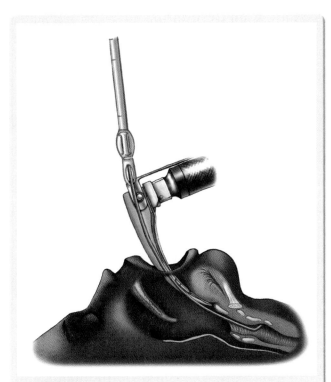

FIGURE 3-18 The gum elastic bougie stylet can assist with an intubation when direct visualization of the airway cannot be accomplished.

Digital intubation is a technique using just the provider's fingers to guide the endotracheal tube past the epiglottis and into the trachea. The provider places the first two fingers on one hand in the patient's mouth, locates the tip of the epiglottis with the middle finger, and slides the ETT down the groove between the two fingers, helped over the epiglottis by the middle finger.

Digital intubation may be a useful tool with patients who have a mandibular fracture or open facial trauma requiring immediate intubation to secure an airway. This technique has several negatives, however, including patients with an intact gag reflex, the chance for the provider to be bitten, and the provider's hand being too short to reach the epiglottis. A blind technique also increases the chance for a misplaced ETT.

Nasotracheal Intubation

Nasotracheal (nasal) intubation is an alternative to orotracheal intubation but with limited applications in the trauma patient **PROCEDURE 10** . The primary indication for nasal intubation is the patient who is expected to have a difficult airway but has spontaneous ventilations.

Nasotracheal intubation requires the patient to be placed into the sniffing position. Suspected cervical spine injury will limit the ability to position the patient to receive the nasal intubation. Contraindications to nasotracheal intubation include:

- Mid-face trauma or suspected basilar skull fracture
- Apnea

Relative contraindications include:

- Combativeness
- Increased intracranial pressure (ICP)
- Suspected hypertension
- Coagulopathy

Nasotracheal intubation should also be avoided in patients who have low oxygen or ventilatory reserves, because the procedure will take more time than the previously discussed procedures.

After lubricating the tube, it is advanced through one of the nares into the hypopharynx. When breath sounds (or whistling through the tube) are heard, the tube should be advanced quickly during inhalation. When the tube enters the trachea the patient will cough. Placement must be confirmed. If no breath sounds are heard, the tube does not advance, or gastric sounds are present, the tube must be repositioned and the procedure attempted again.

An alternative to the standard endotracheal tube is the Endotrol tube. It is more flexible and has an attached line to help the provider curve the end up to enter the trachea when advanced.

Retrograde Endotracheal Intubation

Another technique used to guide a tracheal tube into the trachea is **retrograde endotracheal intubation (REI)**. The technique requires advanced skill and additional time, making it a rarely used technique in the hospital setting and an even less frequently used technique in the prehospital setting. REI requires a catheter to be placed through the cricothyroid membrane and a flexible wire inserted through the catheter, then advanced upward into the mouth. The tracheal tube is then placed over the wire and advanced into the trachea. The wire and catheter are then removed and the tracheal tube advanced slightly into position. There are commercial kits available for the procedure. Given the infrequent use and potential complications, REI should be reserved for when conventional intubation techniques have failed to ventilate the patient and only if local protocols allow.

Pharmacologically Assisted Intubation

Rapid sequence intubations (RSIs) are the standard for intubations in the trauma center. Prehospital systems have begun to investigate this technique and some have developed protocols for usage. Drug-facilitated intubations commonly use a sedative and paralytic agent. Not all patients will require RSI, because many can be intubated with a sedative or an induction agent alone.

Premedication Agents

Several medications may be helpful before intubating a patient. These are referred to as **premedication agents**. The mnemonic LOAD is often used to remember these agents **TABLE 3-2** .

TABLE 3-2   LOAD

Lidocaine

Opiates

Atropine

Defasciculating agents

Lidocaine has two primary potential benefits as a premedication agent in intubation: it can help avoid bronchospasm and lower the chance of increased ICP during intubation. Lidocaine is controversial, however, due to lack of data supporting its effectiveness, and it is not used in all countries.

Sedative and analgesic effects of opiates (eg, fentanyl and morphine) may provide benefit to the injured patient prior to intubation. Fentanyl is more hemodynamically stable than morphine and can blunt airway reactivity during an intubation.

Atropine can be helpful to decrease the amount of airway secretions and to reduce the effect of vagal stimulation. The vagus nerve (or cranial nerve X) follows along the airway on its pathway to the heart. When stimulated, the vagus nerve produces a slowing of the heart rate and subsequent decrease in cardiac output. Vagal stimulation is especially prevalent in children younger than 5 years old, because the smaller airway allows more pressure to be exerted on the vagus nerve.

In RSI, a **defasciculating dose** of a paralytic agent is often given to reduce the amount of increased ICP produced by myoclonal fasciculations caused by standard neuromuscular blocking agents. A defasciculating dose is generally 10% of the paralyzing dose.

Induction Agents

Induction agents are a group of medications used to produce a rapid loss of consciousness to assist in intubation. All agents used to render a patient unconscious have side effects. Careful choice of agent should be based on the patient's presentation and specific characteristics.

Etomidate is a short-acting hypnotic agent used to facilitate intubation. It has rapid onset and clearance and minimal effects on the cardiovascular system. Etomidate is the most often used induction agent in RSI protocols. The only contraindication to etomidate is in patients with known adrenal insufficiency, because it has been associated with increased mortality due to suppression of steroid synthesis. The effect of etomidate on the CNS has led to a small number of cases of masseter spasm or trismus, which would make intubation more difficult or impossible without an additional paralytic agent. Side effects of etomidate may be minimized by administering it via slow IV push (over 30 to 60 seconds).

Propofol is a nonbarbiturate hypnotic agent that rapidly induces deep sedation. It produces a significant relaxation of the laryngeal muscles and produces conditions equal to etomidate. Propofol, however, has a hypotensive effect on the cardiovascular system and should be used with caution in patients with head injuries and patients who are hemodynamically unstable.

Thiopental is an ultra–short-acting barbiturate and is most commonly used in the induction phase of general anesthesia. Thiopental reduces cerebral oxygen consumption and has anticonvulsant effects, making it useful in patients with brain injury. It does, however, reduce myocardial contractility and systemic vascular resistance and can cause laryngospasm. Thiopental is best used for patients who are hemodynamically stable. Another barbiturate with similar effects to those of thiopental is methohexital. Both of these agents have rapid onset of unconsciousness and a short half-life, making them useful in intubation protocols.

Ketamine is a dissociative agent that has rapid onset and anesthetic properties. A sympathomimetic agent, ketamine may produce tachycardia, increased blood pressure, and cerebral vasodilation. It may potentially worsen brain injuries in patients. Caution should be used with patients with documented or suspected injury to the brain. Ketamine is best reserved for patients who have reactive airway disease or hypotension, and for whom brain injury has been excluded.

Neuromuscular Blocking Agents

Pharmacologic paralysis represents an integral component of RSI. If RSI is indicated, the provider must be trained and have a rescue airway available in the event a patient is unable to be intubated. Neuromuscular blocking agents fall into two classes: depolarizing and nondepolarizing. Because paralytic agents produce no sedative or analgesic effects, it is imperative to combine use of a paralytic agent with an appropriate induction agent.

Succinylcholine is a depolarizing acetylcholine dimer that acts noncompetitively at the acetylcholine receptor to produce muscular paralysis at the motor end plate. The ultra-short duration of action renders the rapid return of spontaneous breathing possible if intubation fails. An initial brief period of **fasciculations** (uncontrolled quivering of the skeletal muscles) is followed by sustained motor depolarization. Contraindications include conditions in which potassium is elevated. Thermal burns more than 24 hours old, crush injury, and **rhabdomyolysis** (the breakdown of muscle fibers and release of muscle cell contents) with hyperkalemia are among the traumatic conditions that can create a contraindication. The defasiculations resulting from succinylcholine may also raise intracranial and intragastric pressure. An increase in intraoccular pressure also makes penetrating injuries to the eye a contraindication.

Nondepolarizing muscle blockade agents (NMBA) compete to block acetylcholine at the postjunctional cholinergic receptors. This group of medications can be used in patients with a contraindication to succinylcholine. Common NMBAs include rocuronium, pancuronium, and vecuronium. All the drugs in this class try to approximate the effects of succinylcholine; however, none are able to exactly parallel them. Of the current choices, rocuronium has the shortest onset and produces good intubating conditions.

Complications of RSI

Success rates have shown that RSI is an acceptable method for airway control in prehospital patients, but complications do occur. The primary complication of RSI is airway failure. The most common cause of failure is a misplaced endotracheal tube. In being prepared for airway failure, providers must be familiar with airway rescue maneuvers, including a surgical airway in the event of a failed intubation.

As important as getting the airway into place is keeping it in place. Trauma patients will be moved as they are being secured for spinal precautions, out into an ambulance or air ambulance, transported from the ambulance to the hospital, and then transferred from the ambulance stretcher to the trauma bed. Each of these moves has the ability to dislodge the airway internally, rendering it less effective or completely ineffective. After checking to make sure the airway is in the right position, note the depth markings on the endotracheal tube or other airway device for future reassessments. Secure the airway with tape or a professional device designed to keep the airway in place **FIGURE 3-19**. Commercial devices are often preferred to tape in trauma because airways tend to be wet and it may be hard to find a clean surface on which to tape the airway. Another choice to consider is the addition of a cervical collar to minimize neck flexion or extension, which could lead to airway displacement. The cervical collar used in this manner is not used to secure the neck and may be used with or without a long backboard. It is always wise to print off the ETCO₂ reading from your monitor to show that you had good tube placement at this stage.

Surgical Airways

Cricothyroidotomy may be performed as the first airway maneuver in cases of severe facial trauma precluding intubation, but is most often used after tracheal intubation has failed. Cricothyroidotomy can be completed surgically or through the use of a needle catheter. A number of complications have been described for both methods of cricothyroidotomy. Failure of the procedure, pneumothorax, hemorrhage, and misplaced tube are among the most common; however, age is the single contraindication to surgical cricothyroidotomy. Needle cricothyroidotomy is recommended in children younger than 12 years old.

As with any procedure, preparation is necessary. Evaluation of the anatomy of the neck prior to airway control may facilitate the procedure in the event of a failed intubation. Required equipment will include a scalpel, tissue forceps, or a hemostat. Cuffed endotracheal tubes ranging in sizes from 5 to 7 mm can be used if a commercial device is unavailable **PROCEDURE 12**.

The procedure includes locating the cricothyroid membrane, cleansing the site, and making a vertical incision through the anterior neck. Divide the tissue above the cricothyroid membrane and make a horizontal incision through the membrane. The incision can be dilated digitally (with the small finger) or with a hemostat or other tool. The endotracheal tube should be inserted to a depth of 5 cm using a rigid stylet to avoid the tube turning upward toward the vocal cords. Inflate the cuff and check for tube placement as with other tracheal intubations.

In recent years, a number of commercial devices have been introduced in an attempt to expedite the procedure and reduce the required skill set. These devices are known as cricothyrotomes and use one of two techniques to cannulate the trachea. One type uses the Seldinger technique to thread a tube over a wire inserted through the cricothyroid membrane; the other uses a tube over a puncture-type device to enter the trachea.

Needle cricothyroidotomy uses a large IV-type catheter to puncture the cricothyroid membrane with transtracheal jet insufflation. The technique can be used on adults and children **PROCEDURE 11**. The cricothyroid membrane is located and cleansed as in a cricothyroidotomy. A large-bore catheter (16 g or larger) is attached to a syringe half filled with saline and inserted caudally at an angle of 30° to 60°. The trachea is aspirated, with bubbles in the saline confirming position in the trachea, and the catheter is advanced into the trachea. The needle is removed and the catheter is connected to a jet ventilation system. Alternatively, several homemade devices have been used successfully. Jet insufflation should proceed at 1 second of inspiration (flow) to 3 seconds of expiration (release). It is important to note that, during jet ventilation, oxygen is being supplied to the larger airways but carbon dioxide is not being released from the alveoli. This technique may sustain life for up to 30 minutes while a definitive airway can be arranged.

Ventilation

Many trauma patients are awake and breathing spontaneously. Every patient with a substantial mechanism of injury should have high concentration supplemental oxygen applied to support aerobic activity in the body. A much smaller number will have inadequate ventilations. However, there are many reasons that a patient may begin to ventilate

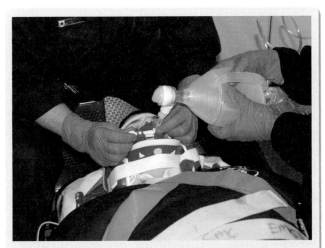
FIGURE 3-19 Securing the airway will help keep it in place.

CONTROVERSIES

The Challenges of Prehospital RSI

PREHOSPITAL RAPID SEQUENCE INTUBATION (RSI) denotes the use of neuromuscular blocking agents to facilitate endotracheal intubation (ETI). RSI is an extremely difficult procedure with strong potential for catastrophic outcomes if performed improperly. Therefore, most EMS medical directors discourage widespread use of prehospital RSI, reserving the technique for only specially trained and experienced EMS personnel.

The intention of RSI is to improve survival. However, no studies have demonstrated improved patient outcomes from prehospital RSI. The San Diego RSI Trial is the only study evaluating patient survival after RSI.[1] The study tested the large scale implementation of ground-based EMS prehospital RSI for traumatic brain-injured patients. The study matched 209 head-injured RSI patients with 600 historical non-intubated controls. The study found that prehospital RSI almost doubled the odds of death compared to no ETI at all.

RSI pharmacologically removes all of the patient's intact airway reflexes. The operator must quickly and successfully accomplish ETI after administration of RSI drug agents, a goal that requires exceptional ETI skill. Failure to quickly, efficiently, and correctly insert an endotracheal tube or other airway may result in hypoxia, cardiac arrest, and death.

Many major trauma victims have severe facial or airway injuries that may complicate laryngoscopy efforts. Even with complete neuromuscular relaxation, identification of airway structures in these patients may be extremely difficult. Unlike healthy operating room patients who may tolerate several minutes without ventilation, victims of major trauma may have significant pulmonary injury or blood loss, severely compromising their oxygen reserves. These patients may experience oxygen desaturation after only brief periods (< 30 seconds) of apnea. These factors further complicate RSI efforts in major trauma patients.

Recent studies highlight that injury or adverse events may occur even with successful RSI efforts. Colloquially speaking, "how the tube got there is as important as whether it's in the right place." In a review of 108 patients from the San Diego RSI Trial, Dunford and associates observed that over half experienced oxygen desaturation, and one fifth experienced bradycardia.[2] These events were attributed to prolonged laryngoscopy efforts occurring after administration of succinylcholine. Another overlooked side effect of RSI is inadvertent hyperventilation, which can harm traumatic brain-injured patients through cerebral vasoconstriction. In the San Diego RSI trial, the investigators found that inadvertent hyperventilation occurred frequently after paramedic RSI.[3]

Unrecognized esophageal intubation is a serious adverse event that may lead to death or catastrophic brain injury. In a series of 108 prehospital ETI patients, Katz and Falk found the endotracheal tube misplaced in 25%.[4] In pharmacologically paralyzed patients, it may be very difficult to recognize endotracheal tube misplacement or dislodgement. For this reason, many medical directors strongly recommend the routine use of waveform end-tidal capnography with RSI cases.[5]

The intention of RSI is to maximize "first-pass" intubation success. To accomplish this goal, EMS personnel must have exceptional *basic* intubation skills. However, several studies highlight limits in paramedic ETI skill, training, and experience. These observations have led medical directors to question the appropriateness of widespread advanced RSI, especially when EMS agencies seem to struggle with even basic ETI skills.

For example, in series of cardiac arrest and RSI patients in Pennsylvania, paramedics often required three or more laryngoscopy attempts to accomplish intubation.[6] In the RSI subset, first-pass success was only 57%.

Paramedics in the United States receive very limited baseline live ETI training. The national paramedic curriculum requires paramedic students to perform only 5 ETI prior to graduation; most students perform less than a total of 10 live ETI.[7,8] Students often gain baseline ETI experience in the operating room under the guidance of anesthesiologists, but a national survey indicated a marked reduction in operating room training opportunities.[9]

Once in clinical practice, paramedics perform few live ETI. In Pennsylvania, paramedics perform only one ETI annually.[10] Studies in Maine and Alabama reveal similar figures.[11,12]

Select air medical and EMS agencies operate successful prehospital RSI programs.[13–15] These agencies emphasize that RSI is "not just about the drugs." Rather, RSI represents one component of a comprehensive effort to optimize all aspects of airway management. Most RSI agencies follow prehospital RSI guidelines prescribed by the National Association of EMS Physicians.[5] Key elements of a successful RSI program include:

- Structured training, including supplemental use of operating room training when available. Some agencies combine live operating room sessions with difficult airway training on mannequins.
- Minimum ETI procedural standards. For example, many RSI agencies require paramedics to perform at least 12 live ETI annually.[13] Individuals not meeting these standards must complete additional operating room training.
- Consistent use of continuous waveform end-tidal capnography to verify endotracheal tube placement.[16]
- Availability of a range of rescue airway devices in the event of failed RSI; for example, Combitube, King LT airway, cricothyroidotomy, etc.[17]
- Close quality assurance and inspection, including individual review of all RSI cases, review of physiologic measures (oxygen saturation, heart rate, blood pressure) during the RSI, and a limited review of patient outcomes.
- Close medical oversight. Some medical directors feel that close oversight is possible only with modestly sized EMS agencies.

Prehospital RSI is an extraordinarily difficult procedure with strong potential to cause injury and death if performed improperly. EMS agencies opting to perform prehospital RSI should adopt the highest standards of airway management skill, training, and oversight.

Henry E. Wang, MD, MS
University of Alabama at Birmingham
Birmingham, Alabama

References

1. Davis DP, Hoyt DB, Ochs M, et al. The effect of paramedic rapid sequence intubation on outcome in patients with severe traumatic brain injury. *J Trauma.* 2003; 54:444–53.
2. Dunford JV, Davis DP, Ochs M, et al. Incidence of transient hypoxia and pulse rate reactivity during paramedic rapid sequence intubation. *Ann Emerg Med.* 2003; 42:721–8.
3. Davis DP, Dunford JV, Poste JC, et al. The impact of hypoxia and hyperventilation on outcome after paramedic rapid sequence intubation of severely head-injured patients. *J Trauma.* 2004; 57:1–8; discussion -10.
4. Katz SH, Falk JL. Misplaced endotracheal tubes by paramedics in an urban emergency medical services system. *Ann Emerg Med.* 2001; 37:32–7.
5. Wang HE, Davis DP, O'Connor RE, Domeier RM. Drug-assisted intubation in the prehospital setting (resource document to NAEMSP position statement). *Prehosp Emerg Care.* 2006; 10:261–71.
6. Wang HE, Yealy DM. How many attempts are required to accomplish out-of-hospital endotracheal intubation? *Acad Emerg Med.* 2006; 13:372–7.
7. National Highway Traffic and Safety Administration: Emergency Medical Technician Paramedic: National Standard Curriculum, Clinical Rotations. Available at: www.nhtsa.gov/people/injury/ems/EMT-P/disk_7%5B1%5D/Clinical.pdf. Accessed March 17, 2009.
8. Wang HE, Seitz SR, Hostler D, Yealy DM. Defining the learning curve for paramedic student endotracheal intubation. *Prehosp Emerg Care.* 2005; 9:156–62.
9. Johnston BD, Seitz SR, Wang HE. Limited opportunities for paramedic student endotracheal intubation training in the operating room. *Acad Emerg Med.* 2006; 13:1051–5.
10. Wang HE, Kupas DF, Hostler D, et al. Procedural experience with out-of-hospital endotracheal intubation. *Crit Care Med.* 2005; 33:1718–21.
11. Burton JH, Baumann MR, Maoz T, et al. Endotracheal intubation in a rural EMS state: procedure utilization and impact of skills maintenance guidelines. *Prehosp Emerg Care.* 2003; 7:352–6.
12. Brown T, Stephens S, Cofield S. Procedural experience of EMTs who attempt endotracheal intubation (abstract). *Prehosp Emerg Care.* 2007; 11:105.
13. Wayne MA, Friedland E. Prehospital use of succinylcholine: a 20-year review. *Prehosp Emerg Care.* 1999; 3:107–9.
14. Wang HE, Davis DP, Wayne MA, Delbridge T. Prehospital rapid-sequence intubation—what does the evidence show? Proceedings from the 2004 National Association of EMS Physicians annual meeting. *Prehosp Emerg Care.* 2004; 8:366–77.
15. Fakhry SM, Scanlon JM, Robinson L, et al. Prehospital rapid sequence intubation for head trauma: conditions for a successful program. *J Trauma.* 2006; 60:997–1001.
16. O'Connor RE, Swor RA. Verification of endotracheal tube placement following intubation. National Association of EMS Physicians Standards and Clinical Practice Committee. *Prehosp Emerg Care.* 1999; 3:248–50.
17. Guyette FX, Greenwood MJ, Neubecker D, et al. Alternate airways in the prehospital setting (resource document to NAEMSP position statement). *Prehosp Emerg Care.* 2007; 11:56–61.

inappropriately. The following situations may interfere with normal ventilation:

- Direct injury to the chest wall or muscles of ventilation, including the diaphragm or intercostal muscles
- Indirect trauma that affects the body's ability to breathe at a normal rate or volume, such as head trauma or oxygen delivery issues (shock)

The provider's goal in treating the patient is to bring the minute volume into the normal range. Normal ventilations for an adult occur at 10 to 16 per minute. Therefore, when ventilations are required they should be provided at 5- to 6-second intervals (10 to 12 per minute). Ventilations should fill the chest and begin to make it expand. Deep ventilations are not required to provide the patient with a good minute volume.

Often a patient who is breathing too fast or too slowly will require additional help to maintain proper ventilation. Respiratory rates above 29 breaths/min or below 10 breaths/min often produce minute volumes that are too low. Each breath moves air into and out of the lungs, but some of this air does not get exchanged in the alveoli. Air in the mainstem bronchus and bronchial tree takes up space, and shallow breaths may not exchange this air with fresh oxygenated air. This space is referred to as *dead space* because the air is not used. The anatomic dead space can be estimated by converting a person's ideal body weight (based on height and body type) in pounds to volume in milliliters. A 150-lb (68-kg) person has a dead space volume of 150 mL. When the ventilatory volume becomes too high or too low, this dead space decreases the amount of available air by even more. Hypoxia and hypercarbia result when the air cannot move into and out of the lungs. Normalizing ventilation is the way to prevent this.

TABLE 3-3 compares two patients: one with a high respiratory rate and one with a low respiratory rate. Notice in the table that Patient A is breathing at a slow rate with normal volume whereas Patient B has an increased rate and decreased volume. Both patients have a minute volume that is too low.

Clinical evaluation to determine when to ventilate these patients requires multiple assessment points. The brain is the most oxygen-sensitive organ in the body. Altered appearance is often seen as anxiety or combativeness. This is the early stage of shock (see Chapter 4). As the hypoxia continues, the body will try to compensate and increase the ventilatory rate and effort. As the ability to exchange the respiratory gasses decreases, carbon dioxide in the blood-

stream increases and the level of consciousness decreases until the patient becomes sleepy and unresponsive. The need for ventilation rests somewhere in between. Monitors such as pulse oximeters and capnometers can measure these changes as they happen. Pulse oximetry and capnography are becoming more widely distributed throughout emergency medical services.

TIP

Lack of oxygen to the brain will make the patient anxious and combative, whereas increased carbon dioxide will decrease the patient's level of consciousness.

Pulse oximetry measures the arterial saturation of **oxyhemoglobin (Hbo_2)**, the oxygen-rich hemoglobin. Oxygen saturation levels obtained from pulse oximetry (Spo_2) are part of a complete assessment of the patient's oxygenation status and are not a substitute for measurement of partial pressure of oxygen (Pao_2) or ventilation. A pulse oximeter is easily applied, noninvasive, and reliable **FIGURE 3-20**. It measures light absorbance at two wavelengths—red and infrared—across the hemoglobin. The ratios of pulsatile absorbance at the two wavelengths determine an estimated value for hemoglobin saturation.

Because pulse oximeters measure absorbance at only two wavelengths, an inaccurate estimate of hemoglobin occurs when more than two types of hemoglobin are present. The two types of hemoglobin typically found are oxyhemoglobin (Hbo_2) and **reduced hemoglobin (RHB)**, the hemoglobin after the oxygen has been released to the cells. In the presence of **methemoglobin (metHb)** (a compound formed by oxidation of the iron on the hemoglobin) or **carboxyhemoglobin (COHb)** (hemoglobin loaded with carbon monoxide), however, normal Spo_2 values may be seen. If the underlying condition goes undiagnosed, relying on Spo_2 may affect the patient adversely. Carbon monoxide binds avidly to hemoglobin, preventing oxygen loading. CO-oximeters have the ability to measure multiple wavelengths

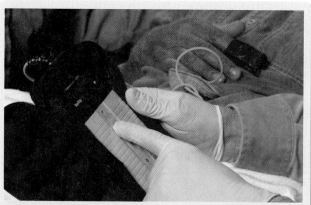

FIGURE 3-20 Pulse oximeters are noninvasive and can help the provider assess the patient.

TABLE 3-3 Minute Volume Comparison		
	Patient A	**Patient B**
Ventilations	8 breaths/min	28 breaths/min
Tidal volume	500 mL	250 mL
Dead space (150 mL)	−1,200 mL	−4,200 mL
Minute volume	2,800 mL	2,800 mL

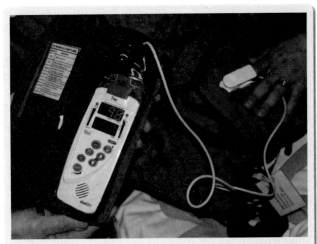

FIGURE 3-21 A CO-oximeter has the ability to measure multiple types of conditions.

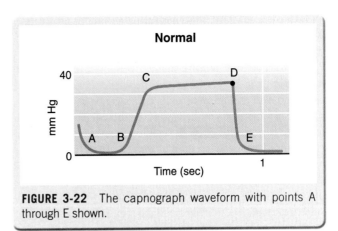

FIGURE 3-22 The capnograph waveform with points A through E shown.

of light and are necessary to measure the concentration of all these types simultaneously **FIGURE 3-21**.

Limitations of pulse oximetry measurement include degradation of signal measurement by ambient light (too much light oversaturates the light of the probe) and low signal-to-noise ratios due to a weak pulse or patient movement. Something that is often forgotten is to ensure the finger probe is cleaned of dirt from a previous patient (bloody finger) and to ensure that the patient is not wearing dark or sparkly fingernail polish. Finally, it is important to remember what pulse oximetry does not measure. It does not measure oxygen transport or delivery, and it does not measure distal perfusion. An anemic patient may have 100% hemoglobin saturation yet have inadequate oxygen to meet metabolic demands because of the lack of hemoglobin.

The body often compensates for lower tidal volume with a higher respiratory rate and vice versa. Increased respiratory rates with normal volume will result in hyperventilation. Current literature has shown this to be potentially detrimental to patients; normal ventilations should be supported. Hyperventilation not only increases the amount of oxygen available in the lower portions of the lungs, but also results in decreasing carbon dioxide (CO_2) levels. CO_2 can have a profound effect on the size of the blood vessels. As CO_2 increases, blood vessels dilate, and when it decreases, they constrict.

End-tidal carbon dioxide ($ETCO_2$) monitors measure the partial pressure of carbon dioxide gas in a sample. The sample taken at the end of the exhalation has a close correlation to arterial Paco$_2$. Typically ETCO$_2$ is 2–5 mm Hg lower than the arterial Paco$_2$. The normal range for ETCO$_2$ in a trauma patient is 30 to 40 mm Hg.

Capnography is the monitoring of the rise and fall of ETCO$_2$ levels over time **FIGURE 3-22**. The important features of the capnographic waveform include contour, baseline level, and rate of rise of CO_2. There are four distinct phases. The first phase (A–B) is the initial stage of exhalation, where the gas sample is dead space gas, free of CO_2. At point B, there is a mixture of alveolar gas with dead space gas and the CO_2 level rises abruptly. The expiratory or alveolar plateau is represented by phase C–D, and the gas sampled is essentially alveolar. Point D is the maximal ETCO$_2$ level, the best reflection of alveolar CO_2. Fresh gas is introduced as the patient inspires (phase D–E), and the trace returns to the baseline level of CO_2, approximately 0.

Exponential decreases in CO_2 waveforms are significant events, often associated with sudden blood loss or other causes of hypotension. Low cardiac output, cardiac arrest, or pulmonary embolism may produce this pattern. Gradual decreases in ETCO$_2$ may reflect hypothermia, hypovolemia, decreasing cardiac output, or decreased metabolic activity (eg, after neuromuscular blockade). A sustained but constant decrease in ETCO$_2$ may be due to hyperventilation or increases in dead space ventilation.

ETCO$_2$ values may rise gradually secondary to hypoventilation, increasing body temperature, increased metabolic activity (eg, fever, sepsis, and malignant hyperthermia), or exogenous CO_2 absorption (laryngoscopy). Transient increases in ETCO$_2$ may be noted after IV bicarbonate administration or release of extremity tourniquets. Chronic obstructive pulmonary disease (COPD) results in a gradually up-sloping of phase B–C.

Common Causes of Traumatic Airways

Difficult Airways

The provider must make many choices while assessing a difficult airway. Does the patient have difficulty breathing with increased work of breathing? Will the patient consent to or allow airway care? Will the patient be a difficult intubation? And, if needed, are advanced airway control methods immediately available?

A patient may require many levels of care. Some will need only basic levels of care, whereas others will need more advanced skill and training levels than may be available at the scene. Most decisions in the care of the difficult airway can follow an algorithm **FIGURE 3-23**. Begin by continuing the administration of high concentration of oxygen. Then determine the best style of airway that will fit the patient's condition. If the level of airway care that the patient requires is above the scope of practice of the provider who is available at the scene, consider requesting additional care to the scene if possible.

Develop a primary and a backup means to maintain an airway. It is extremely important to be able to move to another type of airway quickly when an airway fails. If an oral airway is placed into the oropharynx and bleeding occurs, what will the provider do next? With a difficult airway, an awake and cooperative patient is preferred to one who is sedated as long as they are ventilating well and maintaining a good pulse oximetry saturation. If saturations are above 92%, high-flow oxygen through a nonrebreather is indicated; however, if despite high-flow oxygen the patient cannot maintain Spo_2 readings above 92%, ventilation should be considered. Sedation or paralysis will commit the provider to ensuring an airway, and failure is often lethal. Patients should be evaluated for the ability to be ventilated with a bag mask before advancing to higher level airway control. Several traumatic conditions require additional decision-making ability.

Closed Head Injury

Traumatic injury to the brain is the single most common indication for a definitive airway in patients with blunt trauma. Initial goals focus on airway protection and maintenance. Sustained goals in the management of closed head injury focus on the prevention of secondary injury to

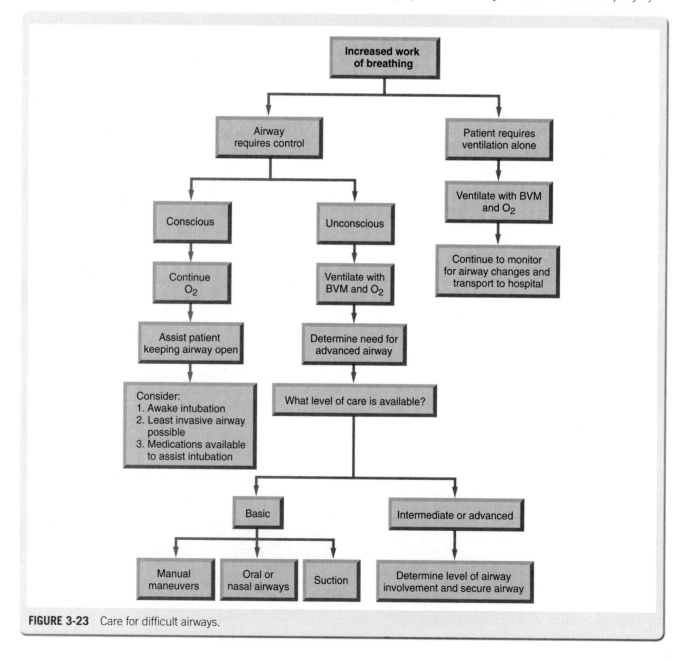

FIGURE 3-23 Care for difficult airways.

the brain by optimizing oxygenation and regulating carbon dioxide **FIGURE 3-24**. Airway management is particularly challenging in patients with traumatic brain injury (TBI) because of the associated problem of intracranial hypertension. It is well recognized that even a single episode of hypoxia can have lethal effects on outcome. Uncontrolled hyperventilation with cerebral vasoconstriction may worsen the outcome as well. Hypoxia (apnea, cyanosis, or oxygen saturation less than 90%) and hypercarbia must be avoided. Hypercarbia results in cerebral vasodilation, effectively increasing intracranial blood volume, with resultant elevated intracranial blood pressure. (See Chapter 5 for more information on head injury.) Early definitive airway control, with the ability to more directly control oxygenation and ventilation, is recommended for a GCS score of less than 9. RSI may help eliminate prolonged awake intubation attempts and, therefore, the risk of hypercarbia.

In patients with an intact gag reflex, insertion of an airway that may cause gagging should be avoided because it will raise ICP. RSI may be appropriate when clinically indicated in TBI, provided preintubation hypoxia and postintubation extreme hyperventilation are avoided.

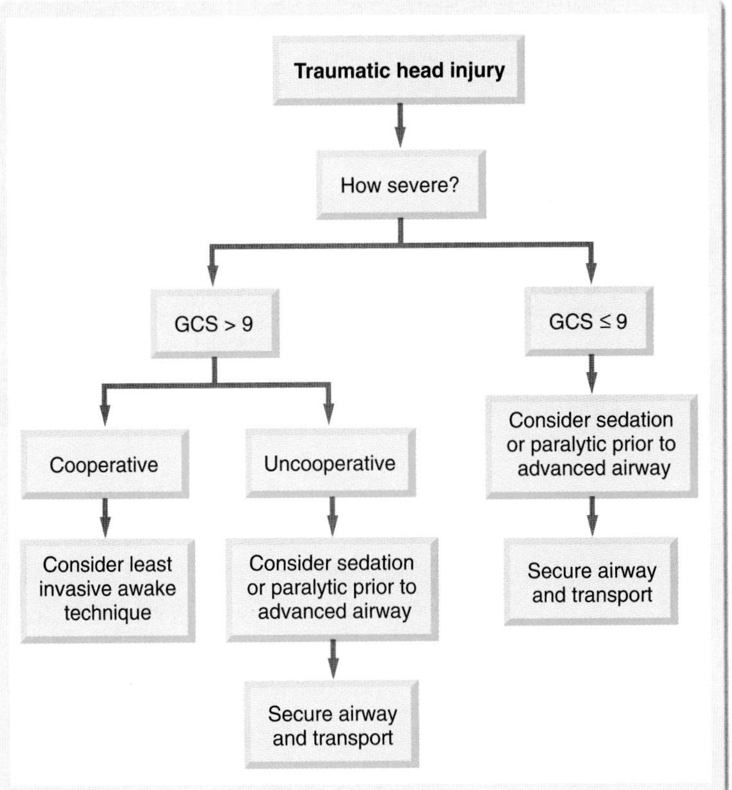

Cervical Spine Trauma

Injury to the spine is common in patients with blunt trauma, and the cervical spine is most often at risk. The critical need to immobilize and protect the cervical spine in virtually all patients with blunt trauma complicates management of the airway. Fear of injury to the spinal cord by cervical manipulation during airway control has led to many local protocols delaying airway control; however, evidence suggests that orotracheal intubation, with strict stabilization of the c-spine, is safe as a standard of care **FIGURE 3-25** **PROCEDURE 8**.

During the intubation attempt, the cervical collar may be loosened to allow better visualization of the vocal cords, as long as c-spine stabilization is maintained by a second provider throughout the procedure. If sufficient time, equipment, and experience exist, alternate techniques to direct laryngoscopy may be considered, such as the Intubating LMA. Given the emergent nature of most intubations performed in the field, constraints of equipment and expertise, and the small degree of extension with proper cervical spine stabilization during laryngoscopy, the tried and true method of airway control in the injured patient remains intubation using direct laryngoscopy with sedation or paralytics.

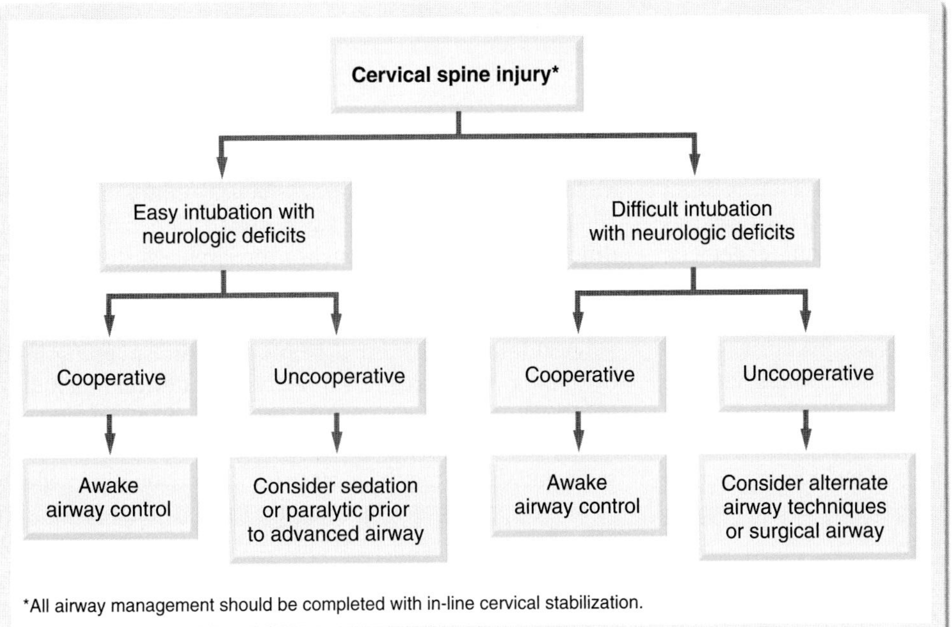

Maxillary-Facial Trauma

Patients with facial, jaw, and anterior neck injuries commonly present with threatened airways.

FIGURE 3-24 Ventilating patients with traumatic head injury.

*All airway management should be completed with in-line cervical stabilization.

FIGURE 3-25 Ventilating patients with cervical spine injuries.

Direct injury to the soft tissues and bony skeleton, tongue, and larynx may cause internal and external obstruction of the airway from edema, hemorrhage, secretions, or loss of bony structure. Many patients require advanced airway tools and techniques or a surgical airway. Most maxillofacial injuries are secondary to blunt mechanisms and are commonly associated with multisystem injuries, including those to the brain. In penetrating trauma, the airway may be no less challenging **FIGURE 3-26**.

Although emergent surgical intervention is often required, many patients with severe injury to bone and soft tissue are able to clear blood and secretions. If the potential for an injury to the spine does not preclude the patient sitting upright, slight forward positioning, suctioning, and calming of the patient frequently allow for forward displacement of bilateral mandible fractures or severe soft-tissue injury and maintenance of a precarious but patent airway. Under these conditions, close observation and rapid transport to a facility prepared to manage the airway are indicated. In the context of massive injury to bone and soft tissue such as a catastrophic self-inflicted gunshot wound, an urgent need for a definitive airway does not necessarily mean that a surgical airway will be necessary. Despite the intimidating appearance of such injuries, many of these patients can undergo orotracheal intubation due to loss of restrictive anatomy. If endotracheal intubation is not plausible or fails, the rescue technique of choice is a surgical airway. Supraglottic airways may or may not be effective when dealing with these types of injuries because they rely on the structure of the airway to be intact. If the style of airway will not allow the airway to be secured, the patient must be moved to more advanced care as a priority.

Airway Compression

Recognition of either direct or indirect injury to the larynx and trachea is important to future and even immediate airway planning. The management of laryngotracheal trauma is based on the status of the airway **FIGURE 3-27**. Clues to the diagnosis of larynx or trachea injury include marked pain, tenderness, and ecchymosis across the anterior neck or larynx; hoarseness or stridor; or the presence of subcutaneous emphysema. Subcutaneous emphysema and crepitus are the chief clinical signs. In most patients with laryngeal fractures, these fractures are caused by penetrating trauma. The need for an advanced airway is an independent predictor of mortality.

Treatment options for these injuries include orotracheal intubation or insertion of a surgical airway depending on the acuity of the presentation. In patients who are oxygenating, ventilating, and protecting their own airway despite a clinical suspicion of laryngotracheal injury, the patient should be transported to the hospital. Under urgent conditions, unless obvious tracheal or laryngeal disruption is evident, orotracheal intubation is the procedure of choice. If there is resistance, intubation should be aborted and a surgical airway performed below the corresponding level of trauma. Temporizing supralaryngeal devices, including bag-mask ventilations, should be avoided in this circumstance due to the risk of worsening subcutaneous emphysema and distorting the airway. For open wounds in which a tracheal injury is visualized, the trachea may be cannu-

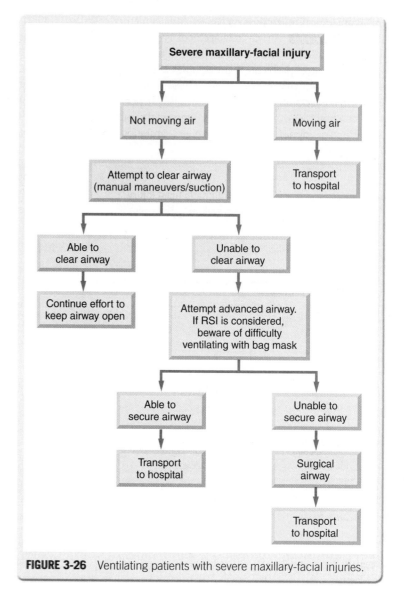

FIGURE 3-26 Ventilating patients with severe maxillary-facial injuries.

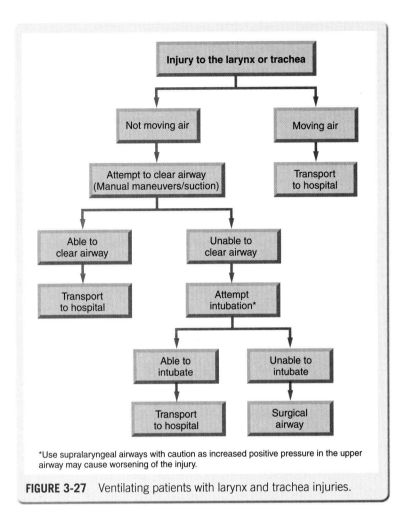

*Use supralaryngeal airways with caution as increased positive pressure in the upper airway may cause worsening of the injury.

FIGURE 3-27 Ventilating patients with larynx and trachea injuries.

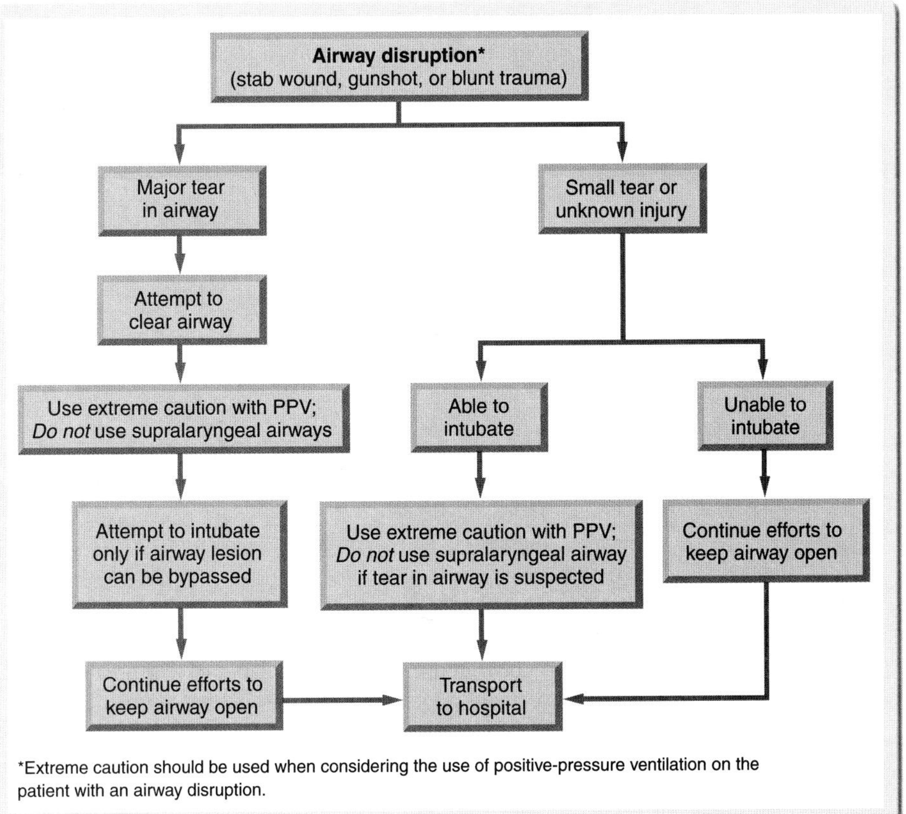

*Extreme caution should be used when considering the use of positive-pressure ventilation on the patient with an airway disruption.

FIGURE 3-28 Ventilating patients with airway disruption.

lated directly, with conversion to orotracheal intubation under controlled conditions.

Airway Disruption

Airway disruption can occur at any level of the airway. An open pneumothorax is an example of a distal airway disruption, whereas a tear of a mainstem bronchus would be a proximal example. Most airway disruption occurs from penetrating trauma, but severe blunt trauma can produce a shearing injury to the airway **FIGURE 3-28**.

Positive pressure ventilation (PPV) delivered to these types of trauma can worsen the injury. Additional air can leak from the airway into the surrounding tissue or internal bleeding and edema can make the patient worse. When the patient is able to move air on their own, high-flow oxygen and rapid transport is indicated. Supralaryngeal airways are all designed to provide PPV at or above the level of the glottis and should be avoided if airway disruption is suspected. If a tension pneumothorax is present, a needle thoracentesis **PROCEDURE 13** is indicated to relieve the pressure. In some cases, a skilled provider will be able to bypass the lesion with the endotracheal tube and provide PPV distal to the injury. One example would be a stab wound to the left side of the chest. If the provider can pass the endotracheal tube into the right mainstem bronchus, the injury would remain above the intubation.

CHAPTER RESOURCES

CASE STUDY ANSWERS

1 What are the priorities for this patient?

Following safety, airway and ventilation control are paramount. Because airway control often requires movement of the cervical spine, mechanisms of injury that suggest spinal injury require spinal stabilization with initial airway care. His fall requires that spinal movements be kept to a minimum throughout his care.

2 Are his ventilations adequate?

His ventilations are inadequate. A rate of 12 breaths/min with shallow breaths will not allow adequate minute volume. His Spo_2 is decreased and increases only slightly with high-flow oxygen.

3 Why does a chest injury affect how you will manage his airway?

The chest wall offers structure to the muscles of ventilation. The flail segment he has on the left side will decrease the ability of the chest to move and create the negative pressures required to move air in and out of the body.

4 What steps should be taken to manage this patient's airway?

Airway care should start with care that requires the least amount of time and equipment and should progress to more advanced airways as time and training allow. His airway requires manual positioning and suctioning immediately. He will require additional airway support to keep the airway open and free of blood. Bleeding in the upper airway can be kept free of the lower airways by using any airway that passes beyond the tongue and seals off the pharynx.

5 What steps should be taken to monitor his airway following placement of an airway adjunct?

Immediately following placement of an airway the placement must be confirmed. Even basic airways should show signs of easier movement of air. Lung sounds, positive change in vital signs, increasing Spo_2 and positive CO_2 return are among the signs of good airway placement. After an advanced airway is placed, he will require positive-pressure ventilations with high concentrations of oxygen. Continued monitoring of vital signs, including Spo_2 and capnometry along with recurring assessment for proper placement of the airway is required.

Trauma in Motion

1. What options are available to your service if a difficult airway is encountered?
2. What tools are available in your service to confirm airway placement and maintenance?
3. What is your local protocol for use of a backup airway?
4. When are backup airways practiced in your service, and is that an appropriate timing interval with which to retain skills?

References and Resources

Abrams KJ, Grande CM. Airway management in the trauma patient with cervical spine injury. *Curr Opinion Anesthesiology.* 1994; 7:184–190.

American Academy of Orthopaedic Surgeons. *Emergency Care and Transportation of the Sick and Injured.* 9th ed. Sudbury, MA: Jones and Bartlett; 2005.

American Academy of Orthopaedic Surgeons. *Nancy Caroline's Emergency Care in the Streets.* 6th ed. Sudbury, MA: Jones and Bartlett; 2007.

American College of Surgeons Committee on Trauma. *Advanced Trauma Life Support for Doctors.* 7th ed. Chicago, IL: American College of Surgeons; 2004.

American Society of Anesthesiologists Task Force. Practice guidelines for management of the difficult airway. *Anesthesiology.* 2003; 98:1269–1277.

Bergen JM, Smith DC. A review of etomidate for rapid sequence intubation in the emergency department. *J Emerg Med.* 1997; 15:221–230.

Bozeman WP, Kleiner DM, Huggett V. A comparison of rapid-sequence intubation and etomidate-only intubation in the prehospital air medical setting. *Prehosp Emerg Care.* 2006; 10(1):8–13.

Brain Trauma Foundation Writing Team. Guidelines for prehospital management of traumatic brain injury, 2nd ed. *Prehosp Emerg Care*. 2007; 12(1).

Bramwell KJ, Haizlip J, Pribble C, et al. The effect of etomidate on intracranial pressure and systematic blood pressure in pediatric patients with severe traumatic brain injury. *Pediatr Emerg Care*. 2006; 22(2):9093.

Crosby E, Lui A. The adult cervical spine: implications for airway management. *Can J Anaesth*. 1990; 37:77–93.

Elling B, Elling K, Rothenberg M. *Anatomy and Physiology: Paramedic*. Sudbury, MA: Jones and Bartlett; 2004.

Feliciano DV, Mattox KL, Moore EE. *Trauma*. 6th ed. New York: McGraw-Hill Medical; 2008.

Frakes MA. Measuring end-tidal carbon dioxide: clinical applications and usefulness. *Criti Care Nurse*. 2001; 21(5):23–35.

Getward JJ, Cook TM, Seller C, et al. Evaluation of the size 4 i-gel airway in one hundred non-paralyzed patients. *Anaesthesia*. 2008; 63:1124–1130.

Grande CM, Barton CR, Stene JK. Appropriate techniques for airway management of emergency patients with suspected spinal cord injury. *Anesth Analg*. 1988; 67:714–715.

Hopson LR, Dronen SC. Pharmacologic adjuncts to intubation. In: Roberts JR, Hedges J, eds. *Clinical Procedures in Emergency Medicine*. 4th ed. Philadelphia: Saunders; 2004.

Jacoby J, Heller M, Nicholas J, et al. Etomidate versus midazolam for out-of-hospital intubation: a prospective, randomized trial. *Ann Emerg Med*. 2006; 47(6):525–530.

Liem EB. Bullard laryngoscope intubation. Available at: http://vam.anest.ufl.edu/airwaydevice/bullard/index.html. Accessed September 16, 2008.

Mock C, Lormand JD, Goosen J, et al. *Guidelines for Essential Trauma Care*. Geneva: World Health Organization; 2004.

Reves JG, Glass PSA, Lubarsky DA, et al. Intravenous nonopioid anesthetics. In: Miller RD, ed. *Miller's Anesthesia*. 6th ed. Philadelphia: Churchill Livingstone; 2005.

Soliz JM, Sinha AC, Thakar DR. Airway management: a review and update. *Internet J Anesth*. 2002; 6(1).

Walls RM. The decision to intubate. In: Thierbach AR, Lipp MDW, eds. Airway Management in Trauma Patients. *Anesth Clin*. 1999; 17:63–81.

Walls RM, ed-in-chief; Murphy MF, Luten RC, Schneider RE, eds. *Manual of Emergency Airway Management*. 2nd ed. Philadelphia: Lippincott Williams & Wilkins; 2004:1–7.

Wharton NM, Gibbison B, Gabbott DA, et al. I-gel insertion by novices in manikins and patients. *Anaesthesia*. 2008; 63:991–995.

Wilson WC. Trauma: airway management, ASA difficult airway algorithm modified for trauma—and five common trauma intubation scenarios. *ASA Newsletter*. 2005; 69(11). Available at: www.asahq.org/Newsletters/2005/11-05/wilson11_05.html. Accessed September 15, 2008.

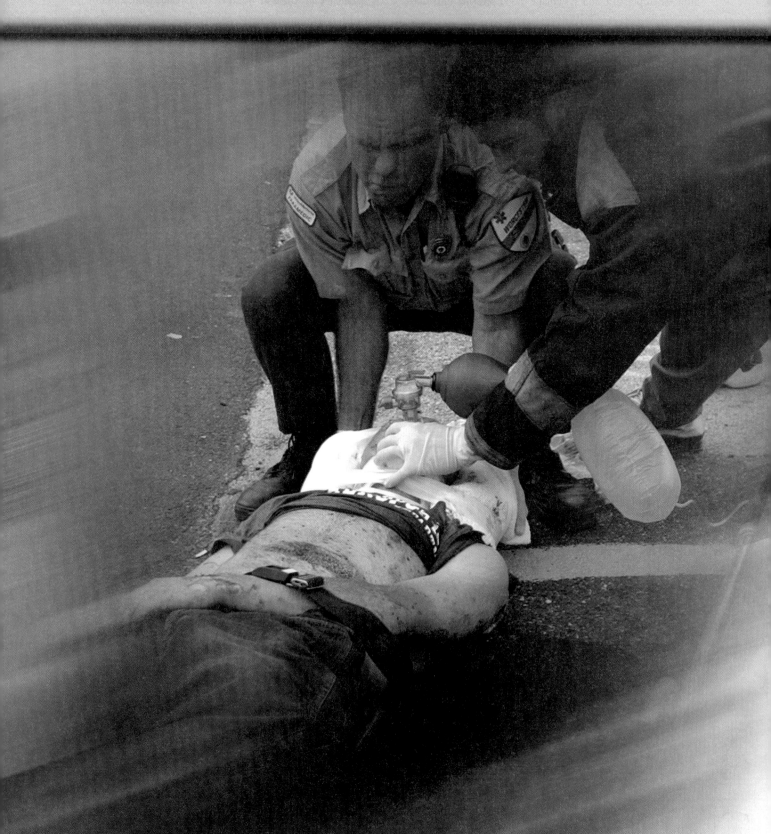

You are dispatched to a pedestrian struck by a truck on a side street. Dispatch advises you that the patient has reportedly lost a lot of blood and police are asking you to expedite your response. Upon your arrival you find a male patient who is unconscious but breathing rapidly. He has a large open wound to his back and left shoulder. Bleeding is slow but a large pool of blood has collected in his shirt. He does not answer or move with your verbal commands.

A quick count of his respirations reveals 48 breaths/min and very shallow. He has a very weak radial pulse at 148 beats/min and feels cool and clammy. He has no jugular venous distension (JVD) or tracheal deviation and equal chest excursion with breaths. You begin ventilating the patient with a bag mask connected to oxygen. Although he fights you at first, you are able to deliver good full breaths that have clear lung sounds when reviewed. The wound on his back is an avulsion that appears to have come from the undercarriage of the truck, because bystanders report the truck ran over him. Inside his shirt you find a large amount of clotted blood but the bleeding from the wound appears to have slowed to a trickle. His left shoulder appears dislocated.

After spinal immobilization and continued ventilations you begin rapid transport to the hospital. Your reassessment shows a patient with no radial pulses but a carotid pulse is present at a rate of 160 beats/min that matches the ECG showing sinus tachycardia. Blood pressure is unobtainable. During transport the patient is intubated and two large IVs are established. A reassessment 5 minutes from the hospital finds the patient with no palpable pulses, and CPR is initiated.

1 Does this patient have symptoms suggesting he is in shock?

2 How does the body try to compensate for shock?

3 What is the etiology for the shock this patient is experiencing?

4 What are the priorities for treatment of this patient?

Introduction

Shock is a condition that results from inadequate flow of oxygen and nutrients to the cells of the body. It is sometimes referred to as **hypoperfusion**. **Perfusion** involves moving oxygen and nutrients from outside the body to the tissues and removing the waste products from the tissues. Aerobic metabolism requires a constant supply of oxygen and nutrients, as well as removal of the simple byproducts of metabolism. Impaired perfusion causes cells to use anaerobic metabolism due to the shortage of oxygen in the tissues. Anaerobic metabolism causes carbon dioxide to build up in the muscles, which creates lactic acid. Lack of oxygen and the increasingly toxic byproducts of anaerobic metabolism will lead to cellular death, then tissue and organ death. Although not usually acknowledged as such, shock is often the final event preceding death. (It is frequently shock that kills the patient rather than the injury itself.) Because tissue perfusion is primarily a function of the cardiovascular system, an examination of that system is key to understanding shock.

Basic Cardiovascular Physiology

The **cardiovascular system** consists of the heart, blood vessels, and circulating blood **FIGURE 4-1**. The heart operates as the pump in the system. It regulates the flow of blood by adjusting the flow rate and volume of fluid it circulates. The muscle layer in the walls of blood vessels also help control the flow of blood through dilation and constriction, which helps direct blood to different areas of the body in times of need (vital body organs). The final factor involved in perfusion is the volume of blood available for circulation. A reduction in the body's total blood volume will reduce perfusion and force the heart and blood vessels to compensate for the loss.

The heart's contractility allows it to increase or decrease the volume of blood it pumps with each contraction, also known as **stroke volume**. The heart can also vary the speed at which it contracts by raising or lowering the heart rate. **Cardiac output** is a measurement of the amount of blood the heart moves over time. Under normal conditions, the heart adjusts well to the needs of the body. If the body is physically active, the heart rate and stroke volume increase to provide the necessary blood flow to support the activity. In times of less activity, the heart rate and stroke volume can be reduced. This eases the workload of the heart.

The arteries and veins in the body contain musculature that allows them to dilate or constrict as needed for proper circulation. Veins are generally somewhat dilated and therefore provide a type of reservoir for the blood. Constriction of the veins decreases the volume of blood contained in this potential reservoir, thus increasing blood return, or **preload**, to the heart (venous return). This contributes to an increase in cardiac stroke volume. Arteries constrict and dilate as well, although to a lesser degree than veins. Constriction of arteries, however, will increase the workload of the heart, even as it helps increase the blood return.

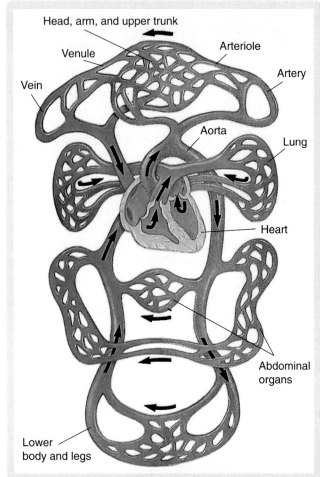

FIGURE 4-1 The circulatory system requires continuous operation of its three components: the heart, the blood and other body fluids, and the blood vessels.

The body contains a relatively fixed volume of blood, which is usually adequate to supply the needs of the tissues without being excessive. The distribution of blood is controlled to a certain extent by the local needs. As oxygen is depleted and waste products accumulate in tissues, the blood vessels supplying that area will be stimulated to dilate, allowing more blood to flow there. Under normal conditions, when one area is active and requires more blood flow, another area is resting and tolerates a decreased flow. This balance is critical to the normal functioning of the body. In situations where the volume of blood available seems to be inadequate, interstitial fluid can be shifted into the blood vessels, increasing the volume to a limited extent. This increase comes at the expense of a dilution of the blood, reducing the number of red blood cells per volume of fluid. Under these conditions, various organs such as the liver and the spleen, which contain stored red blood cells, are stimulated to move the red blood cells back into circulation to restore the **hematocrit** (volume of red blood cells per given volume of blood). During a crisis, the hematocrit level can assist providers in making a more accurate diagnosis of the affecting condition.

Control of the cardiovascular system is a function of the **autonomic nervous system**, which is composed of two competing subsystems **TABLE 4-1**. One of the subsystems, the **sympathetic nervous system**, which is sometimes known as the "fight or flight" system, prepares the body for physical activity during a stressful situation for the body. This preparation includes increasing the heart rate, blood pressure, and respiratory rate while dilating blood vessels in areas required for physical activity and constricting those in areas primarily involved with reproduction and restoration.

The autonomic nervous system is primarily housed in the upper part of the medulla oblongata of the brain. Nerve signals caused by stimulation of the sympathetic nervous system travel between the brain and the body by way of nerves traveling through the spinal cord. These nerves leave the spinal cord between each pair of vertebrae and spread out to affect the tissues in those areas **FIGURE 4-2**. Another mechanism used by the sympathetic nervous system is the chemical release of epinephrine and norepinephrine from the adrenal glands into the bloodstream. These chemicals travel through the bloodstream to all parts of the body to activate a sympathetic response in those areas.

The other subsystem of the autonomic nervous system is the **parasympathetic nervous system**, which is primarily responsible for rest and regeneration. The parasympathetic system opposes every action of the sympathetic system. Where the sympathetic system increases heart rate, blood pressure, and respiratory rate, the parasympathetic system decreases these. The parasympathetic system also constricts

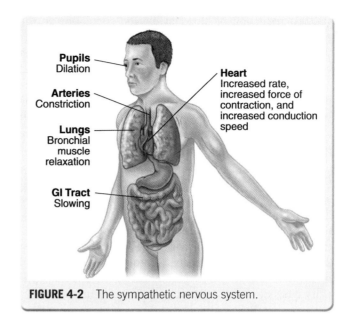

FIGURE 4-2   The sympathetic nervous system.

blood vessels in muscular tissue and dilates those in the digestive system.

Impulses from the parasympathetic nervous system communicate with the body via the 10th cranial nerve, known as the **vagus nerve** **FIGURE 4-3**. The vagus nerves (one on each side of the body) leave the brain through small openings in the base of the skull and travel throughout the body, affecting most of its major systems including the cardiovascular system. The chief chemical involved in the parasympathetic nervous system response is acetylcholine. When acetylcholine is released from the vagus nerves, its effects counteract any sympathetic stimulation that might be occurring in the affected tissues. This can result in effects such as dilating blood vessels that had been constricted. The result of this action is that the vascular system is constantly balancing somewhere between the two extremes of constriction and dilation.

Because the autonomic nervous system is controlled from the medulla of the brain, any change in perfusion of brain tissue will lead to an immediate response. The

TABLE 4-1 Comparison of Sympathetic and Parasympathetic Nervous Systems		
Features	Parasympathetic	Sympathetic
Other name for system	Cholinergic; "rest and digest"	Adrenergic; "fight or flight"
Natural chemical mediator	Acetylcholine	Norepinephrine, epinephrine
Primary nerve(s)	Vagus	Nerves from the thoracic and lumbar ganglia of the spinal cord
Effect of stimulation	Decreases contractility (negative inotropic effect)	Increases contractility (positive inotropic effect)
	Slows conduction velocity (negative dromotropic effect)	Speeds conduction velocity (positive dromotropic effect)
	Slows the heart* (negative chronotropic effect)	Speeds the heart (positive chronotropic effect)
	Constricts pupils	Dilates pupils
	Increases salivation	Slows the gut
	Increases gut motility	Dilates the bronchi

*Slowing occurs mostly in the atria.

smallest reduction of blood or oxygen circulation to the brain results in stimulation of the sympathetic nervous system geared toward restoring normal circulation. The sympathetic nervous system increases the heart rate and constricts blood vessels to restore proper perfusion to the brain quickly. Once this occurs, the excess sympathetic stimulation is reduced by parasympathetic stimulation. If the brain perfusion is not quickly restored, however, the sympathetic stimulation will increase.

Blood Loss Pathophysiology

Blood is lost from the circulatory system when tissue is damaged and blood vessels are broken. Most types of traumatic injuries will result in damage to blood vessels, leading to loss of blood or hemorrhage. The volume of blood lost from traumatic injuries depends on the type of blood vessel injured and also on the extent of the injuries. The three primary types of blood vessels are capillaries, veins, and arter-

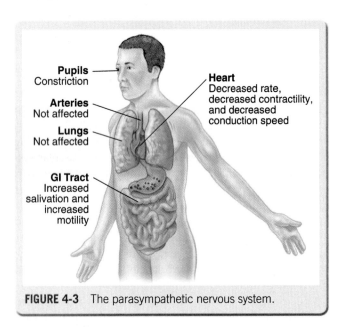

FIGURE 4-3 The parasympathetic nervous system.

ies. Bleeding from each of these has a unique presentation and is treated somewhat differently **FIGURE 4-4**.

Capillary Bleeding

Capillary bleeding is the most common type of hemorrhage resulting from trauma and is also the easiest to control. Because capillaries are only a single cell thick, any trauma applied to them will easily cause them to rupture, releasing the blood within them. Capillaries are so numerous within the body that it is almost impossible to experience a traumatic injury without causing some capillary bleeding. The volume of blood released from a damaged capillary is miniscule due to its size; however, if a large enough number of capillaries are damaged, the bleeding can be of concern. Capillary bleeding is usually easily controlled, allowing the blood clotting process to stop the hemorrhage.

Venous Bleeding

Bleeding from a damaged vein is more serious than capillary bleeding because veins are much larger and contain a significantly greater volume of blood. Veins often act as blood reservoirs, containing over 60% of the total blood volume. As a result, when they are damaged a much greater blood volume loss will be experienced. Venous bleeding is characterized by a steady flow of blood from the site. Bleeding from a vein typically presents with a dark red blood due to the relatively low quantity of oxygen in venous blood.

Arterial Bleeding

Bleeding from an artery is the most serious but fortunately the least common type of hemorrhage. Arteries contain blood under very high pressure. The blood originates at the heart, and as it leaves the heart and continues through the arteries, the arteries expand and then contract, pushing a surge of blood through the artery with almost the same pressure it had when leaving the heart. Because of the blood surges through the arteries, arterial bleeding is characterized by "spurting" blood, which presents with a bright red color due to the high oxygen content of that blood.

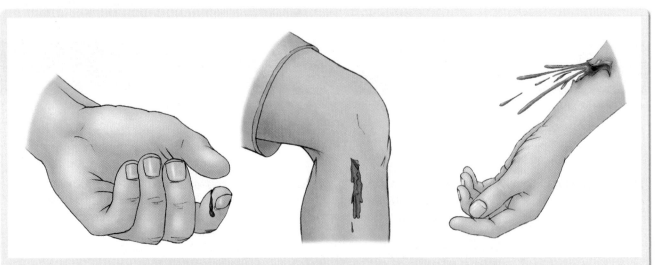

FIGURE 4-4 **A.** Capillary bleeding is dark red and oozes from the wound slowly and steadily. **B.** Venous bleeding is darker than arterial bleeding and flows steadily. **C.** Arterial bleeding is characteristically brighter red and spurts in time with the pulse.

Arterial bleeding is often difficult to control with direct pressure and may require up to 5 minutes of firm direct pressure to be successful. In addition to applying direct pressure, it is helpful to elevate the injured extremity. The combination of direct pressure and elevation, however, may not be sufficient to control powerful arterial bleeding. If these two actions are not adequate to control the bleeding, pressure must be applied to an **arterial pressure point**, often referred to as indirect pressure. Arterial pressure points are locations on extremities where large arteries from the trunk of the body pass near bones as they enter the extremity. By pressing the artery against the bone in this area, the flow of blood through the artery, and therefore the distal pressure within the artery, is reduced. This reduction is usually enough to allow direct pressure in conjunction with elevation to control the bleeding effectively. If a tourniquet was not applied due to catastrophic hemorrhage at the onset of care, then it remains an option. Remember that blood at the point of bleeding starts to clot as soon as direct pressure stops the flow.

Control of Bleeding

Blood clotting, or **coagulation**, is the method by which the body stops bleeding to prevent excessive loss of blood. Coagulation in larger blood vessels begins with a spasm of the vessel wall, which reduces the size of the opening through which the blood is leaking. At the same time, the damage to the endothelium of the blood vessel triggers blood platelets to become adhesive and attach to the injured vessel wall. As these platelets stick together, they form a net across the opening in the vessel, further trapping blood components FIGURE 4-5 . Proteins in the blood plasma respond to form a fibrin mesh to further reinforce the platelet plug. As more blood components are trapped, the clot becomes more solid, allowing only the plasma to leak out. Eventually even the plasma is stopped from leaking as the clot completely closes the leaking blood vessel.

Direct pressure assists in the process of coagulation by slowing the flow of blood out of the vessels and giving the clot time to form. In most cases of external bleeding, if direct pressure is applied quickly to the area of hemorrhage (or to the blood vessel supplying the bleed—indirect pressure), the volume of blood escaping will be greatly reduced.

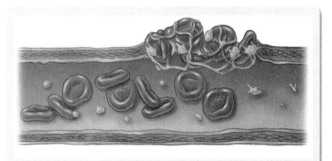

FIGURE 4-5 The forming blood clot continues trapping blood components until the bleeding, and eventually the plasma secretions, have stopped.

To be effective, direct pressure must be at least equal to the pressure of the blood attempting to escape. If this is the case, within just a few minutes the platelet net will be sufficient to hold in the leaking blood and the pressure can be released. If bleeding continues, continue pressure and consider more aggressive treatment.

Because blood loss is a major cause of hypovolemic shock, control of bleeding is one of the most important treatments for a patient in shock (or about to go into shock) due to hemorrhage. The longer bleeding is allowed to continue, the more blood volume will be lost, further reducing perfusion and increasing the likelihood of patient death. If hemorrhage is the cause of shock in a patient, early control of bleeding will give the body an opportunity to reverse the shock through normal compensatory responses. Failure to control the bleeding allows the shock to worsen.

Control of any obvious bleeding should always begin with direct pressure, which forces the blood escaping from the damaged vessel to stop at the opening. Holding pressure for a few minutes is usually enough to control bleeding from most small veins. If the bleeding is from an extremity, the extremity can also be elevated above the level of the heart to decrease the pressure in the blood vessels. The pressure of blood flowing in an elevated extremity is reduced as it moves further from the heart and against gravity. The reduced force of blood attempting to leak from the injury site makes the bleeding easier to control with direct pressure.

Recognition of Shock

Shock is impossible to identify directly because it occurs at the cellular level. Clinical presentation of shock can vary according to the type of shock and the individual patient. In fact, most of the signs and symptoms commonly associated with shock are actually caused by the body's sympathetic response to a decrease in perfusion. The brain, which is extremely sensitive to blood flow, will quickly recognize any situation that reduces its oxygenation. Because of this, one of the earliest signs of shock can be an altered mental status. This early change in mental status is often so minor that it can easily go unnoticed. It may present merely as anxiety, which would be expected in a situation involving a traumatic injury, but it can also present as aggression. The reduced brain perfusion leads to an immediate response from the sympathetic nervous system TABLE 4-2 . If the initial sympathetic response fails to restore adequate brain perfusion, the mental status will continue to deteriorate while the sympathetic stimulation will be increased.

The early sympathetic response to shock includes a release of the **catecholamines** epinephrine and norepinephrine from the adrenal glands. These chemicals stimulate an immediate increase in the heart rate and contractile force. Pulses become quickened and initially slightly stronger from the force of contractions. Blood pressure will remain normal or become slightly increased with the increase of cardiac output. Often this response alone is enough to restore

TABLE 4-2	Responses to Sympathetic Stimulation
Organ	**Sympathetic Stimulation**
Heart	Increased heart rate (positive chronotropic effect) (beta 1)
	Increased force of contraction (positive inotropic effect) (beta 1)
	Increased conduction velocity (positive dromotropic effect) (beta 1)
Arteries	Constriction (alpha)
Lungs	Bronchial muscle relaxation (beta 2)
Liver	Conversion of glycogen to glucose for increased metabolic use
Kidneys	Reabsorption of sodium to retain fluids

TABLE 4-3	Compensated Versus Decompensated Shock
Compensated Shock	**Decompensated Shock**
• Agitation, anxiety, restlessness	• Altered mental status (verbal to unresponsive)
• Sense of impending doom	• Hypotension
• Weak, rapid (thready) pulse	• Labored or irregular breathing
• Clammy (cool, moist) skin	• Thready or absent peripheral pulses
• Pallor with cyanotic lips	• Ashen, mottled, or cyanotic skin
• Shortness of breath	• Dilated pupils
• Nausea, vomiting	• Diminished urinary output (oliguria)
• Delayed capillary refill in infants and children	• Impending cardiac arrest
• Thirst	
• Normal blood pressure	

proper perfusion of the brain, but if not the brain will stimulate the release of more epinephrine and norepinephrine and the signs and symptoms will continue to progress.

The actions of the catecholamines cause a reduction in circulation to the skin and nearby tissues, causing peripheral vasoconstriction. Because blood flow just below the surface causes the normal pink color of the skin, when the peripheral blood flow is reduced the skin becomes pale in appearance. With less blood near the surface of the body releasing its heat, the skin cools. Another effect of the epinephrine and norepinephrine is stimulation of the sweat glands in the skin to produce perspiration. These effects combine to cause the cool, pale, and diaphoretic skin commonly associated with shock patients.

As the sympathetic response increases blood flow, it also needs to increase respirations. Faster respirations attempt to supply the body with more oxygen for the increased demand. The smooth muscle of the airway dilates, allowing air to pass with less resistance. The increased respiratory effort requires an increase in effort from the diaphragm and intercostal muscles. This muscular activity then requires increased metabolism, which is not available due to the shock. Without an increase in blood circulation to support them, the effort of the respiratory muscles becomes weaker. This causes the respirations to become shallow. Rapid and shallow respirations are also commonly associated with shock patients.

The release of epinephrine and norepinephrine stimulates the liver to release stored glucose, causing an increase in blood glucose levels. This glucose is needed to support the metabolic activities of the body (especially the brain) as it responds to the cause of the shock. If the sympathetic system stimulation continues for an extended time, the stores of glucose will be used up and the patient may start to experience hypoglycemia.

When the adrenal glands are stimulated to produce epinephrine and norepinephrine they also secrete aldosterone (an antidiuretic hormone). The aldosterone forces the kidneys to reabsorb sodium and excrete potassium. Water follows the sodium and the fluid level increases in the bloodstream.

The actions of the sympathetic nervous system are intended to contribute to maintaining a normal blood pressure. When these actions are no longer able to maintain an adequate blood pressure, a noticeable drop will occur. Because the sympathetic response is oriented toward compensating for blood pressure, a drop in blood pressure indicates that the body is now decompensating TABLE 4-3 .

Etiology of Shock

Shock has many causes, all of which reduce perfusion. When a patient has suffered a traumatic injury, the most common cause of shock is blood loss. This is known as **hemorrhagic shock**, which is classified as a type of **hypovolemic shock**. All types of hypovolemic shock reduce the total fluid in the body. In hemorrhagic shock this is a direct result of blood loss, whereas in other types of hypovolemic shock (eg, severe burns, heat stroke, or gastroenteritis) the lost fluid is replaced (at least in part) by a shift of fluid from the blood vessels into the tissues. The resulting loss in blood volume then affects the body in the same way as hemorrhage.

There are other types of shock caused by changes to other components of the cardiovascular system. These include **cardiogenic shock**, which results from a weakening pumping action of the heart; and **distributive shock**, which includes **neurogenic shock** (resulting from blood vessel dilation caused by a brain or spinal/nerve injury) and **septic shock** (resulting from fluid shifts associated with massive infections and poisons). There are also other conditions that decrease tissue perfusion, indirectly affecting the cardiovascular system. Among these are conditions that obstruct the flow of oxygen into the bloodstream and into the starving tissue, leading to **obstructive shock**. Conditions that produce an obstructive shock include tension pneumothorax, cardiac tamponade, pulmonary embolism, airway obstruction, and carbon monoxide poisoning. Because each type of shock is unique, each should be examined separately.

Hemorrhagic Shock

Hemorrhagic shock occurs as a direct result of blood loss. Because bleeding is a common event, occurring in all people at various times, a significant volume of blood loss is required for a patient to be considered in hemorrhagic shock. Hemorrhage is often classified by the volume of blood lost, with the lowest category (class I) representing a loss of less than 15% of blood volume and the highest category (class IV) representing a loss of over 40% of blood volume.

Because blood volume loss is almost impossible to measure in the field, treatment must be based on signs and symptoms observed **TABLE 4-4**. If the bleeding is stopped and fluids are added to offset those lost, the body can recover from many cases of hemorrhagic shock. If bleeding cannot be controlled, rapid transport to a trauma facility is of even more importance. Keeping in mind that shock is an evolving condition that continues to worsen without proper treatment, treatment and rapid transport of these patients is critical.

Class I: Blood Volume Loss Less than 15%

A class I hemorrhage is defined as a loss of less than 15% of blood volume in the average adult. Most adults can lose this amount of blood without producing any significant signs or symptoms of shock. A nontraumatic example of this might be a person who donates blood for a local blood drive. Most blood donations consist of approximately 500 mL of blood removed within a 10- to 20-minute time period. After a blood donation, a donor may feel a little lightheaded and is advised to drink plenty of fluids. Within 24 hours, the body has adjusted to the loss of blood volume without any noticeable effects on the donor.

In a class I hemorrhage, the sympathetic nervous system does react, though only to an extent so minor that it is often not obvious to the victim or a casual observer. The primary sympathetic response results in a constriction of the venous system, a slight constriction of the peripheral blood vessels, and a small shift of fluid from the interstitial space

into the circulatory system. If the bleeding is stopped at this level, the body will recuperate completely without recognizable effects. If the bleeding is not controlled at this level, the signs and symptoms of shock will become more obvious.

Class II: Blood Volume Loss 15%–30%

A class II hemorrhage is blood loss between 15% and 30%. At this volume of blood loss, the sympathetic nervous system response is stronger. The heart rate increases noticeably and weakens slightly due to a reduction of stroke volume. The respiratory rate also increases but is slightly shallower due to reduced perfusion of the respiratory musculature. At this level of blood loss, the skin becomes pale, cool, and moist. The level of consciousness of this patient is usually noticeably altered, with nervousness and anxiety the most common symptoms. As fluid continues to shift into the cardiovascular system from the interstitial spaces, the victim begins to experience a slight sensation of thirst. Associated with this, the urinary output begins to reduce slightly.

Response to a class II hemorrhage is critical. Priority should be given to controlling external bleeding and replacing some of the lost fluid volume. It is beneficial to support respiratory effort by providing supplemental oxygen. If possible, place the patient supine and elevate the lower extremities. Cover the patient to prevent heat loss. Failure to respond properly, especially to control bleeding, will eventually lead to a greater deterioration of the patient's condition.

Class III: Blood Volume Loss 30%–40%

Class III hemorrhage (blood loss of 30%–40%) is generally considered the highest class hemorrhage from which a victim can possibly be expected to recover. The sympathetic nervous system response reaches the maximum possible level in a class III hemorrhage. The heart rate is extremely high, with a corresponding reduction of stroke volume resulting in barely palpable pulses. The respiratory volume is significantly diminished, though the rate is rapid. The skin appears extremely pale and diaphoretic and is very cool to the touch. The mental status of the victim at this point is usually anywhere from significant confusion to complete unconsciousness. If conscious, the victim can complain of extreme thirst with the shift of interstitial fluid into the vasculature at the maximum level. Urinary output at this level is reduced to near zero, and as these

TABLE 4-4	Estimated Fluid and Blood Loss and Initial Patient Presentation for an Adult			
	Class I	Class II	Class III	Class IV
Percentage of blood volume lost	Up to 15%	15%–30%	30%–40%	Over 40%
Approximate blood loss (in mL)	Up to 750	750–1,500	1,500–2,000	Over 2,000
Pulse (beats/min)	Less than 100	Over 100	Over 120	Over 140
Blood pressure	Normal	Normal	Decreased	Decreased
Respiratory rate (breaths/min)	Normal	20–30	30–40	Over 36
Mental status	Slightly anxious	More anxious	Anxious/confused	Confused/lethargic

compensatory mechanisms fail, the blood pressure will begin to fall.

The patient who has experienced a class III hemorrhage requires aggressive treatment. All treatment mentioned for class I and class II hemorrhagic shock should be continued, but the most significant treatment for this patient is rapid transportation to a major trauma center. Most patients who have lost this volume of blood will require major surgery to reverse their condition. Generally, many units of blood will have to be transfused to give the patient an opportunity to recover. Failure to respond appropriately will usually result in patient deterioration to the point of death.

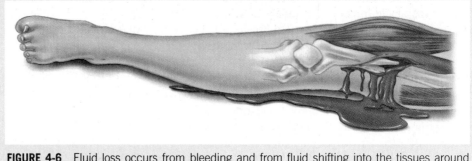

FIGURE 4-6 Fluid loss occurs from bleeding and from fluid shifting into the tissues around the vessels.

Class IV: Blood Volume Loss Greater than 40%

Class IV hemorrhage, or a blood loss of more than 2,000 mL, is usually fatal. A loss of 2,000 mL of blood represents approximately 40% of the total blood volume. At this point, the victim will likely have palpable pulses only at the carotid arteries. Respirations will be rapid but so shallow as to appear almost absent. Respiratory arrest is often followed by cardiac arrest. The patient is usually unresponsive by this time and urinary output is absent. The blood pressure is often too low to measure and death may be inevitable regardless of resuscitation attempts.

Fluid Loss Due to Soft-Tissue Injury

All types of soft-tissue injuries result in fluid loss, the most common being through hemorrhage. Open injuries such as lacerations, abrasions, avulsions, or amputations result in external bleeding. Control of this external bleeding will significantly improve the patient's chance of survival and recovery. Other injuries, such as contusions and fractures, can result in a shift of interstitial fluids around the site of injury (swelling). Long bone fractures have the ability to cause a loss of 500 mL to 1,000 mL, or more of fluid into the tissue surrounding the injury. Multiple long bone fractures can produce enough fluid loss to place the patient into shock.

Burns are another type of soft-tissue injury that can result in loss of fluid without bleeding. As tissue is burned, the adjacent tissues begin to leak interstitial fluid and plasma into the burned area in an effort to cool the area and to begin the healing process. If the burn is serious enough to destroy the upper layers of the skin, the fluid moving into the burned area will evaporate, cooling the skin but also contributing to hypovolemia, which can progress to shock.

Fluid loss, whether from bleeding or fluid shift into the extravascular space, reduces the total blood volume available to perfuse tissues **FIGURE 4-6**. Treatment in these cases consists of two steps. The first action should be to stop any additional fluid loss. The second should be to begin fluid replacement. Although these are considered distinct steps, they should be performed simultaneously for best effect.

Shock associated with fluid loss contributes to impaired perfusion in much the same way as hemorrhage does. Other types of shock not involving a direct loss of fluid can affect perfusion just as powerfully.

Nonhemorrhagic Shock

The nonhemorrhagic causes of shock are commonly grouped by how they reduce perfusion. These types of shock involve either a weakening of the pump, an increase in the size of the container, or a direct mechanical interference with the circulation **TABLE 4-5**. Cardiogenic shock is caused by weakening of the heart. Neurogenic shock is caused by an injury to the head or spinal cord and causes massive vasodilation. Septic shock can be caused by widespread infections, which also result in vasodilation.

Obstructive causes of shock, such as tension pneumothorax and cardiac tamponade, cause compression of the heart and obstruct its normal functioning, whereas pulmonary emboli and carbon monoxide poisoning block the oxygen flow into the circulation. Although fluid infusion is the accepted treatment for hemorrhagic shock, it may be of limited value in nonhemorrhagic shock. In these other types of shock it is important to determine the underlying cause of shock to foster the best outcome.

Cardiogenic Shock

Cardiogenic shock can be caused by damage to the heart muscle itself, dysrhythmias, or structural injury such as a valvular prolapse or ruptured septum. The primary cause of cardiogenic shock is injury to the left ventricle. A myocardial infarction or a cardiac contusion after traumatic injury causes death of cardiac cells. This cellular death weakens the heart muscle and reduces the normal cardiac output.

Cardiac output is a product of the heart rate and stroke volume. Injury to the muscle of the heart or drastic changes in rate will affect the ability of the heart to keep up with demand. When an initial drop in blood pressure is sensed, the brain responds by ordering the sympathetic nervous sys-

TABLE 4-5 Comparison of Types of Shock

Origin	Etiology	Blood Pressure	Pulse	Skin
↓ Pump performance	Cardiogenic	↓	↓→↑	Pale, cool, moist
↓ Fluid volume	Hypovolemic, hemorrhagic	↓	↑	Pale, cool, moist
Vessels or container dilates: maldistribution of blood; low peripheral resistance	Neurogenic	↓	↓	Flushed, dry warm
	Septic	↓	↑	Flushed or pale, hot or cool, moist
Blocked flow of oxygenated blood to the tissues	Tension pneumothorax	↓	↑	Pale, cool, moist
	Cardiac tamponade	↓	↑	Pale, cool, moist
	Pulmonary embolism	↓	↑	Normal skin
	Carbon monoxide poisoning	→	↑	Normal skin

tem to increase the heart rate and the force of contractions. Because of the damage to the heart, the force of contractions may not increase by much or a dysrhythmia may not respond to the chemical stimulation for an increase in heart rate. The vasoconstriction produced by the catecholamine release also increases **afterload** (the pressure against which the heart must pump) on the weakened heart. The weakened heart's inability to pump against this increased afterload can result in a backup of blood from the left ventricle into the pulmonary circulation. This backup eventually leads to a fluid shift from the bloodstream into the alveoli, causing pulmonary edema.

$$\text{Cardiac output} = \text{Heart rate} \times \text{Stroke volume}$$
$$(\text{CO} = \text{HR} \times \text{SV})$$

Infusions of fluid have a diagnostic effect on a patient in cardiogenic shock with hypotension. IV crystalloid fluid boluses will transiently increase the pressure, but the fluid will quickly move out of the vascular space without improving the weakened pump. Fluid infusions in the presence of cardiogenic shock and pulmonary edema may lead to worsened edema. It is therefore necessary to be cautious. Pulmonary edema is a life-threatening condition because it interferes with the transfer of oxygen from the alveoli into the bloodstream. Cardiogenic shock with pulmonary edema affects not only the circulation of the blood, but also its oxygenation. Effective treatment for cardiogenic shock must address the weakened condition of the heart and reduce the pulmonary edema the shock has caused.

Neurogenic Shock

Neurogenic shock is caused by an interruption in the sympathetic nervous system. The spinal cord is the only source of communication between the sympathetic nervous system in the brain and the remainder of the body. When this signal is interrupted, the result is loss of sympathetic control of the heart and control of the blood vessels. The effect on the vessels allows for vasodilation and venous pooling of blood

in the areas below the injury. The heart rate may become slightly slower or stay normal in the face of lower perfusion due to the loss of sympathetic tone. This occurs most often with injuries above T6. (See Chapters 5 and 6.)

The absence of vasoconstriction in the periphery below the level of the injury keeps the skin warm and dry rather than pale, cool, and moist as in other types of shock. Respiratory rates remain normal or low as well, rather than increasing. The low blood pressure is somewhat offset by the patient positioning. A patient with a spinal cord injury is generally unable to stand, and is therefore lying on the ground. Even in the supine position, it is likely that the patient's mental status will be affected by the blood pressure being lower than normal.

The typical presentation of a neurogenic shock victim is that of a spinal cord injury with associated loss of motion and sensation. The patient will usually have an altered mental status, warm and dry skin, normal to slow respirations, and a normal to slow pulse. Finally, the blood pressure will be significantly lower than would be found in the early stages of other types of shock.

Fluid infusions may be of some initial value to increase the vascular volume in an attempt to fill the suddenly enlarged vascular container. As with cardiogenic shock, however, fluid does not address the cause of the condition and is not the long-term treatment of choice for this condition. The best treatment for neurogenic shock is an infusion of sympathomimetic drugs with alpha effects to cause vasoconstriction. Because spinal injuries are often the result of trauma, it is critical to watch for signs of neurogenic shock in spinal injury patients.

TIP

Neurogenic shock is easy to overlook in the field. Any time a patient has a probable spinal injury, as evidenced by absent motion or sensation in the lower (and possibly upper) extremities, anticipate neurogenic shock.

Septic Shock

Septic shock is not seen in an immediate assessment following an acute traumatic event. It is a concern in the days and weeks following a traumatic event. Septic shock occurs when an infection becomes widespread and affects a large area of the body. This can occur when a minor infection grows and spreads through inadequate treatment. It can also occur at a systemic level when an infection spreads into the cardiovascular system and from there throughout the body. The body treats infection with an increase of blood flow to the affected area, allowing more white blood cells to reach the area. The massive influx of white blood cells causes most small infections to be controlled quickly. If an infection affects a very large area, however, the increase of blood flow can lead to shock.

When blood flow is increased to an infected area, the capillaries in that area become much more porous than they would normally be. This effect allows plasma and white blood cells to escape the capillaries and enter the interstitial spaces where the infecting organisms are located. In a small infection, this is a very efficient way to control the infection. In a large or widespread infection, however, this allows excessive leakage of plasma from the vasculature. The movement of large volumes of plasma out of the cardiovascular system can lead to a type of hypovolemic shock similar to hemorrhagic shock.

Septic shock presents similarly to hemorrhagic shock in that the patient will have a weak, thready pulse; shallow, rapid respirations; and altered mental status. One major difference is that septic shock patients usually present with warm or hot skin due to the elevated core body temperature associated with their infection.

Obstructive Causes of Shock

Obstructive causes of shock are those not directly associated with loss of fluid, pump failure, or vessel dilation. Obstructive shock is caused by conditions that obstruct blood flow and lead to reduced perfusion and shock. Two of the most common examples of obstructive shock causes in trauma are tension pneumothorax and cardiac tamponade. Others include a pulmonary embolus, which can block the oxygen from entering the bloodstream through the alveoli, or carbon monoxide poisoning, which can block the oxygen from loading into the red blood cells as they pass through the lungs.

Tension Pneumothorax   A tension pneumothorax is caused by damage to the lung tissue. This damage allows air normally held within the lung to escape into the chest cavity. (See Chapter 6 for more information on pneumothorax.) If a pneumothorax is allowed to continue untreated, a sufficient amount of air will accumulate within the chest cavity and begin applying pressure to the structures in the mediastinum **FIGURE 4-7** . The primary organs in this area are the heart and the great vessels (aorta and vena cava). When the trapped air begins to shift the chest organs toward the uninjured side, a pneumothorax becomes known as a tension pneumothorax, which is a very serious and life-threatening condition. As pressure from one side of the chest cavity

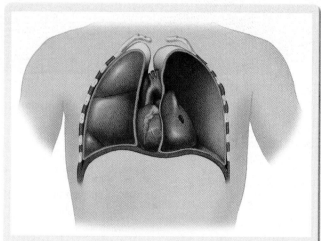

FIGURE 4-7   A tension pneumothorax compresses the mediastinum.

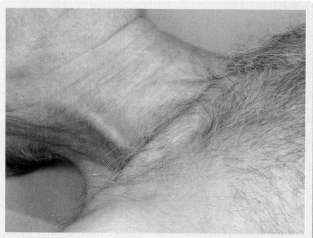

FIGURE 4-8   JVD may be the only visible sign of blood backup in the patient's venous system.

begins to push the mediastinum toward the other side, the vena cava loses its ability to stay fully expanded. This mechanical compression of the vessel leads to reduced preload for the heart. Stroke volume drops, leading to a drop in blood pressure.

A tension pneumothorax will result in a reduced cardiac capacity, causing a backup of blood into the venous system of the body. The only visible sign of this backup is jugular venous distension (JVD) **FIGURE 4-8** . In addition, as the injured lung collapses and the pressure increases toward the uninjured side of the chest, the trachea will begin to shift toward this uninjured side, though this is a late sign. A significant buildup of air from a pneumothorax is required to apply enough pressure to compress the heart and shift the trachea. Once the blood pressure drops, the patient's condition is usually critical.

Usually the only action that can prevent eventual death from a tension pneumothorax is decompression of the injured side of the chest, relieving the pressure in the chest cavity and allowing the heart to expand fully again. Fortunately, needle chest decompression is a skill many providers are allowed to perform **PROCEDURE 13**. The decision to decompress the chest should always be based on good evidence that a tension pneumothorax exists with decreased perfusion.

TIP

Rapid and correct recognition and treatment of a tension pneumothorax in the field can be a matter of life or death. Always assess breath sounds early and often in trauma patients, comparing one side to the other.

Cardiac Tamponade Cardiac tamponade is another traumatic condition that leads to obstructive shock. It is caused by blunt or penetrating trauma and can progress rapidly. Cardiac tamponade occurs when blood leaks into the tough fibrous membrane known as the pericardium, causing an accumulation of blood within the pericardial sac **FIGURE 4-9**.

Blood accumulates quickly within the pericardium. This accumulation of leaked blood leads to compression of the heart. Because the pericardium has minimal ability to stretch, each contraction of the heart allows more blood accumulation between the heart and the sac. This accumulated blood prevents the heart from opening up to allow complete refilling. Continued pressure within the pericardial sac obstructs the flow of blood into the heart, resulting in decreased outflow from the heart. (See Chapter 6 for more information on cardiac tamponade.)

It is important to recognize the possibility of cardiac tamponade early because the only definitive treatment for this condition is surgery; however, **pericardiocentesis**, which involves penetrating the pericardium with a needle and withdrawing the accumulated blood **PROCEDURE 14**, is

the only practical prehospital approach. Pericardiocentesis is rarely performed in the field, so early recognition along with rapid transport is the key treatment available to providers. Vital clues that a cardiac tamponade is present include muffled heart sounds and systolic and diastolic blood pressures starting to merge (ie, the systolic drops and the diastolic rises). This is a very serious and life-threatening condition.

Evaluation of Organ Perfusion

Shock directly affects cells, and by association affects tissues and organs. Direct evaluation of cellular activity is impossible, so the closest assessment that can be performed in the field is evaluation of individual organs or organ systems. In the prehospital environment it is difficult to evaluate perfusion of specific organs with any accuracy. To get an approximation of organ perfusion in the field, the best option is to look at the clinical evidence.

General Assessment
The first organ affected by shock is usually the brain, and the primary measure of brain perfusion is the level of consciousness. An initial slight drop in perfusion of the brain triggers the sympathetic response, which often restores the perfusion to an acceptable level. The initial reduction in brain perfusion, along with the effects of the catecholamines released by the sympathetic system, can lead to restlessness and anxiety in the patient. These early signs can progress to confusion, combativeness, and eventually complete unconsciousness if the perfusion continues to decrease. Because patient assessment starts with a quick evaluation of the level of consciousness, these early signs of inadequate brain perfusion are generally the first signs of shock we notice. As one of the earliest and most accurate indicators of perfusion, the level of consciousness should be monitored constantly on any patient suspected of being in shock.

Another organ whose perfusion can usually be estimated fairly easily is the skin. Skin condition in shock is a result of sympathetic response to inadequate perfusion. In most types of shock, the circulation of blood to the outer layers of the body surface is reduced to perfuse the internal organs better. As the blood vessels near the surface of the skin constrict, the skin becomes pale and cooler. A related sympathetic effect on the skin is the stimulation of the sweat glands, which produce perspiration as the sympathetic response to shock increases. As shock

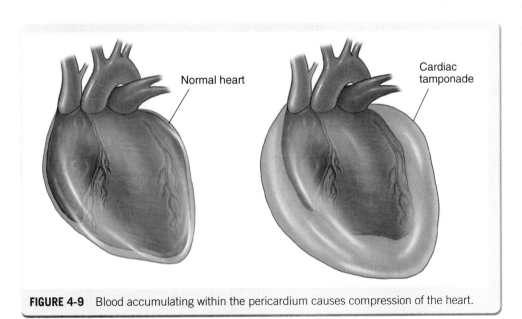

FIGURE 4-9 Blood accumulating within the pericardium causes compression of the heart.

progresses, the skin will become paler, cooler, and more diaphoretic. Like mental status, these signs of shock are easily identified when we first approach the patient and should cause us to recognize quickly the seriousness of the patient's condition. Remember that in some cases, such as neurogenic shock, the skin condition may change little, if at all.

Perfusion of the lungs is impossible to measure in the field, but the effect of reduced perfusion to the musculature required for breathing is more obvious. As circulation is reduced, the blood supply to the muscles supporting respiration becomes progressively less. As these muscles are provided with less and less nutrients and oxygen, they become incapable of strong contraction. In fact, as the demand for contraction of respiratory muscles is increased by the sympathetic nervous system stimulation increasing the respiratory rate, the reduced perfusion of these muscles severely limits their capacity. The resulting rapid but shallow respiratory effort is related to poor perfusion of the respiratory musculature. Rapid, shallow respirations are a classic sign of shock, but unlike altered mental status, they take more time to develop. If a patient has decreased respiratory effort during the primary survey, it is a clear indication that their condition is critical.

Perfusion of the heart itself is not usually affected early in shock, but the response of the heart to reduced systemic perfusion is. The sympathetic stimulation triggered by a reduction in perfusion of the brain will increase the heart rate. As the rate of cardiac contractions increases, the stroke volume can decrease slightly because the ventricular filling time is reduced. The result of these two events is a rapid but weak pulse. As shock progresses, the vascular system continues to constrict. Capillary refill will be greatly extended and distal pulses (radial or pedal) may disappear even though proximal pulses (carotid) remain.

Urinary Output

Urinary output is adversely affected in shock. The kidneys usually require a constant flow of blood secondary only to the heart, lungs, and brain. As overall perfusion is reduced, the blood flow to the heart, lungs, brain, and kidneys is maintained for a while. The sympathetic nervous system response to shock (release of epinephrine and norepinephrine) will cause a reduction of blood flow to the kidneys, but only after a large release of these hormones. As the circulating blood volume is decreased, another hormone, called **angiotensin II**, is released and helps reduce urine production. Vasopressin or **antidiuretic hormone (ADH)** is released from the pituitary gland to stimulate the kidneys to retain water and sodium.

The release of all these hormones creates a condition in which the body conserves as much sodium and water as possible. To conserve this water, the production of urine comes to an almost complete halt. A significant side effect of this protective mechanism is that waste products cannot be eliminated and they build up in the bloodstream, resulting in **acidosis** and other detrimental conditions.

Acid–Base Balance

Reduced perfusion of cells in shock results in greater acid production than normal. As blood flow and oxygen delivery to the tissues is reduced, the cells begin to shift to anaerobic metabolism. Anaerobic metabolism creates large quantities of pyruvic acid, which in the absence of oxygen converts to lactic acid. The reduction of perfusion causes this lactic acid to accumulate in the cell rather than be removed. Another byproduct of decreased perfusion is the accumulation of carbon dioxide in the tissues. The excess carbon dioxide is converted into carbonic acid, which further increases the acidity of the tissues.

The respiratory system attempts to increase respiratory rate and depth in an effort to eliminate CO_2 and thus reduce acidity. In conditions of shock, however, the respirations are already increased and the depth of respirations is limited by reduced perfusion of the respiratory muscles FIGURE 4-10. As a result, the respiratory efforts to balance the excess acidity through elimination of CO_2 are also limited in effectiveness.

The final response to excess acid in the body is for the kidneys to remove hydrogen ions from the bloodstream and eliminate them in the urine. Although this may be somewhat successful early in shock, as we have seen, later in shock the urine production is greatly reduced, eliminating the last option the body has to offset acidosis.

Accumulation of acid, especially lactic acid, and the related accumulation of carbon dioxide in the tissues have numerous negative effects on shock patients. An accumulation of acid in the cells will eventually lead to cellular death. In addition, increased levels of carbon dioxide in the tissues will lead to vasodilation. This vasodilation in the presence of inadequate fluid volume will reduce the blood pressure,

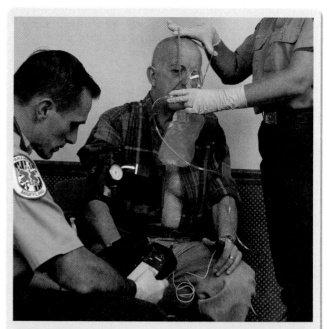

FIGURE 4-10 Effortless tachypnea is a sign of increasing acidosis in the body.

causing further exacerbation of the shock. If this is allowed to continue, the patient will eventually reach a point where death is inevitable.

Special Considerations for Assessing Shock

There are other considerations affecting evaluation and treatment of shock patients. These conditions either increase or decrease the response to shock, often making evaluation more difficult and in some cases making treatment more urgent.

Age

Age is one factor that affects the body's ability to deal with reduced perfusion. As people age, their resting cardiac output becomes lower and their cardiac reserve decreases. It has been suggested that a person's maximum cardiac output may be reduced as much as 50% between the ages of 18 and 80. Maximum heart rate and stroke volume diminish with age, reducing the cardiac reserve. Atherosclerosis in the blood vessels slows the response to vasoconstriction required to compensate for shock.

The main implication of having an elderly patient is the recognition that their natural response to decreased perfusion will be less than optimal. It is important to be aggressive when assessing and treating elderly trauma patients. Elderly patients are also more likely to have complicating medical conditions and medications that may affect their treatment. It is critical that elderly trauma patients receive prompt attention, including treatment and transport.

The very young have the ability to compensate well for blood loss, making the assessment of shock more difficult. Up to approximately age 10, children have an ability to speed up their heart rate and constrict the peripheral vasculature. This allows the maintenance of vital signs in the normal range even in the presence of early shock. Tachycardia and poor skin circulation are often the only signs to alert the provider to shock. Because the heart rate can increase due to fear, pain, or stress, providers must complete a proper assessment to confirm blood loss.

Another confounding factor is that children's normal vital signs are different from those of adults. Children typically have faster normal heart rates and faster respiratory rates (TABLE 4-6). Blood pressure, which is often difficult to obtain in children, will normally be lower in a child than in an adult. The compensation by the heart rate and constriction of the blood vessels will maintain a blood pressure in children with as much as 25% blood loss.

Because of these differences, children who have experienced significant trauma should be treated aggressively. While the common recommendation for treatment of a medical shock in children is to give an IV or IO bolus of 20 mL/kg of body weight of a crystalloid fluid over 10 to 20 minutes, some protocols suggest the use of 5 to 10 mL/kg. This decrease in fluid volume with more frequent assessments decreases the possibility of weakening the clot by placing more pressure against it.

Athletes

In the same way that aging reduces the ability to respond to shock, athleticism increases the ability of patients to handle reduced perfusion. Athletes generally have slower resting heart rates and higher maximum stroke volumes than nonathletes. Exercise strengthens the cardiovascular system of athletes, and also gives them the ability to respond much more effectively to situations that reduce perfusion.

An athlete who experiences a condition that could lead to shock (such as a hemorrhage) will compensate longer than a nonathlete would. This means that if a patient is a well-conditioned athlete, he or she may not present with the classic signs of shock as quickly as might be justified by their condition. This could mislead responders to downplay the seriousness of their condition, possibly leading to disastrous results. Because the compensation hides the signs, an athlete may be much more advanced in shock than he or she appears to be and might not get the appropriate level of care.

Another factor to consider in treating athletes is that when they are injured during competition they may downplay their injuries. The competitive nature of athletes often makes them want to resume competition before getting a thorough evaluation of their condition. It is important to remember that, between the competitiveness and ability of their body to compensate, these patients' conditions may appear less serious than they are.

TABLE 4-6	Normal Adult and Pediatric Vital Signs		
Age	Respiratory Rate (breaths/min)	Pulse Rate (beats/min)	Blood Pressure (mm Hg)
Infants (0–1 year)	25–50	100–160	70–95
Toddlers (1–3)	20–30	90–150	80–100
Preschoolers (3–6)	20–25	80–140	80–100
School-age children (6–12)	15–20	70–120	80–110
Adolescents (13–18)	12–16	60–100	90–110
Adults (19–64)	12–20	60–100	90–140
Elderly adults (≥ 65)	15–20	60–100	100–140

Pregnancy

Pregnancy induces many changes to the female body, including increased total blood volume (mostly plasma with a slight increase in red blood cells by the third trimester) and increased cardiac output. At the end of the first trimester the cardiac output will increase due to the increased plasma volume in the blood. Heart rate increases by 10 to 16 beats per minute over the pregnancy, reaching its maximum by the third trimester. Blood pressure will decrease by 5 to 15 mm Hg (both systolic and diastolic pressures) during the second trimester. This pressure will return to near normal by the third trimester. Blood pressure will also be affected by the increased size and weight of the uterus when a pregnant patient is placed in a supine position. The uterus will press on the inferior vena cava and reduce the blood return to the heart. Supine hypotensive syndrome can be relieved by turning the patient onto the left side **FIGURE 4-11**.

Another consideration in a pregnant woman's response to shock is that her body will respond to protect itself through sympathetic stimulation. Because during shock the sympathetic response normally shunts blood away from the uterus, the blood supply to the fetus is greatly reduced in a pregnant woman experiencing shock. A blood loss of 1,000 to 1,500 mL may result before signs of shock are present. The woman might appear fine, but her fetus could be suffering greatly from reduced perfusion.

Although a pregnant woman will usually be more concerned about her baby than herself, some will have to be convinced to go to the hospital for further evaluation. It is almost impossible to assess the condition of a fetus in the field, so the pregnant patient should be urged to accept transport for further assessment.

Medications

Just as physical conditions can affect a patient's response to shock, a patient's medications can affect their ability to respond as well. Beta-blockers and calcium channel blockers can affect the ability of the body to respond to the sympathetic response to shock. Insulin may be responsible for hypoglycemia, and hypokalemia may be due to diuretic therapy. Aspirin or other nonsteroidal anti-inflammatory drugs (NSAIDs), anti-platelet drugs, or anticoagulants will reduce the ability to clot and make bleeding harder to stop.

Pacemakers

Patients with artificial pacemakers may be unable to increase their heart rate, making it more difficult for them to handle shock conditions. Most people with artificial pacemakers have them because damage to their hearts has limited the ability of the natural pacemakers to control the heart. The artificial pacemaker is usually set to a particular rate, and many of the newer pacemakers sense the natural heart rate and begin pacing only when the natural heart rate drops below the set level. These are known as **demand pacemakers**.

Hypothermia

Hypothermia has profound effects on the primary functions of the body. In general, an increase in body temperature will raise the cardiac output, whereas a decrease will lower it. A cold body develops difficulty forming clots to stop bleeding. The best treatment for hypothermia is prevention. Every effort should be made to keep the shock patient warm.

> **TIP**
>
> Hypothermia can be a deadly complication to patients in shock. When responding to any trauma call in cold weather, you should prepare for handling a hypothermic trauma patient. Gentle treatment is critical, and IV fluids should always be warmed.

▌ Response to Fluid Therapy

Most shock conditions cause either a direct hypovolemia or a relative hypovolemia and often respond to an increase in vascular fluid volume. In the case of hemorrhagic shock, the goal of fluid replacement is to increase the fluid volume to the point where all tissues can be adequately perfused without a significant increase in the blood pressure.

In hypovolemic shock without bleeding, such as is caused by vomiting and diarrhea, larger quantities of crystalloid fluid can be infused without concern for affecting clotting. In cardiogenic shock, the source of the situation is a failure of the heart, so adding fluid may be harmful. Fluid can work initially to increase the preload available to the heart, but it should be used cautiously in the patient with pulmonary edema.

In neurogenic shock, crystalloid fluids will be required as the initial response to hypotension. Neurogenic shock can require sympathomimetics to induce vasoconstriction for proper treatment. Sympathomimetic drugs have no

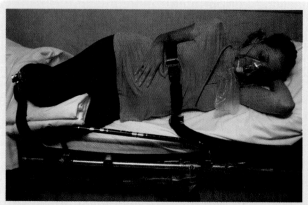

FIGURE 4-11 The pressure of the uterus on the inferior vena cava can result in supine hypotensive syndrome, which can be relieved by turning the patient onto her left side.

benefit in hemorrhagic shock, however, because the sympathetic nervous system response is already in effect.

Rapid Response

The initial response to fluid therapy is an increase in the intravascular volume. The most common fluids used in prehospital treatment are normal saline or lactated Ringer's (or, where applicable, Hartmann's solution). These isotonic crystalloid fluids remain in the vasculature for a short time, increasing the volume in the vessels for increased blood pressure and the ability to move the red blood cells around the body. Crystalloid fluids do not add red blood cells or oxygen-carrying capacity. Because the body in shock has already started moving interstitial fluid into the bloodstream to offset vascular fluid losses, the added isotonic fluids will eventually start to move into the interstitial space to restore this fluid. The final result is that only about one third of infused isotonic crystalloids remain in the bloodstream for more than an hour.

Extended time should not be spent at the scene in the pursuit of IV access. Once en route to the hospital one or two large bore intravenous lines can be established according to local protocols.

In most hypovolemic patients, a rapid infusion of a crystalloid solution will result in an improvement of vital signs by temporarily filling the vascular space and allowing the body's compensatory mechanisms to function. Local protocols will dictate the amount and type of fluid to be infused; however, blood pressures of 80 to 90 mm Hg systolic are often enough to maintain good perfusion to the vital organs. If the total fluid loss is low, such as in an early class II hemorrhage, this may be all that is required to restore the patient to near normal perfusion. Once the vital signs show indications of stabilization, the IV fluid flow should be reduced to minimal flow to avoid increasing the blood pressure and thus inhibiting clotting.

The patient's response to the initial fluid administration should be an improvement of vital signs as well as an improvement in the level of consciousness. Although this early correction is a good indicator, continuous monitoring is necessary because most shock patients have underlying conditions requiring surgical intervention.

Transient Response

Even if a patient has experienced a larger volume loss, such as a large class II or class III hemorrhage, a rapid infusion of crystalloids may have an initial beneficial effect. Because of the total volume lost, however, the volume of crystalloids needed to increase perfusion to an acceptable level will decrease the hematocrit to an inadequate level. Although the initial response is promising, the reduction in the percentage of red blood cells will eventually be detrimental. The best way to avoid this dilution of the blood is to transfuse whole blood. That is impractical in the field, so limiting the volume of fluid used to stabilize the blood pressure is recommended.

Minimal or No Response

When the total volume loss is large, such as in a class IV hemorrhage, the response to fluid infusion will be minimal. As in the transient response, adding fluids to a patient who has lost nearly half their total blood volume is usually ineffective. In these cases, such a large quantity of fluid is required to improve the circulation that the dilution of the hematocrit is extremely serious. Additionally, patients who have lost these quantities of blood typically have traumatic injuries so serious that even major surgical interventions are unlikely to be successful.

PRO/CON

Fluid Therapy

Fluid therapy administered by prehospital providers continues to be controversial in the medical community. Titrate your fluid administration to the patient's condition for best results. Use critical thinking and local protocol to determine the most appropriate IV fluid therapy for your patient.

Blood and Blood Alternatives

Whole blood transfusion is the absolute best treatment for blood loss. The benefit of whole blood transfusion is that along with increasing intravascular volume, red blood cells are also being replaced. This ensures that the increased blood volume has the ability to carry oxygen as well. There is a small drawback to whole blood in that it contains a minimal quantity of anticoagulant, which may result in a slight impairment of the clotting capacity of the patient. Overall, blood transfusions are the best treatment for moderate to large hemorrhages but are not practical in the prehospital setting.

Whole blood transfusions require that the patient's blood type is known and that the matching type of blood is available for transfusion. It is possible to use type O-negative blood if the patient's blood type is unknown, but because that blood type is fairly rare, it would be difficult to keep it available on an ambulance. Another problem with whole blood is that it must be kept refrigerated and then warmed up before transfusion, which also would be difficult in the prehospital setting. Finally, whole blood has a short expiration time: if it is not used within about 2 weeks, it must be discarded.

It is reasonable to expect that in the next few years, technology will allow the development of a reasonable and safe blood alternative for prehospital use. Until that time, however, prehospital treatment of shock patients will continue to rely on the established treatments of bleeding control, oxygen administration, elevation of the extremities, and warming and infusion of isotonic crystalloids.

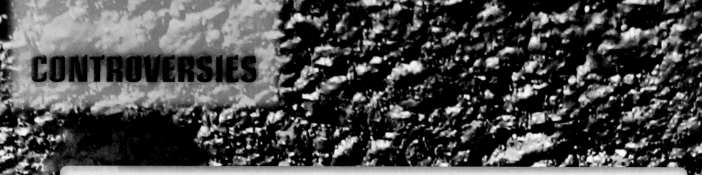

Hemostatic Agents: Evolutionary Adjuncts to Hemorrhage Control

GUNFIRE ERUPTS AS THE EVENING combat patrol passes through the dark city streets. A soldier falls wounded as the bullets tear through flesh not protected by body armor, disrupting soft tissues and blood vessels alike. Blood pools beneath the casualty, and with each successive heartbeat, the hemorrhage continues unabated. If not arrested quickly, this process will lead to certain shock and probable death. This scenario, once common only to a battlefield environment or very large American cities (commonly referred to in the EMS community as the "Knife and Gun Clubs"), is becoming more familiar throughout this country. Even with the best available modern protective equipment, hemorrhage remains the leading cause of death on the modern battlefield.

Statistically, the majority of penetrating wounds are found on the extremities of our soldiers. Although modern body armor worn by all combatants protects the torso relatively well, the exposed areas remain prone to injury. Improved emergency tourniquet devices are currently the preferred method for stopping severe extremity hemorrhage in combat. Military providers are taught to use newly designed compression dressings in conjunction with aggressive wound packing in order to create highly effective pressure bandages in the far-forward setting. However, there are a variety of wound locations (proximal extremities, axilla, groin, torso, and neck) where hemorrhage is difficult to control with direct pressure and tourniquets are not effective. But how do we address wounds that are not amenable to tourniquets when evacuation to surgical capability is not readily available? Even when hemorrhage is controlled, a rigorous casualty movement often defeats the successful intervention during evacuation. This requires a bandage that, when applied to a bleeding wound, actually makes it stop bleeding. This is not some futuristic "Star Wars" device, but rather a sound application of modern technological material development. An effective procoagulant hemostatic agent applied in these situations and injuries will be instrumental in controlling this type of life-threatening bleeding.

Research physicians, physiologists, and bioengineers have developed several new tools and clinical guidelines to address this critical issue. Over the past several years, a number of hemostatic agents, in both bandage and powder form, have been developed that actually make bleeding stop.[1] These products are specifically designed to arrest life-threatening arterial hemorrhage.

These products were developed for military use during combat. Tactical situations often do not lend the time or scene safety required to apply traditional methods of hemorrhage control. What was needed was a relatively quick and effective means to stop red blood cells from leaking out of the injured body.

Initially, there were two products developed and fielded that performed this task better than any previous devices, a bandage and a powder. The bandage is a 4″ × 4″ sponge-like device made from a chitosan-based, freeze-dried paste. This product, when wetted by blood, forms a superglue-like adhesive that actually seals the hole in the damaged blood vessel. The powder is a zeolite material that works by adsorbing the liquid portion of the blood. This concentrates the solid products like clotting factors and blood cells at the site of vessel damage, promoting more rapid clotting. Both of these products worked relatively well in initial clinical evaluations, but as with all modalities were not 100% effective.

The most recent research conducted by both the Army and Navy research centers compared over ten different types of hemostatic agents for controlling arterial hemorrhage in animal models.[2] These two labs found that some work significantly better than others, and some even outperformed the initial products. Several of the newer products are actually procoagulants and promote blood clotting. In addition, the improved efficacy comes with a less expensive price tag.

These agents may seem simple, but they do require a modicum of training in order to maximize their effectiveness. In fact, all hemostatic agents require direct pressure to be exerted on the wound for a period of time, usually 2 to 3 minutes. This can be a long time when you find yourself in a hostile environment, which may delay the use of these agents until the situation becomes more quiescent. Having the ability to stop arterial hemorrhage by applying a bandage or powder to a wound and seeing the bleeding stop in only a few minutes is a wonderful thing. However, none of these agents is intended to be a "stand-alone" product. A successful application must be reinforced with an appropriate pressure dressing to preclude premature dislodgement during casualty movement. This technology is endorsed by the military for use by every combatant on the battlefield.

This measure has been a successful adjunct in saving lives in combat where a paucity of formally trained medics may preclude skilled medical treatment at the time of injury. Each soldier has a first aid kit designed to allow treatment of the preventable causes of death in combat. Since controlling hemorrhage is the priority, having a hemostatic agent with little to no side effects that can be applied to severely bleeding wounds makes sense. If this readily available, effective, and inexpensive agent also requires minimal training resources, the significant benefit to minimal risk ratio makes it a win-win situation.

Does this technology have a place in the civilian community? Although penetrating trauma is seen in both combat and in contemporary civilian environments, it more frequently leads to death from exsanguination on the battlefield. This is not to say that it does not produce significant morbidity within the civilian environment. Every blood product transfusion carries both a risk and a cost. Arresting hemorrhage before the onset of shock also minimizes morbidity. Many EMS services have been using hemostatic agents for some time with excellent results. The newer agents are far superior to the earlier ones and are less costly as well. Why wouldn't we want to place an additional tool in the paramedic's tool kit that requires little training, is cost effective, and has few side effects? While penetrating trauma is less evident in the civilian community than on the battlefield, saving lives remains the paramount factor in providing care in combat or on your local streets.

When a new application for a technological advancement occurs, often the potential benefit is not well understood. Hemostatic agents require an introduction and familiarization at all levels of care, not just among first responders. Emergency personnel will need to become familiar with these products in order to develop appropriate prehospital and hospital intake protocols. Surgeons who must remove these agents from wounds will require an understanding of what has been used and how to mitigate any side effects or problems associated with these agents. An appropriate training package addresses all levels of care providers and allows each to determine how they will interact with this new technology.

Current hemostatic agents are limited by the fact that they are designed for use on external wounds only, and they work very well for this intended purpose. The day will come when we have an injectable hemostatic agent that will travel throughout a casualty's body to the site of the bleeding to arrest local hemorrhage completely. Research currently continues in this field with the use of recombinant factor VIIa. The time is now for prehospital care providers to embrace this technology and incorporate these agents into their tool box for patient care. Casualties with severe life-threatening hemorrhage present a unique problem for the care provider who comes on the scene and must control bleeding while dealing with the multitude of distractions present at the accident site. The safe use of hemostatic agents to control hemorrhage will eventually become as commonplace as applying a bandage to a wound, but will actually be much more effective.

Donald L. Parsons, PA-C, MPAS
Department of Combat Medic Training
Fort Sam Houston, Texas

References

1. Pusateri AE, Holcomb JB, Kheirabadi BS, et al. Making sense of the preclinical literature on advanced hemostatic products. *J Trauma*. 2006;60:674–682.

2. US Army Institute of Surgical Research. Assessment of the efficacy of new hemostatic agents in a lethal model of extremity hemorrhage in swine, study abstract. March 2008.

CHAPTER RESOURCES

CASE STUDY ANSWERS

1 Does the patient have symptoms suggesting he is in shock?

Yes, the patient's symptoms suggest he is in shock. Altered mentation, increased heart rate, rapid shallow respirations, and cool and clammy skin are all signs that suggest shock.

2 How does the body try to compensate for shock?

Through stimulation of hormones and chemicals, the body increases respiration, heart rate, and strength of contraction; causes vasoconstriction of the skin; releases glucose stores from the liver; and retains sodium and water with the kidneys. All of these actions work to maintain adequate metabolism at the cellular level.

3 What is the etiology for the shock this patient is experiencing?

This patient is likely experiencing hemorrhagic shock due to a loss of blood (both external and internal). Other types of shock that should be ruled out include cardiogenic (although his ECG is tachycardic he has no other signs of this), neurogenic (his skin remains cool and moist suggesting that this is not the condition), or obstructive (no JVD suggesting blood backing up from the heart, and lungs are clear and equal suggesting no pneumothorax).

4 What are the priorities for treatment of this patient?

This patient requires spinal immobilization, support of ventilation, and control of external bleeding. Rapid transport to a trauma facility is required. Fluid therapy should be initiated en route to the hospital.

Trauma in Motion

1. Describe the sequence a body goes through to compensate for hemorrhagic shock.
2. Neurogenic shock and septic shock are types of distributive shock. What other types of shock are included in distributive shock?
3. Priapism (a condition in which the patient experiences an uncontrolled erect penis) is caused by what factor of neurogenic shock?
4. Describe how a tension pneumothorax causes shock.
5. If a small blood loss is found in a patient and stopped and the fluid is replaced, will the perfusion be worse due to lost red blood cells, be the same because the volume is replaced, or be improved because the fluid reduces the viscosity of the blood traveling in the system, improving movement of the red blood cells?

References and Resources

American Academy of Orthopaedic Surgeons. *Nancy Caroline's Emergency Care in the Streets.* 6th ed. Sudbury, MA: Jones and Bartlett; 2007.

American Academy of Pediatrics. *Pediatric Education for Prehospital Professionals (PEPP).* 2nd ed. Sudbury, MA: Jones and Bartlett; 2006.

American College of Surgeons Committee on Trauma. *Advanced Trauma Life Support for Doctors, Student Course Manual.* Chicago, IL: American College of Surgeons; 2004.

American Geriatrics Society, National Council of State Emergency Medical Service Training Coordinators. *Geriatric Education for Emergency Medical Services.* Sudbury, MA: Jones and Bartlett; 2003.

Head and Neck Trauma

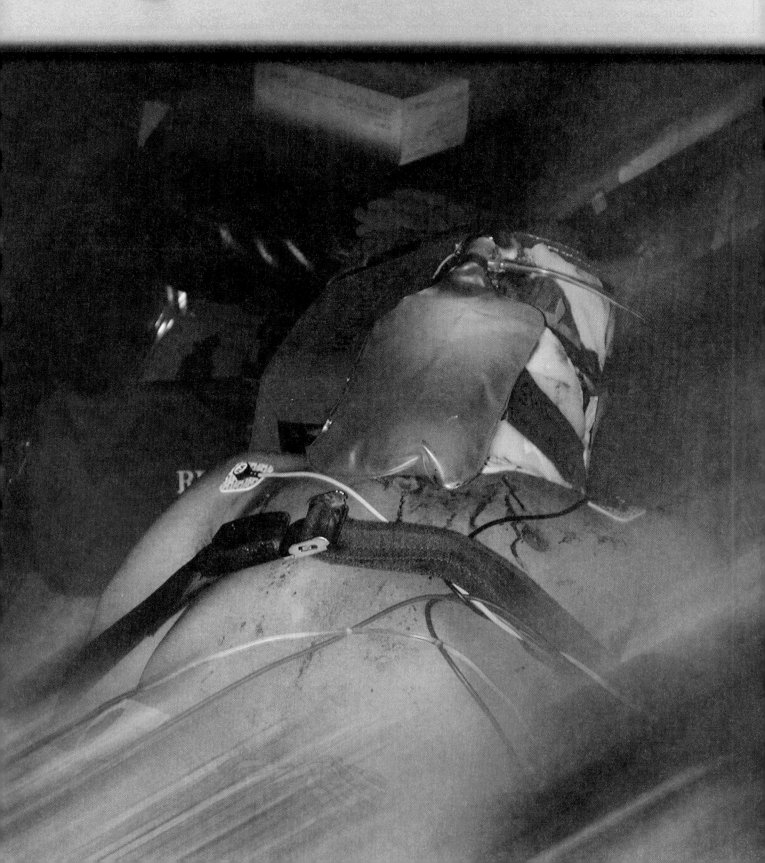

CASE STUDY

You have been dispatched to a fight at a local pub. As you arrive, the police are in the process of locating the patient. An onlooker yells out that the victim stumbled down an alley next to the business. With police assistance, you arrive at the side of a 25-year-old man with multiple wounds around his face and head. A friend of the victim is on the scene and tells you three men hit and kicked the man following an argument.

Your patient is unconscious but moans with any physical stimuli. His airway appears clear, however you notice a broken tooth and a lacerated upper lip. His breathing is deep and regular and you notice the smell of alcohol on his breath (his friend readily admits "he had a lot to drink tonight"). His radial pulse is bounding and although there is blood from several cuts on his head and face, none of the cuts are actively bleeding. His left eye is swollen shut but the pupil in the right eye responds briskly to light.

Your assessment reveals the patient has abrasions on his hands, but his chest and abdomen do not appear to be injured. His vital signs are respirations of 12 breaths/min, pulse of 64 beats/min, blood pressure of 160/92 mm Hg, Sao_2 of 96% on ambient air, and his skin is warm and dry. He does not open his eyes to your contact, moans when you touch him, and withdraws to painful stimuli. You rapidly immobilize the patient on a backboard with a cervical collar, place him on high-flow oxygen, and begin transport to the trauma center. An IV is placed as transport begins. Minutes into your trip, the patient appears to gag and then begins to have a seizure. Your driver informs you that the drive time to the trauma center will be 20 minutes.

1 What is the mechanism of injury (MOI)? Does knowing he was hit and kicked make a difference in your assessment of forces involved?

2 What is his Glasgow Coma Scale score (GCS)? Does it differ because he cannot open his swollen eye?

3 What is his main injury? What are the clues?

4 What could have caused him to have a seizure?

5 How should you manage this patient? Would your management change if the trip were 2 minutes instead of 20 minutes?

Introduction

Injuries to the head and neck are among the most devastating, with death and long-term disability the worst outcomes. An estimated 1.4 million traumatic brain injuries (TBIs) occur every year in the United States, accounting for 50,000 trauma deaths. In the United Kingdom, up to 700,000 people may be seen in the emergency department for head injury, but less than 10% are considered moderate to severe. More than 13,000 hospitalizations occur every year in Australia due to TBI, and 55,000 Canadians incur a brain injury each year. But injury to the brain is only part of the long-term disability problem faced by trauma casualties.

Spinal cord injuries (SCIs) affect 11,000 Americans each year, with 52% suffering paraplegia (affecting the lower extremities) and 47% quadriplegia or tetraplegia (affecting all four extremities). An average of 900 Canadians experience SCIs every year, primarily due to vehicle collisions. In the United Kingdom, 600 to 700 persons are hospitalized each year with a traumatic SCI, with falls barely surpassing motor vehicle trauma as the leading cause of injury.

The prehospital provider is in a unique position to alter the outcome in many of these patients. Early stabilization and immobilization have been shown to be beneficial to both individuals suffering a TBI and individuals suffering SCI. Airway control, ventilatory support, control of spinal movement, and management of bleeding and perfusion reduce the risk of secondary injury.

Anatomy and Physiology

Skull

The skull consists of 28 bones in three anatomic groups: the auditory ossicles, the cranium, and the face. There are six auditory ossicles, three located on each side of the head;

the remaining 22 bones constitute the cranium and the face **FIGURE 5-1**. Protection for the skull itself is provided by the scalp, which consists of several layers—skin, subcutaneous tissue, the galea aponeurotica, loose connective tissue (alveolar tissue), and periosteum **FIGURE 5-2**.

The <u>cranium</u>, or cranial vault, encases and protects the brain; it consists of eight bones, including the parietals, temporals, frontal, occipital, sphenoid, and ethmoid bones. The <u>foramen magnum</u> allows the brain to connect to the spinal cord.

The <u>occipital condyles</u> on the occipital bone, which are the points of articulation between the skull and the vertebral column, lie on either side of the foramen magnum. Portions of the maxilla and the <u>palatine bone</u>, the irregularly shaped bone in the posterior nasal cavity, form the <u>hard palate</u>, which is the bony anterior part of the palate, or roof of the mouth. The <u>zygomatic arch</u> is the bone that extends along the front of the skull below the orbit(s).

Facial Bones

The frontal and ethmoid bones are part of the cranium and the face. The 14 facial bones form the structure of the face without contributing to the cranium. They include the maxillae, vomer, inferior nasal concha, and the zygomatic, palatine, nasal, and lacrimal bones (see Figure 5-1A).

The facial bones protect the eyes, nose, and tongue; they also provide attachment points for the muscles that allow chewing. The zygomatic process of the temporal bone and the temporal process of the zygomatic bone form the zygomatic arch (Figure 5-1B), which lends shape to the cheeks.

Orbits

The orbits are cone-shaped fossae (cavities) that enclose and protect the eyes. In addition to the eyeball and muscles that move it, the orbits contain blood vessels, nerves, and fat.

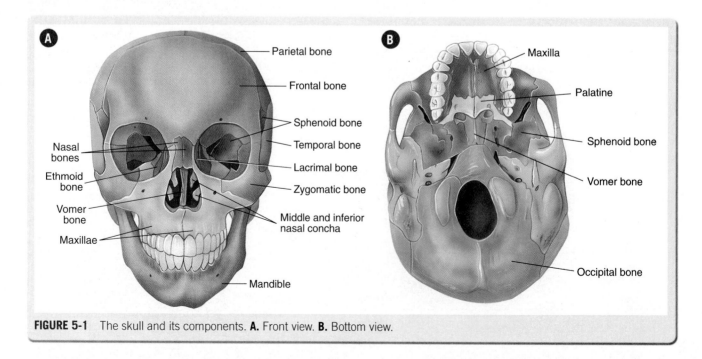

FIGURE 5-1   The skull and its components. **A.** Front view. **B.** Bottom view.

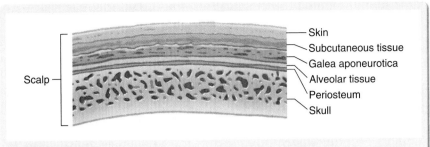

FIGURE 5-2 Protection for the skull itself is provided by the scalp, which consists of several layers—skin, subcutaneous tissue, the galea aponeurotica, loose connective tissue (alveolar tissue), and periosteum.

Nose

The nose is one of the two primary entry points for oxygen-rich air to enter the body. The **nasal septum**—the separation between the nostrils—is located in the midline. The external portion of the nose is formed mostly of cartilage.

Mandible and Temporomandibular Joint

The **mandible** is the large movable bone forming the lower jaw and containing the lower teeth. Numerous muscles of chewing attach to the mandible and its rami (branches). The posterior condyle of the mandible articulates with the temporal bone at the temporomandibular joint (TMJ), allowing movement of the mandible.

Hyoid Bone

The **hyoid bone** "floats" in the superior aspect of the neck just below the mandible. Although it is not actually part of the skull, it supports the tongue and serves as a point of attachment for many important neck and tongue muscles.

Cervical Spine

The **cervical spine** includes the first seven bones of the vertebral column and its supporting structures. In addition to protecting the vital cervical spinal cord, the cervical spine supports the weight of the head and permits a high degree of mobility in multiple planes.

Bones of the Cervical Spine

Like the rest of the spinal column, the cervical spine consists of irregular bones called vertebrae, which articulate to form the **vertebral column**—the major structural component of the axial skeleton. These skeletal components are stabilized by both ligaments and muscle. Together, these components support and protect neural elements while allowing for fluid movement and erect structure.

The cervical spine starts where the first vertebra (C1, also called the *atlas*) articulates with the bottom of the skull. The cervical spine curves slightly inward and ends where the last vertebra (C7) joins the top of the thoracic spine **FIGURE 5-3** .

The **vertebral body**, the anterior weight-bearing structure, is made of bone that provides support and stability. Components of the vertebra include the lamina, pedicles, and spinous processes **FIGURE 5-4** .

Each vertebra is unique in appearance but, with the exception of the atlas (C1) and axis (C2), shares basic structural characteristics. The atlas and axis are uniquely suited

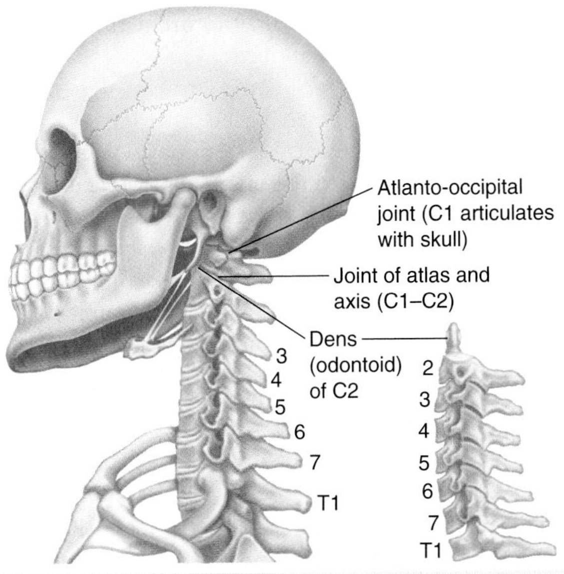

FIGURE 5-3 The cervical vertebrae.

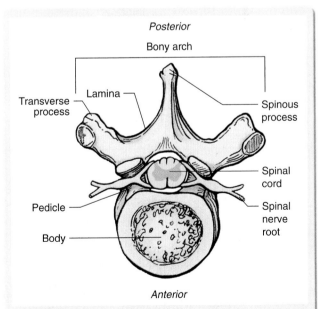

FIGURE 5-4 Vertebrae in different sections of the spinal column vary in shape; this is a general representation. The space through which the spinal cord passes is called the *canal* (or *vertebral foramen*), and the space through which a nerve root passes is called a *foramen* (or *transverse foramen*).

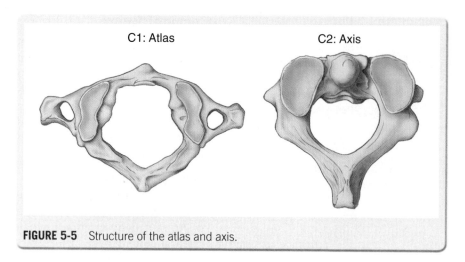

FIGURE 5-5 Structure of the atlas and axis.

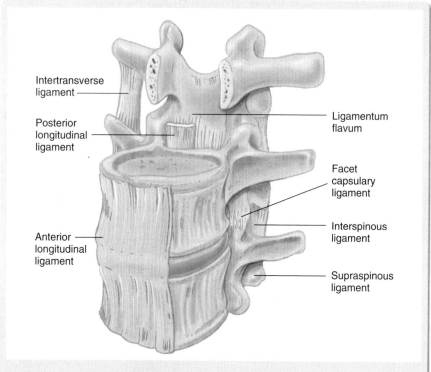

FIGURE 5-6 Several long ligaments connect on the anterior and posterior sections of the spinal vertebrae.

to allow for rotational movement of the skull FIGURE 5-5 . The atlas articulates with the skull at the atlanto-occipital joint.

Spinal Ligaments

Ligaments are strong connective tissues that connect bones to other bones. Several long ligaments connect on the anterior and posterior sections of the spinal vertebrae FIGURE 5-6 . The anterior longitudinal ligament extends down the front

of the vertebral bodies. The posterior longitudinal ligament attaches on the back of the vertebral bodies. The **ligamentum flavum** is a long elastic band that connects to the anterior surface of the lamina bones.

Spinal Cord

The spinal cord transmits nerve impulses between the brain and the rest of the body. Originating at the base of the brain, it represents the continuation of the central nervous system. The spinal cord exits the skull through the foramen magnum and extends through the torso downward to the lumbar spine. Spinal nerves extend past the end of the cord, making up the cauda equina or horse's tail. This collection of nerves continues through the spinal column exiting in pairs through the levels of the sacrum FIGURE 5-7 .

A cross-section of the spinal cord reveals a butterfly-shaped central core of gray matter that is composed of neural cell bodies and synapses. This gray matter is divided into posterior (dorsal) horns, which carry sensory input, and anterior (ventral) horns, which innervate the motor nerve of each segment. Surrounding the gray matter on each side are three columns of peripheral white matter composed of myelinated ascending and descending fiber pathways. Messages are relayed to and from the brain through these spinal tracts.

Specific groups of nerves are named based on their origin and point of termination. Ascending tracts carry information to the brain, and descending tracts carry information to the rest of the body.

Nerve impulses travel to and from the brain through the spinal cord to a specific location via the **peripheral nervous system (PNS)**. The PNS is the complex system of nerves that arise from the spinal nerve roots. There are 31 pairs of spinal nerves that emerge from each side of the spinal cord and are named for the vertebral region and level from which they arise. The eight cervical nerve roots control different functions in the scalp, neck, shoulders, and arms as follows:

- **C1–C2:** Head and neck
- **C3–C5:** Diaphragm
- **C4:** Upper body muscles (eg, deltoids and biceps)
- **C5–C6:** Wrist extensors
- **C7:** Triceps
- **C8:** Hands

Nerve roots occasionally converge in a cluster called a **plexus** that permits peripheral nerve roots to rejoin and function as a group. The cervical plexus includes C1 through C5; the phrenic nerve (C3–C5) arises from this plexus and innervates the diaphragm. The brachial plexus (C5–T1) joins nerves that control the upper extremities; the main nerves arising from this plexus are the axillary, median, musculocutaneous, radial, and ulnar.

Anterior Neck

The principal structures of the anterior part of the neck include the thyroid and cricoid cartilage, trachea, and numerous muscles and nerves **FIGURE 5-8**. The major blood vessels in this area are the internal and external carotid arteries and the internal and external jugular veins **FIGURE 5-9**. The vertebral arteries run laterally to the cervical vertebrae in the posterior part of the neck.

The major arteries of the neck—the carotid and vertebral arteries—supply oxygenated blood directly to the brain. The internal and external jugular veins drain deoxygenated blood from the head.

Other key structures of the anterior part of the neck that may sustain injury from blunt or penetrating mechanisms include the vagus nerves, thoracic duct (which connects the lymphatic system to the left subclavian vein), esophagus, thyroid and parathyroid glands, lower cranial nerves, brachial plexus (which is responsible for function of the lower arm and hand), soft tissue and fascia, and various muscles.

Muscle Structure

The muscles in the neck that enable head movement are located in the anterior, posterior, and lateral aspects

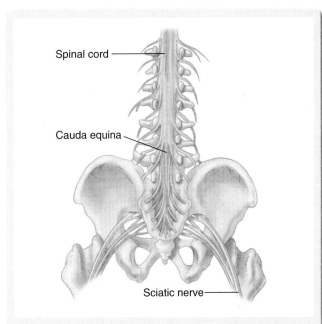

FIGURE 5-7 Spinal nerves extend past the end of the cord making up the cauda equina or horse's tail.

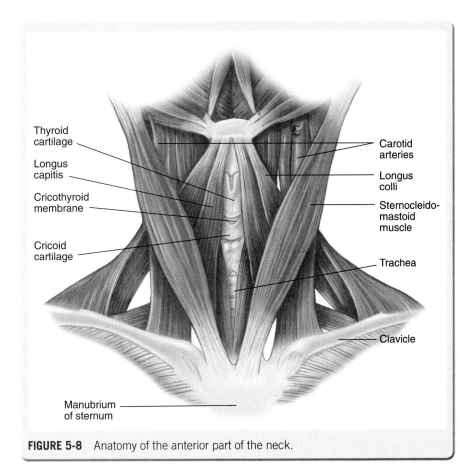

FIGURE 5-8 Anatomy of the anterior part of the neck.

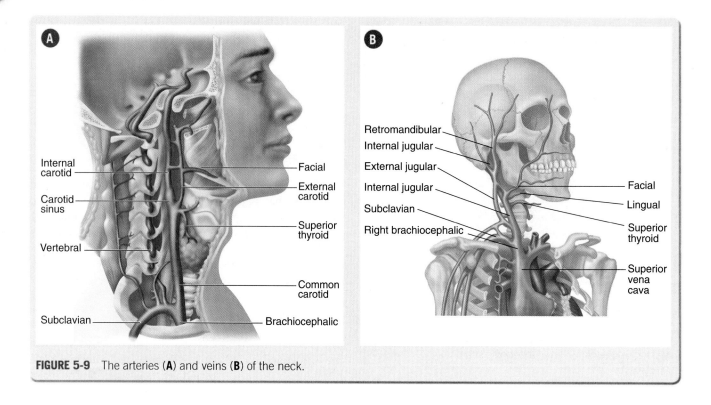

FIGURE 5-9 The arteries (**A**) and veins (**B**) of the neck.

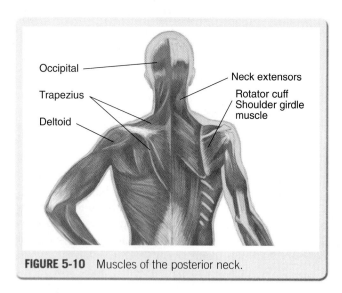

FIGURE 5-10 Muscles of the posterior neck.

of the skull (**FIGURE 5-10**). Most of these muscles originate at the upper cervical vertebrae and insert into the skull, usually at the occipital bone. Innervation is provided by cervical roots C1 and C2, as well as the spinal accessory nerve.

Eyes, Ears, and Mouth
Eye

The eye is composed of many structures (**FIGURE 5-11**). The **sclera** (white of the eye) is a tough, fibrous layer that helps maintain the shape of the eye and protects its contents.

The **cornea** is the transparent anterior portion of the eye that overlies the iris and pupil. The **conjunctiva** is a delicate mucous membrane that covers the sclera and internal surfaces of the eyelids (except the iris). The **iris** is the pigmented part of the eye that surrounds and protects the pupil; it contains muscles and blood vessels that contract and expand to regulate pupillary size. The **pupil** is a circular, adjustable opening within the iris through which light passes to the lens. The **lens** is a transparent structure behind the pupil; it can alter its thickness to focus light on the retina at the back of the eye. The **retina**, which lies in the posterior aspect of the internal globe, receives light impulses and converts them to nerve signals that are conducted to the brain by the optic nerve and interpreted as vision.

The **globe**, or eyeball, is a spherical structure measuring about 1" (2–3 cm) in diameter that is housed within the eye socket, or **orbit**. The eyes are held in place by loose connective tissue and several muscles. These muscles also control eye movements. The **oculomotor nerve** (third cranial nerve) innervates the muscles that cause motion of the eyeballs and upper eyelids. It also carries parasympathetic nerve fibers that cause constriction of the pupil and accommodation of the lens. The **optic nerve** (second cranial nerve) transmits nerve impulses necessary for the sense of vision.

The anterior chamber is the portion of the globe between the lens and the cornea. It is filled with **aqueous humor**, a clear watery fluid. If aqueous humor is lost through a penetrating injury to the eye, it will gradually be replenished.

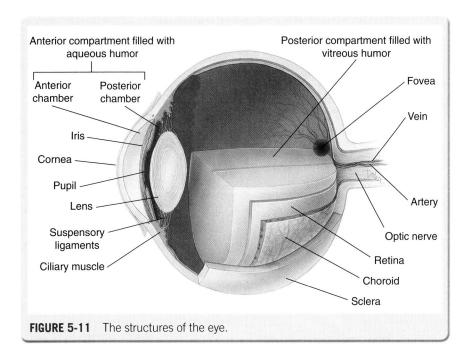

FIGURE 5-11 The structures of the eye.

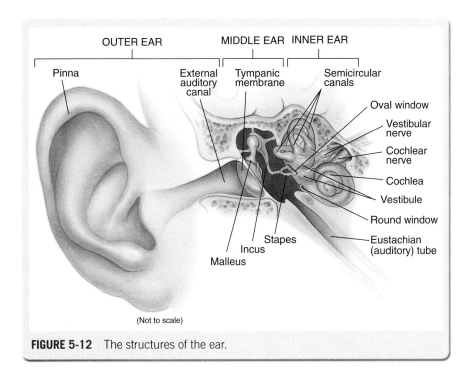

FIGURE 5-12 The structures of the ear.

of the pinna, the external auditory canal, and the exterior portion of the tympanic membrane (eardrum). The middle ear consists of the inner portion of the tympanic membrane and the ossicles, and the inner ear consists of the cochlea and semicircular canals.

Sound waves enter the ear through the auricle, or pinna, the large cartilaginous external portion of the ear. They then travel through the external auditory canal to the tympanic membrane. Vibration of sound waves against the tympanic membrane sets up vibration in the ossicles, the three small bones on the inner side of the tympanic membrane.

Mouth

Digestion begins in the mouth with **mastication**, or the chewing of food by the teeth. During mastication, food is mixed with secretions from the salivary glands.

The tongue, a muscular organ in the floor of the mouth, is the primary organ of taste; it is also important in the formation of speech and in chewing and swallowing of food. The tongue is attached at the mandible and hyoid bone, is covered by a mucous membrane, and extends from the back of the mouth upward and forward to the lips.

The normal adult mouth contains 32 permanent teeth, which are distributed around the maxillary and mandibular arches. The teeth on each side of the arch are mirror images of each other and form four quadrants: right upper, left upper, right lower, and left lower.

The top portion of the tooth, external to the gum, is the crown. Below the crown lie the neck and the root. The pulp cavity fills the center of the tooth and contains blood vessels, nerves, and specialized connective tissue, called pulp.

Brain

The brain, which occupies 80% of the cranial vault, contains billions of neurons (nerve cells) that serve a variety of vital functions **FIGURE 5-13**. The major regions of the brain are the cerebrum, diencephalon (thalamus

The posterior chamber is the portion of the globe between the iris and the lens. It is filled with **vitreous humor**, a jellylike substance that maintains the shape of the globe. If vitreous humor is lost, it cannot be replenished and blindness may result.

Ear

The ear is divided into three anatomic parts: external, middle, and inner **FIGURE 5-12**. The external ear consists

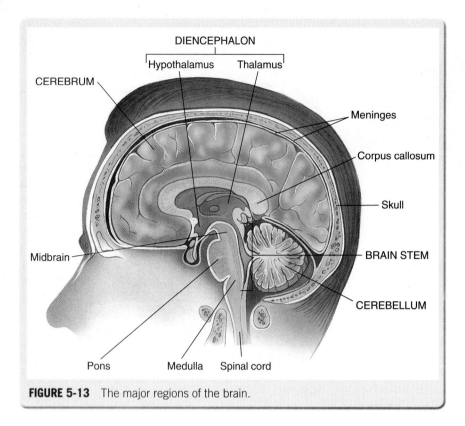

DIENCEPHALON
Hypothalamus   Thalamus

CEREBRUM

Meninges

Corpus callosum

Skull

BRAIN STEM

CEREBELLUM

Midbrain

Pons   Medulla   Spinal cord

FIGURE 5-13 The major regions of the brain.

Cerebellum

The **cerebellum** is located beneath the cerebral hemispheres in the inferoposterior part of the brain. It is sometimes called the "athlete's brain" because it is responsible for the maintenance of posture and equilibrium and the coordination of skilled movements.

Brain Stem

The **brain stem** consists of the midbrain, pons, and medulla. It is located at the base of the brain and connects the spinal cord to the remainder of the brain. The brain stem houses many structures that are critical to the maintenance of vital functions. High in the brain stem, for example, is the reticular activating system (RAS), which is responsible for maintenance of consciousness, specifically one's level of arousal. The centers that control basic but critical functions—heart rate, blood pressure, and respiration—are located in the lower part of the brain stem. Damage to this area can easily result in cardiovascular derangement, respiratory arrest, or death.

The midbrain lies immediately below the diencephalon and is the smallest region of the brain stem. The **pons** connects the midbrain and the medulla and contains numerous important nerve fibers, including those for sleep, respiration, and the medullary respiratory center.

The inferior portion of the midbrain, the **medulla**, is continuous within the spinal cord (see Figure 5-13). It serves as a conduction pathway for ascending and descending nerve tracts. It also coordinates heart rate, blood vessel diameter, breathing, swallowing, vomiting, coughing, and sneezing. The **vagus nerve** (10th cranial nerve) is a bundle of nerves that primarily innervates the parasympathetic nervous system; it originates from the medulla.

Cranial Nerves

Cranial nerves are not mediated by the spinal cord; they originate in the medulla and go directly to and from the brain. They innervate the face, head, and parts of the neck, with the exception of the vagus nerve, which runs down the neck and into the chest and abdomen. There are 12 pairs of cranial nerves in total. They play roles in a wide variety of motor and sensory functions that involve both the somatic and autonomic nervous systems `TABLE 5-1`.

When assessing the cranial nerves, a number of simple maneuvers can be employed to determine the presence

and hypothalamus), brain stem (medulla, pons, midbrain [mesencephalon]), and cerebellum. The remaining intracranial contents include cerebral blood (12%) and cerebrospinal fluid (8%).

The brain accounts for only 2% of the total body weight, yet it is the most metabolically active and perfusion-sensitive organ in the body. The brain metabolizes 25% of the body's glucose, burning approximately 60 mg/min, and consumes 20% of the total body oxygen (45 to 50 L/min). Because the brain has no storage mechanism for oxygen or glucose, it is totally dependent on a constant source of both fuels via cerebral blood flow provided by the carotid and vertebral arteries. As such, the brain will continually manipulate the physiology as needed to guarantee that a ready supply of oxygen and glucose is available.

Cerebrum

The largest portion of the brain is the **cerebrum**, which is responsible for higher functions, such as reasoning. The cerebrum is divided into right and left cerebral hemispheres by a longitudinal fissure. The hemispheres of the cerebrum are not entirely equivalent functionally. In a right-handed person, for example, the speech center is usually located in the left cerebral hemisphere, which is then said to be the dominant hemisphere. This crossing over occurs as the nerve impulses enter the spinal cord and are not actually a brain function.

TABLE 5-1 Cranial Nerves

Number	Name	Motor vs Sensory	Functions
I	Olfactory	Sensory	Smell
II	Optic	Sensory	Light perception and vision
III	Oculomotor	Motor	Pupil constriction, eye movements
IV	Trochlear	Motor	Eye movements
V	Trigeminal	Motor and sensory	Motor: chewing Sensory: face, sinuses, teeth
VI	Abducens	Motor	Eye movements
VII	Facial	Motor	Face movements
VIII	Vestibulocochlear	Sensory	Hearing, balance perception
IX	Glossopharyngeal	Motor and sensory	Motor: throat and swallowing, gland secretion Sensory: tongue, throat, ear
X	Vagus	Motor and sensory	Heart, lungs, palate, pharynx, larynx, trachea, bronchi, GI tract, external ear
XI	Spinal accessory	Motor	Shoulder and neck movements
XII	Hypoglossal	Motor	Tongue, throat, and neck movements

and degree of disability **TABLE 5-2**. The provider should be able to conduct the entire cranial nerve examination in less than 3 minutes.

Meninges

The meninges are protective layers that surround and enfold the entire central nervous system—specifically the brain and spinal cord **FIGURE 5-14**. The outermost layer is a strong, fibrous wrapping called the dura mater (meaning "tough mother"). The dura mater covers the entire brain, folding in to form the tentorium, a structure that separates the cerebral hemispheres from the cerebellum and brain stem. The dura mater is firmly attached to the internal wall of the skull. Just beneath the suture lines of the skull, the dura mater splits into two surfaces and forms a venous sinus. When the veins connecting the brain and the central sinus are disrupted during a head injury, blood can collect beneath the dura mater to form a subdural hematoma.

The meningeal arteries are located between the dura mater and the skull. When one of these arteries (usually the middle meningeal artery) is disrupted, bleeding occurs above the dura mater, resulting in an epidural (extradural) hematoma.

The second meningeal layer is a delicate, transparent membrane called the arachnoid mater. It is so named because the structure of the membrane resembles a tightly woven spiderweb. The third meningeal layer, the pia mater ("soft mother"), is a thin, translucent, highly vascular membrane that firmly adheres directly to the surface of the brain.

TABLE 5-2 Tests for Disability in Cranial Nerves

Cranial Nerve	Test
I	Check smell
II	Check visual acuity
III	Check pupil size, shape, symmetry, response to light, and eye movements
IV	Check eye movements
V	Check jaw clench; touch both sides of face at forehead, cheeks, and jaw
VI	Check eye movements
VII	Check facial symmetry; look for abnormal movements; have patient raise eyebrows, grin broadly, frown, shut eyes tightly, and puff out cheeks; note any asymmetry
VIII	Check hearing and balance
IX, X	Check swallowing; perform general physical exam
XI	Check shoulder shrug; turn head from left to right and back
XII	Check swallowing; turn head from left to right and back

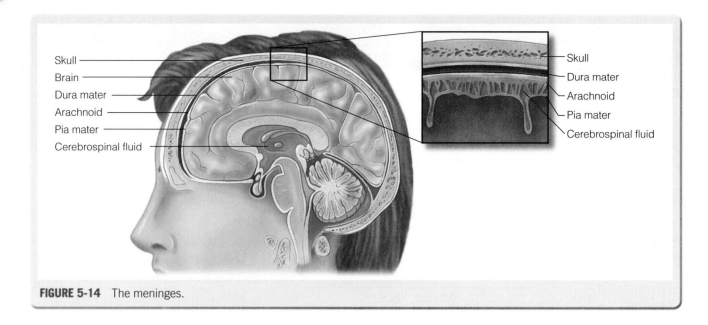

FIGURE 5-14   The meninges.

The meninges float in cerebrospinal fluid (CSF). CSF flows in the subarachnoid space, located between the pia mater and the arachnoid. Together, the meninges and CSF form a fluid-filled sac that cushions and protects the brain and spinal cord.

Face Injuries

Soft-Tissue Injuries

Although open soft-tissue injuries to the face—lacerations, abrasions, and avulsions—by themselves are rarely life threatening, their presence, especially following a significant mechanism of injury, suggests the potential for more severe injuries (eg, closed head injury or cervical spine injury). Furthermore, massive soft-tissue injuries to the face can compromise the patient's airway.

Maintain a high index of suspicion when a patient presents with closed soft-tissue injuries to the face, such as contusions and hematomas **FIGURE 5-15**. These indicators of blunt force trauma suggest the potential for more severe underlying injuries.

Impaled objects in the soft tissues or bones of the face may occur in association with facial trauma. Although these objects can damage facial nerves, the risk of airway compromise is of far greater consequence. This is especially true when an impaled object penetrates the cheek, because massive oropharyngeal bleeding can result in airway obstruction, aspiration, and ventilatory inadequacy. In addition, blood is a gastric irritant; swallowing even small quantities of blood can cause vomiting, further increasing the risk of aspiration.

Facial Fractures

Facial fractures commonly occur when the facial bones absorb the energy of a strong impact. The forces involved may be massive. General signs and symptoms of facial

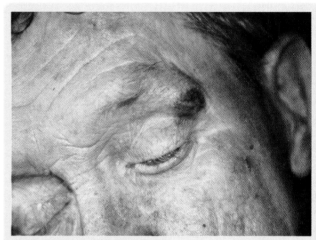

FIGURE 5-15   Closed soft-tissue injuries to the face may indicate more severe underlying injuries.

fractures include ecchymosis, swelling, pain to palpation, crepitus, dental malocclusion, facial deformities or asymmetry, instability of the facial bones, deep facial lacerations, impaired ocular movement, and visual disturbances.

Mandibular Fractures

Second only to nasal fractures in frequency, fractures of the mandible typically result from massive blunt force trauma to the lower third of the face; they are particularly common following an assault injury. Because significant force is required to fracture the mandible, it may be fractured in more than one place and, therefore, unstable to palpation. The fracture site itself is most commonly located at the angle of the jaw.

Mandibular fractures should be suspected in patients with a history of blunt force trauma to the lower third of the face who present with dental malocclusion (misalignment of the teeth), numbness of the chin, and inability to open the

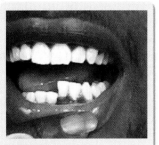

FIGURE 5-16 Malocclusion of the bottom teeth often indicates a mandible fracture.

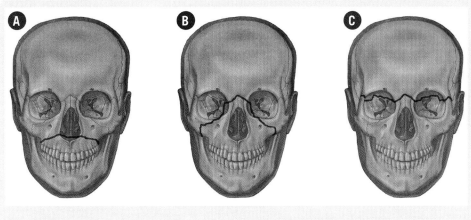

FIGURE 5-17 Le Fort fractures. **A.** Le Fort I. **B.** Le Fort II. **C.** Le Fort III.

mouth FIGURE 5-16 . There will likely be swelling and ecchymosis over the fracture site, and teeth may be partially or completely avulsed.

Midface Fractures

Midface fractures are most commonly associated with mechanisms that cause substantial blunt facial trauma, such as motor vehicle crashes, falls, and assaults. They produce massive facial swelling, instability of the midfacial bones, dental malocclusion, and an elongated appearance of the patient's face. Midfacial structures include the maxilla, zygoma, orbital floor, and nose.

Le Fort fractures FIGURE 5-17 are classified into three categories:

- **Le Fort I fracture**: A horizontal fracture of the maxilla that involves the hard palate and inferior maxilla
- **Le Fort II fracture**: A pyramidal fracture involving the nasal bone and inferior maxilla
- **Le Fort III fracture** (**craniofacial disjunction**): A fracture of all midfacial bones, separating the entire midface from the cranium

Le Fort fractures can occur as isolated fractures (Le Fort I) or in combination (Le Fort I and II), depending on the location of impact and the amount of trauma.

Fractures of the zygoma (cheek bone) commonly result from blunt trauma secondary to motor vehicle crashes and assaults. When the zygoma is fractured, that side of the patient's face appears flattened and there is loss of sensation over the cheek, nose, and upper lip; paralysis of upward gaze may also be present. Other injuries commonly associated with zygomatic fractures include orbital fractures, ocular injury, and epistaxis (nosebleed).

Orbital fractures are another potential midface injury. A blow to the eye may result in fracture of the orbital floor because the bone is extremely thin and breaks easily. A blowout fracture results in transmission of forces away from the eyeball itself to the supporting bony structure that gives way under pressure and fractures. Blood and fat then leak into the maxillary sinus.

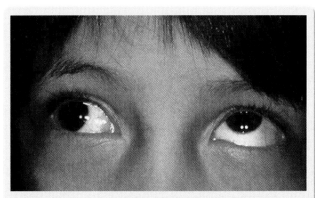

FIGURE 5-18 In a patient with an orbital blowout fracture, the eyes may not move together because of ocular muscle entrapment.

The patient with an orbital fracture may complain of double vision (**diplopia**) and lose sensation above the eyebrow or over the cheek secondary to associated nerve damage. Massive nasal discharge may occur, and vision is often impaired. Fractures of the inferior orbit—the most common type—can cause paralysis of upward gaze (the injured eye will not be able to follow your finger above the midline) because of associated ocular muscle entrapment, or **dysconjugate gaze** (both eyes are not fixated on the same point) FIGURE 5-18 .

Because the nasal bones are not as structurally sound as the other bones of the face, nasal fractures are the most common facial fracture. These fractures are characterized by swelling, tenderness, and crepitus when the nasal bone is palpated. Deformity of the nose, if present, usually appears as lateral displacement of the nasal bone from its normal midline position.

TIP

Assess eye movements in all visual fields in any patient with possible facial fractures.

Nasal fractures, like any maxillofacial fracture, are often complicated by the presence of anterior or posterior epistaxis, which can compromise the patient's airway if blood is aspirated.

Assessment and Treatment of Facial Injuries

TABLE 5-3 summarizes the characteristics of various maxillofacial fractures. It is impractical to attempt to distinguish among the various maxillofacial fractures in the prehospital setting; this determination requires radiographic evaluation. Rapid patient assessment, management of life-threatening conditions, full spinal precautions, and prompt transport are far more important considerations.

Management of the patient with facial trauma begins by protecting the cervical spine. Because many severe facial injuries are complicated by a spinal injury, the provider must assume that one exists.

If the patient has a reduced level of consciousness, open the airway with the jaw-thrust maneuver while manually stabilizing the head in a neutral position. Inspect the mouth for fragments of teeth, dentures, or any other foreign bodies that could obstruct the airway, and remove them immediately. Suction the oropharynx as needed to keep the airway clear of blood and other liquids. If the provider is unable to open the airway effectively with the jaw-thrust maneuver, he or she must carefully perform the head tilt–chin lift maneuver; regardless of the situation, the patient's airway must be open.

Insert an airway adjunct as needed to maintain airway patency. Do not, however, insert a nasopharyngeal airway or attempt nasotracheal intubation in any patient with suspected mid-face fractures or in patients with CSF rhinorrhea. These are often the signs of a basilar skull fracture, which may have weakened the posterior wall of the nasopharynx. After establishing and maintaining a patent airway, assess the patient's breathing and intervene appropriately. Apply high-flow oxygen via nonrebreathing mask if the patient is breathing adequately (see Chapter 2). If the patient is breathing inadequately, assist ventilations with a bag-mask device and high-flow oxygen. Monitor the patient's oxygen saturation, and, if needed, his or her cardiac rhythm.

Airway management can be especially challenging in patients with massive facial injuries. Oropharyngeal bleeding poses an immediate threat to the airway, and unstable facial bones can hinder the provider's ability to maintain an effective mask-to-face seal for bag-mask ventilation. Therefore, tracheal intubation is often required, especially if the patient is unconscious, to protect the airway from aspiration and to ensure adequate oxygenation and ventilation. Pharmacologic agents (ie, sedation, paralytics) are often needed to facilitate intubation in patients who have a reduced level of consciousness and/or have an intact gag reflex. Patients with extensive maxillofacial injuries may require cricothyrotomy (surgical or needle) when endotracheal intubation is extremely difficult or impossible to perform (ie, unstable facial bones, massive swelling, severe oral bleeding) (Chapter 3).

Treat facial lacerations and avulsions as you would any other soft-tissue injury. Control all bleeding with direct pressure and apply sterile dressings. If you suspect an underlying facial fracture, apply just enough pressure to control the bleeding. Leave impaled objects in the face in place and stabilize them appropriately unless they pose a catastrophic threat to the airway.

For severe oropharyngeal bleeding in patients with inadequate ventilation, suction the airway for 15 seconds and provide ventilatory assistance for 2 minutes; alternate suctioning and ventilating until the airway is clear or the airway has been secured with an appropriate device. Monitor the patient's oxygen saturation throughout this process.

Epistaxis following facial trauma can be severe and is most effectively controlled by applying direct pressure to the nares. If the patient is conscious and spinal injury

TABLE 5-3	Summary of Maxillofacial Fractures
Injury	**Signs and Symptoms**
Multiple facial bone fractures	• Massive facial swelling • Dental malocclusion • Palpable deformities • Anterior or posterior epistaxis
Zygomatic and orbital fractures	• Loss of sensation below the orbit • Flattening of the patient's cheeks • Paralysis of upward gaze
Nasal fractures	• Crepitus and instability • Swelling, tenderness, lateral displacement • Anterior or posterior epistaxis
Maxillary (Le Fort) fractures	• Mobility of the facial skeleton • Dental malocclusion • Facial swelling
Mandibular fractures	• Dental malocclusion • Mandibular instability

TIP

Although the patient's airway must be opened regardless of the situation, take care if you suspect a patient has mid-face fractures or CSF rhinorrhea. In these cases, *do not* insert a nasopharyngeal airway or attempt nasotracheal intubation. These signs often indicate a basilar skull fracture, which may have weakened the posterior wall of the nasopharynx.

is not suspected, instruct the patient to sit up and lean forward as you pinch the nares together. Unconscious patients should be positioned on their side, unless contraindicated by a spinal injury. Proper positioning of the patient with epistaxis is important to prevent blood from draining down the throat and compromising the airway. If the conscious patient with severe epistaxis is secured to a backboard, pharmacologically assisted intubation (eg, rapid-sequence intubation [RSI]) may be needed to gain definitive airway control.

Although facial lacerations and avulsions can contribute to hemorrhagic shock, they are rarely the sole cause of this condition in adults. Severe epistaxis, however, can result in significant blood loss. Therefore, the patient should be assessed carefully for signs of hemorrhagic shock; administer crystalloid fluid boluses as needed to maintain adequate perfusion.

If the facial fracture is associated with swelling and ecchymosis, cold compresses may help minimize further swelling and alleviate pain **FIGURE 5-19**. Do not apply a compress to the eyeball (globe) if injury following an orbital fracture is suspected; doing so may increase intraocular pressure (IOP) and further damage the eye. Other than protecting the airway, little can be done to treat facial instabilities; however, firmly applying a self-adhering roller bandage (such as Kerlix or Kling) can stabilize the mandible. Make sure you do not compromise the airway when stabilizing the mandible.

After addressing all life-threatening injuries and conditions, the provider should attempt to ascertain the events that preceded the injury and determine whether the patient has any significant medical problems. The incident that caused the injury may have been preceded by exacerbation of an underlying medical condition (eg, acute hypoglycemia, cardiac arrhythmia, or seizure). For unconscious patients, medications that the patient is taking may provide information about his or her medical history. Determine the approximate time the injury occurred and ask about any drug allergies and the last oral intake during the SAMPLE history.

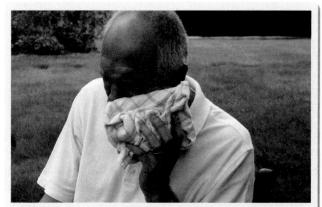

FIGURE 5-19 Cold compresses will help decrease swelling and pain.

Eye Injuries

Lacerations, Foreign Bodies, and Impaled Objects

Lacerations of the eyelids require meticulous repair to restore appearance and function. Bleeding may be heavy, but it usually can be controlled by gentle, manual pressure. If there is a laceration to the globe itself, apply no pressure to the eye; compression can interfere with the blood supply to the back of the eye and result in permanent loss of vision from damage to the retina. Furthermore, pressure may squeeze the vitreous humor, iris, lens, or even the retina out of the eye and cause irreparable damage or blindness **FIGURE 5-20**.

The protective orbit prevents large objects from penetrating the eye; however, moderately sized and smaller foreign objects can still enter the eye and, when lying on the surface of the eye, produce severe irritation. The conjunctiva becomes inflamed and red (conjunctivitis) almost immediately, and the eye begins to produce tears in an attempt to flush out the object. Irritation of the cornea or conjunctiva

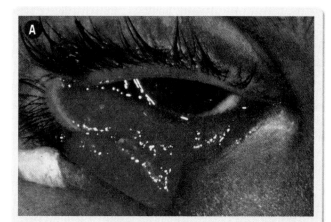
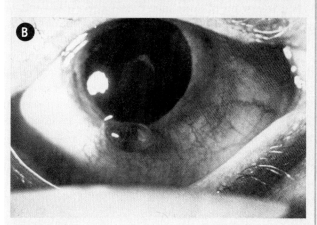

FIGURE 5-20 Eye lacerations are serious injuries that require prompt transport. **A.** Although bleeding can be heavy, never exert pressure on the eye. **B.** Pressure may squeeze the vitreous humor, iris, lens, or retina out of the eye.

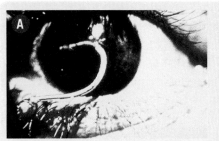
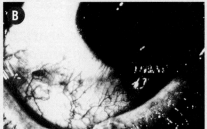
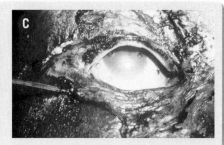

FIGURE 5-21 Any number of objects can be impaled in the eye. **A.** Fishhook. **B.** Sharp, metal sliver. **C.** Knife blade.

causes intense pain. The patient may have difficulty keeping the eyelids open because the irritation is further aggravated by bright light.

Foreign bodies ranging in size from a sliver of metal to a pencil may become impaled in the eye **FIGURE 5-21**. Clearly, these objects must be removed by a physician. Prehospital care involves stabilizing the object and preparing the patient for transport. The greater the length of the foreign object sticking out of the eye, the more important stabilization becomes in avoiding further damage. Whenever possible, cover both eyes to limit unnecessary movement as the patient tries to use the uninjured eye to compensate for the loss or limited vision of the injured eye **PROCEDURE 29**.

Blunt Eye Injuries

Blunt trauma can cause serious eye injuries, ranging from swelling and ecchymosis to rupture of the globe. **Hyphema** is bleeding into the anterior chamber of the eye that obscures vision, partially or completely **FIGURE 5-22**. It often follows blunt trauma and may seriously impair vision. Approximately 25% of hyphemas are associated with globe injuries.

In orbital blowout fractures, fractured bone fragments can entrap some of the muscles that control eye movement. Any patient who reports pain, double vision, or decreased vision following a blunt injury near the eye should be assumed to have a blowout fracture and should be transported promptly to an appropriate medical facility.

Another potential result of blunt eye trauma is **retinal detachment**, or separation of the inner layers of the retina from the underlying **choroid** (the vascular membrane that nourishes the retina). Retinal detachment is often seen in sports injuries, especially boxing. This painless condition produces flashing lights, specks, or "floaters" in the field of vision and a cloud or shade over the patient's vision. Because it can cause devastating damage to vision, retinal detachment is an ocular emergency and requires immediate medical attention.

Burns of the Eye

Chemicals, heat, and light rays can all burn the delicate tissues of the eye, often causing permanent damage.

Chemical burns, which are usually caused by acid or alkali solutions, require immediate emergency care **FIGURE 5-23**. Flush the eye with copious amounts of sterile

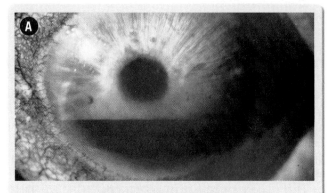

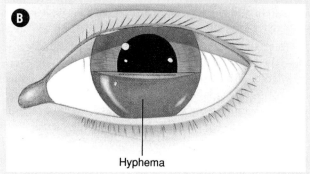

Hyphema

FIGURE 5-22 A hyphema, characterized by bleeding into the anterior chamber of the eye, can occur following blunt trauma to the eye and should be considered a sight-threatening emergency. **A.** Actual hyphema. **B.** Illustration.

water or saline solution. If these are not available, use any clean water. Specific techniques for irrigating the eyes are discussed later in this chapter.

Thermal burns occur when a patient is burned in the face during a fire, although the eyes usually close rapidly because of the heat. This reaction is a natural reflex to protect the eyes from further injury. However, the eyelids remain exposed and are frequently burned **FIGURE 5-24**.

Infrared rays, eclipse light (if the patient has looked directly at the sun), and laser burns can cause significant damage to the sensory cells of the eye when rays of light become focused on the retina. Retinal injuries caused by

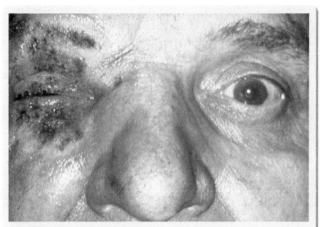

FIGURE 5-23 Chemical burns typically occur when an acid or alkali is splashed into the eye.

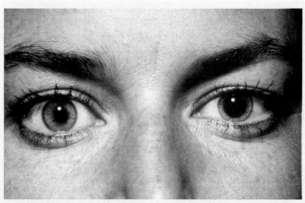

FIGURE 5-25 Asymmetric pupils suggest injury to the papillary sphincter muscle, optic nerve, or globe.

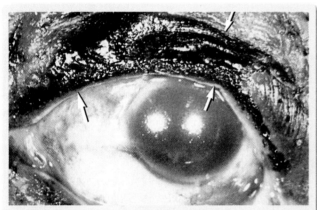

FIGURE 5-24 Thermal burns occasionally cause significant damage to the eyelids. Arrows show areas of full-thickness burns.

exposure to extremely bright light are generally not painful but may result in permanent damage to vision.

Superficial burns of the eye can result from ultraviolet rays from an arc welding unit, prolonged exposure to a sunlamp, or reflected light from a bright snow-covered area (snow blindness). This kind of burn may not be painful initially but may become so 3 to 5 hours later, as the damaged cornea responds to the injury. Severe conjunctivitis usually develops, along with redness, swelling, and excessive tear production.

Pupillary Response

The pupils are normally round, black, and of approximately equal size. When assessing the pupils, check for size (in millimeters), shape, symmetry, reaction to light, and accommodation.

The pupil should constrict immediately when a light is shone directly into it (direct response); the contralateral (opposite) pupil should constrict at the same time (consensual response). Both pupils should be equal in their response and should dilate simultaneously when the light source is removed.

Pupillary accommodation is a reflex action of the eye in response to focusing on objects that are near and far. To assess pupillary accommodation, ask the patient to fixate on an object (eg, a penlight). The pupils should constrict bilaterally as you move the object closer to the eyes and dilate when you move the object further away.

In the context of an eye injury, an abnormal pupillary response such as asymmetric pupils (anisocoria) or accommodation abnormalities suggests injury to the pupillary sphincter muscle, optic nerve, or globe **FIGURE 5-25**. Abnormal pupillary responses may also be seen with conditions such as physiologic anisocoria (a benign condition affecting about 20% of the population), cataracts, brain injury, drug use, ocular prosthesis, and certain drugs.

Assessment of Eye Movements

Voluntary extraocular muscles are controlled by cranial nerves III, IV, and VI; when intact, they should allow the patient to move his or her eyes voluntarily in six directions of gaze without experiencing double vision.

Extraocular movement (EOM) is assessed by asking the patient to track an object visually—without moving his or her head—up, down, to the left, and to the right. Ask the patient if he or she experiences double vision in any direction of gaze and observe for dysconjugate gaze. Abnormal EOM suggests edema of the orbital structures, muscle entrapment from a fracture, or cranial nerve injury.

Assessment and Treatment of Eye Injuries

The first step in assessing a patient with an eye injury is to note the mechanism of injury (MOI). If it suggests the potential for a spinal injury, use spinal motion restriction precautions. Ensure a patent airway and adequate breathing, and control any external bleeding. Perform a rapid trauma assessment if the MOI or patient's clinical status dictates it.

When obtaining the history, determine how and when the injury happened, when the symptoms began, what symptoms the patient is experiencing, and whether one or both eyes are affected. Ascertain if the patient has any eye diseases (eg, glaucoma or cataracts) and whether he or she is taking medication for his or her eyes. Additional history should include if the patient was wearing glasses, contact lenses, or protective eyewear at the time of the injury.

A variety of symptoms may indicate serious ocular injury:

- Visual loss that does not improve when the patient blinks is the most important symptom of an eye injury. It may indicate damage to the globe or to the optic nerve.
- Double vision suggests trauma to the extraocular muscles, such as an orbital fracture.
- Severe eye pain is a symptom of a significant eye injury.
- A foreign body sensation usually indicates superficial injury to the cornea or the presence of a foreign object trapped behind the eyelids.

During the physical examination of the eyes, evaluate each of the visible ocular structures and ocular function **TABLE 5-4**.

Treatment for specific eye injuries begins with a thorough examination to determine the extent and nature of any damage. Always perform your examination using body substance isolation precautions, taking great care to avoid aggravating the injury.

TABLE 5-4	Examination of the Eyes
Part to Be Examined	**Clinical Findings**
Orbital rim	Ecchymosis, swelling, lacerations, and tenderness
Eyelids	Ecchymosis, swelling, and lacerations
Corneas	Foreign bodies
Conjunctivae	Redness, pus, inflammation, and foreign bodies
Globes	Redness, abnormal pigmentation, and lacerations
Pupils	Size, shape, equality, and reaction to light
Eye movements in all directions	Paralysis of gaze or dysconjugate gaze
Visual acuity	Make a rough assessment by asking the patient to read a newspaper or a hand-held visual acuity chart. Test each eye separately and document the results.

Although isolated eye injuries are usually not life threatening, they should be evaluated by a physician. More severe eye injuries often require evaluation and treatment by an ophthalmologist.

Injuries to the eyelids—lacerations, abrasions, and contusions—require little in the way of prehospital care other than bleeding control and gentle patching of the affected eye. No eyelid injury is trivial, so every patient with eyelid trauma should be transported to the hospital.

Most significant injuries to the globe—including contusions, lacerations, foreign bodies, and abrasions—are best treated in the emergency department, where specialized equipment is available. Aluminum eye shields or other bandaging material that can bridge the orbit of the eye applied over both eyes are generally all that is necessary in the field **PROCEDURE 29**. Follow these three important guidelines in treating penetrating injuries of the eye:

1. Never exert pressure on or manipulate the injured globe in any way.
2. If part of the globe is exposed, gently apply a moist, sterile dressing to prevent drying.
3. Cover the injured eye with a protective metal eye shield, cup, or sterile dressing. Apply soft dressings to both eyes, and provide prompt transport to the hospital.

If hyphema or rupture of the globe is suspected, take spinal motion restriction precautions. Such injuries indicate that a significant amount of force was applied to the face and, thus, may include a spinal injury. Elevate the head of the backboard approximately 30° to decrease IOP and to discourage the patient from performing activities that may increase IOP (eg, coughing).

On rare occasions following a serious injury, the globe may be displaced (avulsed) out of its socket **FIGURE 5-26**. Do not attempt to manipulate or reposition it in any way. Cover

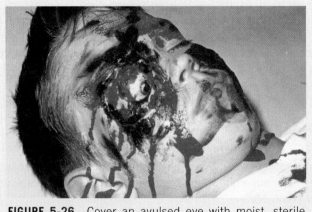

FIGURE 5-26 Cover an avulsed eye with moist, sterile dressings and protect it from further injury.

the protruding eye with a moist, sterile dressing and stabilize it along with the uninjured eye to prevent further injury due to **sympathetic eye movement**, the movement of both eyes in unison. Place the patient in a supine position to prevent further loss of fluid from the eye, and transport promptly.

Burns to the eye that are caused by ultraviolet light are most effectively treated by covering the eye with a sterile, moist pad and an eye shield. The application of cool compresses lightly over the eye may afford the patient pain relief. Place the patient in a supine position during transport and protect the patient from further exposure to bright light.

Chemical burns to the eye—acid or alkali—can rapidly lead to total blindness if not immediately treated. The most important prehospital treatment in such cases is to begin immediate irrigation with sterile water or saline solution **PROCEDURE 30**. Never use any chemical antidotes (such as vinegar or baking soda) when irrigating the patient's eye; use sterile water or saline only.

The goal when irrigating the eye is to direct the greatest amount of solution or water into the eye as gently as possible. Because opening the eye spontaneously may cause the patient pain, you may have to force the lids open to irrigate the eye adequately. Ideally, you should use a bulb or irrigation syringe, an IV through the tubing or connected to a nasal cannula, or some other device that will allow you to control the flow. In some circumstances, you may have to pour water into the eye by holding the patient's head under a gently running faucet, or you can have the patient immerse his or her face in a large pan or basin of water and rapidly blink the affected eyelid.

Irrigate the eye for at least 5 minutes. If the burn was caused by an alkali or a strong acid, irrigate the eye continuously for 20 to 30 minutes because these substances can penetrate deeply. One common chemical burn occurs where anhydrous ammonia is used during the process of cooking methamphetamine. If the eyes are not irrigated promptly and efficiently, permanent damage is likely. Whenever you have to irrigate the eye(s), continue to irrigate en route to the hospital if possible.

Irrigation with a sterile saline solution will frequently flush away loose, small foreign objects lying on the surface of the eye. Always flush from the nose side of the eye toward the outside to avoid flushing material into the other eye. You may also consider using a nasal cannula to flush both eyes at the same time **FIGURE 5-27**. After its removal, a foreign body will often leave a small abrasion on the surface of the conjunctiva, which leads to continued irritation; further evaluation may be required.

Gentle irrigation usually will not wash out foreign bodies that are stuck to the cornea or lying under the upper eyelid. To examine the undersurface of the upper eyelid, pull the lid upward and forward (eyelid inversion) **FIGURE 5-28**. If you spot a foreign object on the surface of the eyelid, you may be able to remove it with a moist, sterile,

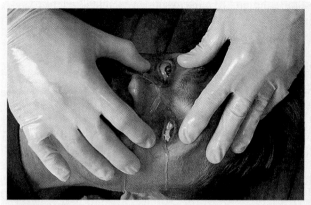
FIGURE 5-27 Flush from the nose side of the eye toward the outside to avoid flushing material into the other eye.

cotton-tipped applicator. Never attempt to remove a foreign body that is stuck or embedded in the cornea.

When a foreign body is impaled in the globe, do not remove it. Stabilize it in place. Cover the eye with a moist, sterile dressing; place a cup or other protective barrier over the object and secure it in place with a bulky dressing **FIGURE 5-29**. Cover the unaffected eye and promptly transport the patient to the hospital.

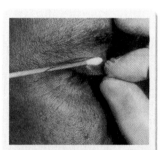
FIGURE 5-28 To examine the undersurface of the upper eyelid, pull the lid upward and forward.

Removal of contact lenses should be limited to patients with chemical burns to the eye. To remove hard contact lenses, use a specialized suction cup (if available) moistened with sterile

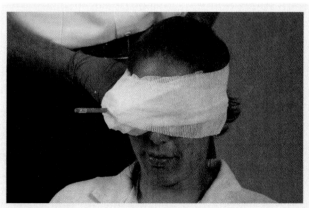
FIGURE 5-29 Secure an impaled object in the eye with a protective barrier and bulky dressing.

saline solution. To remove soft (hydrophilic) contact lenses, instill 1 or 2 drops of saline or irrigating solution, and gently pinch off the lens with your gloved thumb and index finger.

Ear Injuries

Soft-Tissue Injuries

Lacerations, avulsions, and contusions to the external ear can occur following blunt or penetrating trauma. The pinna can be contused, lacerated, or partially or completely avulsed **FIGURE 5-30**. Trauma to the earlobe can result in similar injuries.

The pinna has an inherently poor blood supply, so it tends to heal poorly. Healing of the cartilaginous pinna is often complicated by infection.

Ruptured Eardrum

Perforation of the tympanic membrane (ruptured eardrum) can result from foreign bodies in the ear or barotrauma (eg, blast injuries, diving-related injuries). Signs and symptoms of a perforated tympanic membrane include loss of hearing and blood drainage from the ear. Although the injury is

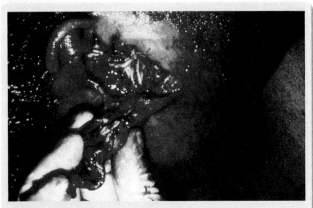

FIGURE 5-30   A major laceration to the ear.

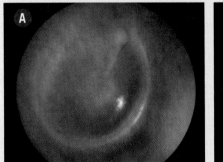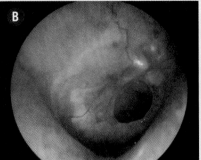

FIGURE 5-31   Inspect the ear canal and tympanic membrane with an otoscope. **A.** Normal eardrum. **B.** Ruptured eardrum.

extremely painful for the patient, the tympanic membrane typically heals spontaneously and without complication. Nevertheless, a careful assessment should be performed to detect and treat other injuries, some of which may be life threatening.

Assessment and Treatment of Ear Injuries

Assessment and management of the patient with an ear injury begins by ensuring airway patency and breathing adequacy. If the mechanism of injury suggests a potential for spinal injury, apply full spinal motion restriction precautions.

Assessing the ears involves checking for new aberrations in hearing perception and inspecting and palpating for wounds, swelling, or drainage. If possible, visualize the external ear canal and tympanic membrane with an otoscope—especially if the patient experienced a blast injury **FIGURE 5-31**. A perforated tympanic membrane is characterized by a visible tear; bleeding may or may not be present.

In general, the ears' poor blood supply limits the amount of external bleeding. If manual direct pressure does not control this bleeding, first place a soft, padded dressing between the ear and the scalp because bandaging the ear against the tender scalp can be extremely painful. Then apply a roller bandage to secure the dressing in place. An ice pack can also help reduce swelling and pain.

If the pinna is partially avulsed, carefully realign the ear into position and gently bandage it with sufficient padding that has been slightly moistened with normal saline. If the pinna is completely amputated, attempt to retrieve the avulsed part, if possible, for reimplantation at the hospital. If the detached part of the ear is recovered, treat it as any other amputation; wrap it in saline-moistened gauze, place it in a plastic bag, and place the bag on ice. If a chemical ice pack is used, shield the avulsed part with several gauze pads to diffuse the cold; chemical ice packs are actually colder than ice, and inadvertent freezing of the part can occur.

If blood or CSF drainage is noted, apply a loose dressing over the ear—taking care not to stop the flow—and assess the patient for other signs of a basilar skull fracture.

Do not remove an impaled object from the ear. Instead, stabilize the object and cover the ear to prevent gross movement and to minimize the risk of contamination of the inner ear.

Because isolated ear injuries are typically not life threatening, you must perform a careful assessment to detect or rule out potentially more serious injuries. You may then proceed with specific care of the ear, provide emotional support, and transport the patient to an appropriate medical facility.

Oral and Dental Injuries

Soft-Tissue Injuries

Lacerations and avulsions in and around the mouth are associated with a risk of intraoral hemorrhage and subsequent airway compromise **FIGURE 5-32**. Fractured or avulsed teeth and lacerations of the tongue may cause profuse bleeding into the upper airway. A conscious patient with severe oral bleeding is often unable to speak unless he or she is leaning forward; this position facilitates drainage of blood from the mouth.

Patients may swallow blood from lacerations inside the mouth, so the bleeding may not be grossly evident. Because blood irritates the gastric lining, the risks of vomiting and aspiration are significant. Objects that are impaled in or through the soft tissues of the mouth (such as the cheek) can also result in profuse bleeding and, once again, the threat of vomiting with aspiration and airway compromise.

Assessment and Treatment of Oral Soft-Tissue Injuries

Ensuring airway patency and adequate breathing are the priorities of care when managing patients with soft-tissue injuries of the mouth. Place the patient in a position that will facilitate drainage of blood from the mouth and suction the oropharynx as needed. Apply c-spine motion restriction precautions as dictated by the mechanism of injury. If profuse oral bleeding is present and the patient cannot spontaneously control his or her own airway (ie, decreased level of consciousness), pharmacologically assisted intubation may be necessary.

Impaled objects in the soft tissues of the mouth should be stabilized in place unless they interfere with the

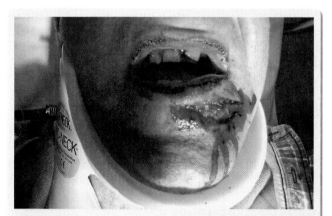

FIGURE 5-32 Soft-tissue injuries in and around the mouth can be associated with profuse intraoral bleeding and airway compromise.

patient's breathing or your ability to manage the patient's airway. In those cases, remove the impaled object from the direction that it entered, and control bleeding with direct pressure.

Dental Injuries

Fractured and avulsed teeth—especially the anterior teeth—are common following facial trauma. Dental injuries may be associated with mechanisms that cause severe maxillofacial trauma (eg, motor vehicle crashes), or they may occur in isolation (eg, direct blow to the mouth from an assault).

> **TIP**
>
> When assessing a patient with fractured or avulsed teeth following an assault, you should also assess the individual who struck the patient if it is safe to do so. The human mouth is filled with bacteria and other microorganisms, and lacerations to the person's hands or knuckles can easily become infected.

You should always assess the patient's mouth following a facial injury, especially in cases of fractured or avulsed teeth. Teeth fragments (or even whole teeth) can become an airway obstruction and should be removed from the patient's mouth immediately.

Assessing a Tooth for Reimplantation

When assessing a tooth for possible reimplantation, it is important to remember that trauma to the oral cavity may result in airway complications. Handle the tooth by the crown only and avoid touching the root surface of the tooth. Assess the tooth for possible fractures and examine the socket for any remaining fragments of the tooth.

Care of a Tooth for Reimplantation

An avulsed tooth may be successfully reimplanted even if it has been out of the mouth for up to 1 hour. In the United States, medical control may ask you to reimplant the tooth in its socket and hold it in place with you fingers or have the patient gently bite down. Conversely, this clinical decision will be at the discretion of the provider in the United Kingdom, although advice may be sought from the identified receiving facility. If prehospital reimplantation of a tooth is not possible, follow the guidelines established by the American Association of Endodontists and the American Dental Association, which is universal and contemporary in other countries as well **TABLE 5-5**.

Retrieval and reimplantation or storage of an avulsed tooth is a low priority if the patient is in a clinically unstable condition (such as compromised airway or shock). In such cases, aggressive airway management, spinal immobilization, and rapid transport of the patient are obviously more important, with the dental problem being addressed at a later time.

TABLE 5-5   Care for an Avulsed Tooth

- Handle the tooth by the crown only. Avoid touching the root surface of the tooth.
- Gently rinse the tooth with sterile saline or water. Avoid the use of soap or chemicals and do not scrub the tooth.
- Do not allow the tooth to dry. Place it in one of the following:
  - Emergency tooth preservation system (such as EMT Tooth Saver, 3M Save-a-Tooth): a break-resistant storage container with soft inner walls and a pH-balanced solution (such as Hanks Balanced Salt Solution) that nourishes and preserves the tooth.
  - Cold whole milk
  - Sterile saline solution (for storage periods less than 1 hour)
- Transport the tooth with the patient and notify the hospital of the situation.

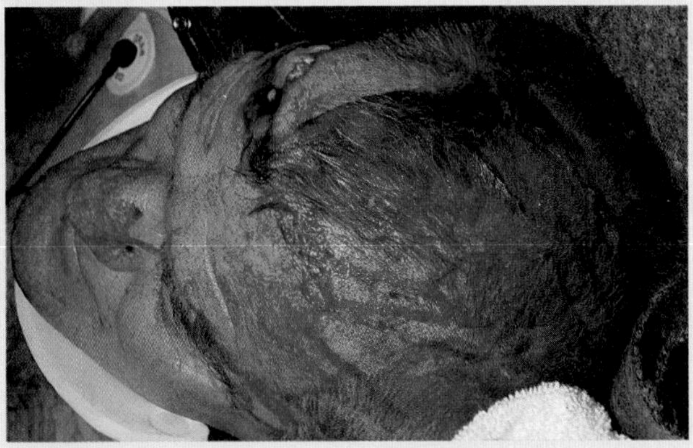

FIGURE 5-33 The scalp has a rich blood supply, so even small lacerations can lead to significant blood loss.

Head Injuries

A head injury is a traumatic insult to the head that may result in injury to soft tissue, bony structures, or the brain. More than 70% of head trauma victims worldwide are male and nearly one third of all head injuries are reported in children under the age of 15. More than half of all traumatic deaths result from a head injury.

Motor vehicle collisions are the most common mechanism of injury, with more than two thirds of people involved in motor vehicle collisions experiencing some form of head injury. Head injuries also occur commonly in victims of assault, with falls, during sports-related incidents, and in a variety of incidents involving children.

There are two general types of head injuries: open and closed. A closed head injury (the most common type) is usually associated with blunt trauma. Although the dura mater remains intact and brain tissue is not exposed to the environment, closed head injuries may result in skull fractures, focal brain injuries, or diffuse brain injuries. Furthermore, these injuries are often complicated by increased ICP.

With an open head injury, the dura mater and cranial contents are penetrated and brain tissue is open to the environment. Gunshot wounds—one of the most common penetrating mechanisms of injury—have a high mortality rate, and for those who survive there is almost always significant neurologic deficit and a decreased quality of life.

Soft-Tissue Injuries

Scalp lacerations can be minor or very serious. Because of the scalp's rich blood supply, even small lacerations can quickly lead to significant blood loss **FIGURE 5-33**. Hypovolemic shock in adults is rarely caused by scalp lacerations alone; this is more common in children. However, bleeding from the scalp can contribute to hypovolemia in any patient, especially one with multiple injuries. In addition, because scalp lacerations usually result from direct blows to the head, they often indicate deeper, more severe injuries. Because the skin is pulled tight around the scalp, wounds are often stretched open, allowing bleeding to occur unimpeded. Bleeding control is best done with direct pressure to either side of the wound, not directly above the wound.

Skull Fractures

There are four basic types of skull fractures: linear, depressed, basilar, and open **FIGURE 5-34**. The significance of a skull fracture is directly related to the type of fracture, the amount of force applied, and the area of the head that was struck. Skull fractures are most commonly seen following motor vehicle collisions and significant falls. They may or may not be associated with soft-tissue scalp injuries. Potential complications of any skull fracture include intracranial hemorrhage, cerebral damage, and cranial nerve damage, among others.

Linear Skull Fractures

Linear skull fractures (nondisplaced skull fractures) account for approximately 80% of all fractures to the skull; approximately 50% of linear fractures occur in the temporal-parietal region of the skull. Radiographic evaluation is required to diagnose a linear skull fracture because there are often no gross physical signs (such as deformity or depression). If the brain is uninjured and the scalp is intact, linear fractures are relatively benign. However, if a scalp laceration occurs in conjunction with a linear fracture—making it an open fracture—there is a risk of infection. In addition, if the fracture occurs over the temporal region of the skull, injury to the middle meningeal artery may result in epidural (extradural) bleeding.

Depressed Skull Fractures

Depressed skull fractures result from high-energy direct trauma to a small surface area of the head with a blunt

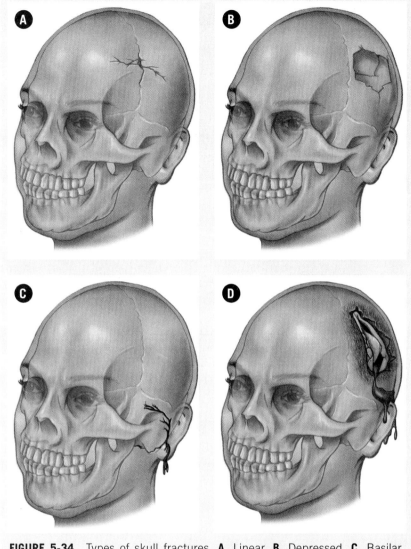

FIGURE 5-34 Types of skull fractures. **A.** Linear. **B.** Depressed. **C.** Basilar. **D.** Open.

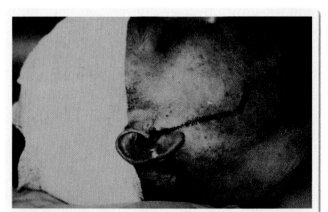

FIGURE 5-35 Blood draining from the ear after a head injury may contain CSF and suggests a basilar skull fracture.

object (such as a baseball bat to the head). The frontal and parietal regions of the skull are most susceptible to these types of fractures because the bones in these areas, compared with other bones of the skull, are relatively thin. As a consequence, bony fragments may be driven into the brain, resulting in underlying injury. The overlying scalp may or may not be intact. Patients with depressed skull fractures often present with changing neurologic signs (such as loss of consciousness).

Basilar Skull Fractures

Basilar skull fractures also are associated with high-energy trauma, but they usually occur following diffuse impact to the head (eg, falls or motor vehicle crashes). These injuries generally result from extension of a linear fracture to the base of the skull and can be difficult to diagnose without radiography.

Signs of a basilar skull fracture include CSF otorrhea (CSF drainage from the ears), which indicates rupture of the tympanic membrane and freely flowing CSF through the ear **FIGURE 5-35**. Rhinorrhea with CSF can occur as the CSF combines with blood to flow from the nose. Patients with leaking CSF are at risk for bacterial meningitis.

Other signs of a basilar skull fracture include **periorbital ecchymosis** (raccoon eyes) that develops under or around the eyes or **retroauricular ecchymosis** (Battle's sign), bruising behind the ear over the mastoid process **FIGURE 5-36**. Depending on the extent of the damage, raccoon eyes and Battle's sign may appear relatively quickly, but in many cases, they may not appear until up to 24 hours following the injury, so their absence in the prehospital setting does not rule out a basilar skull fracture.

Open Skull Fractures

Open fractures of the cranial vault result when severe forces are applied to the head, and often are associated with trauma to multiple body systems. Brain tissue may be exposed to the environment, which significantly increases the risk of a bacterial infection (such as bacterial meningitis). Open cranial vault fractures have a high mortality rate.

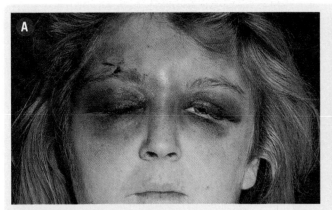
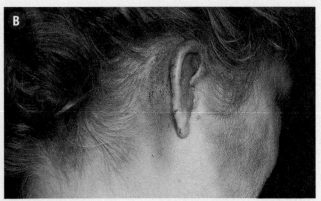

FIGURE 5-36 **A.** Ecchymosis under or around the eyes (raccoon eyes). **B.** Ecchymosis behind the ear over the mastoid process (Battle's sign).

Traumatic Brain Injury

The Brain Trauma Foundation in the United States defines a traumatic brain injury (TBI) as "a traumatic insult to the brain capable of producing physical, intellectual, emotional, social, and vocational changes." The National Collaborating Centre for Acute Care in the United Kingdom recognizes TBI as among the most important causes of death in young adults, with an overall mortality rate for severe TBI of over 50%. TBIs are classified into two broad categories: primary (direct) injury and secondary (indirect) injury.

Primary Brain Injury

Primary brain injury is injury to the brain and its associated structures that results instantaneously from impact to the head. The brain can be injured directly by a penetrating object, such as a bullet, knife, or other sharp object. More commonly, however, such injuries occur as a result of blunt external forces exerted on the skull.

For example, when the passenger's head hits the windshield of a motor vehicle on impact with a fixed object, the brain continues to move forward until it comes to an abrupt stop by striking the inside of the skull. This rapid deceleration results in compression injury (or bruising) to the anterior portion of the brain along with stretching or tearing of the posterior portion of the brain FIGURE 5-37. As the brain strikes the front of the skull, the body begins its path of moving backward. The head falls back against the headrest and/or seat, and the brain slams into the rear of the skull. This type of front-and-rear injury is known as a *coup-contrecoup* injury. The same type of injury may occur on opposite sides of the brain in a lateral collision.

Secondary Brain Injury

Secondary brain injury refers to physiologic impairments that result from the primary injury. These include processes such as cerebral edema, increased ICP, cerebral ischemia and hypoxia, and infection. Secondary brain injury can occur anywhere from a few minutes to several days following the initial injury.

STATS

TBI care consumes 1 million acute hospital bed days and over 15,000 intensive care unit bed days annually in the United Kingdom, and patients who do survive significant TBI experience an enormous burden of long-term physical disability, neurocognitive deficits, and neuropsychiatric sequelae. The financial impact is significant: The National Health Service spends over £1 billion on just the acute hospital care of the 10,000 patients with significant TBI. The costs of rehabilitation and community care are difficult to estimate, but likely total many times that number.

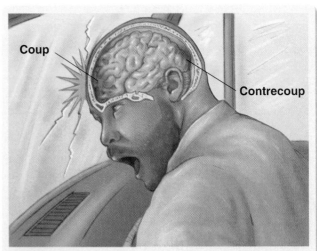

FIGURE 5-37 During rapid deceleration, the brain continues its forward motion and strikes the inside of the skull, resulting in compression injury to the anterior portion of the brain and stretching or tearing of the posterior portion.

Intracranial Pressure

The adult skull is a rigid, unyielding structure that allows little, if any, expansion within the brain. It also provides a hard and somewhat irregular surface against which brain tissue and its blood vessels can be injured following a head injury.

Accumulations of blood within the skull or swelling of the brain can rapidly lead to an increase in **intracranial pressure (ICP)**, the pressure within the cranial vault. Increased ICP squeezes the brain against bony prominences within the cranium.

Normal ICP in adults ranges from 0 to 15 mm Hg. Increases in ICP (such as from cerebral edema or intracranial hemorrhage) decrease cerebral blood flow and cerebral perfusion pressure. **Cerebral perfusion pressure (CPP)**, the pressure required to make blood flow through the brain, is the difference between blood pressure and ICP. The **mean arterial pressure (MAP)**, the average (or mean) blood pressure against the arterial wall during a cardiac cycle, must be higher than the ICP (CPP = MAP − ICP) to have blood flowing through the brain. Obviously, decreasing cerebral blood flow is a potential catastrophe because the brain depends on a constant supply of blood to furnish the oxygen and glucose it needs to survive.

The critical minimum threshold, or the minimum CPP required to adequately perfuse an adult brain, is 60 mm Hg. A CPP of less than 60 mm Hg will lead to cerebral ischemia, potentially resulting in permanent neurologic impairment or death. In fact, according to the Brain Trauma Foundation (BTF), a single drop in CPP below 60 mm Hg is associated with a doubling of mortality in the brain-injured patient. A patient with a normal ICP of 10 mm Hg requires a MAP of 70 mm Hg to maintain blood flow to the brain. (A blood pressure of 96/60 mm Hg would result in a MAP of 72 mm Hg.)

The body responds to a decrease in CPP by increasing MAP through a process known as autoregulation (also known as Cushing's reflex). This is a sympathetic release in an attempt to increase arterial blood pressure and peripheral vascular resistance. However, an increase in cerebral blood flow causes blood vessels in the brain to swell, and a further increase in ICP results. As ICP continues to increase, blood pressures must continue to increase to maintain flow to the brain.

Clearly, the patient with increased ICP is caught in the midst of a vicious cycle. As ICP increases, cerebral blood flow increases secondary to autoregulation, which in turn leads to a potentially fatal increase in ICP. Conversely, if cerebral blood flow decreases, CPP decreases as well, and the brain becomes ischemic.

CPP cannot be calculated in the prehospital setting. Therefore, prehospital treatment must focus on maintaining cerebral blood flow, while mitigating ICP as much as possible—a very fine balance to maintain.

If increased ICP is not promptly treated in a definitive care setting, cerebral herniation may occur. Because the skull is a closed box and usually contains 80% brain tissue, 12% blood volume, and 8% CSF, an increase in the volume of one requires a decrease in the volume of another. This is known as the Monro-Kellie doctrine. At first the body allows CSF to move from around the brain down through the foramen magnum to swell around the spinal column. This allows only a limited amount of room in the skull. In herniation, brain tissue is forced from the cranial vault, either through the foramen magnum or through the tentorium **FIGURE 5-38**.

Diffuse Brain Injury

Brain injuries are broadly classified as diffuse or focal. A diffuse brain injury is any injury that affects the entire brain. These injuries include cerebral concussion and diffuse axonal injury.

Cerebral Concussion

A cerebral concussion occurs when the brain is jarred around in the skull. This kind of mild diffuse brain injury is usually caused by rapid acceleration-deceleration forces

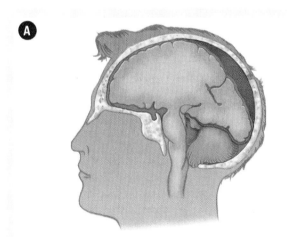 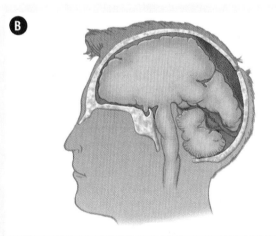

FIGURE 5-38   Herniation of the brain through the foramen magnum (**A**) and tentorium (**B**).

(coup-contrecoup), such as those seen following motor vehicle collisions or falls.

A concussion injury results in transient dysfunction of the cerebral cortex; its resolution is usually spontaneous and rapid and is not associated with structural damage or permanent neurologic impairment. Signs of a concussion range from transient confusion and disorientation to confusion that may last for several minutes. Loss of consciousness may or may not occur. **Retrograde amnesia**, a loss of memory relating to events that occurred before the injury, or **anterograde (posttraumatic) amnesia**, a loss of memory relating to events that occurred after the injury, may follow a concussion.

Diffuse Axonal Injury

Diffuse axonal injury (DAI) is often associated with a concussion. Unlike a concussion, however, this more severe diffuse brain injury is often associated with a poor prognosis. DAI involves stretching, shearing, or tearing of nerve fibers with subsequent axonal damage. An **axon** is a long, slender extension of a **neuron** (nerve cell) that conducts electrical impulses away from the **neuronal soma** (cell body) in the brain.

DAI most often results from high-speed, rapid acceleration-deceleration forces, such as motor vehicle collisions and significant falls. The severity and prognosis of

DAI depends on the degree of axonal damage (ie, stretching versus shearing or tearing); DAI is classified as being mild, moderate, or severe **TABLE 5-6**.

Focal Brain Injury

A focal brain injury is a specific, grossly observable brain injury (ie, it can be seen on a CT scan). Such injuries include cerebral contusions and intracranial hemorrhage.

Cerebral Contusion

In a **cerebral contusion**, brain tissue is bruised and damaged in a local area. Because a cerebral contusion is associated with physical damage to the brain, greater neurologic deficits (such as prolonged confusion or loss of consciousness) are more commonly observed than with a concussion. The same mechanisms of injury that cause concussions—acceleration-deceleration forces and direct blunt head trauma—also cause cerebral contusions.

The area of the brain most commonly affected by a cerebral contusion is the frontal lobe, although multiple areas of contusion can occur, especially following coup-contrecoup injuries. As with any bruise, the reaction of the injured tissue will be to swell. Significant swelling leads to increased ICP and the negative consequences that accompany it.

TABLE 5-6   Diffuse Axonal Injury

Pathophysiology	Incidence	Signs and Symptoms	Prognosis
Mild DAI			
Temporary neuronal dysfunction; minimal axonal damage	Most common result of blunt head trauma; concussion is an example	Loss of consciousness (brief, if present); confusion, disorientation, amnesia (retrograde and/or anterograde)	Minimal or no permanent neurologic impairment
Moderate DAI			
Axonal damage and minute petechial bruising of brain tissue; often associated with a basilar skull fracture	20% of all severe head injuries; 45% of all diffuse axonal injuries	Immediate loss of consciousness: secondary to involvement of the cerebral cortex or the reticular activating system of the brain stem; residual effects: persistent confusion and disorientation, cognitive impairment (eg, inability to concentrate), frequent periods of anxiety, uncharacteristic mood swings, sensory/motor deficits (such as altered sense of taste or smell)	Survival likely, but permanent neurologic impairment common
Severe DAI			
Severe mechanical disruptions of many axons in both cerebral hemispheres with extension into the brain stem; formerly called "brain stem injury"	16% of all severe head injuries; 36% of all diffuse axonal injuries	Immediate and prolonged loss of consciousness; posturing and other signs of increased ICP	Survival unlikely; most patients who survive never regain consciousness but remain in a persistent vegetative state

Intracranial Hemorrhage

The closed box of the skull allows no extra room for accumulation of blood, so bleeding inside the skull also increases ICP. Bleeding can occur between the skull and dura mater, beneath the dura mater but outside the brain, within the parenchyma (tissue) of the brain itself (intracerebral space), or into the cerebral spinal fluid CSF (subarachnoid space).

An **epidural (extradural) hematoma** is an accumulation of blood between the skull and dura mater **FIGURE 5-39**. It is usually the result of a blow to the head that produces a linear fracture of the thin temporal bone. The middle meningeal artery courses along a groove in that bone, so it is prone to disruption when the temporal bone is fractured. In such a case, brisk arterial bleeding into the epidural (**extradural**) space results in rapidly progressing symptoms.

It is common for the patient with an epidural hematoma to lose consciousness immediately following the injury; this is often followed by a brief period of consciousness (lucid interval), after which the patient lapses back into unconsciousness and begins experiencing the deleterious effects of increased ICP. Death may follow very rapidly without surgery to evacuate the hematoma.

A **subdural hematoma** is an accumulation of blood beneath the dura mater but outside the brain **FIGURE 5-40**. It usually occurs after falls or injuries involving strong deceleration forces. Subdural hematomas are more common than epidural (extradural) hematomas and may or may not be associated with a skull fracture. Bleeding within the subdural space typically results from rupture of the veins that bridge the cerebral cortex and dura.

A subdural hematoma is associated with venous bleeding, so this type of hematoma—and the signs of increased ICP—typically develops more gradually than an epidural hematoma. The patient with a subdural hematoma often experiences a fluctuating level of consciousness, focal neurologic signs (such as unilateral hemiparesis), or slurred speech.

Subdural hematomas are classified as acute (clinical signs developing within 24 hours following injury) or chronic (symptoms may not appear for as long as 2 weeks). Chronic subdural hematomas are more common in elderly patients, patients with alcoholism, patients with bleeding diatheses (such as hemophilia), and patients taking anticoagulants (such as warfarin).

An **intracerebral hematoma** involves bleeding within the brain tissue (parenchyma) itself **FIGURE 5-41**. This type of injury can occur following a penetrating injury to the head or because of rapid deceleration forces.

Many small, deep intracerebral hemorrhages are associated with other brain injuries, such as DAI. The progression of increased ICP and neurologic deficit depends on several factors, including the presence of other brain injuries, the region of the brain involved (frontal and temporal lobes are most common), and the size of the hemorrhage. Once symptoms appear, the patient's condition often deteriorates quickly. Intracerebral hematomas have a high mortality rate, even if the hematoma is surgically evacuated.

In a **subarachnoid hemorrhage**, bleeding occurs into the subarachnoid space, where the

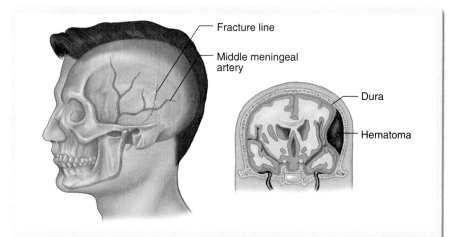

FIGURE 5-39 In an epidural hematoma, arterial blood rapidly accumulates between the dura mater and the skull.

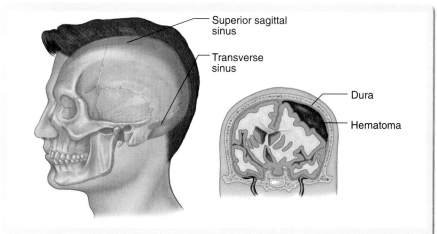

FIGURE 5-40 In a subdural hematoma, venous bleeding occurs beneath the dura mater but outside the brain.

CSF circulates. It results in bloody CSF and signs of meningeal irritation (such as nuchal rigidity or headache). Common causes of a subarachnoid hemorrhage include trauma or rupture of an aneurysm or arteriovenous malformation (AVM).

The patient with a subarachnoid hematoma typically presents with a sudden, severe headache (sometimes described as a "thunder clap" headache). This headache is often localized initially but later becomes diffuse due to increased meningeal irritation. As bleeding into the subarachnoid space increases, the patient experiences the signs and symptoms of increased ICP: decreased level of consciousness, pupillary changes, posturing, vomiting, and seizures.

A sudden, severe subarachnoid hematoma often results in death. People who survive often have permanent neurologic impairment.

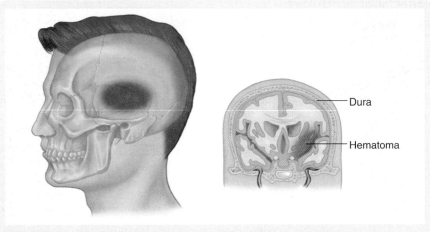

FIGURE 5-41 An intracerebral hematoma involves bleeding within the brain tissue itself.

Assessment of Traumatic Brain Injury

Motor vehicle collisions, direct blows, falls from heights, assaults, and sports-related injuries are common causes of head and traumatic brain injuries. A patient who has experienced any of these events should immediately elevate your index of suspicion and prompt a search for signs and symptoms of these types of injuries **TABLE 5-7**.

Level of Consciousness

A change in the level of consciousness is the single most important observation you can make when assessing the severity of a TBI. The level of consciousness usually indicates the extent of brain dysfunction; assessing it frequently allows you to detect subtle changes in the patient's clinical status. Whenever you suspect a head injury, you should perform a baseline neurologic assessment using the AVPU scale (Alert; responsive to Verbal stimuli; responsive to Pain; Unresponsive) and record the time.

Assessing Intracranial Pressure

Although ICP cannot be quantified (assigned a numeric value) in the prehospital setting, its severity can be estimated based on the patient's clinical presentation **TABLE 5-8**. You must monitor the head-injured patient closely for signs and symptoms of increased ICP. The exact clinical signs encountered depend on the amount of pressure inside the skull and the extent of brain stem involvement. Early signs and symptoms include vomiting (often without nausea), headache, an altered level of consciousness, and seizures. Later, more ominous signs include hypertension (with a widening pulse pressure), bradycardia, and irregular respirations (Cushing's triad). Pupillary abnormalities, coma, and posturing are also ominous signs.

As ICP increases, the body tries to compensate for the decreasing blood flow to the brain. As the ICP rises to the

TABLE 5-7   Signs and Symptoms of Head Injury
• Lacerations, contusions, or hematomas to the scalp
• Soft area or depression noted on palpation of the scalp
• Visible fracture or deformities of the skull
• Battle sign or raccoon eyes
• CSF rhinorrhea or otorrhea
• Cushing's triad: hypertension, bradycardia, and irregular or erratic respirations
• Dizziness
• Nausea or vomiting
• Pupillary abnormalities
• Unequal pupil size
• Sluggish or nonreactive pupils
• Visual disturbances, blurred vision, or double vision (diplopia)
• Seeing "stars"
• Severe headache ("worst ever")
• Confusion or disorientation
• Repeatedly asking the same question(s) (perseveration)
• Amnesia (retrograde and/or anterograde)
• Combativeness or other abnormal behavior
• A period of unresponsiveness
• Numbness or tingling in the extremities
• Loss of sensation and/or motor function
• Focal neurologic deficits
• Seizures
• Posturing (decorticate and/or decerebrate)

TABLE 5-8	Signs and Symptoms of Increasing ICP
Mild elevation	• Cheyne-Stokes respirations (respirations that are fast and then become slow, with intervening periods of apnea • Decreased pulse rate • Increased blood pressure • Pupils still reactive • Patient initially attempts to localize and remove painful stimuli; this is followed by withdrawal and extension • *Effects are reversible with prompt treatment*
Moderate elevation	• Central neurogenic hyperventilation (deep, rapid respirations; similar to Kussmaul, but without an acetone breath odor) • Widened pulse pressure • Bradycardia • Pupils are sluggish or nonreactive • Decerebrate posturing • *Survival possible, but not without permanent neurologic deficit*
Severe elevation	• Ataxic respirations (Biot respirations; characterized by irregular rate, pattern, and volume of breathing with intermittent periods of apnea) or absent respirations • Irregular pulse rate • Fluctuating blood pressure; hypotension common • Changes in the QRS complex, ST segment, or T wave • Ipsilaterally fixed and dilated ("blown") pupil • Flaccid paralysis • *Most patients do not survive this level of ICP*

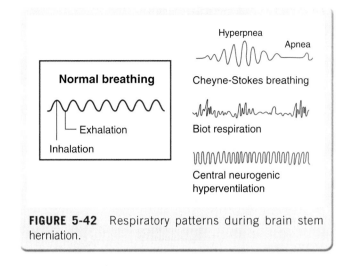

FIGURE 5-42 Respiratory patterns during brain stem herniation.

GLASGOW COMA SCALE

Eye Opening

Spontaneous	4
To Voice	3
To Pain	2
None	1

Verbal Response

Oriented	5
Confused	4
Inappropriate Words	3
Incomprehensible Words	2
None	1

Motor Response

Obeys Command	6
Localizes Pain	5
Withdraws (pain)	4
Flexion (pain)	3
Extension (pain)	2
None	1

Glasgow Coma Score Total	**15**

FIGURE 5-43 Glasgow Coma Scale scores should be assessed frequently in head-injured patients. The lower the score, the more severe the extent of brain injury.

point of herniation, respirations increase in rate and depth to decrease the amount of carbon dioxide in the blood. (Hyperventilation decreases the size of the blood vessels and therefore the amount of space required in the skull.) When the ICP decreases, the brain allows the chemoreceptors to work normally to stimulate breathing based on the CO_2 level in the bloodstream. Because the levels are decreased from the brief period of hyperventilation, the respiratory pattern slows and becomes shallow, allowing the CO_2 to rise again to normal levels. This rise in carbon dioxide allows the ICP to rise and the pattern starts again. This pattern is recognized as Cheyne-Stokes breathing **FIGURE 5-42**. When the ICP increases and the respiratory cycle does not allow it to decrease, the body continues trying to compensate and produces a pattern of hyperventilation called central neurogenic hyperventilation. This pattern is characterized by rapid, deep breaths attempting to blow off carbon dioxide. This respiratory pattern is similar in function to the Kussmaul breathing seen in diabetic ketoacidosis (DKA), but the pattern appears more exaggerated. Biot respirations are much more irregular by nature and represent damage to the medulla oblongata. They are sometimes called "clustered breathing" because the patient has bursts of irregular breaths followed by an apneic period. Biot's breathing has little or no pattern to it and requires ventilation assistance when encountered.

Glasgow Coma Scale

When performing serial neurologic assessments of a head-injured patient, the **Glasgow Coma Scale (GCS)** should be used **FIGURE 5-43**. The GCS—a widely accepted method of assessing level of consciousness—is based on three independent measurements: eye opening, verbal response, and motor response.

Prehospital measurement of the GCS is a significant and reliable indicator of the severity of TBI and should be assessed frequently to identify improvement or deterioration over time. The adult GCS should be used for patients older than 5 years. Brain injuries with a GCS of 13–15 are considered mild, 9–12 are moderate, and below 9 are considered severe **PROCEDURE 3** **PROCEDURE 4**.

Posturing

<u>Posturing</u> is an abnormal response to painful stimuli associated with increases in ICP. **Decorticate (flexor) posturing** involves rigidity and flexion of the arms toward the chest as well as extension of the legs. **Decerebrate (extensor) posturing** involves rigid extension of the arms and legs and is usually accompanied with downward pointing of the toes and arching of the head **FIGURE 5-44**.

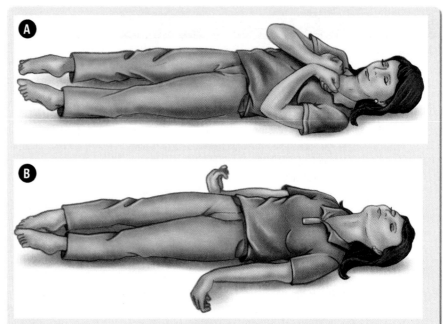

FIGURE 5-44   Posturing indicates significant ICP. **A.** Decorticate (flexor) posturing. **B.** Decerebrate (extensor) posturing. You can remember the difference by thinking of the arms being pulled into the "core" of the body.

Pupillary Assessment

Frequently monitor the size, symmetry, and reactivity of the head-injured patient's pupils. The pupillary response depends on a properly functioning retina, optic nerve, brain stem, and oculomotor nerve (third cranial nerve). Localized injury to the eye can cause the pupil not to respond, but deeper brain function is often the cause of altered pupillary response.

Shining a light into the pupil should cause it to constrict briskly (direct response); the contralateral pupil should constrict simultaneously as well (consensual response). Both pupils should constrict to the same size and then dilate simultaneously when the light source is removed. The direct pupillary response assesses unilateral oculomotor nerve function, and the consensual pupillary response assesses contralateral nerve function.

A pupil that is slow or sluggish to constrict is a relatively early sign of increased ICP; a sluggish pupil could also indicate cerebral hypoxia. Asymmetric (unequal) or bilaterally fixed and dilated ("blown") pupils are later, more ominous signs of increased ICP and indicate pressure on one or both oculomotor nerves **FIGURE 5-45**.

Asymmetry is defined as greater than 1 mm difference in pupillary diameter. A fixed pupil is defined as less than 1 mm constriction in response to light.

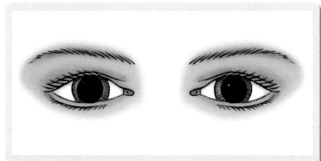

FIGURE 5-45   Asymmetric or bilaterally fixed and dilated (shown above) pupils in a head-injured patient are ominous signs and indicate a significantly increased ICP.

Confounding Factors

When assessing a patient with a TBI, be aware of the underlying factors that could potentially complicate your assessment. Although these patients may be difficult to assess regardless of confounding factors, it is important that you consider these factors in your assessment.

Alcohol/Drugs

Changes to the level of consciousness are common with patients experiencing some form of head trauma. Patients who have alcohol and/or illicit drugs in their system may also present with an altered mental status regardless of whether a head injury took place. It may be unclear if the patient has a decreased level of consciousness due to the head injury or from the effects of alcohol/drugs. High blood alcohol levels may also cause pupillary abnormalities and dysconjugate gaze.

Age
Head injuries to pediatric patients are significant injuries. The anatomy of the child's brain and skull make head trauma more likely. Their compensatory mechanisms are not as developed, making a slower response to lower CPP than in adults.

Elderly patients are subject to significant head injuries as well. These patients are prone to falls and other accidents; therefore, assessing for a possible head injury is imperative when treating these patients. As people age, brain tissue begins to atrophy; this allows for larger potential spaces inside the skull for intracranial bleeding. Elderly patients do possess compensatory mechanisms; however, many are inhibited by preexisting medical conditions and medication use. Getting a clear understanding of the patient's baseline mental status, medical history, and medication use is essential to the assessment and treatment of this population.

Previous Medical Conditions
Underlying medical conditions should be considered in any head trauma patient. Conditions that cause altered levels of consciousness may add to the difficulty when assessing a head injury. Patients with dementia or brain diseases such as Alzheimer's may have an altered mental status as their baseline. If possible, ask the patient or family questions regarding previous medical conditions, such as a cerebrovascular accident (CVA) or diabetes, when assessing their mental or neurologic status.

When considering the underlying medical conditions, consider the possibility that an underlying condition may have precipitated the traumatic injury. Patients with a history of transient ischemic attacks or hypoglycemia may have sustained a traumatic injury as a direct result of an underlying medical condition. Make sure you complete a thorough assessment of your patient to look for possible medical causes of the traumatic injury.

Treatment of the Traumatic Brain Injury
As with any patient, airway management is always the first priority when initiating treatment of the traumatic brain injury patient. If the patient is unable to maintain his or her airway due to an altered level of consciousness, open the airway with the most appropriate method for the situation (see Chapter 3).

Vomiting is common with head injury patients and often occurs without nausea. Swelling or injury can stimulate centers along the medulla that cause a violent and often projectile vomiting episode. Be prepared to manage the airway aggressively if your patient begins to vomit. Rolling the patient on the side—while maintaining spinal stabilization—may be

necessary to prevent aspiration. Use suction to clear secretions, such as blood or thin secretions from the oropharynx. It is important to note that mortality significantly increases if aspiration occurs.

Ventilation/Hyperventilation
Cerebral edema and ICP are aggravated by hypoxia and hypercarbia (CO_2 is a potent vasodilator); therefore, you must continually assess the ventilatory status of a head trauma patient to ensure adequate oxygenation and ventilation.

Research has demonstrated that prompt administration of supplemental oxygen can reduce the amount of brain damage and improve neurologic outcome. An injured brain is even less tolerant of hypoxia than a healthy one; therefore, administration of high-flow oxygen should be applied as early as possible.

If the respiratory center of the brain (pons and medulla) has been injured, the rate, depth, or regularity of breathing may be ineffective. Ventilation may also be impaired by concomitant chest injuries or, if the spinal cord is injured, by paralysis of some or all of the respiratory muscles. Patients with signs of inadequate ventilation such as shallow ventilations or slow respiratory rates, especially if associated with a decreased level of consciousness, should receive bag-mask ventilation and 100% oxygen.

Ventilate a brain-injured adult at a rate of 10–12 breaths/min or as dictated by local protocol. Avoid routine hyperventilation of brain-injured patients. Although hyperventilation causes cerebral vasoconstriction, which will shunt blood from the cranium and lower ICP, this outcome will merely provide additional room for the injured brain to swell or for more blood to accumulate in the skull. Most importantly, cerebral vasoconstriction shunts oxygen away from the brain, resulting in a drop in CPP and increasing cerebral ischemia. Overaggressive ventilations may result in a secondary ischemic brain injury. Patients should be hyperventilated (20 breaths/min for adults, 25 for children, and 30 for infants) only if signs of cerebral herniation are present:

- Asymmetric pupils or pupils that are nonreactive
- Decorticate or decerebrate posturing
- Decrease in GCS of 2 or more points if the original score was 9 or less

Management of increasing ICP should begin with simple efforts to decrease any backup of venous flow from the head. If no spinal injury is suspected, raise the head of the stretcher to 30°. If the patient is immobilized on a long backboard, raise the head of the backboard by placing a rolled blanket or towel underneath it. The patient should be placed into a cervical collar to keep the head upright to avoid positioning that would place pressure on the venous structures of the neck. Proper cervical collar sizing and placement should be ensured to avoid external obstruction of the structures **PROCEDURE 16**.

When available, end-tidal carbon dioxide (ETCO$_2$) is the preferred method for monitoring ventilation and should be assessed with digital capnometry. Optimally, you should ventilate the patient to maintain ETCO$_2$—an approximation of arterial Paco$_2$—between 35 and 40 mm Hg. Under no circumstances should the Paco$_2$ be allowed to drop below 30 mm Hg during hyperventilation, because the subsequent vasoconstriction will almost assuredly result in brain injury due to hypoxia.

Endotracheal intubation of a head-injured patient requires special precautions or it may precipitate dangerous increases in ICP. If intubation of the head-injured patient is required (ie, unresponsive patient, unable to ventilate with a bag-mask device), observe the following guidelines:

- Preoxygenate the patient with 100% oxygen for at least 2–3 minutes or an oxygen saturation (Sao$_2$) reading of 100%.
- Consider administering 1–1.5 mg/kg of lidocaine IV push. Lidocaine may blunt an acute increase in ICP during intubation. Follow your local protocol or consult medical control when considering lidocaine for these patients.
- Perform intubation with the patient's head in a neutral position. Intubation of the head-injured or any patient with significant trauma should be performed by two people: one to maintain manual stabilization of the patient's head and the other to intubate.
- Closely monitor the patient's Sao$_2$ and maintain it at 95% or higher.
- Monitor capnometry and maintain an ETCO$_2$ level between 35–40 mm Hg.

TIP

Effectively managing a brain-injured patient's airway and ensuring adequate oxygenation and ventilation are absolutely critical to the patient's survival.

Fluid Administration

An isolated closed head injury will not cause hypovolemic shock in an adult because the skull does not have enough room to accommodate large volumes of blood. If signs of shock are present (ie, persistent hypotension, tachycardia, diaphoresis), carefully assess the patient for occult injuries such as intra-abdominal or intrathoracic hemorrhage.

Establish at least one large-bore IV with normal saline or lactated Ringer's or Hartmann's solution. Use caution when administering dextrose-containing solutions (such as 5% dextrose in water [D$_5$W]) because osmolarity of the solution may worsen cerebral edema.

Brain-injured patients are often hypertensive—a sign of the body's autoregulatory response. IV fluid infusions should be restricted to 25–50 mL/h to minimize cerebral edema and ICP. However, if hypotension develops, infuse fluids as needed to maintain a systolic blood pres-

TIP

When assessing and managing an adult with a severe head injury, use the "90-90-9 rule":
- A single drop in the patient's oxygen saturation (Sao$_2$) to less than 90% doubles his or her chance of death.
- A single drop in the patient's systolic blood pressure to less than 90 mm Hg doubles his or her chance of death.
- A single drop in the patient's GCS score to less than 9 doubles his or her chance of death. A drop in the GCS score of two or more points, at any time, also doubles mortality.

sure of at least 90 mm Hg. Hypotension in a brain-injured patient can be lethal because it may decrease CPP with resultant cerebral ischemia, permanent brain damage, and death.

Thermal Regulation

Regulating body temperature is important in any trauma patient. Patients with head injuries, however, unlike those with shock, can develop a very high body temperature (**hyperpyrexia**). This can worsen the condition of the brain, resulting in further permanent damage; therefore, do not allow the patient to become overheated. If the ambient temperature is 70°F (21°C) or higher, refrain from covering the patient with a blanket.

Associated Injury Treatment

Associated injuries are quite common with head injury patients. If the patient has any external hemorrhaging or leakage of CSF from the ears or nose, cover the areas with a sterile dressing and apply direct pressure to any uncontrolled bleeding. Lightly cover open skull fractures with exposed brain tissue with a sterile dressing that has been moistened with sterile saline. Objects impaled in the skull should be stabilized in place and protected from movement.

Pharmacologic Therapy

Pharmacologic therapy, other than that used to facilitate intubation or treat seizures, is usually not indicated for brain-injured patients in the prehospital setting. If transport will be prolonged, however, medical control may order the administration of certain medications.

Steroids   The use of steroids has been shown to be detrimental to TBI patients and is associated with increased mortality.

Diuretics   Mannitol is widely accepted for use in TBI. It is a sugar compound that elevates blood plasma osmolarity, resulting in enhanced flow of water from tissues, including the brain and cerebrospinal fluid, into interstitial fluid and plasma. Its osmotic properties take up to 15 to 30 minutes to create the pressure gradient that will draw water out of the neurons. As a result, cerebral edema, elevated ICP, and cerebrospinal fluid volume and pressure may be reduced. Mannitol should not be used for extended periods. It is best used by bolus to manage acute changes associated with increasing ICP and herniation of brain tissue. Dosing is between 0.3 and 1 g/kg IV over 5 minutes. Higher dose mannitol has become controversial following review of the literature.

Furosemide (Lasix) is another diuretic that can be given in the setting of increasing ICP and cerebral herniation. Dosing is 0.5 to 1 mg/kg by IV. Lasix is a loop diuretic and creates a generalized diuresis, but there is little evidence that cerebral tissue is directly affected.

Anticonvulsants Seizures in a brain-injured patient must be terminated as soon as possible so they do not provoke further increases in ICP or body temperature. Use benzodiazepines, such as diazepam (Valium) or lorazepam (Ativan), to control seizure activity in brain-injured patients. Follow local protocol or contact medical control regarding the doses of these medications.

Phenytoin (Dilantin) or fosphenytoin (Cerebyx) are preferred treatments for some areas. Dosing is 15 to 20 mg/kg IV given at a rate of no more than 50 mg/min. Carbamazepine and phenobarbitol can also be useful in management of seizures.

Injury to the Anterior Neck

Situated in the neck are the critical portion of the airway (ie, larynx, trachea), the major blood vessels to and from the head, and the spinal cord; this makes it extremely susceptible to life-threatening injuries. Any injury to the anterior part of the neck—blunt or penetrating—must be considered critical until proven otherwise. Other structures contained within the neck that are also vulnerable to injury include muscles, nerves, and glands.

Soft-Tissue Injuries

Blunt and penetrating mechanisms can damage the soft tissues of the anterior neck and its associated structures. In both cases, you must be aware of the potential for cervical spine injuries and airway compromise.

Blunt trauma to the soft tissues of the neck often results in swelling and edema, particularly injury to the trachea, larynx, esophagus, or cervical spine. Less commonly, blunt injuries may damage the vasculature of the anterior neck. Carefully assess the patient and be prepared to initiate aggressive management; blunt trauma to the neck is associated with a high incidence of airway compromise and ventilatory inadequacy.

The primary threats from penetrating neck trauma are massive hemorrhage from major blood vessel disruption and airway compromise secondary to soft-tissue swelling or direct damage to the larynx or trachea. Although lacerations or puncture wounds may be superficial and involve

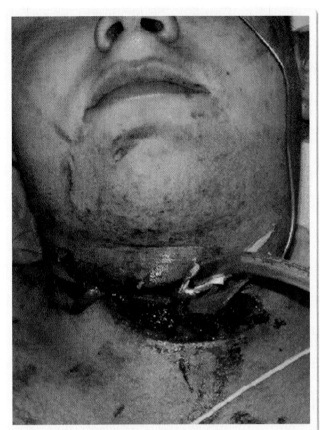

FIGURE 5-46 Open injuries to the neck can be very dangerous. If vital structures are exposed, airway, breathing, and circulation can all be at risk.

only the fascia or fatty tissues of the neck, assessment for deep and involved injury to the larynx, trachea, esophagus, nerves, or major blood vessels of the neck needs to be considered.

A special danger associated with open neck injuries is the possibility of a fatal air embolism. If the large veins of the neck are exposed to the environment, they may pull air into the vessel and occlude the flow of blood to the lungs **FIGURE 5-46** .

Impaled objects in the neck can present several life-threatening problems for the patient, including injury to major blood vessels with massive hemorrhage; damage to the larynx, trachea, or esophagus; or injury to the cervical spine **FIGURE 5-47** . Impaled objects should not be removed but rather stabilized in place and protected from movement. The only exception is if the object is obstructing the airway or impeding your ability to effectively manage the airway. In some cases, an emergency cricothyrotomy may be necessary to establish and maintain a patent airway **PROCEDURE 11** **PROCEDURE 12** .

Injuries to the Larynx, Trachea, and Esophagus

It is important to maintain a high index of suspicion and perform a careful assessment of any patient with blunt trauma to the anterior part of the neck. Significant injuries

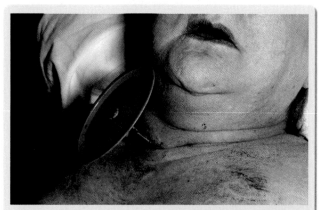

FIGURE 5-47 Impaled objects in the neck can cause profuse bleeding if the major blood vessels are damaged, as well as direct injury to the larynx, trachea, esophagus, or cervical spine.

TABLE 5-9 Signs and Symptoms of Injuries to the Anterior Part of the Neck	
Injury	**Signs and Symptoms**
Laryngeal fracture, tracheal transaction	• Stridor • Hoarseness, voice changes • Labored breathing or reduced air movement • Hemoptysis (coughing up blood) • Subcutaneous emphysema • Swelling, edema
Vascular injury	• Gross external bleeding • Signs of shock • Hematoma, swelling, edema • Pulse deficits
Esophageal perforation	• Dysphagia (difficulty swallowing) • Hematemesis • Hemoptysis (suggests aspiration of blood)
Neurologic impairment	• Signs of a stroke (suggests air embolism or cerebral infarct) • Paralysis or paresthesia • Cranial nerve deficit • Signs of neurogenic shock

to the larynx or trachea pose an immediate risk of airway compromise due to the disruption of normal air passage, soft-tissue swelling, or aspiration of blood into the lungs. The larynx and its supporting structures (ie, hyoid bone, thyroid cartilage) may be fractured, the trachea may be transected from the larynx, or the esophagus may be perforated. Esophageal perforation can result in mediastinitis, an inflammation of the mediastinum often due to leakage of gastric contents into the thoracic cavity. Mediastinitis is associated with a high mortality rate if not surgically repaired in a timely manner.

Many injuries to the larynx, trachea, and esophagus are occult; because they are not as obvious and dramatic as penetrating neck injuries, they can be easily overlooked. Therefore, it is imperative that a complete assessment of the neck is conducted and high index of suspicion is maintained when dealing with anterior neck injuries.

> **TIP**
>
> Any blunt force that is powerful enough to disrupt the larynx, trachea, or esophagus is powerful enough to injure the cervical spine, so the use of spinal motion restriction is important. Carefully assess the patient for signs of a spinal injury: vertebral deformities (step-offs), paralysis, paresthesia, or signs of neurogenic shock (hypotension, normal or slow heart rate, lack of diaphoresis).

Patients with injuries to the anterior part of the neck may experience concomitant maxillofacial fractures, which can make bag-mask ventilation difficult (usually because of an inadequate mask-to-face seal). Likewise, endotracheal intubation may be extremely challenging, if not impossible,

owing to distortion of the normal anatomic structures of the upper airway. If basic and advanced techniques to secure the patient's airway are unsuccessful or impossible, a surgical or needle cricothyrotomy may be your only means of establishing a patent airway and ensuring adequate oxygenation and ventilation.

Bruising, redness to the overlying skin, and palpable tenderness are common signs associated with all injuries to the anterior part of the neck. **TABLE 5-9** summarizes the signs and symptoms of specific injuries.

Treatment of Injuries to the Anterior Neck

The primary focus is always on treating injuries that will be the most rapidly fatal. Because death following trauma to the anterior neck is usually the result of airway compromise or massive bleeding, aggressive airway management and external bleeding control are the highest priorities of care. After addressing any life-threatening or other serious problems with the ABCs during the initial/primary assessment, you may perform a rapid trauma/secondary assessment to detect and treat other injuries.

Immediately cover open wounds to the neck with an occlusive dressing to control bleeding and prevent air embolism **FIGURE 5-48**. Apply manual direct pressure over

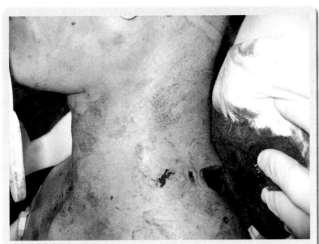

FIGURE 5-48 Cover open neck wounds with an occlusive dressing and apply manual pressure to control bleeding.

TIP

Avoid using positive-pressure ventilation on a patient with trauma to the anterior part of the neck and signs of laryngeal or tracheal injury when possible. The pressure delivered by such devices can cause barotrauma and potentially exacerbate the patient's injury.

the occlusive dressing with a bulky dressing. Do not circumferentially wrap bandages around the neck to secure the dressing in place; this may impair cerebral perfusion by occluding the carotid arteries or interfere with the patient's breathing, which could have fatal consequences. Monitor the patient's pulse for reflex bradycardia, which may indicate parasympathetic nervous stimulation due to excessive pressure on the vagus nerve within the carotid artery sheath.

If signs of shock are present, keep the patient warm; establish vascular access with at least one large-bore IV en route to the hospital if possible, or on-scene if indicated; and infuse an isotonic crystalloid solution (such as lactated Ringer's [Hartmann's Solution]or normal saline) as needed to maintain adequate perfusion.

If the patient has experienced an open tracheal wound, you may be able to pass a cuffed ET tube directly through the wound to establish a patent airway. Use caution, however, because the trachea may be perforated anteriorly and posteriorly, which could increase the risk of false passage of the ET tube outside the trachea. It is critical to use multiple techniques for confirming correct tube placement: frequently monitor breath sounds, use capnometry, assess for adequate chest rise, and assess for vapor mist in the ET tube during exhalation.

Injury to the Cervical Spine

Cervical spine injuries are some of the most devastating injuries found in the prehospital environment. Although prehospital practitioners have limited treatment options for spinal cord injuries in the field, participating in preventive measures for reducing the number of annual spinal cord injuries is the provider's best option for decreasing the morbidity and mortality associated with spinal cord injuries.

Acute injuries of the cervical spine are classified according to the associated mechanism, location, and stability of the injury. Vertebral fractures can occur with or without associated spinal cord injury. Because stable fractures do not involve the posterior column, they pose less risk to the spinal cord. Unstable injuries involve the posterior column of the spinal cord and typically include damage to portions of the vertebrae and ligaments that directly protect the spinal cord and nerve roots. Unstable injuries carry a higher risk of complicating spinal cord injury and progression of injury without appropriate treatment.

Flexion Injuries

Flexion injuries result from forward movement of the head, typically as the result of rapid deceleration or from a direct blow to the occiput. At the level of C1-C2, these forces can produce an unstable dislocation at the atlanto-occipital joint with or without an associated fracture. Loss of more than half the original size of the vertebral body or multiple levels of injury suggests involvement of the posterior column.

Hyperflexion injuries of greater force can result in teardrop fractures—avulsion fractures of the anterior-inferior border of the vertebral body. The injuries to ligaments associated with teardrop fractures raise concern for possible spinal cord injury and qualify as unstable fractures. Severe flexion can also result in a potentially unstable dislocation of vertebral joints. This situation does not involve fracture, but can severely injure the ligaments. Strong forces can result in the anterior displacement of facet joints. A bilateral facet dislocation is an extremely unstable fracture.

Rotation With Flexion

The only area of the spine that allows for significant rotation is C1–C2. Injuries to this area are considered unstable due to its high cervical location and scant bony and soft-tissue support. Rotation-flexion injuries often result from high acceleration forces. Rotation with abrupt flexion can produce a stable dislocation in the cervical spine.

Vertical Compression

Vertical compression forces are transmitted through vertebral bodies and directed either inferiorly through the skull or superiorly through the pelvis or feet. They typically result from a direct blow to the crown (parietal region) of the skull or rapid deceleration from a fall through the feet, legs, and

Clearing a C-spine in the Field

TO BE INVOLVED IN A ROAD collision or a fall and to end up tetraplegic is a tragedy, but to be neurologically intact initially and develop tetraplegia minutes, hours, or days later is an even greater tragedy because this should be preventable. If a health care professional is in any way involved (eg, by moving the neck or by allowing the patient to move the neck), that professional (and his or her employer) have a problem too because he or she may face severe and expensive medicolegal consequences. Even if the patient has a neurologic injury when first seen, careful handling may prevent worsening of a spinal cord injury (eg, deteriorating from a C6 level, which enables the patient to flex the elbows and rotate the forearms, to a C5 level signifies a major loss of function). For this reason, it is essential to have a low threshold for immobilizing the cervical spine if there is any possibility of spinal or cord injury. It is better to immobilize 100 spines than to miss one significant fracture.

Admittedly, this requirement to immobilize the spine is not evidence-based,[1] and it has been argued that it is unlikely that a patient with a fracture would cause a cord injury by moving the neck because the forces a patient will exert by movement will be minimal compared to those that occurred at the time of the injury. Sometimes, in the hospital, the assessment of the stability of a known spinal fracture is done by moving the neck and taking radiographs in flexion and extension. However, few would dispute the need for a low threshold in immobilizing the neck.

The current UK national guidelines for paramedics state: "All patients should be initially immobilized if the mechanism of injury suggests the possibility of SCI [spinal cord injury]."[2] The guidelines then go on to say that: "following assessment it is *possible* [emphasis added] to remove the immobilization" depending on certain criteria.

In any road collision or significant fall there is the *possibility* of a spinal cord injury, and so when faced with this advice and the consequences of mismanaging such an injury, many prehospital care providers play it safe by applying and maintaining spine immobilization even when there is no *evidence* of such an injury. They are unlikely ever to be criticized for immobilizing the spine, but might be criticized if they don't.

Unfortunately, spine immobilization is not without problems. Immobilization with a rigid collar, sandbags, and tape on a backboard is uncomfortable and even painful, and moving a neck from a position of comfort, or forcing a deformed neck (eg, in ankylosing spondylitis) into a neutral position to put on a collar may damage the spinal cord. Immobilization may raise intracranial pressure, cause dysphagia, restrict ventilation, and increase the risk of aspiration. Prolonged immobilization also risks pressure sores.[1]

Injuries of the cervical spine and cord are uncommon, and only a very small percentage of patients who have had immobilization applied will turn out to have an injury. It is known that simple neck sprains do better when treated with early mobilization than when treated with a soft collar. The effects of several hours' rigid immobilization on these injuries are unknown but may not be negligible. There is also a cost to this. If an uninjured patient has full spinal immobilization applied just because he or she has been involved in a car collision and is then transported to the hospital, there is a cost to the patient and health service for both transport and hospital assessment. Inexperienced doctors may be unhappy to "clear the cervical spine" clinically in a patient who is immobilized, and by the time the patient reaches the emergency department he or she may be complaining of pain leading to the additional costs of radiography. When the radiographs are normal and the collar is removed, it is not uncommon for the patient to then say, "Now that the collar has been removed, I feel much better and the pain has gone."

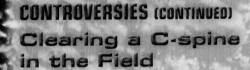

CONTROVERSIES (CONTINUED)
Clearing a C-spine
in the Field

Once a patient's neck has been immobilized, somebody needs to "clear the cervical spine" (ie, make the decision that the patient does not have a cervical spine injury and that it is safe to remove the immobilization). Traditionally this has been done in the hospital by using radiographs and, increasingly, CT scanning. This decision is not always easy, and the consequences of getting it wrong may be serious. Difficult decisions (eg, in patients with arthritic and deformed spines) are frequently referred to a specialist, not only because they have greater experience but because they get paid to make such difficult decisions. Even a normal CT scan does not exclude a potentially unstable ligamentous injury, and clearing the cervical spine of those who remain unconscious remains controversial.

Two well-validated guidelines have been drawn up to enable emergency department doctors to reduce the number of radiographs taken by clearing the cervical spine of some patients clinically without using radiographs. The first was from the NEXUS study.[3] This concluded that in blunt trauma, patients with a mechanism or force consistent with a neck injury do not need cervical spine radiographs (ie, one can clear the cervical spine) if they can satisfy all of the following five criteria:

- No midline cervical tenderness
- No focal neurologic deficit
- Normal alertness
- No intoxication
- No painful distracting injury

The other study produced the Canadian Cervical Spine Rules.[4] They state that in some patients there are low risk factors, which means it is safe to assess the range of movement of the neck. These are:

- Simple rear-end motor vehicle collision (excluding cars pushed into oncoming traffic; cars hit by a high-speed vehicle, a bus, or a large truck; and collisions resulting in a rollover)
- Sitting position in the emergency department
- Ambulatory at any time since the injury
- Delayed onset of neck pain
- Absence of midline cervical spine tenderness

The Canadian rules say that patients with any one of the following risk factors should have radiographs requested:

- GCS less than 15 at the time of assessment
- Paresthesia in the extremities
- Focal neurologic deficit
- Not possible to test for range of motion in the neck
- Patient not able to actively rotate neck 45° to the left and right (if assessment is possible)

Cervical spine imaging should also be requested in patients with the following risk factors, provided they have some neck pain or tenderness:

- Age greater than or equal to 65 years
- Dangerous mechanism of injury (fall from greater than 1 meter or five stairs; axial load to head (eg, from diving); high-speed motor vehicle collision of greater than 65 miles per hour; rollover motor accident; ejection from a motor vehicle; accident involving motorized recreational vehicles; bicycle collision). A lower threshold for height of falls should be used when dealing with infants and young children (ie, younger than 5 years old)

Absence of any requirement for radiographs will constitute clearing the cervical spine. Both sets of guidelines are very sensitive and pick up all significant fractures, but the Canadian Cervical Spine Rules may be more specific and lead to more patients being cleared clinically.

Can this decision to clear the spine be made before the patient gets to the hospital? Undoubtedly EMTs and paramedics can be taught to follow protocols based on these guidelines with the aim of clearing the cervical spine prehospital. One study has shown that 67% of patients had their spines cleared at the scene;[5] however, this study of 103 patients was not big enough to give any assurance on safety. In addition, guidelines that have been validated for use in an emergency department by doctors cannot automatically be assumed to be valid when used by EMTs and paramedics much earlier after the injury and when working in the cold, wet, and dark at the roadside.

A study of 504 patients with spinal injury showed that a different guideline was 99% sensitive for immobilizing patients later shown to have spinal fractures. However, those researchers recommended care at the extremes of age because of the five patients missed by the guideline, four were elderly and one was a child of 9 months.[6] It is not clear how many patients were cleared at the scene, but only 1.2% of patients immobilized turned out to have a fracture; however, there is the possibility that this study could have missed some patients.[7]

Although accepting that one should have a low threshold for immobilizing a patient who might have a cervical spine injury, it can be quite clear, at the scene, that some patients do not have a spinal injury despite a high-risk mechanism. Inexperienced providers might be cautious and immobilize the cervical spine, but experienced paramedics should be allowed to remove spine immobilization on such patients (or even not apply it in the first place). However, some paramedics are inexperienced and others may be overcautious or risk-takers, and so guidelines are needed to assist them in making this decision. Validated guidelines for use in the prehospital setting do not currently exist, so further research is needed. Prehospital care systems already using guidelines to allow prehospital clearance of the cervical spine should continue to use them, but their guidelines should be audited.

Henry Guly, MD, FCEM, FRCP
Consultant in Emergency Medicine
Derriford Hospital
Plymouth, United Kingdom

References

1. Kwan I, Bunn F, Roberts I, on behalf of the WHO Pre-Hospital Trauma Care Steering Committee. Spinal immobilisation for trauma patients. *Cochrane Database of Systematic Reviews.* 2001, Issue 2. Art. No.: CD002803. DOI: 10.1002/14651858. CD002803.

2. Joint Royal Colleges Ambulance Liaison Committee. *UK Ambulance Service Clinical Practice Guidelines.* Pub JRCALC. London, UK: 2006.

3. Hoffman JR, Wolfson AB, Todd K, Mower WR. Selective cervical spine radiography in blunt trauma: methodology of the National Emergency X-Radiography Utilization Study (NEXUS). *Ann Emerg Med.* 1998; 32:461–469.

4. Stiell IG, Wells GA, Vandemheen KL, et al. The Canadian c-spine rule for radiography in alert and stable trauma patients. *JAMA.* 2001; 286:1841–1848.

5. Armstrong BP, Simpson HJ, Crouch R, Deakin CD. Prehospital clearance of the cervical spine: does it need to be a pain in the neck? *Emerg Med J.* 2007; 24:501–503.

6. Stroh G, Braude D. Can an out-of-hospital cervical spine clearance protocol identify all patients with injuries? An argument for selective immobilization. *Ann Emerg Med.* 2001; 37:609–615.

7. Hoffman JR, Mower WR. Out-of-hospital cervical spine immobilization: making policy in the absence of definitive information. *Ann Emerg Med.* 2001; 37:632–634.

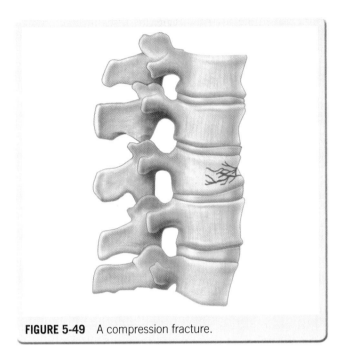

FIGURE 5-49 A compression fracture.

pelvis. Forces transmitted through the vertebral body cause fractures, ultimately shattering and producing a "burst" or compression fracture without associated spinal cord injury **FIGURE 5-49**. Compression forces can cause the herniation of disks, subsequent compression of the spinal cord and nerve roots, and fragmentation into the canal.

Most fractures resulting from these injuries are stable; however, primary spinal cord injury can occur when the vertebral body is shattered and fragments of the bone become embedded in the cord. Some compression injuries may be associated with significant retropharyngeal edema, and serious airway compromise is a consideration.

Hyperextension

Hyperextension of the head and neck can result in fractures and ligamentous injury of variable stability. The hangman's fracture (C2) or dislocation results from hyperextension due to rapid deceleration of the skull, atlas, and axis as a unit. The resulting bilateral pedicle fracture of C2 is an unstable fracture; however, it is rarely associated with a spinal cord injury. A teardrop fracture of the anterior-inferior edge of the vertebral body results from hyperextension, resulting in rupture or tear of the anterior longitudinal ligament. The injury is stable with the head and neck in flexion, but unstable in extension due to loss of structural support.

Spinal Cord Injuries

Complete disruption of all tracts of the spinal cord, with permanent loss of all cord-mediated functions below the level of injury, is commonly called a **complete spinal cord injury**. When the injury affects the patient high in the cervical spine, the result is tetraplegia or quadriplegia (loss of function in all extremities). A similar injury in the high thoracic area would result in paraplegia (loss of function in the lower extremities). Brown-Sequard syndrome is a unique

situation that occurs when only one side of the spinal cord is injured following penetrating trauma, leaving the patient with hemiparesis.

Patients who retain some degree of cord-mediated function 24 hours following an injury are classified as having an **incomplete spinal cord injury**. The initial neurologic dysfunction may be temporary, and there is some potential for recovery.

Assessment of the Cervical Spine

Limiting the progression of a spinal cord injury is the major goal of prehospital management. You should be familiar with the circumstances that commonly produce spinal cord injury and try to determine, through history taking and examination of the scene, whether any of these circumstances exist:

- Motor vehicle collision
- Collision with pedestrian/bicyclist
- Falls (greater than 1 meter [3′] or 5 steps)
- Assault (struck by fist, foot, or object)
- Contact sports
- Diving/fall onto head
- Recreational vehicle accident
- Penetrating trauma to the spine

Initial Assessment

While completing the scene size-up, determine the need for c-spine immobilization **PROCEDURE 15**. While maintaining the head and neck in a neutral position, manually stabilize the cervical spine and assess the level of consciousness. Airway maneuvers should be made with consideration for c-spine stabilization. Remember not to manipulate the cervical spine by opening the airway with a head tilt–chin lift maneuver. A jaw-thrust maneuver is a preferable method of opening an airway **PROCEDURE 6**. (For additional information on airway control see Chapter 3.)

Evaluate the patient's breathing, noting the rate, depth, and symmetry of each respiration. The diaphragm is innervated by the phrenic nerve (nerve roots C3-C5). Injury above the level of C3–C4 may present with apnea and requires immediate ventilations to survive. Lesions occurring below C5 may consequently lead to paralysis of the intercostal muscles at the level of the injury, leaving the patient dependent on the diaphragm and accessory muscles of the neck for breathing. This is seen clinically as abdominal breathing with the use of accessory muscles of the neck. Patients with inadequate respirations require assisted ventilations with a bag-mask device.

To assess perfusion, compare the radial and carotid pulses for their presence, rate, quality, regularity, and equality. Then examine the patient's skin color, temperature, and moisture. Patients with significant sensory loss from a spinal cord injury may equilibrate to the surrounding environmental temperature due to the lack of input from the periphery for temperature control. In neurogenic shock, the skin is usually warm, dry, and flushed due to vasodilation and the absence of sweating. These findings should be correlated with the patient's mental status.

Focused History and Physical Exam

An accurate history and physical examination are critical for directing management of patients with potential spinal cord injuries. Pay particular attention to the level of consciousness and mechanism of injury when assessing these patients. A patient's reliability as a historian must always be assessed before performing a focused or detailed assessment. The patient should appear calm, cooperative, nonimpaired, and able to perform cognitive functions appropriately. Patients who present with an acute stress reaction, distracting injuries (eg, long bone fractures, rib fractures, pelvic fractures, or clinically significant abdominal pain), or an alteration in mental status due to brain injury or intoxication from drugs and/or alcohol should be considered unreliable in terms of the neurologic exam. These patients should have continuous spine protection (spinal immobilization) until the presence of an injury can be excluded radiographically at the receiving hospital.

In case of potential spine injuries, the exam includes rapid inspection and palpation of the head, neck, and back for injuries. Perform a brief motor and sensory exam in all four extremities in patients with potential spinal cord injury.

You will need to expose the patient for your exam. Cut away the clothes to minimize motion of the spine during the exam or treatment. Directly observe the back to assess for penetrating trauma. Most patients can be log rolled to allow visualization of the deformity or injury. Palpate the spine to assess for deformity or displacement (step-off) of vertebral bodies. Once the exam is complete, cover the patient with a blanket to maintain normal body temperature.

The absence of pain or tenderness along the spine, coupled with a normal neurologic exam and low-risk mechanism of injury, may eliminate the need for manual in-line spinal immobilization (check local protocol). Paralysis or paresthesia of a limb, however, should always include stabilization and immobilization of the spine.

Neurologic Exam

The primary focus of the neurologic exam in the prehospital environment is to assess the need for immobilization and to determine a baseline neurologic status for later comparison. This will aid the hospital staff in assessing changes to the neurologic status and conclude if immediate surgery is needed.

The neurologic exam begins by assessing the level of consciousness. Once the initial assessment is complete, determine the GCS level of the patient. It is important to remember that patients who have limb paralysis do not receive a "1" for motor response. Instead, have the patient blink their eyes and move other muscles to assess motor response.

Continue with your neurologic exam in a head-to-toe fashion by assessing the cranial nerves. Observe the patient for drooping of the upper eyelid (ptosis) and a small pupil (Horner's syndrome) that could indicate an injury to the sympathetic pathway at the C3–C4 level.

Bilaterally assess each major motor group from the top down to identify the lowest spinal segment associated with normal voluntary motor function. Because of the possibility of incomplete spinal cord injury, it is important to determine the extent of function in segments below this level. Monitor for possible ascending lesions, paying special attention to alterations in respiratory patterns with cervical lesion.

Ask the patient to flex (C5) and extend (C7) both elbows and then both wrists (C6). Have the patient curl all four fingers while the examiner applies opposite force with his or her finger to determine strength against resistance **FIGURE 5-50**. This will test the finger flexors (C8).

Treatment of Cervical Spine Injuries

Current principles of spine trauma management include recognition of potential or actual injury, appropriate immobilization, and reduction or prevention of the chance for secondary injury. The primary goal of spinal immobilization is to prevent further injuries. Unfortunately, studies have shown that complete spinal immobilization can be painful, especially at pressure points on the occiput and lumbosacral areas, and can produce a restriction of ventilation.

The decision to immobilize the spine of a patient with a suspected spinal cord injury is based on the mechanism of injury and the clinical presentation of the patient. The NEXUS (National Emergency X-Radiography Utilization Study, 1998) study developed criteria to aid practitioners in their decision regarding radiographic study of the c-spine in the emergency department. It progressed further to the NEXUS Low-Risk Criteria (NLC) to assist prehospital providers in determining the need for c-spine immobilization **TABLE 5-10**. The criteria focus on level of consciousness, neu-

TABLE 5-10 NEXUS NLC and Canadian C-Spine Rule Protocols	
NEXUS Low-Risk Criteria	**Canadian C-Spine Rule**
Cervical spine immobilization is indicated for patients with trauma unless they meet all of the following criteria: • No posterior midline c-spine tenderness • No evidence of intoxication • A normal level of alertness (GCS = 15) • No focal deficit • No painful distracting injuries	Patients should be further evaluated (immobilized) if they: • Are over 65 • Have a severe mechanism of injury • Have paresthesias • Have tenderness to midline spine • Are walking at scene • Have decreased ROM ($< 45°$) following minor injury • Patients with delayed onset of neck pain are not evaluated.

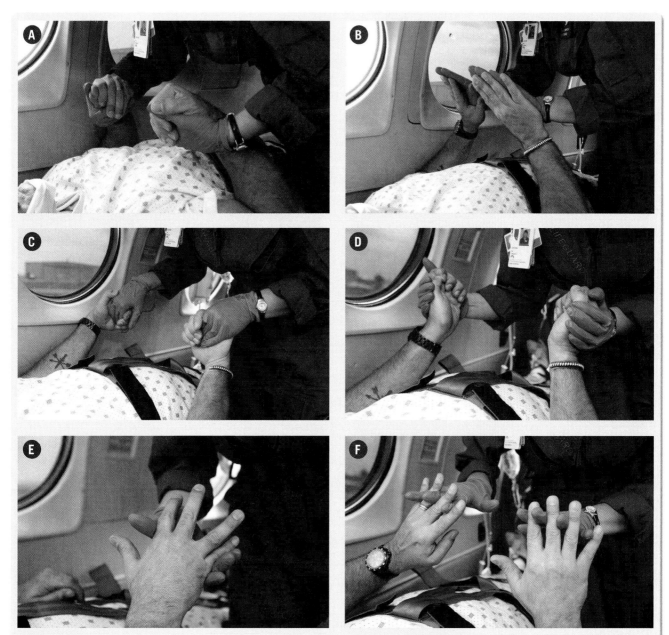

FIGURE 5-50   Ask the patient to flex (**A**) and then extend (**B**) both elbows. Ask the patient to flex (**C**) and then extend (**D**) both wrists. Have the patient abduct the fingers and keep them open against resistance (**E**), then adduct the fingers and attempt to close them against resistance (**F**).

rologic deficits, pain or deformity to the spine, mechanism of injury, presence of alcohol/drugs, distracting injuries, and communications. The Canadian Cervical Spine Rule (CCR) is also used in the emergency department, but has been found to be slightly more specific to spinal injury.

Whether the patient is suffering from blunt or penetrating trauma to the head/neck, any patient with an altered mental status or any neurologic impairment warrants immediate immobilization of the cervical spine, followed by complete spinal immobilization. Patients with an altered mental status are not reliable historians and may not be aware of their injury. In addition to neurologic deficits, tenderness or pain to the cervical vertebrae suggests significant risk of cervical spine injury. These patients require immobilization and transportation to a hospital for further assessment. Remember to assess the peripheral pulses, motor response, and sensation bilaterally before and after any immobilization of the spine.

If the patient is alert and oriented, is not exhibiting any neurologic deficits, and denies pain during the exam, consideration of the mechanism of injury should be reviewed. Not all mechanisms of trauma require spinal immobilization. However, injuries involving falls, rapid acceleration/deceleration, lateral bending forces to the neck or torso, ejection, shallow-water diving, or violent impact to the head, neck, or torso are deemed significant enough to cause spinal cord injuries. These patients should be immobilized for further evaluation of possible injury.

If the mechanism of injury is not deemed significant and the patient has no neurologic deficits, the patient may not require spinal immobilization based on the criteria. At this point, consider additional factors that may alter your assessment findings in these patients. Patients who present with alcohol or drugs may not be able to feel pain or decipher paresthesias due to the effects of the alcohol/drugs.

Consideration should be given to patients with distracting injuries and language barriers. Distracting injuries are often the focus of the patient's attention. These patients should receive full spinal immobilization precautions. The patient may not be aware of a head or neck injury due to the distracting injury; as a result, they may not verbalize pain or neurologic deficits during the assessment. In addition, patients with an inability to communicate with health care providers should be considered for spinal immobilization even when the mechanism of injury is not significant. Communication is key when determining level of consciousness and neurologic deficits. If the provider is not able to communicate with the patient and the mechanism of injury suggests the possibility of a cervical spine injury, immobilization is indicated.

Penetrating trauma that does not cause neurologic deficits may not require spinal immobilization. Neurologic changes are unlikely to occur if no injury to the spine is evident during the examination.

Cervical Spine Immobilization

If your assessment reveals that your patient meets the criteria for spinal immobilization, immediately begin the immobilization process. The word *process* indicates there is a systematic approach to spinal immobilization. By following a systematic approach, health care providers can ensure that the head, torso, and pelvis move as a unit and are properly immobilized.

Manual Stabilization Immobilization of the spine begins with manual in-line stabilization of the head and cervical spine. Explain the procedure to the patient. Hold the patient's head firmly on each side and instruct the patient not to move their head. Once manual stabilization is initiated, it must continue until the immobilization is complete with an immobilization device in place. Support the lower jaw with your index and long fingers and support the head with your palms. If the patient is supine, kneel at the head of the patient to accomplish this. Make sure the patient's head lies in a neutral position FIGURE 5-51 . Never twist, flex, or extend the head or neck excessively. If the patient is not able to move their head into a neutral position, do not force it. The patient may experience muscle spasm, numbness, tingling, or a compromised airway. Instead, immobilize the patient in the position in which you found him or her.

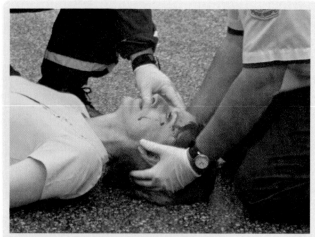

FIGURE 5-51 Bring the head and neck into neutral position while holding manual immobilization.

Occasionally, safety devices used to reduce injury will need to be removed to allow access for providers to care for the patient. Sport helmets such as those used for bicycling are easily removed and are often clear of the patient before EMS arrives. Helmets that wrap around the head to provide coverage to the entire skull can make airway care or immobilization impossible without the removal of the helmet. Patients who are wearing full-face helmets should have the helmets removed to facilitate complete assessment of the head, neck, and airway. Helmet removal will also allow the provider to move the patient's neck into neutral alignment from the flexion caused by most large helmets.

Some local protocols require helmets to be left in place if the helmet is tightly fitted to the patient, there is no airway compromise, and the patient is in a neutral position. However, if there is risk for airway deterioration, the helmet is improperly fitted and loose on the patient's head, or the patient cannot be moved into neutral position (even through use of padding), the helmet must be removed. Helmet removal requires two providers to accomplish without compromising the patient's spine FIGURE 5-52 PROCEDURE 21 .

Cervical Collar Cervical collars are soft or rigid devices used to aid in the immobilization of the cervical spine. They work to decrease flexion-extension (neck to chest) but do not completely immobilize the cervical spine; therefore, continued manual stabilization of the head is necessary until the head can be completely secured to an immobilization device (eg, long backboard, short board, vacuum mattress). Assess the cervical vertebrae for deformities and tenderness before applying the collar and assess the distal PMS function in each extremity. Apply an appropriately sized cervical collar to the patient. Use the manufacturer specifications when selecting an appropriate size for your cervical collar. An improperly sized collar could potentially cause further injury. Make sure the chin rests comfortably in the chin sup-

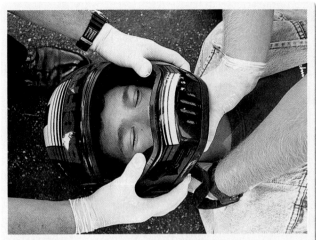

FIGURE 5-52 Helmets should be removed if they are loose fitting, the c-spine cannot be moved into a neutral position, or the airway is unstable.

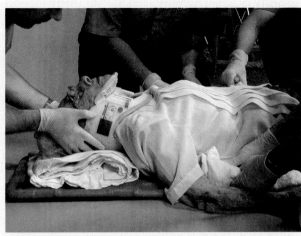

FIGURE 5-54 Patients may require additional padding to fill the voids when on a long backboard.

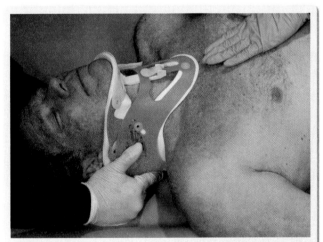

FIGURE 5-53 Each manufacturer has a different way to size a c-collar, but all should fit firmly under the chin and sit on the chest.

port and wrap the collar around the neck while maintaining manual immobilization. Secure the collar and check that the neck is in a neutral position **FIGURE 5-53**.

Additional Immobilization Devices   Once manual stabilization and a cervical collar are in place, the patient will need to be secured to a definitive immobilization device. Because the spine is mobile from end to end, it must be immobilized completely. Patients found in the supine or standing position will most likely benefit from a long backboard device or other whole body stabilization device for spinal immobilization. These devices allow for complete body immobilization and serve as a convenient mode for transporting your patient **PROCEDURE 23**.

Most boards are composed of plastic and are typically x-ray translucent. One downfall to long backboards is that they are flat and do not contour to the body. The body will be forced into this shape and pressure sores can develop where bony prominences compress the skin, blanching blood from the area. Another issue develops when the muscles in the back relax in an attempt to allow the body to give up its normal curves and flatten to the shape of the board. Spasms can develop and may cause the patient more pain when lying on the long backboard for extended periods. Providing padding between the patient and the board (blanket or commercial pad) can help reduce the risk of sores. In addition, padding may also be needed in the void areas between the board and the patient, particularly in the pediatric and geriatric populations **FIGURE 5-54**.

Conversely, the use of a vacuum mattress alleviates a number of the concerns associated with the long backboard, because the mattress conforms to the body shape placed on it. Once the patient is lowered onto the device, air is evacuated from it to form a rigid platform **PROCEDURE 19**. This not only provides the immobilizing support, but also offers a comfortable surface for the patient, reducing the risks associated with pressure sores. Moreover, contemporary research indicates that this methodology of immobilization may be more stable during transportation than the traditional application of long backboard devices.

The short board is another device used to immobilize the spine. Its smaller size allows EMS providers the flexibility of utilizing it in tight spaces. Typically used for the seated patient, the short board is versatile in its spinal immobilization functions. Most short boards are a flexible vest design. This allows the device to be manipulated into tight spaces where an otherwise rigid board would not fit. The convenience and practicality of this device enables it to be used in a variety of arenas of patient care **PROCEDURE 18**. While the spine is completely immobilized by this device, the patient should have the leg straps released and be placed on a long backboard or vacuum mattress for transport **FIGURE 5-55**.

Ongoing Assessment

Every patient who undergoes spinal immobilization must have a thorough neurologic assessment completed before and after the maneuver. Any changes such as weakness, numbness, tingling, or paresthesias that develop should be documented. As with any patient, continued assessment of airway, breathing, and circulation is essential for spinal cord injury patients. Vital signs and oxygenation should be monitored every 5 minutes in an unstable patient and every 15 minutes in a stable patient. Patients with hypotension without other signs of shock (eg, rapid pulse, pale skin) may be in neurogenic shock. (See Chapter 4 for more information on shock.) If neurogenic shock is present, reassess the peripheral neurologic status for any changes. A spinal cord injury causing the hypotension generally produces a loss of sensation or completely flaccid paralysis below the level of injury.

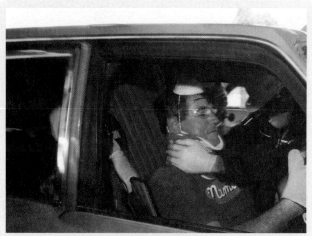

FIGURE 5-55 Short backboards are often shaped like vests to make it easier to access patients in a seated position.

CHAPTER RESOURCES

CASE STUDY ANSWERS

1 What is the mechanism of injury (MOI)? Does knowing he was hit and kicked make a difference in your assessment of forces involved?

His MOI is significant for head injury from an assault. Knowing he was both kicked and struck by fists does make a difference. Legs can impart a much greater force than hands. It also makes a difference knowing that another object was not used to strike your patient, such as a bat, pipe, or stick.

2 What is his Glasgow Coma Scale score (GCS)? Does it differ because he cannot open his swollen eye?

His GCS is a 7. He would receive a 1 for eye opening, 2 for best verbal response, and 4 for withdrawing from pain ($1 + 2 + 4 = 7$). When a patient cannot open his eyes due to swelling or other mechanical obstruction, you should not apply a score to the eye opening segment but total the others and place them with a notation of swelling of the eyes to indicate the test was unable to be completed. To decrease the score when it is not a neurologic problem could affect your patient's care.

3 What is his main injury? What are the clues?

His main injury is the head or brain injury. The clues to localizing the injury include: altered level of consciousness, GCS < 9, wounds to the outside of the head and face, increased blood pressure, and seizure.

CASE STUDY ANSWERS

4 What could have caused him to have a seizure?

The seizure could have been caused by traumatic brain injury, hypoxia, alcohol or drugs, or another medical cause.

5 How should you manage this patient? Would your management change if the trip were 2 minutes instead of 20 minutes?

With any acute change in patient status a reassessment is required. After ensuring the ABCs are adequate, the seizure should be stopped pharmacologically. Look for underlying causes of the seizure and correct any abnormalities. Hypoglycemia, hypoxia, and increasing ICP should be ruled out. The 20-minute trip might require additional advanced airway control, whereas a much shorter trip might be manageable with much simpler maneuvers. Longer transport times can require an alternate means of transportation such as aeromedical resources.

Trauma in Motion

1. What are your local protocols regarding determining which patients require spinal immobilization?
2. Do you have local hospitals with specialty care for head or spinal injury?
3. Have you reviewed and practiced the use of the spinal immobilization tools carried by your agency in the last year?
4. What specialty tools do you carry for treating injury to the eyes? For assessing the eyes? For flushing the eyes? For bandaging the eyes?
5. What are the local protocols regarding treatment in the patient with increasing ICP and potential brain herniation?

References and Resources

American Academy of Orthopaedic Surgeons. Pollak AN, ed. *Nancy Caroline's Emergency Care in the Streets*. 6th ed. Sudbury, Mass: Jones and Bartlett; 2007.

American College of Surgeons Committee on Trauma. Thoracic trauma. In: *Advanced Trauma Life Support for Doctors. Instructor Course Manual*. Chicago: American College of Surgeons; 2004.

Frakes MA. Measuring end-tidal carbon dioxide: clinical applications and usefulness. *Crit Care Nurse*. 2001; 21:23–35.

Guidelines for prehospital management of traumatic brain injury. 2nd ed. *Prehosp Emerg Care*. 2007; 12(1):S1–S52.

Guidelines for the management of severe traumatic brain injury. 3rd ed. *J Neurotrauma*. 2007; 24(Supp 1).

Hesdorffer DC, Ghajar J. Marked improvement in adherence to traumatic brain injury guidelines in United States trauma centers. *J Trauma Inj, Infect Crit Care*. 2007; 63:841–848.

National Collaborating Centre for Acute Care. Head injury: triage, assessment, investigation and early management of head injury in infants, children and adults. Available at: www.nice.org.uk/guidance/index.jsp?action=download&o=36260. Accessed November 26, 2008.

Stiell IG, McKnight RD, Schull MJ, et al. The Canadian C-Spine Rule versus the NEXUS Low Risk Criteria in patients with trauma. *N Engl J Med*. 2003; 349:2510–2518.

Stiell IG, Wells GA, Vandemheen K, et al. The Canadian C-Spine Rule for radiography in alert and stable trauma patients. *JAMA*. 2001; 286:1841–1848.

Trauma: Who cares? A report of the National Confidential Enquiry into Patient Outcome and Death. 2007.

Wakai A, Roberts IG, Schierhout G. Mannitol for acute traumatic brain injury. *Cochrane Database of Systematic Reviews*. 2007, Issue 1. Art. No.: CD001049. DOI: 10.1002/14651858.CD001049.pub4.

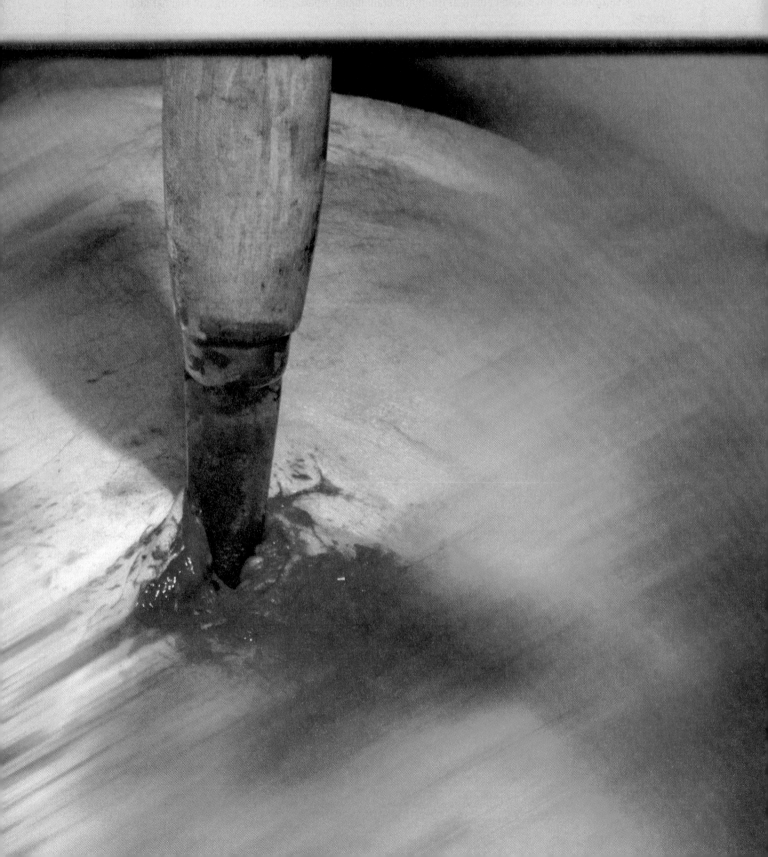

6 Torso Trauma

CASE STUDY

You are dispatched to a single-family home for a man in respiratory distress. It is early afternoon and the neighborhood where you are going is middle class. Upon your arrival, a woman in her mid-30s greets you at the door and hurries you into the kitchen where you find a 36-year-old man with a knife in his chest. The woman is the patient's wife. She tells you that her husband and his brother got into an argument and his brother stabbed him with a knife and then ran from the home.

The wife tells you that the brothers were drinking when an argument started. She went out of the room and when she returned her husband was pushing his brother around. The brother then turned around and grabbed the knife off the counter and stabbed her husband. He fell backwards and started coughing blood. She called EMS but didn't tell the dispatcher that her husband had been stabbed because he didn't want the police involved. You try to call for the police, who were not sent because it was a medical call, but the patient says "no police." He tries to get up from the floor but cannot lift himself up. There is a large amount of blood on the floor around the patient.

The man speaks in single-word sentences and complains that he cannot breathe. As he pulls a towel away from his chest, bubbles come from around the knife and blood has clotted in the towel. Lung sounds reveal decreased sounds on the right. He has weak and rapid radial pulses with cool and clammy skin. His respirations are 40 breaths/min, pulse is 148 beats/min and blood pressure is 80/40 mm Hg. Pulse oximetry shows 88% prior to oxygen administration and 92% with high-flow oxygen applied.

1 What concerns are there for scene safety?

2 Are there times when EMS should report injuries to law enforcement even though the patient may not approve?

3 How should the knife be secured?

4 Does this patient have a pneumothorax? Hemothorax?

5 Will your patient require ventilation, IV fluids, or both? What are the dangers of aggressive management in either?

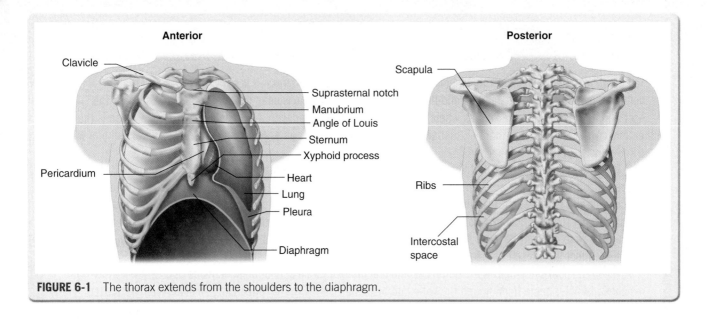

FIGURE 6-1 The thorax extends from the shoulders to the diaphragm.

Introduction

The largest mass of the human body is the chest (thorax) and the abdomen, collectively called the torso. The torso contains and protects all the vital organs responsible for breathing, circulation, digestion, filtration, and reproduction. These vital organs require large amounts of blood to function adequately, making them vulnerable to trauma.

Anatomy and Physiology

Thorax

The thorax extends from the neck and shoulders downward to the **diaphragm** **FIGURE 6-1**. The diaphragm is the thin muscle responsible for respirations and serves as a partition between the chest and the abdominal cavities. The thorax contains the lungs, heart, and large blood vessels, all of which are pressure sensitive. The contents of the thorax are protected by the rib cage and the small, tough intercostal muscles that connect them. There are 12 sets of ribs, which are all connected to the spinal column dorsally (posteriorly): seven pairs are connected to the sternum, three more pairs connect by cartilage anteriorly, and two pairs are floating with no other connection. The ribs provide framework for the lungs to do their job and provide effective respirations.

The diaphragm is the main muscle used to breathe, but the body can call on other muscles to help. The scalene, the parasternal portion of the external intercostal muscles, the sternocleidomastoid, and the trapezius make up the accessory muscles. When the accessory muscles contract, the chest expands upward and outward. At the same time, the diaphragm contracts, pulling downward and increasing the volume inside the chest **FIGURE 6-2**. During periods of increased work of breathing (WOB) all of the accessory muscles are used for breathing, whereas during normal breathing the accessory muscles are used only minimally. When the pressure inside the thorax becomes lower than atmospheric

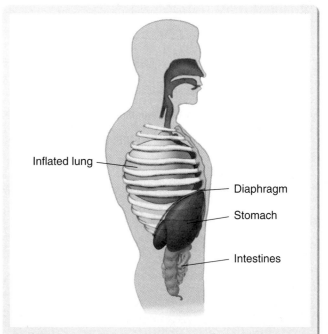

FIGURE 6-2 During inspiration, the diaphragm flattens downward while the intercostal muscles and the respiratory accessory muscles pull the chest outward to create more chest volume.

pressure, air rushes in, filling all the open spaces with inhaled air (inspiration). On relaxation, the internal intercostal muscles pull the ribs downward and contract inward while the diaphragm relaxes, decreasing the chest volume and causing an increase in pressure in the thorax that pushes air out (expiration). This expansion and contraction of the chest wall represents one complete cycle and is counted as one respiration.

Any injury of the rib cage can cause a disruption in the continuity of the chest wall to act as a pressure vessel. This causes less effective respirations, which will lead to hypoventilation and hypoxia.

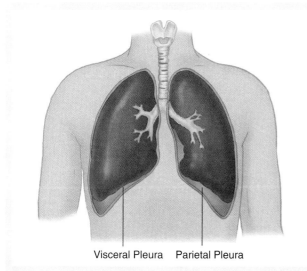

FIGURE 6-3 A thin layer of fluid holds the visceral pleura on the lung to the parietal pleura on the chest wall, keeping the lung moving with the chest wall.

Visceral Pleura   Parietal Pleura

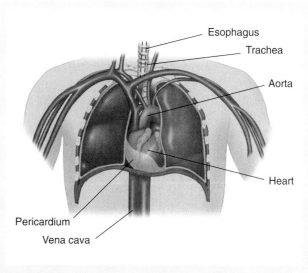

FIGURE 6-4 The heart, great vessels, esophagus, and trachea are separated from the lungs into an area called the mediastinum.

Esophagus · Trachea · Aorta · Heart · Pericardium · Vena cava

The lungs occupy the majority of the space in the thorax. Each lung is composed mostly of small air sacs (**alveoli**) and airways that get smaller until they enter the alveoli (**bronchi** and **bronchioles**). To allow for efficient gas exchange, the lungs are very vascular. Around the outside of each alveolus is a series of capillaries where the exchange of gases takes place. The capillaries represent the end of the arterial flow of blood and the beginning of the venous flow. This transition is at such a microscopic level that only one blood cell is able to pass at a time. The walls of the alveoli and the capillaries stretch on inspiration, becoming thin and permeable and allowing gas molecules to pass from high concentrations to lower concentrations. Through diffusion, high concentrations of oxygen in the alveolus move across into the capillary and carbon dioxide crosses back from the hemoglobin to the alveolus to be exhaled to the atmosphere. Trauma transferred through the rib cage into the lungs can cause bruising on the lung tissue from rupture of the capillaries, which will disrupt the exchange of gases in the affected area.

The entire lung surface is covered with **visceral pleura**, a sticky membrane that allows the lungs to stay connected to the rib cage but also to move with it. The inside of the chest wall is lined by the **parietal pleura**. Between the two layers of pleura is a small amount of fluid that acts as a lubricant to reduce friction and create suction between the chest wall and the moving lungs **FIGURE 6-3**. If blood, air, or fluid collects outside the lung tissue it can end up in the space between the pleurae.

In the center of the chest (the **mediastinum**) lies the heart, the great vessels, the esophagus, and the trachea **FIGURE 6-4**. These structures are all held together by loose connective tissue that surrounds and separates them from the lungs. Bringing deoxygenated blood back to the right side of the heart is the superior and inferior **vena cava**. The

vena cava, a thin-walled vessel that remains open due to the blood pressure inside it, lies along the right side of the spine. The pulmonary arteries exit the right ventricle and cross under the ascending aorta and in front of the descending aorta. Pulmonary veins bring oxygenated blood back to the left side of the heart through the same window under the aortic arch. The aorta exits the heart, loops upward, and then turns downward along the left side of the spine. At the top of the arch, the aorta is connected tightly to the spine with fibrous tissue. The aorta is a thick-walled vessel capable of withstanding the higher pressures of the arterial blood flow and pressure that can be placed on it from outside the vessel.

The heart lies between the lungs and just to the left of the midsternal chest line. The heart consists of three distinct layers: the **pericardium**, **myocardium**, and **endocardium**. The pericardium is a very strong fibrous sac that surrounds the heart. It contains a thin film of fluid, which serves as a lubricant to prevent the myocardium (heart muscle) and pericardium from rubbing and becoming irritated when the heart beats. In cases of trauma, there is a potential for blood or excess fluid accumulation within the pericardium. The endocardium is the innermost layer of the heart, forming a lining on the inside of the ventricles.

Abdomen

The abdominal (peritoneal) cavity is bordered superiorly by the diaphragm and extends to the pelvic floor. Because the diaphragm divides the chest from the abdomen and the diaphragm changes its shape during each phase of ventilation, the external markings for the abdomen change as the patient breathes **FIGURE 6-5**. Abdominal organs assist in filtering blood, digestion, and reproduction. The liver, spleen, and kidneys all filter blood for waste products, damaged blood cells, toxins, and excess fluid. The esophagus, stomach, and small and large intestines are responsible for

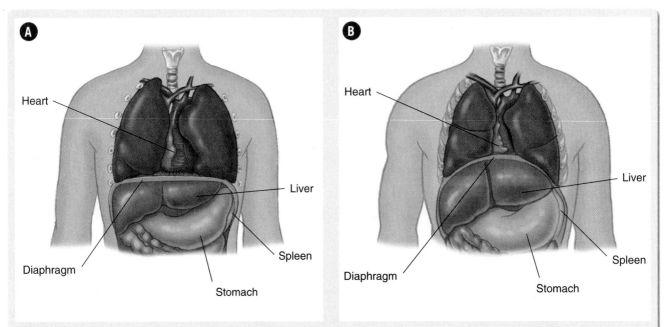

A. Heart, Liver, Spleen, Diaphragm, Stomach

B. Heart, Liver, Spleen, Diaphragm, Stomach

FIGURE 6-5   The diaphragm divides the chest from the abdomen. **A.** During inspiration, the diaphragm flattens downward, lengthening the chest. **B.** During expiration, the diaphragm relaxes and moves upward into its domed shape, pulling the abdomen upward.

the digestion and absorption of nutrients from food. The stomach, pancreas, and liver all contribute enzymes, which help break down food into its basic properties so the intestines can absorb the nutrients. Reproductive organs in females, including the uterus, ovaries, and fallopian tubes, are located within the abdominal cavity.

The descending aorta passes through the diaphragm along the left side of the spinal column down to the second lumbar vertebra. All of the abdominal blood flow branches from, and is anchored by, the aorta **FIGURE 6-6**. Returning blood travels from the organs back to the inferior vena cava to be returned to the heart. The vena cava sits opposite the aorta on the right side of the spine.

Like the thoracic organs, all the abdominal organs are covered with a thin visceral covering call the **visceral**

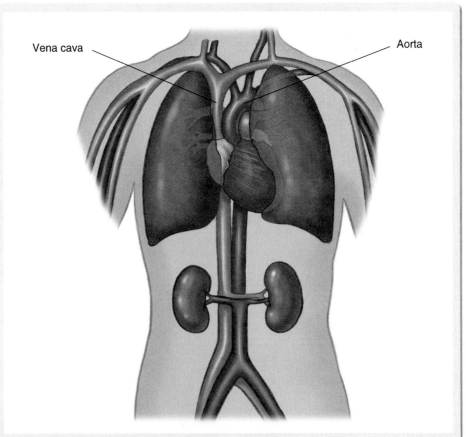

Vena cava   Aorta

FIGURE 6-6   Blood flows to the organs through the aorta and returns through the vena cava.

peritoneum. The visceral peritoneum creates a capsule around each organ, protecting them from friction when rubbing against other organs and the inside of the abdominal wall. The abdominal wall is covered with __parietal peritoneum__, which also serves as connective tissue (__mesentery__). The mesentery is basically a double thickness of parietal peritoneum that connects the small intestine to the posterior abdominal wall. The mesentery has many nerve endings and is very vascular, making it vulnerable to trauma.

Several organs often referred to as abdominal organs are actually located outside of the peritoneum. The renal system is located in the __retroperitoneal space__, which is posterior and just inferior to the 12th rib. The ureters, renal arteries and veins, and adrenal glands make up the renal system, which balances fluid requirements, filters waste products, and retains important electrolytes from the blood. The external genitalia of the male and female are both very vascular and contain erectile tissue that can become temporarily engorged with blood; these tissues are at risk of significant hemorrhage when traumatized.

The abdominal organs can also be classified into either solid or hollow organs. The liver, spleen, pancreas, and kidneys are solid organs and the stomach, intestines, and bladder are all hollow organs. Solid and hollow organs react differently under different types of trauma. Solid organs fracture or break apart when blunt or penetrating forces are applied; hollow organs compress and do not suffer the same damage as solid organs. Both can tear under blunt, penetrating, shearing, or stretching forces.

Spine

The thoracic spine consists of 12 vertebrae, stacked vertically and numbered from top to bottom starting below the cervical spine. Each of these vertebral bodies connects to a pair of ribs; the column is encased in muscle to protect it from injury. There are five lumbar vertebrae that connect the thoracic spine to the sacrum. The spinal cord passes through the vertebral channel, which lies posterior to each of the vertebral bodies.

Innervation of the intercostal muscles begins at the spinal cord and exits the vertebra at the level following the ribs around to the anterior chest. These nerves follow along the bottom of the ribs along with the intercostal arteries and veins. The body can be divided into regions primarily supplied by dorsal nerve pairs. Indeed, the sensory nerve roots can be mapped to areas along the body surface referred to as *dermatome distribution*. __Dermatomes__, areas of the skin supplied by particular nerves, are useful in locating the site of damage in a spinal injury **FIGURE 6-7**.

Pelvis

The pelvis is a basin-shaped structure that supports the spinal column and protects the abdominal organs. The pelvic girdle is actually three separate bones: the sacrum and the two innominate bones. Three bones—the ischium, ilium, and pubis—fuse together to form the innominate bone and the sacrum **FIGURE 6-8**. The two iliac bones are joined

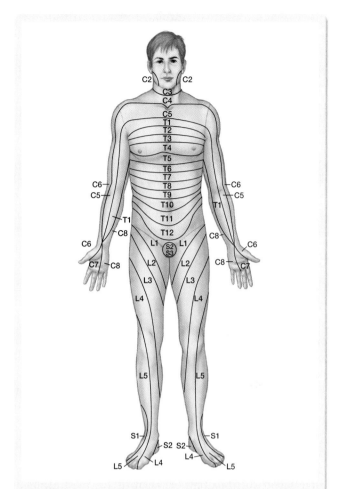

FIGURE 6-7 The dorsal nerve routes exit along the spine and follow patterns that can be mapped as dermatomes along the skin.

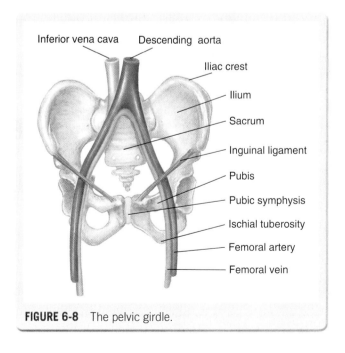

FIGURE 6-8 The pelvic girdle.

posteriorly to the sacrum by tough ligaments at the sacroiliac joints; the two pubic bones are connected to each other anteriorly by equally tough ligaments at the symphysis pubis. These joints allow very little motion, making the pelvic ring strong and stable.

The aorta divides as it enters the pelvis and splits again, leaving several large vessels to supply blood to the organs and lower extremities.

Mechanism of Injury

Any time energy is absorbed by the human body, injury is going to occur. The amount of energy and how it is delivered determines the type and severity of injury. Blunt and penetrating trauma are the two basic ways in which energy is delivered; each can be further divided into more specific subclasses.

Blunt Trauma

Blunt trauma results in compression and shearing of organs. Abrupt deceleration injuries are produced by a sudden stop of a body's forward motion. Whether from a fall or a high-speed vehicle crash, decelerating forces can induce shearing, avulsing, or rupturing of organs from their restraining fascia, vasculature, nerves, and other soft tissues. Solid, dense organs like the liver and spleen can fracture and break apart under compressive force, and blood vessels and hollow organs like the lungs and intestines will tear under shearing force.

The chest is vulnerable to aorta injury. The aorta, the large blood vessel exiting the heart, is the most common site of deceleration injury in the chest. The aorta may be torn away from its points of fixation in the body. Shearing of the aorta can result in rapid loss of all the body's blood and immediate death. The parietal peritoneum is very vascular and is susceptible to the same shearing forces that can lead to intra-abdominal hemorrhage. Irritation of the mesentery from blood, stomach or intestinal contents, or bacteria from infection of the abdomen will result in inflammation and pain. When any of these organs or the blood vessels that service these organs is damaged, there is real potential for blood loss, resulting in hypovolemic shock.

Compression injuries of the chest may produce fractured ribs or internal injuries of the lungs and heart. Almost all abdominal organs can be affected by hitting an external object. For example, compression against a seatbelt may result in bowel rupture, bladder rupture, diaphragm tearing, and spinal injuries. The major blood vessel in the abdomen is the descending or abdominal aorta, which supplies oxygen-enriched blood to the abdominal organs and lower extremities. A possible injury is the rupture of the aortic valve, caused by blood being forced the wrong way through the abdominal aorta following external compression of the abdominal cavity. External compressive trauma also can cause pelvic fractures, potentially injuring the bladder, vagina, rectum, lumbar plexus, and pelvic floor and leading to severe bleeding in the large arteries near the femoral head.

Use the mechanism of injury along with a thorough physical assessment, visual indicators, palpation, the patient's complaints, and vital signs to identify and confirm the presence of abdominal injuries. Bruising and abrasions are the external indicators of where energy was in contact with the body. In cases of potential indirect blunt trauma, consider referred pain (eg, spleen injury may present as pain in the left shoulder, known as *Kehr's sign*).

Penetrating Trauma

The severity of a stab wound depends on the anatomic area involved, depth of penetration, blade length and dimension, and angle of penetration. Chest wounds can involve critical anatomic structures such as arteries, the lungs, the trachea, the esophagus, or the thoracic duct. Wounds of sufficient energy can result in spinal cord involvement.

The most important factor for determining the seriousness of a gunshot wound is the type of tissue through which the projectile passes. Tissue of high elasticity (eg, muscle) is better able to tolerate stretch (temporary cavitation) than tissue of low elasticity, like the liver **FIGURE 6-9**. A high-velocity bullet fired through a fleshy part of the leg may do much less damage than a relatively low-velocity bullet that punctures the aorta or the liver.

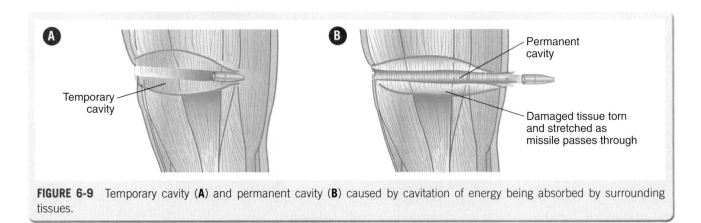

FIGURE 6-9 Temporary cavity (**A**) and permanent cavity (**B**) caused by cavitation of energy being absorbed by surrounding tissues.

TIP

Any penetrating trauma between the nipple line and the lower margin of the ribs should be considered both chest and abdominal injuries, until proven otherwise.

Bowel, muscle, and lung are relatively elastic, resulting in fewer permanent effects of temporary cavitation. Liver, spleen, and brain are relatively inelastic, however, and the temporary cavity may become a permanent defect.

Any penetrating trauma to the chest should be considered a very serious injury. A hole in the chest wall may ruin the integrity of the thorax by allowing air to enter the chest cavity during the negative pressures created during inspiration and exit during expiration. There is less resistance for air to enter and exit the thorax through the hole in the chest wall than through the bronchial tree.

Blast Injury

Pressure waves from an explosion create injury to air-containing organs such as the lungs, intestines, and inner ears due to the sudden change in atmospheric pressure. The blast wave's impact on the lung tissue results in tearing of the bronchioles and alveoli, hemorrhage, contusion, and edema. The injury can create a ventilation-perfusion mismatch, which is caused when air enters the lungs while blood flow is interrupted through the lungs. Another often fatal lung injury caused by an explosion is an air embolism that occurs when air leaking from the lung enters into a ruptured blood vessel. Unless there are objects thrown by the explosion (or the patient is pushed into an object, creating outward injury to the chest), a blast causes little external trauma. The internal injury, however, can be immense.

The amount of injury is affected by the level of pressure change. The closer the patient is to the blast, the more injury will occur. Pressure changes are greater when they occur indoors. Pressure changes of 40 psi are needed to create injury; changes of 80 psi often create severe trauma.

Torso Assessment

During the initial/primary assessment, the chest and abdomen are quickly assessed for immediately life-threatening conditions that would affect the ABCs **PROCEDURE 1**. The assessment process must be completed when time and conditions permit. The rapid trauma/secondary assessment should be systematic to avoid missing potential injuries **PROCEDURE 2**. The torso exam usually follows examination of the head and neck in the process of assessing from head to toe. Keep in mind that assessment of the torso in special populations (eg, pregnant women) requires some different considerations (see Chapter 10).

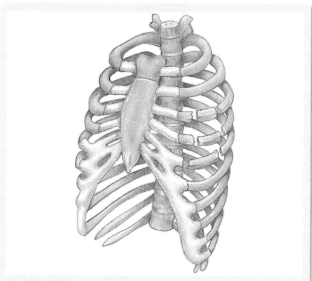

FIGURE 6-10   Rib fractures cause pain and muscle spasm that alter the chest wall movement.

Chest Assessment

To examine the chest, it must be exposed enough to inspect the skin for any outward signs of trauma such as abrasions, bruising, or deformity. Begin by looking for symmetry. As the chest moves through the ventilation sequence, observe it for equal movement and for depth of ventilation. When ribs are injured, the muscle surrounding them tightens to guard the injury, and less movement is noted **FIGURE 6-10**. Occasionally, paradoxical movement or movement opposite the movement of the chest will be seen with a flailed segment of ribs. This segment consists of two or more consecutive ribs broken in two or more spots, creating a floating portion of the rib cage. During inspiration, when the chest expands, the pressure inside the chest is lower and this segment will be pulled inward. When the patient expires, the chest diameter decreases and pressure in the chest is high, pushing the segment outward. This opposing movement of the chest wall is very painful and is not seen until the body has stopped splinting the area with muscle spasm.

Open wounds of the chest should be observed for air movement through the wound. Bleeding may appear to bubble or suck as air moves with the pressure changing in the chest. These wounds are often referred to as **sucking chest wounds**.

After observing the chest, assess for additional injury by palpating the structure of the musculoskeletal system. Palpate the clavicles, sternum, and ribs, giving attention to tenderness or deformity. Visually examine for lacerations, punctures, or deformities. An additional sign that may be found while palpating the chest wall is subcutaneous emphysema. Caused by air leaking into the skin from inside the chest, the bubbles formed in the skin crackle under the touch.

Auscultation for lung sounds and heart tones should be done after palpating the chest. During the initial/primary assessment, lung sounds were assessed for their presence or absence. Additional assessment of the chest warrants listening for a full set of lung sounds and the conditions that may go with them. Immediately following a blast injury, the presence of equal lung sounds is of major importance, but careful assessment after treating the threats to life often reveals crackles and worsening difficulty breathing. Percussion can assist the provider in determining the presence of air or blood in the chest; however, the ambient noise levels encountered on trauma scenes and in the ambulance may make it hard to use. The chest should have a hollow sound when percussed. A hyperresonant pitch is indicative of a pneumothorax, whereas a pitch that is dull indicates blood filling the chest. While the tone when percussed is important, the inequality or non-symmetry of the sounds from side to side is more indicative of trauma.

Abdomen Assessment

Moving down from the chest into the abdomen should be seamless. Observe the abdomen, looking for signs of trauma such as abrasions from seatbelts, bruising from blunt trauma, or wounds associated with penetrating injury. Seatbelts often cause injury when they are worn incorrectly, and abrasions or bruising seen across the lower abdomen are indicators for internal trauma. **Cullen's sign** is a bruise-type marking around the umbilicus. It may be seen in patients with a delay after the trauma, as it usually presents after 12 to 48 hours following internal bleeding. **Grey Turner's sign** is also a delayed sign of internal bleeding and presents as a dark discoloration along the flanks.

When assessing the abdomen it is important to establish whether the patient is moving their abdominal wall. Normally the front abdominal wall moves with the chest wall when the patient breaths and talks. When the patient does not move their abdominal wall, this may indicate one of the following problems:

- The front abdominal wall has been traumatized.
- The abdominal muscles are trying to stabilize the rib cage.
- The diaphragm has been paralyzed.
- Muscle guarding and rigidity are present secondary to peritonitis.

Eviscerations to the abdominal cavity allow the internal organs to be exposed to the outside of the body. Usually a loop of intestine is the presenting organ because of the flexibility of the organ to move through an opening. Although these injuries are very eye catching, the patient must be evaluated for shock and additional internal bleeding. Impaled objects in either the chest or abdomen are of great concern. Injury from an impaled object is related to the path and length of the object. Secure the object from movement before moving the patient for further assessment or treatment FIGURE 6-11.

Palpate the abdomen systematically to evaluate for tenderness. If the patient complains of a painful area, examine that area of the abdomen last to avoid referring pain throughout the abdomen. The most sensitive indicator of tenderness is the patient's facial expression (so watch the patient's face, not your hands). Voluntary or involuntary guarding may also be present. Examine superficially and then more deeply. Push a bit more firmly so you are assessing the deeper aspects of the upper abdomen, particularly if the patient has a lot of subcutaneous fat. Pushing up and in while the patient takes a deep breath may make it easier to feel the liver edge because the downward movement of the diaphragm will bring the liver toward your hand.

The main concern when palpating the abdomen is to prevent voluntary muscle contractions, which make further palpation impossible or can mistakenly be assumed to be muscle guarding. These steps can help the provider:

1. Distract the patient's attention by asking them questions.
2. Perform palpation by flexing your fingers mainly at the metacarpophalangeal joint, keeping your wrist joint light with no tension in it. To avoid tension in the wrist when palpating an obese patient, apply additional pressure with the other hand over the palpating one (Hausmann's maneuver).
3. Perform fast but gentle palpation. (A rough hand will produce voluntary contractions.)
4. Gradually increase the pressure to perform deep palpation.
5. Do not take your hand off to move to the next region. Instead, gradually decrease the pressure and slide your hand to the adjacent region, preparing it to accept your hand without muscle contractions.

Rebound tenderness is used to assess peritoneal irritation. It is especially useful when looking for blood or bowel contents that have spilled into the abdominal

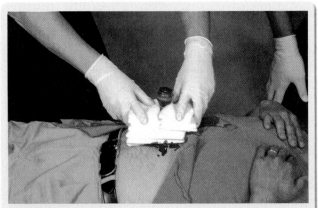

FIGURE 6-11 Impaled objects should be secured before moving the patient.

cavity and irritated the intestinal linings. To check for rebound tenderness, press deeply on the abdomen with your hand. After a moment, quickly but smoothly release the pressure. If it hurts when you release, the patient has rebound tenderness. The tenderness occurs from inflammation of the intestinal walls moving over themselves or other organs.

Auscultation of the abdomen has limitations in the acutely injured patient. Catecholamine release following trauma will slow the activity of the bowel, so slower than normal bowel sounds will be present. Percussion also has its limitations in assessment of trauma due to environmental noises and time of onset. Both tools may be helpful in evaluating the patient who has a delayed presentation for care.

Back and Spine Assessment

When completing the examination of the torso, do not leave out the back and spine. This examination will often require the provider to roll the patient prior to placing them on a spinal immobilization device. Inspect the back for signs of trauma. In multisystem trauma, this is an often overlooked area. Victims with penetrating wounds should always have the back examined to determine all sites of entry or exit. Victims who are obese may have wounds hidden by folds of skin. Listen to posterior lung sounds if given the opportunity, to confirm the previous assessment. Palpate the posterior rib cage and along the vertebral column, looking for tenderness or deformity **FIGURE 6-12**. The spinous process along each vertebra should line up without a significant "step off" or drop between them.

When the initial/primary assessment indicates spinal injury, assess sensation along the torso to determine the level of involvement. In a more controlled environment, this is done with a pointed and a dull instrument, but accuracy

TIP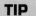

> When a spinal cord injury is suspected, an approximate level of injury can be estimated by finding the level to which the patient still has sensation. Light, painful stimuli can help determine the level.

in the trauma environment will produce only gross results; sensation to palpation is appropriate. Continue the assessment, looking for additional signs of spinal injury including incontinence; priaprism; loss of sensation in the lower torso or extremities; or decreased or lack of movement of the extremities.

Pelvis Assessment

Contained within the pelvis are elements of the urinary system, reproductive system, GI system, and the neurovascular components that control the legs. Assessment begins by visually scanning the area. Mechanism of injury will help the provider to determine the suspicion of trauma to the pelvic area. Bruising from seatbelts can be an indicator of bladder injury or dislocation of the symphysis pubis. Signs of penetrating trauma can be overlooked in the skin folds that are formed as the abdomen and the legs meet the pelvis. For obese patients, the excess folds of skin need to be lifted to assess for trauma that may go unnoticed.

Palpate the lowest segment of the abdomen, just above the symphysis pubis, for pain or tenderness. External genitalia require assessment only when the visual scan indicates trauma as noted by blood on the clothing or tenderness on palpation. The pelvis is palpated only once in the rapid trauma/secondary assessment because additional bleeding can be caused by further movement of an unstable bony structure. If the visual assessment of the pelvis indicates deformity, the physical exam should be deferred, allowing the pelvis to remain in place. Gentle pressure with the heel of the hand should be placed on the symphysis pubis in an anterior to posterior direction. The iliac crests should then be compressed medially and laterally with gentle but steady pressure. If instability is noted, the exam should be ended immediately and the patient prepared for transport.

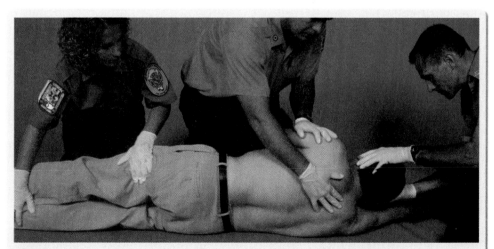

FIGURE 6-12 Palpate along the spine looking for tenderness and continuity of the spinous processes.

CONTROVERSIES

Ambulance Sonogram Utilization

PICTURE YOURSELF IN THE BACK of an ambulance en route to the hospital, code 3 with a critically ill or injured patient. In addition to vital signs, assessment skills, and monitoring, you wish you had all the help you could get to evaluate the extent and severity of the patient's illness or injuries. One new modality now opening important doors for EMS personnel to enhance their physical assessment is the use of ultrasound in the field.

In essence, ultrasound allows the EMS provider to image or "see" inside the patient as you assess them. Probably everybody has seen an ultrasound used to examine the status of a fetus during pregnancy.[1] The transducer is placed on the mother's abdomen and the baby is visible on the screen as a grayscale image. Even most laypeople can now make out this image as a baby.

Now let's return to the scenario in the back of the ambulance with our critical patient. Let's say, for example, that this is a blunt trauma patient, and the patient's blood pressure is very low. Using assessment with the ABCs, the airway is open; the patient is breathing; there are no obvious external bleeding sites; and the pulse is weak, rapid, and thready.

After carrying out routine resuscitation maneuvers according to medical protocol, ultrasound could next be used to examine some very basic issues within the body of the patient. These issues include vital areas of assessment, including the movement and contraction of the heart[2] and the location and evidence of internal bleeding. How can this be accomplished in the back of a moving ambulance running code 3 with this critically injured patient? And, very importantly, can EMS personnel be trained to routinely perform ultrasound examinations while en route with critically ill patients?

We believe that the answer to these questions is already being answered. Equipment and training are now available that can provide this view into the patient that will greatly expand the knowledge base and sophistication within EMS systems.[3] An important goal to achieving the training level needed to prove a "value added" for ultrasound in EMS is to keep the learning process as simple as possible for the field paramedic.

Ultrasound in the field uses simple imaging. Today's ultrasound machines have built-in capabilities far exceeding the need in EMS applications. For example, in the hands of a cardiologist, this same ultrasound machine could acquire a full echocardiogram. In the hands of a paramedic, the use of the sonogram in the evaluation of a patient's heart is to visualize basic images such as the movement of the heart during a code. This is a straightforward concept of imaging the chest to see *if* the heart is contracting and *how* it is contracting. If this seems simple to the reader, the concept demonstrates just how much information can be gained from the basic use of an ultrasound examination as well as how appropriate it is to place this equipment in the hands of the EMS provider.

The message is clear: EMS providers could be screening for a few basic diagnoses that would suggest the possibility of life-threatening conditions. We could screen for obvious abnormalities, not performing a formal ultrasound like a radiologist would. EMS ultrasound—at least into the foreseeable future—should become a part of the armamentarium of the evaluation of critically ill and injured patients.

An important key to field ultrasound use will be keeping the exams very basic in nature. Questions to be answered with this type of ultrasound are also basic:

- Is the heart beating? This is an important point, especially in the setting of a potential field termination of a cardiac arrest patient who has not responded to resuscitation.
- Is the patient bleeding within the abdomen? We are referring to the FAST examination, which gives views of "free blood or fluid" in the areas surrounding the heart, liver, spleen, kidneys, and bladder.
- Is this patient pregnant?
- Is a patient's abdominal pain being caused by an abdominal aortic aneurysm?

Finally, one last area of prehospital ultrasound usage could be for peripheral venous access. Patients often need an IV for therapy (fluid or medications), but they can be a tough IV or "tough stick." Perhaps the patient is too large for an intraosseous, and intranasal medication administration is insufficient to fix the problem. We routinely use ultrasound in the emergency department to assist us with the starting of difficult intravenous access. Experienced trauma nurses who are skilled at ultrasound IVs can place a large IV in a patient's brachial vein as fast as an intraosseous can be placed. Maybe one day, as ultrasound becomes the standard of care in EMS, we will see highly skilled ultrasound-trained professionals who will be able to use ultrasound imaging for those patients who absolutely require urgent intravenous access because no other route is available.

We believe that this window into the future is already quite clear, and we challenge both EMS educational programs and equipment manufacturers alike to move quickly into this rapidly evolving area of patient assessment and management. Prehospital ultrasound can improve patient care, increase patient safety, and reduce patient discomfort.

Dave Spear, MD, FACEP
Clinical Assistant Professor
Emergency Ultrasound Programs
Parkland Hospital
Dallas Children's Medical Center
Dallas, Texas

Raymond L. Fowler, MD, FACEP
Professor of Emergency Medicine, Surgery
Associate Professor of Allied Health Professions
Chief of EMS Operations
Co-Chief in the Section on EMS, Disaster Medicine, and Homeland Security
University of Texas Southwestern Medical Center
Attending Faculty, Parkland Memorial Hospital Emergency Department
Dallas, Texas

References

1. Woo J. A short history of the development of ultrasound in obstetrics and gynecology. Available at: http://www.ob-ultrasound.net/history1.html. Accessed June 16, 2009.

2. Bahner DP. Trinity: A hypotensive ultrasound protocol. *J Diag Med Sonography.* 2002; 18(4):193–198.

3. Ma OJ, Mateer JR. *Emergency Ultrasound*, 2nd ed. New York: McGraw-Hill; 2008.

Chest Injuries

Rib Fractures and Flail Segment

The ribs are flat, curved bones, making them inherently stronger and more resilient to trauma than other bones. Because the ribs work in unison, if one rib is fractured it may cause a disruption to the respiratory system. Not only would the integrity of the rib cage be disrupted, but the sharp edges of the broken bones have the potential to puncture other tissues, including the lungs or liver. If more than one rib is fractured, the continuity of the rib cage is compromised and hypoxia becomes a concern. The muscles between the ribs can be damaged by blunt or penetrating trauma. Muscle injury from the mechanism of injury and secondarily through movement of the fractured bone edges cutting additional muscle with movement further reduces the continuity of the rib cage. The intercostal nerves and blood vessels run just below each rib; this neurovascular bundle is not immune to injury.

Perhaps the most serious rib fractures are <u>flail segments</u>, where more than two consecutive ribs are fractured in two or more areas. It takes a lot of energy to cause a flail segment. This injury can occur anywhere: anterior, posterior, sternal, or in the lateral areas of the thorax. Any time the chest wall absorbs enough energy to cause a flail segment, any tissue surrounding the rib cage is at risk of injury. With the amount of energy required to create the multiple fractures that cause a flail segment, the underlying lung tissue is particularly at risk of serious injury. The associated pulmonary contusion underlying the fractures is the most clinically significant finding. Obviously, the larger the injury, the greater the chance of hypoxia. The lung injury impedes oxygenation in the affected portion of the lung, while the pain from the rib fractures causes less effective ventilations by forcing the chest wall to limit movement and lessen the depth of breath.

Bruising and abrasions indicate potential rib fracture. There may also be pain upon inspiration, resulting in shallow respirations, and pain upon palpation of the injured area. Although deformity is a possibility, intercostal muscles are very strong and may splint the injured area. <u>Crepitus</u> (bone ends grating together) may also indicate a rib fracture. A late sign of flail segment, however, is paradoxical movement.

Treatment of Rib Fractures and Flail Segments

Splinting rib fractures may be difficult due to their location; however, the goal is to reduce the patient's discomfort. Apply oxygen to maximize the patient's F_{IO_2} and maintain Spo_2 and end-tidal CO_2 measurements at normal levels. If a flail segment is suspected, splint the injured site with wide tape stretched from a noninjured area of the chest over the injured area to a noninjured area of the chest wall. An alternate method includes using a trauma dressing to cover the injured area and taping in place. By splinting the flail segment you are returning the unity of the chest to allow ventilations to occur as normally as possible. This procedure is not supported in all organizations, however. Please follow local protocol.

Positive-pressure ventilation does not require splinting the injured chest wall. It allows the lungs to fill with air without creating negative pressure inside the thorax, eliminating paradoxical movement. Positive-pressure ventilation allows the lungs to fill, despite the damaged chest wall, and also prevents hypoxia from the contused lung tissue, thus preventing fluid and/or blood accumulation in the alveoli. Constant vigilance is required when ventilating an intubated patient with a flail segment, because pneumothorax is always a risk when inflating the damaged lung tissue with positive pressure.

Sternum Fracture

Most sternal fractures are caused by blunt chest trauma **FIGURE 6-13**. Motor vehicle collisions involving patients using seatbelts with no air bag deployment account for most

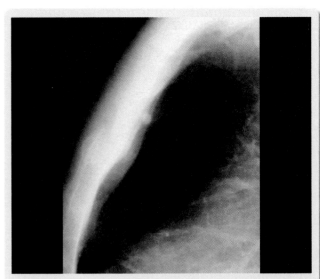

FIGURE 6-13 This lateral radiograph of the chest shows a minimally displaced fracture of the sternum in a patient who sustained direct blunt trauma to the chest. Cardiac and lung injury commonly occur in conjunction with these injuries.

TIP

The intercostal muscles will spasm and splint any serious rib injury; therefore, paradoxical movement is a late sign in assessing for a flail segment. Place your hands with fingers spread wide on the anterior thorax with thumbs together over the midsternum, then feel for chest movement. If there is any nonmovement or paradoxical movement, a flail segment may be indicated. You will be more likely to feel any reduction in movement than to visualize it.

fractures; however, direct-impact sports, falls, pedestrian injuries, and assaults can create fractures. The mortality rate from isolated sternal fracture is extremely low. Death is usually related to injury to the internal structures.

Sternal bruising or abrasions may indicate a fracture. The patient may also be experiencing pain on inspiration, resulting in shallow respirations, and pain on palpation of the injured area. Deformity and crepitus may also be present.

Treatment of Sternum Fracture

Treatment of sternal injury is symptomatic. Treat with oxygen for hypoventilation due to the pain. Assess for cardiac arrhythmias and treat with standard advanced cardiac life support (ACLS) or local protocols. Pain management should be provided based on local protocols and available medications.

Pulmonary Contusion

A **pulmonary contusion**, a bruise of the lung tissue, can impair gas exchange due to the direct injury response of edema and blood leakage into the alveoli **FIGURE 6-14**. The lung tissue becomes irritated and inflamed in the presence of free blood. These findings further complicate gas exchange through an increase in pulmonary vascular resistance, less tissue for the exchange of gases, and decreased lung compliance. Gas exchange is affected even with adequate tidal volume, and the alveoli and the bronchioles may collapse without internal pressure to keep them open. A patient may require airway support and positive end-expiratory pressure (PEEP) to keep the alveoli from collapsing during expiration.

Indicators of pulmonary contusion include external bruising or abrasions to the chest wall; low or decreasing O_2 saturations, even with supplemental O_2; diminished breath sounds in the affected area; and adventitious lung sounds (crackles, rhonchi).

Treatment of Pulmonary Contusion

Identifying a pulmonary contusion in the field is difficult at best; however, a high index of suspicion must be maintained for a contusion anytime a traumatic injury causes rib fractures. It may take 24–48 hours for a pulmonary contusion to develop fully. Splinting fractured ribs as described earlier and maximizing ventilation with the aid of appropriate analgesia and high concentration oxygenation for any patient who has sustained any chest trauma are the first steps to effec-

tive treatment. If you are having difficultly maintaining good O_2 saturations, you may want to add PEEP, about 5 cm H_2O to start, titrated to the patient's condition.

Simple Pneumothorax

Pneumothorax refers to the presence of air in the pleural cavity between the parietal and visceral pleura, which results in creating a void between the normally contacted pleural surfaces **FIGURE 6-15**. A pneumothorax is caused by lung trauma that allows air to leak from the alveoli into the space. Air may also enter the pleural space coming from the atmosphere when the thoracic wall is injured. **Simple pneumothoraces** are defined by air in the pleural space that does not build up pressure and is contained to 10%–30% collapse of the lung. The lung injury often seals itself, stopping the leakage of air. A simple pneumothorax can be large

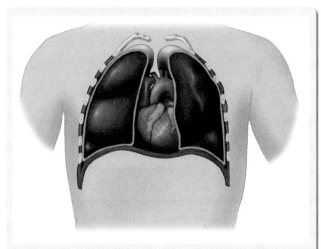

FIGURE 6-14 Pulmonary contusions occur when the lung tissue becomes injured.

TIP

Positive end-expiratory pressure (PEEP) keeps small amounts of back pressure in the airways, causing the alveoli and bronchioles to remain open and requiring less ventilatory pressure to open the alveoli on the next ventilation.

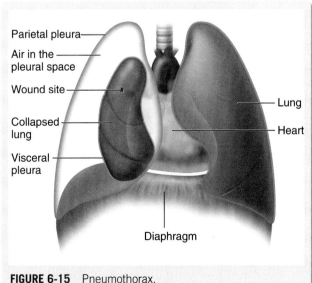

FIGURE 6-15 Pneumothorax.

enough to cause hypoxia due to decreased lung volume, but will not cause cardiovascular symptoms.

External bruising or abrasions to the chest wall may indicate simple pneumothorax. Other indicators include diminished breath sounds in the affected area, tachypnea, and tachycardia. The patient may also experience low or decreasing O_2 saturations, even with supplemental O_2.

Treatment of Simple Pneumothorax

Treatment of the patient with a simple pneumothorax consists of mostly supportive care. Maximize the oxygenation capability of the patient by giving high-flow oxygen. Reassess the patient frequently. Pulse oximetry and ECG should be monitored. If the patient suddenly becomes more short of breath or vital signs show sudden signs of shock, this has likely become a tension pneumothorax.

Open Pneumothorax

An **open pneumothorax** occurs when a pneumothorax is associated with an open chest wall injury and air can enter and exit the chest through the exterior wound opening. During inspiration, when negative intrathoracic pressure is generated, air can enter into the chest cavity not only through the trachea, but also through the hole in the chest wall. This is because the passage through the chest wall injury is much shorter than the trachea and provides less resistance to flow. Once the size of the hole is more than three quarters the size of the trachea, air will preferentially enter through the injury site. This results in inadequate oxygenation and ventilation and a progressive buildup of air in the pleural space. A tension pneumothorax may develop if a flap has been created that allows air in but not out. A wound in the chest wall that appears to be "sucking air" into the chest and may be visibly bubbling indicates an open pneumothorax.

An external laceration or puncture to the chest wall may indicate an open pneumothorax. Patients may also present with diminished breath sounds in the affected area, bubbling of blood or visible movement of air in a chest wound, dyspnea or tachypnea, tachycardia, low or decreasing O_2 saturations (even with supplemental O_2), and signs of shock.

Treatment of Open Pneumothorax

Any penetrating chest wound must be covered with a nonporous dressing to prevent air from being drawn into the thorax through the wound **PROCEDURE 26**. The nonporous dressing can be anything from commercially acquired chest seals, to plasticized paper wrappers from bandaging material, to bio-occlusive skin barrier dressings. Many of the commercially available devices have a one-way valve built in to prevent air pressure from building up under the dressing and causing a tension pneumothorax. Where they are not available, use an alternative occlusive dressing and secure the edges of the dressing on three sides to facilitate air escape and to help minimize the risk of causing a tension pneumothorax.

Apply high-flow oxygen as soon as the chest defect has been secured and prepare to secure an airway. Provide

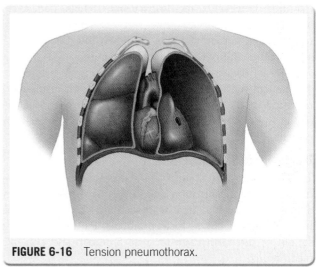

FIGURE 6-16   Tension pneumothorax.

adequate ventilatory support to maintain near normal physiologic levels. Caution may be required with regards to a suspected pneumothorax that could develop quickly into a tension pneumothorax. Frequent reassessments and monitoring of pulse oximetry and ECG are required.

Tension Pneumothorax

A **tension pneumothorax** develops when there is an oblique opening into the pleura that occludes and acts as a one-way valve. Consequently, air enters the pleural cavity during inspiration but cannot escape during expiration. As pressure continues to increase from the escaping air, the patient develops air hunger. Because they are oxygen starved, they breathe harder and faster. This increases the work of breathing, causing more air to escape from the damaged lung. In time, the pressure of the trapped air will push the damaged lung against the mediastinum and eventually against the uninjured lung. As the mediastinum and the uninjured lung start to be compressed, blood vessels, bronchi, and the vena cava are being kinked, causing the life-threatening chest injury known as a tension pneumothorax **FIGURE 6-16**. Once the vena cava has become compressed, the result is poor blood return to the right side of the heart. The resultant drop in preload causes a drop in cardiac output, leading to shock. Along with the shock, one lung is completely collapsed and the other is being compressed against the chest wall. Ventilation and oxygenation is now significantly compromised; rapid intervention is needed.

Indicators of a tension pneumothorax include bruising or abrasions to the external chest wall, diminished breath sounds in the affected area, and low or decreasing O_2 saturations, even with supplemental O_2. The patient may also have tachycardia, distended neck veins, subcutaneous emphysema, and difficulty ventilating. Hyperresonance to percussion is also an indication, as is a deviated trachea (though this is a late sign).

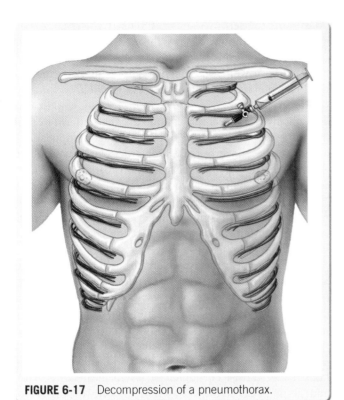

FIGURE 6-17 Decompression of a pneumothorax.

Treatment of Tension Pneumothorax

High-flow oxygen should be applied early to decrease hypoxia. Determining which finding you have is paramount. After establishing that a tension pneumothorax is present, decompression of trapped air is clearly indicated. Decompression must occur on the side with the pneumothorax. Absent breath sounds indicate the affected side. If tracheal deviation is noted, select the side opposite the direction of the tracheal deviation, because the pressure from the pneumothorax will push the trachea away from it. If the trachea is deviated to the right, the pneumothorax will be on the left side. Two sites are acceptable to decompress: the second or third intercostal space at the midclavicular line and the fifth intercostal space at the midaxillary line **FIGURE 6-17**.

Decompression is an aseptic technique, so use of alcohol or betadine swabs is required. Use the biggest gauge angiocatheter or over-the-needle cannula possible (at least

TIP

Rely on your local protocols and scope of practice for proper placement for a needle decompression. The midaxillary site has a few drawbacks: it is not immediately visible on arrival in the trauma room, it can be occluded by strapping the arm down to the side of the body, and it can be occluded by blood in the case of a hemo/pneumothorax.

1.5″ in length for the average adult). Insert the angiocatheter or over-the-needle cannula over the top of the rib to avoid the nerves and blood vessels that run under each rib. While inserting the angiocatheter, feel for the "pop" as the needle enters the pleural space. Remove the needle, leaving the catheter in place. Leave the open end of the catheter open to the atmosphere or place a commercially purchased one-way valve over the top of the catheter. Placing a one-way valve over the catheter will prevent air leaking back into the thorax once pressure in the thorax drops below barometric pressure. Air may or may not be heard escaping through the catheter. The patient should feel relief and breathing will become easier. Reassessment following the procedure should include pulse oximetry, ECG, and ETCO$_2$ if an advanced airway has been placed before the decompression. In the intubated patient, the provider ventilating the patient will notice that the resistance of ventilation will decrease and bag-mask ventilations will require less work.

Hemothorax

A **hemothorax** occurs when blood enters the pleural space **FIGURE 6-18**. In fact, laceration of any of the costal blood vessels can lead to a hemothorax. Blood may also come from an injured lung. Blood accumulates in the thorax, eventually displacing lung tissue (not to mention the loss of circulating blood volume), thus leading to impaired oxygenation and shock. The potential of a large hemorrhage in the chest cavity is so great that shock will occur without much warning or other symptoms. Blood will accumulate in dependent areas above the posterior section of the diaphragm in an upright patient and along the posterior chest wall in a supine patient.

Bruising or abrasions to the external chest wall; diminished breath sounds in the affected area; and low or decreasing O$_2$ saturations, even with supplemental O$_2$, may indicate hemothorax. Other indications include flat neck veins, dull percussion, tachypnea, tachycardia, and signs of shock, which may be profound in the presence of a massive hemothorax (> 1,500 mL).

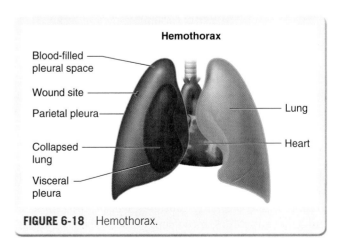

FIGURE 6-18 Hemothorax.

Treatment of Hemothorax

Treating a hemothorax like a pneumothorax could complicate the patient's condition. Maximizing the amount of oxygenation and ventilations in either case should be a priority. Avoid decompressing a hemothorax because lowering the thoracic pressure could lead to more bleeding. A pneumothorax will often be accompanied by a small hemothorax; the provider must weigh the risks to benefits of relieving a pneumothorax in the presence of a potential hemothorax. At least two large-bore IVs should be started and the provider should be prepared to administer crystalloid fluids to support systolic blood pressure to around 90–100 mm Hg or as dictated locally. Frequent reassessments are required and should include pulse oximetry and ECG monitoring.

Cardiac Contusion

Similar to other contusions, a **cardiac contusion** is a bruise on the heart. Bruises cause damage to tissue and bleeding within the tissue. In the case of a cardiac contusion, the bleeding within the tissue can disrupt the heart's mechanical function and electrical conduction. When there is bleeding within the cardiac tissue, the cells often are unable to conduct the electrical impulses required for proper functioning of the heart muscle. The result of the electrical conduction difficulties is ectopic arrhythmias, often tachycardias; however, specific types of arrhythmia are dependent on the location of electrical conduction problems.

Often the only prehospital indicator of cardiac contusion is coronary electrical abnormality and ectopy. The type of ectopy is dependent on the location of the contusion. Ventricular contusion results in possible ventricular dysfunction and premature ventricular contractions (PVCs) or runs of ventricular tachycardia. When the ventricular wall is injured, the muscle does not squeeze well (or at all), resulting in compromised cardiac output.

Other possible indications of cardiac contusion are bruising and abrasions, chest pain, jugular venous distension (JVD), and decreased cardiac output.

Treatment of Cardiac Contusion

After caring for the ABCs, including administering oxygen, supporting cardiac output with fluids and monitoring for lethal arrhythmias should be the first order of business. Watch for other physiological signs of decreased profusion, including JVD, quality of pulses, color of patient's skin, and blood pressure. If the patient is lying supine and has no JVD, fluids may be required to increase the preload, which will ultimately increase the cardiac output. Arrhythmias should be treated according to standard ACLS algorithms.

Cardiac Tamponade

The heart lies in the middle of the pericardium. Cardiac tamponade can be caused by either blunt or penetrating trauma where bleeding from the myocardium, aorta, or any other supporting blood supply accumulates inside the pericardium. As the collection of blood inside the pericar-

dium starts to exert pressure on the heart, the compression decreases the amount of flow through the heart. Because the fluid building inside the pericardium does not expand outward very well, this mechanism eventually squeezes the heart muscle, causing a decrease in stroke volume. If rapidly accumulating, as little as 106–150 mL could cause enough myocardial compression to impede diastolic filling, thus dropping cardiac output. Cardiac tamponade is an obstructive shock because it obstructs the flow of blood through the heart, blocking perfusion to the end organs. Slower bleeds will allow more accumulation of fluid or blood due to the pericardium stretching, at times accumulating up to 1,000 mL of fluid before any compromise in cardiac output. Blunt and penetrating chest trauma can cause cardiac tamponade.

Indicators of cardiac tamponade include bruising and abrasions, distant heart tones, **pulsus paradoxus** (weakening pulse with inspiration), **Kussmaul's sign** (increased jugular filling pressure with inspiration), and narrowing pulse pressures. JVD is also an indication of cardiac tamponade; however, if a patient is hypotensive, JVD might not be present. The three points in Beck's triad (used to diagnose tamponade) consist of muffled or distant heart tones, JVD, and decompensated shock (as noted by blood pressure of less than 90 mm Hg).

Pulsus paradoxus is a good indicator of cardiac tamponade, being a condition in which the distal pulses decrease in strength on inspiration. Kussmaul's sign is when the jugular veins bulge on inspiration. These two findings are caused by the expanding lungs pushing on the engorged pericardium, which then pushes on the heart muscle. On the left side, decreased cardiac output shows pulsus paradoxus; on the right side, decreased diastolic filling causes Kussmaul's sign.

Treatment of Cardiac Tamponade

Increasing cardiac output should be the provider's priority in treating cardiac tamponade. As the heart is being squeezed by the increasing pressure in the pericardium, the preload must be increased. Oxygen should never be withheld from a patient who needs it; however, you must weigh the need for positive-pressure ventilations against the possibility of hypoventilation.

Pericardiocentesis is a technique to remove blood and fluid from the pericardium and relieve the squeezing pressure on the heart **PROCEDURE 14**. The procedure (which is not used in all jurisdictions) is to advance a 16-gauge, 6″ angiocatheter, with a 30- to 60-mL syringe (20-mL or 50-mL syringe in the UK) attached, from just to the right and inferior to the xiphoid process, aiming toward the midclavicle on the left. After entering the thorax with a "pop," draw back on the syringe slightly until a second "pop" is felt and blood returns to the syringe. When placement is confirmed, remove the needle from the angiocatheter and attach a three-way stopcock to the hub of the catheter to help facilitate future removal of blood. One method to confirm that pericardial blood (and not ventricular blood) was withdrawn is to place a small amount of the blood in a basin or dish and allow sufficient time to clot; if it does not clot, you are evacuating pericardial blood. Please consult your protocol and/or medical director prior to implementing this procedure.

Myocardial Rupture

Blunt cardiac trauma, most commonly in the setting of a motor vehicle collision, may cause myocardial rupture as a result of cardiac compression between the sternum and the spine, direct impact (sternal trauma), or deceleration injury. It may result in rupture of the papillary muscles, cardiac free wall, or ventricular septum.

Cardiac injury is the possible result of penetrating chest wounds and blunt chest traumas. Traumatic myocardial rupture is observed more commonly in males 15–63 years old. Delayed myocardial rupture has been reported as a result of cardiac contusion. Acute mitral or tricuspid regurgitation, ventricular septal defect, or pericardial tamponade may result from myocardial rupture secondary to blunt cardiac trauma.

Penetrating myocardial injury occurs most commonly as a result of stab or gunshot wounds. Unlike blunt trauma, penetrating cardiac injury always involves the pericardium. Consequently, ventricular free-wall rupture in this setting may result in either pericardial tamponade or intrathoracic hemorrhage. Although pericardial tamponade is more common with stab wounds, gunshot wounds more frequently are associated with hypovolemic shock.

Indicators of myocardial rupture include tachycardia, dyspnea and tachypnea, bruising or tenderness of the anterior chest wall, cardiogenic or hypovolemic shock, and pericardial tamponade or exsanguination. Patients with pericardial tamponade may present with dyspnea, chest pain, hypotension, cold peripheries, and mental status changes. Myocardial rupture can also be indicated in cases of sudden death, acute pulmonary edema following papillary muscle rupture, congestive heart failure following ventricular septal rupture, and hypotension following free-wall rupture.

Treatment of Myocardial Rupture

Prehospital treatment of a myocardial rupture consists of high-flow oxygen and transport to an appropriate facility. Early surgical intervention is essential for the treatment of myocardial rupture. Symptomatic medical therapy may be used in some cases to stabilize the patient based on the presentation during transport to the surgical team.

Commotio Cordis

Commotio cordis typically involves Caucasian boys between the ages of 4 and 16 years old. It occurs when blunt, non-penetrating, and innocuous-appearing trauma to the anterior chest results in immediate cardiac arrest and sudden death from ventricular fibrillation. Baseball, softball, hockey, lacrosse, and football are the sports activities most commonly involved. Cases have also been reported from bas-

ketball, cricket, martial arts, boxing, street fights, and motor vehicle collisions.

Ventricular fibrillation can be triggered by chest wall impact immediately over the heart and occurs most frequently with impact over the center of the left ventricle. Chest wall impact that does not overlie the heart fails to produce ventricular fibrillation or any other ECG abnormalities.

Patients who are unresponsive, apneic, and pulseless may be experiencing commotio cordis. Many such patients are cyanotic, and tonic-clonic (grand mal) seizures have been evident in some. Chest wall contusions and localized bruising that correspond to the site of chest impact are also indicators.

Treatment of Commotio Cordis

ACLS protocols for cardiac arrest should be initiated, although survival after an event is unusual. Efforts at resuscitation occur frequently; however, the onset of CPR is often delayed because observers underestimate the severity of the trauma or believe that the wind has been knocked out of the person. A 25% survival rate has been associated with effective CPR efforts that are begun within 1–3 minutes of the collapse and are associated with early defibrillation. The survival rate drops dramatically to 3% when resuscitative efforts are delayed longer than 3 minutes.

Aortic Tear or Transection

Blunt aortic injury is part of the spectrum of blunt or deceleration polytrauma. Injury to the thoracic aorta accounts for up to 15% of all deaths resulting from motor vehicle collisions; many are dead on scene from complete aortic transection. Patients who survive transport frequently have tears of the aortic wall with pseudoaneurysm formation.

Penetrating injury (eg, stabbing or gunshot injury) is a different clinical entity from blunt or deceleration trauma. Blunt or deceleration injury to the aorta is mostly confined to the thoracic aorta, except for a seatbelt injury, which involves the abdominal aorta.

The way the heart and aorta are secured to the spinal column leads to a potentially lethal injury. Most blunt aortic injuries occur in the proximal thoracic aorta, although any portion of the aorta is at risk. The descending aorta is tightly adhered to the spinal column where it is at greatest risk from the shearing forces of sudden deceleration. Thus the aorta is at greatest risk in frontal or side impacts and falls from heights.

Large tears result in the patient quickly exsanguinating. Like all arteries, the aorta is made up of several different layers **FIGURE 6-19**:

- The endothelial **tunica intima** is the innermost layer, where the blood flows.
- The **tunica media** is the smooth, muscular middle layer.
- The external layer, the **tunica adventitia**, is made of connective and elastic tissue.

In any deceleration incident in which the heart swings forward, stress can cause the intima to tear. This tearing allows blood to leak, resulting in a weakened bubble in the

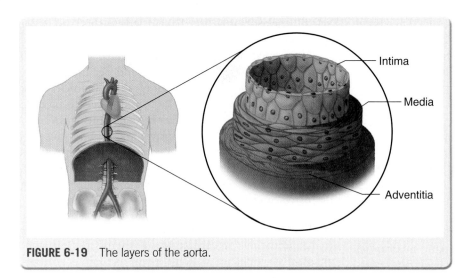

FIGURE 6-19 The layers of the aorta.

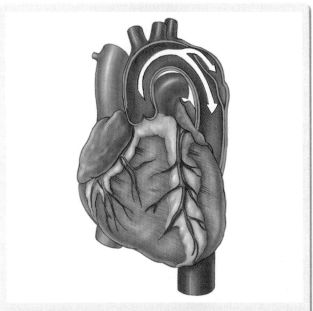

FIGURE 6-20 An aortic tear can produce an aneurysm by allowing blood to leak into the space between the layers of the arterial wall.

arterial wall **FIGURE 6-20**. Partial tears of the aorta have the potential to become an aneurysm over time. These tears often start in the intima and increase in size under pressure of the heart pumping. As the aneurysm expands, the layers of the aorta start to separate, splitting the layers; this is a dissecting aneurysm. An aortic aneurysm is a ticking time bomb unless discovered and treated prior to rupturing.

An aortic tear is usually transverse and involves the layers of the aorta to varying degrees. A complete tear through the intima, media, and adventitia usually leads to rapid exsanguination and death. In aortic rupture survivors, the pseudoaneurysm is contained by the adventitia and occasionally mediastinal structures.

Traumatic aortic disruption or traumatic aortic injury (TAI) syndrome are time-sensitive injuries requiring rapid and accurate diagnosis to prevent mortality. TAI syndrome may be clinically silent, include contained rupture (pseudoaneurysm), and be quickly followed by uncontained pseudoaneurysm rupture, exsanguination, and death.

Indicators of aortic tear include bruising and abrasions of the chest, high index of suspicion, unequal pulses in the upper extremities, change in blood pressure between the upper extremities (> 15 mm Hg), sensation of cutting or tearing through the chest or into the back, and hypotension.

One of the best field findings for an aortic tear or dissecting aneurysm is unequal blood pressures and pulses in the upper extremities. These findings result from the anatomy of the aorta; the subclavian arteries are the third and fifth arteries. Often tears start at the arch where the aorta is anchored and these other arteries exit. The aneurysm restricts flow or occludes the flow into the subclavian arteries, resulting in weaker pulses and blood pressures.

Treatment of Aortic Tear

Recognition of a potential aortic tear is absolutely necessary to prompt aggressive resuscitative treatment. High-flow oxygen is indicated to reduce the chance of shock. Fluid therapy and short-acting antihypertensive agents should be used to keep the systolic blood pressure normal. Be prepared to flow high volumes of crystalloid through large IV or IO catheters to resuscitate the aortic tear victim. Closely monitor the patient's heart rate, ECG, and blood pressure to maintain systolic pressure around 90 mm Hg.

Diaphragm Injuries

The diaphragm is the most important muscle of respiration and functions as a vital pump, moving air into and out of the pulmonary gas-exchange units. The diaphragm is innervated by cervical motor neurons C3–C5 by means of the phrenic nerves. Diaphragmatic contraction decreases chest pressure during inspiration to facilitate the movement of gases into the lungs.

TIP

Excessive fluid resuscitation in the presence of continued uncontrolled bleeding may be detrimental to trauma patients. Research has also proven that attempting to bring the patient's blood pressure to normal may very well worsen hemorrhage.

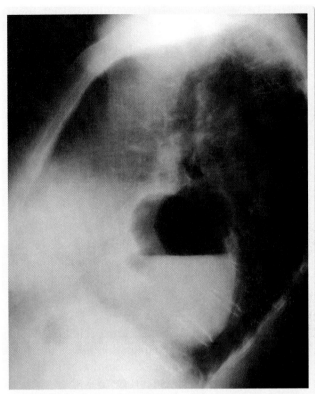

FIGURE 6-21 Radiograph of a diaphragmatic rupture. Notice the dark area of air inside the bowel in the chest cavity.

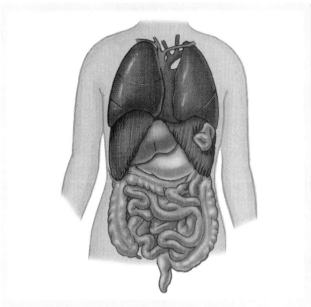

FIGURE 6-22 Diaphragmatic tear with bowel in the chest cavity.

Tears of the diaphragm can be caused by both penetrating and blunt torso trauma **FIGURE 6-21**. Diaphragmatic injury is thought to arise from the abrupt increase in intra-abdominal pressure during blunt trauma. Motor vehicle collisions account for the majority of these events, but falls or crush injuries are also possible causes. A lateral-impact automobile collision is three times more likely than any other impact to result in diaphragmatic rupture. Direct laceration may result from a penetrating object or from a fragment of a fractured rib. It is not a common finding in blunt abdominal trauma, and it may be overlooked because the dominant clinical symptoms may be related to other associated injuries.

Trauma patients with large diaphragmatic tears will present rather quickly with compromised cardiorespiratory function. The cardiorespiratory difficulty may be due to large herniation of abdominal contents including bowel, blood, air, or GI contents into the pleural space. Other patients may be asymptomatic or have vague symptoms. With smaller tears, negative thoracic pressure during respiration causes gradual herniation of the abdominal organs into the thorax. The patient is at risk of strangulation, obstruction, and other life-threatening disorders if the diaphragmatic injury is not repaired. Penetrating injuries can produce small lacerations in the diaphragm, but organ herniation is uncommon.

Due to the proximity of the diaphragm, the spleen and liver are often injured as well. The diaphragm is the primary muscle used in respiration and when it becomes injured, dyspnea and an increase in the work of breathing is often the result. As the patient becomes more dyspneic and the work of breathing increases, there is a greater chance of hernia of the small bowel and other abdominal contents into the thorax. If the bowel is herniated through the tear, there could be some interesting findings when breath sounds are assessed and bowel sounds are heard in an area where they should not be heard. As more and more abdominal contents are herniated into the chest, a tension can form, with the lungs, great vessels, and heart being compressed against the opposite side of the thorax. Eventually, if this injury is missed, the bowel (which is now in the chest) will become confined or kinked, compromising blood supply and leading to an ischemic bowel **FIGURE 6-22**.

Diaphragmatic paralysis may present as either bilateral or unilateral. Bilateral diaphragmatic paralysis typically presents with compromised pulmonary and respiratory-muscle function. If the patient lies supine, the lung capacity is further reduced. Another cause of diaphragmatic paralysis is traumatic injury to the thorax or cervical spine, affecting the phrenic nerve.

In bilateral diaphragmatic paralysis, the accessory respiratory muscles increase the strength and intensity of their contractions to assume some or all of the work of respiration. This extra workload may result in muscle fatigue and respiratory failure.

Treatment of Diaphragmatic Tears

There are many different injuries that could cause difficulty breathing and diminished ventilations, so priority care should be directed to airway and breathing. High-flow oxygen is indicated for all suspected traumatic injuries of the diaphragm. When a tear in the diaphragm is noted early, endotracheal intubation may be indicated. Endotracheal intubation causes an increase in transthoracic pressure, preventing additional herniation of abdominal contents. Positive-pressure ventilation relieves the muscular activity needed by the diaphragm to create the negative pressures in the chest during normal ventilation. To decrease the negative pressures that may pull bowel into the chest, the provider should use a bag-mask device early and maintain airway control. With the possibility of other injuries that are equally critical, IV access and fluid resuscitation should be aimed at maintaining the patient's blood pressure around 90 mm Hg systolic. The earlier the diagnosis of a diaphragmatic tear, the better the patient's outcome will be.

Esophageal Rupture

Esophageal rupture or perforation usually occurs from penetrating injury, but occasionally follows blunt trauma to the chest. The esophagus is the tube through which food and nutrients pass from the pharynx to the stomach. Any disruption of the esophagus allows abdominal contents to leak out into the chest cavity.

Patients who have received a severe blow to the lower sternum or epigastrium, and are in pain or shock out of proportion to the apparent injury, are at risk for esophageal rupture.

Retrosternal pain and pain in the lower anterior chest or upper abdomen indicate esophageal rupture. The patient may also experience difficulty in swallowing, vomiting, hematemesis, tachypnea, tachycardia, and subcutaneous emphysema in the neck.

Treatment of Esophageal Rupture

Patients who experience an esophageal rupture are at high risk of death due to the additional trauma sustained to the chest. Maintain airway and breathing including high-flow oxygen, because a pneumothorax is possible. Frequent suctioning to maintain a clear airway may be required. Nasogastric (NG) or orogastric suctioning is contraindicated in the preshopital setting due to the risk of inserting the NG tube through the wound. Treat shock-like symptoms with fluids and transport all suspected cases to a trauma center.

Tracheobronchial Injury

Anatomic construction and common mechanisms of injury account for the possibility of tracheal or bronchial tearing. The trachea and proximal bronchi have varying amounts of structural support. Distal bronchi and lungs tend to be more mobile than the stronger proximal cartilage framework. This framework helps the trachea and mainstem bronchi stay fixed. Because of this difference, deceleration injuries from blunt trauma often are seen at the area between the fixed and mobile bronchi. Occasionally, blunt trauma to the anterior neck results in rupture of the trachea.

Tracheobronchial tears can be caused by the following:

- A deceleration injury in which there are shearing forces between the fixed trachea and the mobile distal bronchi/lungs
- Rapid chest compression causing traction on the lungs and causing the bronchus to tear from the fixed carina
- Rupture resulting from a sudden increase in pressure against a closed glottis (paper bag syndrome)
- Compression of the trachea between the sternum and spinal column
- Perforation, sometimes by a stylet or an endotracheal tube (ETT)
- Other penetrating injuries

Dyspnea, cough, hemoptysis, and cyanosis are all indicators of tracheobronchial injury. The patient may also present with cervical subcutaneous emphysema, tracheal shift, and signs of airway obstruction.

Treatment of Tracheobronchial Injury

Treatment and transport decisions for this condition depend on the patient's condition and any associated injuries. If a tracheobronchial tear is suspected, consider performing an emergency bronchoscopic examination to confirm the diagnosis. Keep in mind that placing an airway above the tear to provide positive-pressure ventilations may worsen the condition. When conditions permit, allow the patient to continue to breathe on their own with supplemental oxygen.

Traumatic Asphyxia

Compressive asphyxia refers to the mechanical limitation of the expansion of the chest. In trauma situations, the term traumatic asphyxia is usually used to describe compressive asphyxia resulting from being crushed or pinned under a large weight or force FIGURE 6-23 . An example of compressive asphyxia includes cases in which an individual has been using a car jack to repair a car from below, only to be crushed under the weight of the vehicle when the car

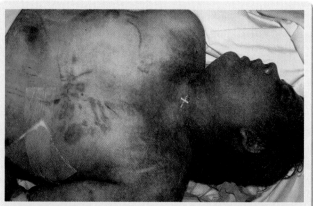

FIGURE 6-23 Traumatic asphyxia results from a victim being crushed or pinned under a large weight or force.

jack slips. Other examples include victims entrapped in an earthen cave-in and fatal crowd disasters from the compression of victims against other victims or the walls of the stadium.

The cause of death of detainees who have been restrained and left prone, for example in police vehicles, and are unable to move into safer positions, has been referred to as *positional asphyxia* or *restraint asphyxia*, which is a form of traumatic asphyxia.

Traumatic asphyxia is caused by sudden and violent compression of the chest or abdomen. Prolonged compression of the thorax results in increased superior vena cava (SVC) pressure and obstruction of flow through the valveless veins of the innominate and jugular venous system. This increased pressure causes backup in the capillary beds in the head, neck, and upper extremities, producing discoloration of the skin.

Indicators of traumatic asphyxia include craniocervical cyanosis and edema, subconjunctival hemorrhage or petechia, JVD, pulmonary contusion, and hemothorax.

Treatment of Traumatic Asphyxia

Treatment is directed at reversing the asphyxia. Release the patient from the confined position or reposition the patient to support blood flow into the chest. Standard ACLS protocols are indicated with attention given to airway and ventilation support. Mortality in cases involving traumatic asphyxia is more often due to associated injuries; additional assessment should be geared to identifying these.

Evisceration

In an evisceration, an organ has spilled outside of its intended cavity, usually the small intestine through the abdominal wall or rectum **FIGURE 6-24**. Intestinal evisceration through the abdominal wall is most often caused by penetrating trauma. Blunt trauma following falls from great distances or crush mechanisms is the most likely cause of

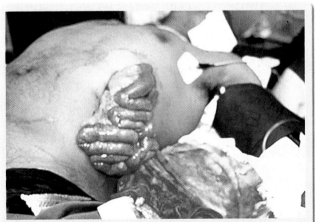

FIGURE 6-24 Eviscerations allow abdominal organs to be exposed to the outside of the body.

evisceration through the rectum or perineum. Generally little pain is associated with this type of injury; however, you may notice a rigid abdomen, bleeding, and shock in addition to the bowel outside of the abdomen.

Treatment of an Evisceration

Although these injuries are usually very visual, considering the mechanism of injury, a high index of suspicion, and good assessment technique will allow the provider to recognize this injury. Begin by keeping the patient calm to avoid internal pressure causing more bowel to become displaced externally. Administer high-flow oxygen and cover the injury with a moist sterile dressing. Protect the protruding bowel from hanging because gravity or movement can cause additional displacement of bowel. Follow local protocols to determine whether you should cover with an occlusive dressing. Secure the bandage, making it snug but not tight to avoid further injury. Resist the temptation to try to push the evisceration back into the wound; this will cause more injury to the already damaged bowel and increase the risk of infection. Prepare to support the patient's circulation by having an IV in place for fluid resuscitation.

Liver Injury

The liver is the largest intra-abdominal solid organ. The most common cause of liver injury is blunt trauma, because the liver is relatively large and in a fixed position **FIGURE 6-25**. In most occurrences, this injury is secondary to motor vehicle collisions. Although the liver is the second most commonly injured organ in abdominal trauma, liver damage is the most common cause of death after abdominal injury.

Deceleration injuries with shear forces may tear the liver and may involve the inferior vena cava and hepatic veins. Liver injury occurs more easily in children than in

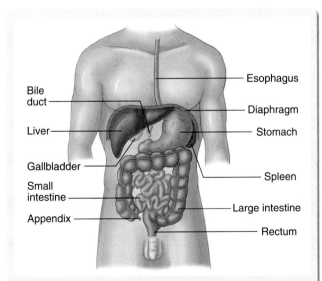

Esophagus
Bile duct
Diaphragm
Liver
Stomach
Gallbladder
Spleen
Small intestine
Large intestine
Appendix
Rectum

FIGURE 6-25 The liver is the largest solid abdominal organ and is prone to blunt trauma.

adults. A child's undeveloped liver and more flexible rib cage allow more force to be transmitted internally. The liver is one of the most common abdominal organs injured by penetrating trauma. Penetrating trauma of the liver may be caused by bullets, shrapnel, knives, and other sharp objects. Suspect liver laceration when penetrating trauma involves the right lower chest or right upper abdomen, or when upper right abdominal tenderness accompanies blunt trauma.

Suspect liver injury if the patient experiences signs of blood loss, such as shock, hypotension, tachycardia, tachypnea, or pallor; right upper quadrant tenderness and guarding; or peritoneal irritation. Remember, however, that rebound sensitivity and guarding will not be present until blood has been in the abdomen long enough to cause peritoneal irritation.

Treatment of Liver Injury

Treatment of injury to the liver is based on the level of blood loss and shock. Because liver injuries produce large amounts of blood loss, supplemental oxygen is required. Fluid replacement should be directed to the level of shock present (see Chapter 4). Rapid transport to a trauma center is indicated for all suspected liver injuries.

Spleen Injury

The spleen is the most vascular organ of the body and contains approximately 1 unit (400–500 mL) of blood at a given time. The functionally complex spleen, located in the left upper abdomen, is a commonly injured organ when torso trauma occurs. Penetrating injuries also frequently involve the spleen. Like the liver, the spleen is protected by the rib cage and its position is maintained by several ligaments, making deceleration injury common.

Signs of blood loss, such as shock, hypotension, tachycardia, tachypnea, or pallor, indicate possible splenic injury. The patient may also present with left upper abdominal or flank tenderness and guarding, as well as peritoneal irritation. Rebound sensitivity and guarding will not be present, however, until blood has been in the abdomen long enough to cause peritoneal irritation.

Treatment of Spleen Injury

Treatment of blood loss and shock is the key when treating injury to the spleen. Because splenic injuries result in large amounts of blood loss, assessment and treatment of shock with high-flow oxygen and fluids is indicated. Splenic trauma is a surgical emergency and transport to a trauma center is indicated for all suspected cases.

Pancreatic Injury

Pancreatic injury is very difficult to diagnose and has a high mortality. Additionally, duodenal or biliary duct injury often accompanies the injury. Because of the anatomic position of the pancreas in the retroperitoneum, it is relatively well protected. It typically takes a high-energy force to damage the pancreas. These high-energy forces are most commonly produced by penetrating trauma. Blunt injury should be suspected after a localized blow to the midabdomen, such as from motorcycle handlebars or a steering wheel.

Suspect an injury to the pancreas with any localized blow to the abdomen. The patient will likely experience vague upper and midabdominal pain that radiates into the back. Hours after the injury, generalized peritoneal irritation may reveal the presence of traumatic pancreatitis.

Treatment of Pancreatic Injury

Injuries to the pancreas have subtle or absent signs and symptoms initially and should be suspected after a localized blow to the midabdomen. Over the course of hours to days, pancreatic injuries result in the spillage of enzymes into the retroperitoneal space, which can damage surrounding structures and lead to gross systemic infection and retroperitoneal abscess. These patients usually experience a vague upper and midabdominal pain that radiates to the back. Peritoneal signs may develop several hours after the injury. Repeated abdominal examinations are the key to discovering a patient's worsening condition before vital signs change.

Gastrointestinal Tract Injury

Injuries that break the wall of the bowel are usually due to penetrating injury. In penetrating trauma, the small bowel is most frequently injured, followed by the stomach and large intestine. Blunt trauma can occur from vehicular accidents, falls, and assaults **FIGURE 6-26**.

Rupture can occur when a localized crush occurs, such as when the steering wheel pinches the duodenum against the spine. The location of the duodenum and its ligamentous attachments make it one of the most commonly injured areas of the abdomen. Shearing injury also can occur adjacent to the ligament of Treitz. When the colon is injured, compressive injury to the transverse colon, the sigmoid colon, or the cecum is common.

The physical forces involved in the mechanism of injury to the bowel in blunt abdominal trauma can be divided into two categories: compression forces and deceleration forces.

- *Compression forces* increase the pressure in the bowel and compress the fluid-filled bowel against the spine or other solid structures.
- *Deceleration forces* can stretch and tear the bowel loops at points of attachment, such as the ligament of Treitz or the phrenocolic ligament.

Each anatomic region of the GI tract is associated with characteristic patterns of injury. Blunt abdominal gastric trauma can occur after a full meal. Most full-thickness gastric injuries result from penetrating trauma. Symptoms may result from the intestinal contents and not from blood loss.

Swelling, bruising, skin penetration, and lack of bowel sounds may indicate a GI injury. Other indicators are guarding and direct or rebound tenderness and burning epigastric pain with rigidity and rebound sensitivity. If the small bowel and colon are injured, vague generalized pain may be present, with peritonitis occurring hours later. A patient with back pain may have a duodenal injury. Suspect kidney injury as well.

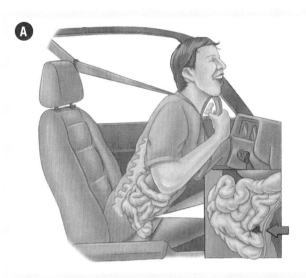
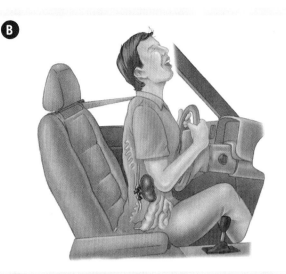

FIGURE 6-26 Blunt trauma to the GI tract can be from **A.** compression forces or **B.** shearing forces.

Treatment of Gastrointestinal Tract Injury

Repeated abdominal examinations are the key to discovering a patient's worsening condition before vital signs change. While en route to the hospital, continue to reassess the location, intensity, and quality of pain; whether or not nausea or vomiting is present; the contour of the abdomen; any ecchymosis or open areas present on the soft-tissue inspection; and the presence or absence of rebound tenderness, guarding, rigidity, spasm, or localized pain. A common misconception is that patients without abdominal pain or abnormal vital signs are unlikely to have serious intra-abdominal injuries. Keep in mind that peritonitis can take hours to days to develop. Similarly, nonspecific symptoms such as hypotension, tachycardia, and confusion may not develop until the patient has lost more than 40% of his or her circulating blood volume.

IV fluids and oxygen should be initiated to treat for early stages of shock. Administering pain medication is somewhat controversial because it may mask symptoms and often is contraindicated because of the patient's hypotension. In some instances, it may be appropriate to consult with medical direction en route to the hospital to discuss analgesia.

Because older adults usually have a more flaccid abdominal wall (containing less muscle and more fat) than younger people, apply increased pressure when palpating the abdomen to assess for injury. You should suspect that any older trauma patient who complains of abdominal pain has an internal organ injury.

Kidney Injury

Kidney injury is seen commonly with falls, causing a shearing injury, and automobile collisions. Where there is fracture of the 11th–12th ribs or flank tenderness, suspect kidney injury. If any hematuria is present, note the nature of the injury because kidney lacerations may bleed heavily into the retroperitoneal space. Additional indicators of kidney injury include pain, specifically in the abdomen and flank on inspiration, and costovertebral angle (CVA) tenderness. Flank discoloration may be found later.

Treatment of Kidney Injury

The contused kidney is easily noted. What is not simply observed is whether the kidney lacerations can be managed nonsurgically or will bleed, producing shock. Treat for shock if present and continue frequent reassessments. All patients with suspected kidney trauma should be transported to a center capable of performing surgery if needed.

Bladder Injury

The likelihood of bladder injury varies according to the bladder's distension. A full bladder is more likely to be injured than an empty one. Patients with a bladder injury have a history of pelvic trauma, usually from motor vehicle collisions, deceleration injuries, or assaults to the lower abdomen. In an automobile collision, bladder injury may occur from direct impact with the car or indirectly from the steering wheel or seatbelt. Falling many feet onto an unyielding surface can result in deceleration injuries to the bladder. Bladder perforation usually results from blunt trauma to the lower abdomen or penetrating trauma to the suprapubic area.

STATS

Males have a higher incidence of bladder injury than females. The position of the female pelvis protects the bladder from injury better than the male pelvis.

Gross hematuria, suprapubic pain and tenderness, difficulty urinating, abdominal distension, and guarding or rebound tenderness all indicate a bladder injury.

Treatment of Bladder Injury

Bladder injuries require surgical intervention. Be alert for signs of shock because outward signs of bleeding may not be present. Treat the patient symptomatically and provide transport to a facility with surgical capabilities.

Pelvic and Genital Injuries

Pelvic Fractures

The pelvis is best thought of as a ring, with its sacral, iliac, ischial, and pubic bones held together by ligaments. Large forces are required to damage this ring. The majority of pelvic fractures are a result of blunt trauma from motor vehicle collision or from vehicles striking pedestrians **FIGURE 6-27**. Because of the forces required to break the pelvis, suspect multisystem trauma if your patient has a pelvic injury (until proven otherwise).

Anteroposterior compression, which can result from a head-on collision, may lead to an "open-book" pelvic fracture in which the pubic symphysis spreads apart. The subsequent increase in volume of the pelvis means a patient with internal pelvic bleeding may lose a much larger amount of blood than someone without an open-book fracture. Vertical shear is seen in falls from heights. It results in one side of the pelvis moving superiorly or inferiorly compared to the other, disrupting the bony or ligamentous structures. This unstable fracture results in an increased pelvic volume. Lateral compression of the pelvis results from a side impact. It generally does not result in an unstable pelvis. Because the volume in the pelvis is not increased, life-threatening hemorrhage is less of a concern in such cases.

Saddle injuries result from falling on an object. They may result in fractures of the bones that are directly under the female and male genitalia (pubic rami fractures).

Although penetrating trauma to the pelvis may result in bony fractures, the more worrisome injury is to the major vascular structures, which can cause life-threatening hemorrhage. Open fractures (not to be confused with open-book fractures) may result from either penetrating or blunt trauma and frequently result in chronic pain and disability that persist for years after the initial injury **FIGURE 6-28**.

If there has been enough energy applied to fracture the pelvis, other structures like the femoral arteries and veins, bladder, uterus, and internal female reproductive organs are at risk of injury. Pelvic fractures are associated with a high risk of blood loss. A ruptured bladder and tears of the femoral artery or veins top the list of these potential pelvic injuries.

Indicators of pelvic fracture include pain in the pelvis, groin, or hips; hematomas or contusions to the pelvic region; obvious external bleeding including bleeding at the

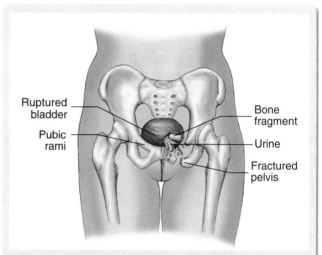

FIGURE 6-27 Pelvic fractures commonly cause laceration of the bladder as a result of penetration by bony fragments. Externally, pelvic fractures can cause severe bruising and swelling.

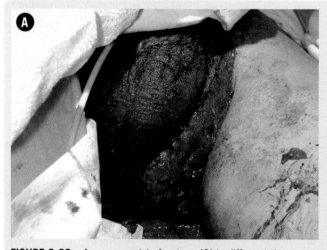
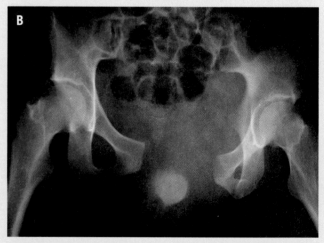

FIGURE 6-28 An open pelvic fracture (**A**) is different than an open book pelvic fracture (**B**).

urethra; hypotension without obvious external bleeding; unstable pelvis; and pain with compression of the iliac crest.

Treatment of Pelvic Fracture

Splint the pelvis to help minimize blood loss from the fracture. A pelvic strap or a bed sheet wrapped around the pelvis at the iliac crest and secured appropriately will help tamponade the bleeding **PROCEDURE 35**. It is essential to tie the strap or sheet correctly for the splint to work properly. For an open-book pelvic fracture in a patient with hypotension, tie a sheet around the patient's hips at the level of the superior anterior iliac crests, thereby decreasing the pelvic volume. There are several devices specific to the treatment of this type of injury that provide superior immobilization and are faster to apply **FIGURE 6-29**. For example the SAM sling or the Hip Hugger system from Morrison Medical wrap around the hips to provide stabilization of hip fractures.

With the potential for large volumes of blood loss, there may be a need for fluid resuscitation to maintain systolic blood pressure of 90–100 mm Hg. Such patients will require IV fluids with lactated Ringer's or Hartmann's solution or normal saline but may still remain hypotensive in the field. Respiratory compromise is common after splinting the pelvis; intubation may be required.

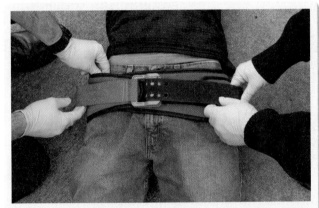
FIGURE 6-29 Several pelvic straps/splints are available or a sheet can be used to bring the bones of the pelvis back into closer alignment.

PRO/CON

The pneumatic antishock garment (PASG) is a controversial treatment that can be used to stabilize the pelvis during rapid transports. It can potentially decrease pain by causing less movement of the fractured bones and decrease bleeding by reducing pelvic volume, although some emergency medicine specialists believe that the PASG may increase bleeding by putting pressure on pelvic vessels.

Genital Injuries
Male

Male external genital injuries result from violence, accidents, sports injuries, or sexually related trauma. In young boys, one of the most common causes of genital injury is having the seat slam down while they are using the toilet or entrapment of the scrotum, penis, or foreskin in a zipper. Injury to the genitals can be very painful and bleed heavily. It can affect the reproductive organs as well as the bladder and urethra. The amount of damage can range from minimal to severe. Temporary as well as permanent damage can be done.

Penetrating trauma of the penis can occur from gunshot wounds but is more often a self-inflicted attempt at amputation or complete amputation. Victims with gunshot wounds usually have associated injury to the thigh, scrotum, pelvis, or buttock **FIGURE 6-30**. The most common reason for penile amputation is self-mutilation. The majority of these patients are actively psychotic at the time of injury and almost all have some form of psychiatric illness.

Motorcycle injuries where the victim has slid forward over the gas tank are one cause of injury. Kicking, biting, or beating is possible during an assault. Another common cause of genital injuries in younger males is having the feet slip while they are climbing or playing (such as on monkey bars) and landing with the legs on each side of the bar (straddle injury). This can also happen by falling onto the crossbar of a bicycle. Blunt trauma can occur to the penis or testicles, resulting in internal bleeding. This bleeding is usually confined to the penis or scrotum, but a degloving injury can occur.

Burns to the genitals are uncommon, but when they do occur they are accompanied by a larger burn surface area, and should be referred to a specialist burn center. Burns to the genitals in children should leave the provider with a suspicion of child abuse. The child can suffer a burn when a parent or caregiver tries to teach the child a lesson about not touching themselves by applying hot water or oil.

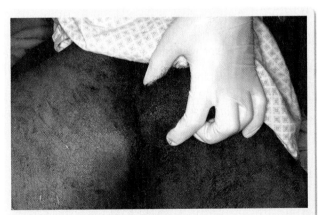
FIGURE 6-30 Penetrating trauma to the penis or scrotum may result from a gunshot.

Female

Injury to the external female genitalia is much less common. Sexual assault is a more common cause of blunt trauma and in cases of rape or sexual abuse, a medical examination is necessary—it is essential for the victim's health and to prevent the spread of infectious diseases.

The following are indicators of genital trauma:

- Abdominal pain
- Bleeding
- Bruising
- Affected area has changed in shape
- Faintness
- Object embedded in a body opening
- Groin pain or genital pain (can be extreme)
- Swelling
- Urine drainage, painful urination, or inability to urinate
- Vomiting
- Genital wound

Treatment of Genital Injuries

Treatment of genital injury is largely symptomatic. Control external bleeding with direct pressure. If vaginal bleeding is present following trauma, place a sanitary pad at the vaginal opening to collect the blood, but do not attempt to locate the bleeding. Have the patient remain with her legs closed to keep internal pressure in the vagina. Assaults are a law enforcement case. Remember to keep all articles of clothing for evidence and advise the patient not to shower or change clothes until after an exam is completed at the hospital.

In the case of penile amputations, place the amputated penis in a bag and keep it cool. Transport it with the patient to the hospital for reimplantation. Cases of genital trauma are not only physically traumatic, but also have a psychological stigma for victims. Care for these patients requires first aid for both injuries. For less serious cases, such as the foreskin caught in a zipper, reassurance and pain management are both indicated. Various techniques exist which involve either breaking the zipper "teeth" pattern, or cutting through the bridge of the movable part to allow the zipper to part.

CHAPTER RESOURCES

CASE STUDY ANSWERS

1 What concerns are there for scene safety?

Scenes of family violence can be very volatile. EMS providers should be alert for sudden changes that could endanger them or their partners.

2 Are there times when EMS should report injuries to law enforcement even though the patient may not approve?

Patient privacy is something that EMS providers should respect. There are several situations that often require mandatory reporting. Calls such as child abuse, animal bites, and penetrating trauma often have mandatory reporting requirements. You should know your local laws and protocols and how they relate to your patients.

3 How should the knife be secured?

The knife should be secured with bulky dressings to keep it from moving. Often stacking several bandages one above the other and making a cut halfway across the bandages will allow you to slide the bandages around the object. The bandages should then be taped securely in place.

4 Does this patient have a pneumothorax? Hemothorax?

The bubbling coming through the wound indicates an open pneumothorax. This pneumothorax has the possibility of becoming a tension pneumothorax if the wound becomes clotted and excess air is not allowed to exit the chest. The high pulse and low blood pressure most likely indicate bleeding into the chest. A hemothorax is likely unless additional injury is noted.

CASE STUDY ANSWERS

5 Will your patient require ventilation, IV fluids, or both? What are the dangers of aggressive management in either?

Your patient will require high-concentration oxygen and may require ventilation if his condition does not stabilize or worsens. Aggressive ventilation in the setting of a pneumothorax can make the pneumothorax worse. When positive pressure is placed into the lung, air can leak into the pleural space, making a larger pneumothorax or allowing a simple pneumothorax to become a tension pneumothorax.

Due to the low blood pressure and signs of shock, fluid therapy should be initiated. Many local protocols are based on maintaining a minimum blood pressure that will preserve organ function but not over-resuscitate the patient. When the patient is bleeding into the chest, there is little that will help tamponade that bleeding. Aggressive fluid therapy could increase the blood pressure, allowing more blood to accumulate in the chest.

Trauma in Motion

1. What is your local protocol regarding tension pneumothorax and decompression? What equipment do you have available?
2. What is your local protocol regarding open pneumothorax? What equipment do you have available?
3. What tools does your organization have to manage unstable pelvic fractures?
4. What are your local protocols regarding pain management and abdominal trauma?
5. Recognizing that some patients are too unstable to withstand a long trip or that a trauma center may be a great distance away, what facilities are available in your area to manage:
   - Emergent chest trauma requiring skills above your level?
   - Abdominal trauma based on mechanism of injury but not confirmed by physical exam?
   - Uncontrolled shock from a pelvic fracture?

References and Resources

Ahmed Z, Mohyuddin Z. Management of flail chest injury: internal fixation versus endotracheal intubation and ventilation. *J Thorac Cardiovasc Surg.* 1995; 110:1676.

American College of Surgeons Committee on Trauma. Thoracic trauma. In: *Advanced Trauma Life Support for Doctors. Instructor Course Manual.* Chicago: American College of Surgeons; 1997:147–163.

Bandi G, Santucci RA. Controversies in the management of male external genitourinary trauma. *J Trauma.* 2004; 56:1362–1370.

Britten S, Palmer SH, Snow TM. Needle thoracocentesis in tension pneumothorax: insufficient cannula length and potential failure. Available at: www.brooksidepress.org/Products/OperationalMedicine/DATA/operationalmed/Manuals/FMSS/INJURYMECHANISMSFROMCONVENTIONALWEAPONSFMST0424.htm. Accessed February 6, 2009.

Cohn SM. Pulmonary contusion: review of the clinical entity. *J Trauma.* 1997; 42:973–979.

Dubinsky I, Low A. Non–life-threatening blunt chest trauma: appropriate investigation and treatment. *Am J Emerg Med.* 1997; 15:240.

Eckstein M, Suyehara D. Needle thoracostomy in the prehospital setting. *Prehospital Emerg Care.* 1998; 2(2):132–135.

McKenzie D. To breathe or not to breathe: the respiratory muscles and COPD. *J Appl Physiol.* 2006; 101:1279–1280.

Nagy KK, Fabian T, Rodman G, et al. Guidelines for the diagnosis and management of blunt aortic injury. 2000. Available at: www.east.org/tpg/chap8.pdf. Accessed February 6, 2009.

Pelosi P, Cereda M, Foti G. Alterations of lung and chest wall mechanics in patients with acute lung injury: effects of positive end-expiratory pressure. *Am J Resp Crit Care Med.* 1995; 152:531.

Tadler SC, Burton JH. Intrathoracic stomach presenting as acute tension gastrothorax. *Am J Emerg Med.* 1999; 17:370–371.

Welsford M. Diaphragmatic injuries. Available at: www.emedicine.com/emerg/TOPIC136.HTM. Accessed February 6, 2009.

Williams M, Carlin AM, Tyburski JG, et al. Predictors of mortality in patients with traumatic diaphragmatic rupture and associated thoracic and/or abdominal injuries. *Am Surg.* 2004; 70(2):157–162.

Yarlagadda C, Hout WM. Cardiac tamponade. Available at: www.emedicine.com/med/TOPIC283.HTM. Accessed February 6, 2009.

7 Musculoskeletal and Extremity Trauma

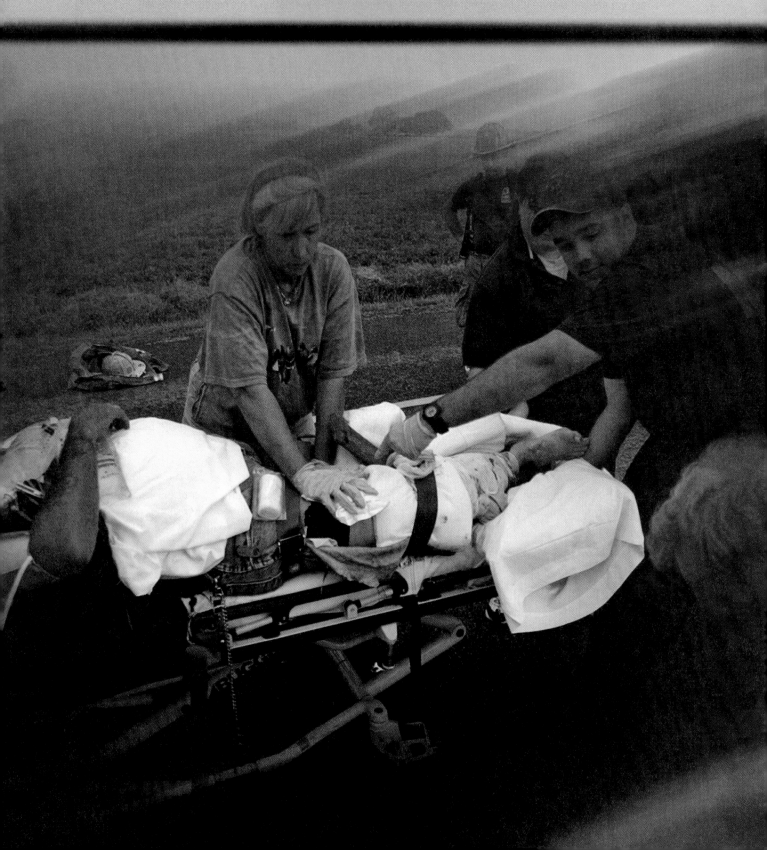

You are dispatched to a collision involving a motorcycle and an automobile. En route, dispatch informs you that the motorcyclist has been thrown some distance and is badly injured. The roadway you are sent to is a straight stretch of highway that often sees vehicles traveling faster than the speed limit.

Your initial observation of the scene reveals a patient lying on the side of the roadway. The automobile has front right-sided damage and the motorcycle, which has extensive damage, is off the roadway in the grass. The driver of the car tells you that he did not see the motorcycle until the last moment and he tried to swerve, but was unable to avoid the motorcycle.

The patient is a 32-year-old man who complains of extreme pain in his right leg. He tells you that the car moved into his lane of traffic and when they struck, the bike went down on his right leg. He is very anxious and keeps telling you he cannot feel his right foot. He does not think he lost consciousness and states he took off his own helmet but his leg hurt too much to move. He is alert and is able to maintain his own airway. His breathing is slightly tachypneic at 22 breaths/min. His skin is pale and radial pulses are weak at a rate of 110 beats/min. Further questioning reveals he has no pertinent medical history, takes no medication, and is allergic to morphine.

As you review the patient, you notice pooled blood around his right femur. After exposing the leg, heavy and steady bleeding is noted from a large laceration crossing the upper leg. Direct pressure with a trauma bandage is able to control the bleeding. The only injury noted during your rapid trauma assessment is of the right leg. The femur is deformed above the knee and there is an open fracture of the lower leg proximal to the ankle. There is no pedal pulse and capillary refill in the right foot is delayed. After applying high-flow oxygen and spinal immobilization, the patient is moved to the ambulance for further treatment and transport to the trauma center.

1 What are the priorities for assessment of this patient?

2 If direct pressure to the wound on the leg did not control the bleeding, what other options are available?

3 Would realignment and splinting of the leg be appropriate?

4 Describe your assessment for a lower extremity and an upper extremity.

Introduction

Injury to the extremities is usually the most common single system trauma call for an emergency medical service (EMS) system. This type of injury causes decreased locomotion and significant pain for the patient. Because the human body uses the arms and legs for stability and movement, they are often the site where outside energy impacts the body. Mechanisms of injury (MOIs) often include loss of balance resulting in localized trauma in an attempt to try to support a falling body.

To supply the oxygen and nutrients to support the muscular activity, large amounts of blood must pass through the extremities. Nervous structure is required to produce movement and return sensory information to help position the body. The circulatory and nervous systems are at great risk when an extremity is injured by either direct or indirect trauma. Direct trauma can cut through the structures or break bones, and indirect trauma can occur due to a loss of circulation following swelling or pinching of pulses. These traumas can cause permanent disability. Treatment of extremity trauma is best served by early immobilization in the prehospital setting. Pain control should also be handled through pharmacological and nonpharmacological means.

Anatomy and Physiology

The term **musculoskeletal system** refers to the bones, tendons, ligaments, and voluntary muscles that give the body its form and movement. The adult human skeleton consists of 206 bones of various shapes and sizes. The skeleton, or scaffolding, gives us our upright posture and also protects the vital organs. The tendons attach the muscles to the bone and the bones are attached to each other by the ligaments.

Skeletal Structure

Bones are rigid structures that give the body shape and protection **FIGURE 7-1** . They protect the vital organs in the abdomen and pelvis, as well as the brain and lungs. They also allow for movement of the body where muscles lever articulating bones called **joints**. **Osseous tissue**, or bone tissue, is the three-dimensional honeycomb-like structure that gives the bone rigidity and shape. Bone marrow, found in the center of the bone, produces red and white blood cells and stores calcium and phosphorus.

There are two bone forms: the hard outer shell, or cortex, called **cortical bone** (or compact bone) and the inner spongy bone called **cancellous bone**. In long bones, the innermost space is called the marrow cavity or **intramedullary canal**. Other types of tissue found in bones include endosteum and periosteum, which line the inner and outer cortex, respectively, and cartilage, a specialized connective tissue. The tough, fibrous periosteum contains blood vessels, lymphatic vessels, and nerves **FIGURE 7-2** .

The bones of the body come in a variety of sizes and shapes. The four principal types are long, short, flat, and irregular bones. Long bones are located mainly in the skel-

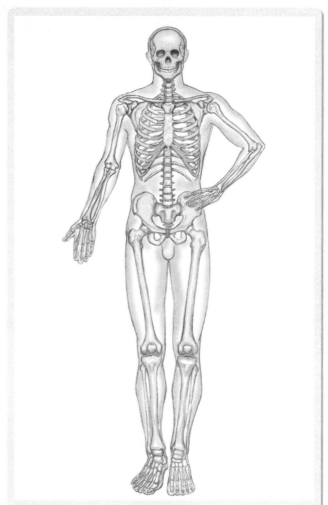

FIGURE 7-1   The skeleton gives the body structure and protects the internal organs.

eton of the arms and legs, whereas most short bones are in the hands, feet, wrists, and ankles. Long bones consist of a long shaft, called the **diaphysis**, with two bulbous ends with shorter bones consisting of little or no diaphysis. Flat bones are thin, flattened, and usually curved. The bones of the skull and rib cage are flat bones. Bones that do not fit in any of the other categories are irregular bones. The vertebrae and some bones of the skull are irregular bones.

Because increasing age decreases bone density, the bones of the elderly tend to be more fragile. The condition of decreased bone density is called osteoporosis. Poor diet without sufficient amounts of calcium and vitamin D also contribute to weakening bones.

Structure of the Shoulder and Upper Extremities

The shoulder girdle consists of three joints comprising the humerus, scapula, clavicle, and sternum. The joints are therefore termed the sternoclavicular, acromioclavicular, and glenohumeral joints. The **scapula** is a large, triangular, flat bone on the back side of the rib cage, commonly called the shoulder blade. The shoulder blade overlays the second through the seventh rib and serves to attach several muscles.

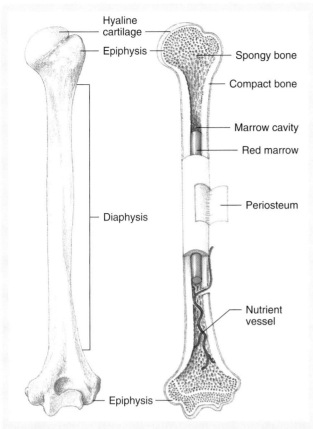

FIGURE 7-2 Bone has blood vessels along the periosteum and in the intramedullary canal.

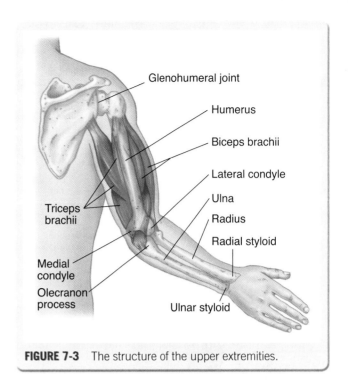

FIGURE 7-3 The structure of the upper extremities.

joint. The tibia and fibula make up the lower leg. Extending from the femur to the talus, the tibia supports the weight of the body while the fibula articulates with the tibia to add stability to the body. Tarsals, metatarsals, and phalanges make up the bones of the feet and toes FIGURE 7-4.

Joints

Joints are where two or more bones articulate. Ligaments provide structure to connect the bones across the joint. Tendons connect muscle to the bones on either side of a joint, allowing for movement of the skeleton. Some joints are fixed, like those in the skull, and allow for no movement. Other joints that are tightly supported by ligaments, like those in the spine, allow for limited movement. Many joints, especially in the extremities, allow for greater movement, providing the ability for locomotion.

Types of Joints

The shoulder and hip are ball-and-socket joints and allow a wide range of movement and rotation. The **condyloid joints** of the jaw and fingers allow for movement, but no rotation. **Gliding joints**, such as those in the wrists, ankles, and spine, allow bones to glide past each other. The knee and elbow are **hinge joints** and allow movement much like that of a door hinge. The **pivot joints** of the neck allow bones to pivot or twist around one another. The thumb has a **saddle joint**, which allows movement back and forth and side to side, but very little rotation. All movable joints are lubricated by synovial fluid within the joint. Many joints also have a **bursa**, a synovial-like membrane around the joint to protect it and to decrease the friction of rubbing tendons over their bony prominences.

A shallow depression called the glenoid cavity holds the head of the humerus to form the glenohumeral joint (shoulder joint). The clavicle, or collarbone, is a slender S-shaped bone that connects the upper arm to the body and holds the shoulder joint away from the body by keeping the scapula on the posterior aspect of the thorax and preventing the glenoid from turning anteriorly. This ultimately allows for a greater range of motion. The proximal end of the clavicle is connected to the sternum, forming the sternoclavicular joint and the distal end to the acromion (most superior aspect) of the scapula and making the **acromioclavicular joint**. These structures are readily exposed and easily dislocated or fractured. The lower arm contains the radius and ulna, whereas the carpals, metacarpals, and phalanges make up the wrist, hand, and fingers, respectively FIGURE 7-3.

Structure of the Pelvis and Lower Extremities

The pelvis is made up of three separate parts: the ilium, ischium, and pubis bones. In an adult, these three bones are rigidly connected together to form the pelvic girdle. The large bone in the upper leg is called the femur. At the distal end of the femur, the lateral and medial condyles articulate with the tibia. These condyles support the attachment of muscles and ligaments. The patella, or kneecap, lies within the major anterior tendon of the thigh muscles, articulates with the trochlear groove in the femur, and covers the knee

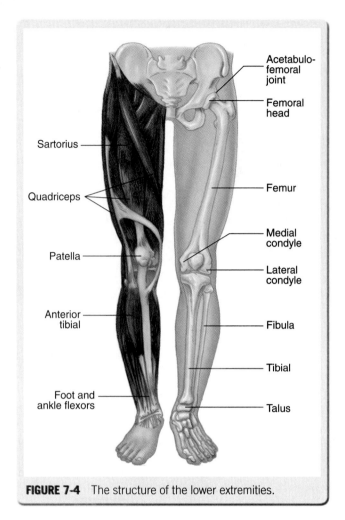

FIGURE 7-4 The structure of the lower extremities.

Labels (Figure 7-4):
Acetabulo-femoral joint
Femoral head
Sartorius
Femur
Quadriceps
Patella
Medial condyle
Lateral condyle
Anterior tibial
Fibula
Tibial
Foot and ankle flexors
Talus

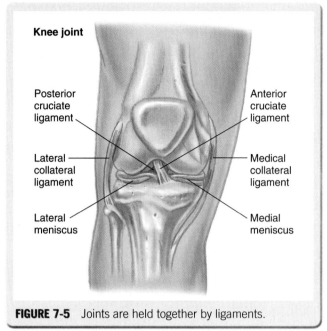

Knee joint

Posterior cruciate ligament
Anterior cruciate ligament
Lateral collateral ligament
Medical collateral ligament
Lateral meniscus
Medial meniscus

FIGURE 7-5 Joints are held together by ligaments.

Skeletal Connecting and Supporting Structures

Joints are held together by **ligaments** FIGURE 7-5 . Ligaments are tough bands of tissue made up of collagen fibrils that bind the bones on either side of the joint. These ligaments control the range of motion and stabilize the joint so the bones move in the proper alignment. A sprain occurs when the joint is forced apart and the ligament is stretched or torn. **Tendons** also help stabilize the joint but are the source of movement to the joint. Tendons are also made up of collagen, a very tough, yet flexible band of fibrous tissue that connects the muscle to the bone. When a muscle contracts, the tendon pulls on the bone on the opposite side of the joint to provide movement. A strain occurs when the muscle is stretched or torn.

Skeletal Muscle

Skeletal muscles are the engine that your body uses to propel itself. Muscles turn energy into motion. Muscle fibers, connective tissue, blood vessels, and nerves form the body of the muscle. The number of muscle cells in the body of a muscle remains constant throughout life. Size and strength of the muscle depend on the individual muscle fibers or cells. Absolutely everything that your brain conceives is expressed as muscular motion. Skeletal muscle operates in pairs or groups: one muscle that contracts to move the joint in one direction and another that contracts to move the joint in the opposite direction. The head, or origin, of a muscle connects to the more stationary of the two bones it connects. The insertion is at the opposite end of the muscle and attaches to the more mobile of the bones of the joint. The largest point between the origin and the insertion is referred to as the belly of the muscle. Some muscles can have multiple origins.

Skeletal muscles are **voluntary muscles**, meaning that we think about moving them and the nervous system tells them to move. Smooth muscles are **involuntary muscles** and are found in the digestive system, blood vessels, bladder, and airway. These muscles have the ability to stretch and hold tension for long periods of time and are controlled by the autonomic or involuntary nervous system. Cardiac muscle is found only in the heart and is the strongest muscle in the body as far as endurance and consistency.

The body can make muscles work together to form a movement, called synergy, or make muscles work in opposition to each other, making them antagonists. We often use synergy of muscles in movement to produce locomotion while having muscles working in opposition to provide stability, such as for standing upright.

Blood Supply

The upper extremities' blood supply originates from the subclavian artery. When the subclavian artery reaches the axilla, it is referred to as the axillary artery. After giving off several branches that supply the shoulder region with

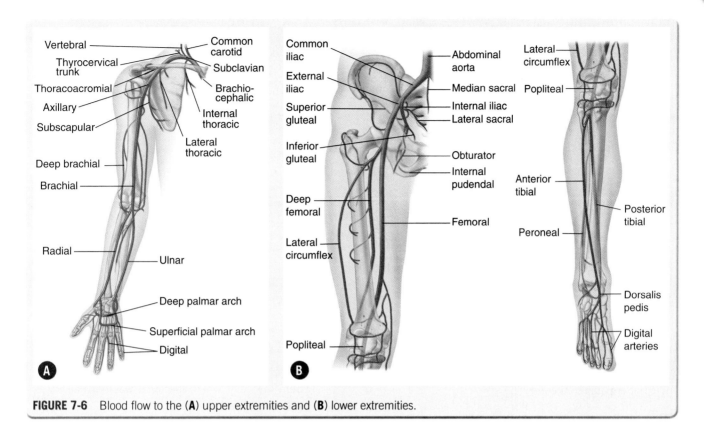

FIGURE 7-6 Blood flow to the (**A**) upper extremities and (**B**) lower extremities.

blood, the artery leaves the axilla and becomes the brachial artery. After the brachial artery passes through the elbow, it divides into the radial artery and ulnar artery. In the hand, the radial and ulnar arteries form superficial and deep arcades of blood vessels that branch to form the arteries of each finger, the **digital arteries** `FIGURE 7-6`.

In the lower extremities, the blood supply originates from the external iliac artery. When the external iliac artery reaches the leg, it becomes the femoral artery. When it reaches the knee, the femoral artery turns posteriorly and laterally and is referred to as the popliteal artery. The popliteal artery divides into the anterior tibial artery and posterior tibial artery. The anterior tibial artery travels along the anterior and lateral surface of the tibia until it reaches the ankle, where it proceeds along the dorsal surface of the foot toward the great toe and becomes the dorsalis pedis artery. The posterior tibial artery travels along the posterior aspect of the tibia until it reaches the ankle, where it follows a path just behind the medial malleolus until it reaches the plantar aspect of the foot. Within the foot, many arteries supply the various structures with blood and give off branches that form the digital arteries of the toes.

Nervous Structure

Skeletal muscle is innervated by **somatic motor neurons**. These neurons transmit electrical stimuli to a muscle that cause it to contract. The combination of the muscle and the neuron that innervates it constitutes a motor unit. A motor unit that receives a signal to contract responds as forcefully as possible or does not contract at all: It is an all-or-nothing response. To generate a more forceful contraction, more neurons need to signal more muscle cells to contract, a process called **recruitment**.

Innervation of the upper extremities arises from the brachial plexus. The brachial plexus is formed by a network of nerves that originate from the spinal cord at the C5–T1 levels. After the fibers of these nerves network with one another, five distinct nerves are formed: the axillary, radial, musculocutaneous, ulnar, and median. Innervation of the lower extremities is provided by the lumbar and lumbosacral plexuses, which are formed by the spinal nerves that originate from L1–S4. The networking of nerves within these two plexuses leads to the formation of multiple distinct nerves, including the sciatic nerve, which branches in the popliteal fossa to form the peroneal and tibial nerves, and the femoral nerve exits the next level of the spine.

Mechanism of Injury

Trauma is the principal cause of musculoskeletal disorders. Optimal patient care requires an understanding of the different mechanisms of trauma and the predictable pattern of injuries that may result. By obtaining a complete and accurate account of the mechanism of injury (MOI), one

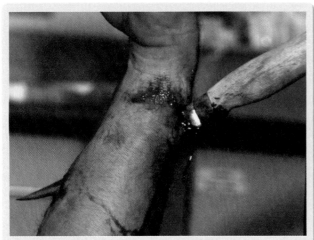

FIGURE 7-7 Direct injury from penetrating trauma can become worse if not immobilized.

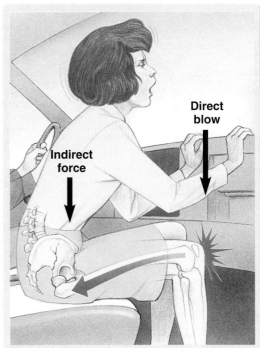

FIGURE 7-8 Indirect force causes injury away from the point where the force was originally applied.

can anticipate the injuries before even touching the patient. Remember, however, that the MOI is not always an accurate indicator of patient outcome.

Direct Force

An object that strikes a person will transfer its energy to its point of impact. This energy is first absorbed by the soft tissues in the region of the impact. When the amount of force is so great that the soft tissues cannot fully dissipate it, a fracture occurs.

Penetrating injuries may also lead to a fracture or other musculoskeletal injury **FIGURE 7-7**. A high-velocity injury, such as that caused by a high-power rifle, typically shatters bone and causes extensive soft-tissue damage.

An impalement injury commonly causes a soft-tissue injury similar to that seen in a low-velocity penetrating injury. If the impaled object happens to strike a bone, it may cause a fracture. In any case of impalement, it is essential to stabilize the object to protect the soft tissues from further injury.

Indirect Force

An indirect injury occurs when a force is applied to one region of the body but causes an injury in another region of the body. In this type of injury, the force is transmitted through the skeleton until, at some point, it reaches an area that is structurally weaker in comparison to the other parts of the musculoskeletal system through which the force has traveled.

For example, a hip fracture may occur when a person's knee strikes the dashboard during a motor vehicle crash **FIGURE 7-8**. In this case, the force is applied to the knee and travels proximally along the femur. When this force reaches the femoral neck, it causes the femoral neck to fracture.

Forces may be transmitted along the entire length of a bone or through several bones in series and may cause an injury anywhere along the way. Thus, a person falling on an

outstretched hand may have one or more injuries as the result of forces transmitted proximally from the point of impact:

- Fracture of the scaphoid bone of the hand (direct blow)
- Fracture of the distal ulna and radius (**Colles fracture**)
- Fracture/dislocation of the elbow
- Fracture/dislocation of the shoulder
- Fracture of the clavicle

Twisting injuries, like those that commonly occur in football or skiing, result in fractures, sprains, and dislocations. Typically, the distal part of the limb remains fixed (as when cleats or a ski hold the foot to the ground) while torsion develops in the proximal section of the limb. The resulting force causes tearing of tendons and ligaments and spiral fractures of bone. Older people, particularly those with osteoporosis, are more susceptible to fractures than younger people.

Fractures

Fracture Classification

A **fracture** is a break in the bone, which may also involve the vital organs they protect and/or their surrounding tissue, including vital neurovascular structures. Fractures can be classified as complete, where both cortices of the bone are fractured, or incomplete, where one cortex has been fractured. They may also be classified as open or closed. A **closed fracture** is any fracture that does not penetrate overlying skin or mucous membrane to the outer air. An **open** (or compound) **fracture**, which is far more severe, is when bone at the fracture site penetrates through soft tissue and skin to become exposed to the outside environment. The bone fragment will not always stay exposed and the skin wound may vary from a small puncture to a large soft-tissue defect. Open fractures are considered a true orthopaedic emergency, and therefore emergency care providers should turn to careful skin inspection of areas of suspected fracture or focal tenderness and swelling. The contamination caused by the open fracture significantly increases the risk of infection, and without immediate treatment may lead to a persistent bone infection (<u>osteomyelitis</u>) that could be life or limb threatening.

Types of Fractures

There are several types of fractures FIGURE 7-9 . A <u>hairline fracture</u> is a small crack in the bone with no displacement of the ends. This would show no deformity, although there would be an area of generalized pain, possibly slight swelling, and increased pain with weight bearing. A <u>comminuted fracture</u> is when the bone is crushed, splintered, or broken into multiple fragments. These fragments may need surgical repair for proper healing. An <u>oblique fracture</u> results from the ends of the bone compacting at an oblique angle to the long bone itself. Often these fractures result in an open fracture due to the sharp ends piercing the skin. A <u>spiral fracture</u> occurs when the bone is twisted apart by a torsional force. The spiral fracture line runs obliquely, encircles the shaft of long bones, and may resemble a corkscrew on a radiograph. A <u>transverse fracture</u> forms a line or break at a right angle to the axis of the bone. The fractured ends are not stable and easily displace, putting them at high risk for open fracture.

<u>Pathologic fractures</u> occur at a point where the bone is weakened from another disease process. Causes of weakened bone include tumors, infection, and certain inherited bone disorders. There are also many other diseases and conditions that can cause a pathologic fracture. When evaluating the patient with a suspected pathologic fracture, remember that the amount of force needed to cause the fracture will be much less than in a healthier patient.

An <u>avulsion fracture</u> is an injury to the bone where a tendon or ligament attaches to the bone. When an avulsion fracture occurs, the tendon or ligament pulls a piece of the bone free. Children are at higher risk for an avulsion fracture because the ligaments are often stronger than the bones and growth plates are also at risk. In adults the ligament often receives the injury before the bone gives way. Avulsion fractures often present much like a sprain or strain and require the same treatments.

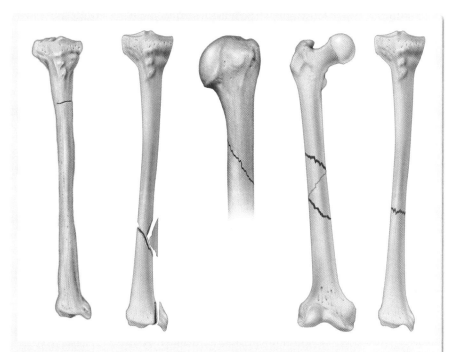

FIGURE 7-9 Types of fractures. **A.** Hairline fracture. **B.** Comminuted fracture. **C.** Oblique fracture. **D.** Spiral fracture. **E.** Transverse fracture.

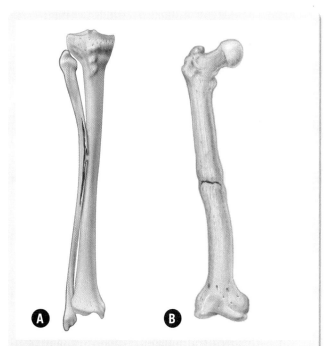

FIGURE 7-10 (**A**) Greenstick and (**B**) torus fractures are more common in children.

In addition to the fractures noted above, there are partial or incomplete fractures that are more common in the pediatric patient FIGURE 7-10 . A <u>greenstick fracture</u> is a partial break in which the bone does not break through the skin. It is more common in children because their bones are more pliable. These fractures are usually due to direct trauma to the bone. Most greenstick fractures have slight angular deformity with local pain and swelling. Because one cortex remains intact, the fractured ends do not move, allowing the pain from the injury to improve quickly. Greenstick fractures almost always heal without incident. A **torus fracture** (or buckle fracture) is another type of incomplete fracture commonly seen in the pediatric patient. A buckle fracture is the result of compression force, which leads to a buckling of the pliable cortex.

Injuries That May Accompany Fractures

Amputations

Amputation is the complete separation or loss of a body part, usually a finger, toe, arm, or leg. If the body part is recovered, it can sometimes be reattached. Fingertip amputations are common and are often the result of crush injury or laceration **FIGURE 7-11**. Time is critical in amputations. Transportation of the patient and amputated part to a hospital with replantation capabilities should be as rapid as possible. Muscle is susceptible to permanent damage from ischemia in as little as 6 hours at room temperature. Because digits do not have muscle, their ischemia time is much longer. Although the earlier replantation takes place the better, successful digit replantations have been done after 30 hours with warm ischemia and 90 hours with cold ischemia.

Amputations closer to the body core are associated with risks for additional trauma. Larger blood vessels are located closer to the body core. Bleeding from these injuries may be extreme. Bleeding control (preventing excessive blood loss and maintaining central pressures) can be a major concern of large extremity amputations. In catastrophic injury with gross uncontrolled bleeding, a tourniquet may provide rapid immediate bleeding control **PROCEDURE 27**. For control of most forms of bleeding, attempt direct pressure for at least 5 continuous minutes, adding additional dressings if bleeding soaks through. Indirect pressure to points above

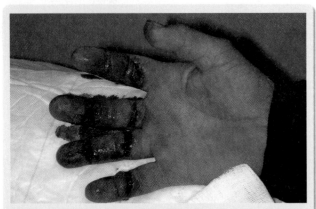

FIGURE 7-11 Fingertip amputations are often the result of crush injury or laceration.

TIP

Patients who have had an amputation above the wrist or ankle should be transported to trauma centers.

the wound along the arteries, added to direct pressure, can decrease the pressure in the wound, allowing time for clotting to take place. Pressure dressings may be helpful when personnel are scarce, but do not replace direct pressure for the first 5 minutes. Tourniquets can be used to stop bleeding in catastrophic cases.

Once the severed part is recovered, place it in a cool, dry container (like a plastic bag) or place a towel or blanket over the part, and pack it in ice. Wrap digits and smaller parts in sterile gauze soaked in normal saline, place in a plastic bag, and then place on ice. Keep the amputated part cool but do not allow it to freeze. Do not waste time trying to recover digit amputations that are distal to the distal interphalangeal (DIP) joint because these injuries are not indicated for replantation.

Lacerations

A **laceration** is an injury to the skin and its underlying soft tissue. **Avulsions** and **incisions** can be grouped with lacerations. An avulsion is a three-sided cut that leaves a flap of skin and soft tissue attached to the body on the fourth side. An incision is a clean, possibly surgical-type laceration with smooth, straight edges that can be stitched back together easily. As with any soft-tissue injury, injury to the underlying tendons, arteries, and nerves is the major concern. Venous damage or bleeding will present with dark red blood oozing from the wound. This bleeding can be significant depending on the location and size of the wound, but typically this bleeding can be controlled with direct pressure and pressure dressings. Arterial bleeding will present with bright red blood spurting from the wound. Large arteries can spurt as far as 15′ and can be a source of blood loss in large volumes. These are life-threatening injuries, and bleeding must be controlled.

Bite wounds are another type of injury to the soft tissue. Bite wounds are partly pressure or crushing injury to the localized tissue and can also puncture, avulse, or lacerate the skin. When bites penetrate the skin the risk for infection increases. The mouths of animals contain bacteria normal to that animal. Human bites can be worse than some animals and all bite wounds require cleansing and follow-up care.

In all laceration injuries, active range of motion should be examined to assess tendon involvement. Lack of ability to flex or extend a body part can indicate tendon laceration or nerve injury. Splint these injuries to help prevent motion that can lead to a tendon contracting, which would make repair more difficult.

Ligament Injuries and Dislocations

Dislocations, Subluxations, and Diastasis

Joints are very susceptible to traumatic injury, which can be classified as **dislocation**, **subluxation**, or **diastasis**. A dislocation is a complete disruption of a joint with total loss of contact between the joint's articular surfaces. A subluxation is a joint malalignment where some of the opposing joint surfaces remain in contact. A diastasis is a separation or dislocation between two bones that are attached but have no true joint. An example is diastasis of the pubic symphysis or distal tibiofibular syndesmosis. As with fractures, dislocations and subluxations can be open or closed. Like open fractures, the possibility of infection in open dislocations warrants emergent evaluation. Unlike subluxations, which typically reduce on their own, a dislocation of any joint will usually need help to relocate or reduce. Shoulders, hips, fingers, and knees are joints prone to dislocations. Recognition of dislocations and fractures is very important because the movement of the bone ends can sever, shear, or occlude nearby vascular structures. Always check for distal pulses and nerve function, before and after splinting, for any fracture or dislocation **FIGURE 7-12**.

Inflammatory Processes

Inflammation is our body's reaction to tissue damage caused by injury, disease, or a foreign substance such as bacteria and viruses. The response at the injury site involves cellular, vascular, neurologic, and humoral responses. The hallmarks of inflammation are pain, swelling, redness, and warmth. In some diseases, however, the body's defense system inappropriately triggers the inflammatory response when there are no foreign substances to fight off. In autoimmune disorders such as arthritis, tendinitis, and bursitis, the body's normally protective immune system now causes damage to its own tissue, causing the characteristic signs and symptoms.

Tendinitis and bursitis are very common in adults and may develop from repetitive motion or injury. If untreated, these conditions often worsen over time with increasing pain and stiffness. The mainstays of treatment include rest, immobilization, ice, and medications like nonsteroidal anti-inflammatory drugs (NSAIDs). In extreme cases, a corticosteroid injection can be beneficial.

Muscle and Tendon Injuries

Sprains and **strains** are soft-tissue injuries specific to the type of tissue affected. A sprain is the result of stretching or partial tearing of a ligament, the supporting structures of a joint that connect bone to bone. A strain is a stretching or partial tearing of a muscle or musculotendinous unit. The complete tearing of a ligament, tendon, or muscle is typically referred to as a rupture.

Strains and ruptures of muscle and tendon usually occur from sudden movement, quick heavy lifting, sports, or even normal daily activities. A sprain injury usually occurs from sudden trauma and overstretching of a joint. Ankle sprains are the most common and can be serious. A serious ankle sprain can be more painful and take longer to heal than a fracture in the same area. Another well-known sprain is to the anterior cruciate ligament (ACL) of the knee, which is common among athletes. The severity of a sprain can be graded as in **TABLE 7-1**.

Signs and symptoms of sprains generally include tenderness, swelling, stiffness, and pain with weight bearing. Tearing a muscle can damage small blood vessels, causing

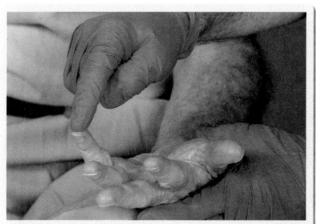

FIGURE 7-12 Check for distal pulse, motor, and sensation when assessing a dislocation.

TABLE 7-1	Severity of Sprains
Degree of Severity	**Description**
First degree	A partial tearing of a ligament that results in local swelling and tenderness but no instability of the joint. Treatment is for symptomatic relief only.
Second degree	A partial tearing of a ligament that causes some instability of the joint and a greater loss of function. Management includes immobilization to protect and support the injured joint.
Third degree	A complete tear of a ligament with resulting instability of the joint. These injuries require immobilization and possibly repair.

Current Concepts in the Use of Tourniquets in the Prehospital Environment

USE OF TOURNIQUETS BY EMS PROVIDERS to control bleeding from extremity wounds in a civilian patient population is relatively uncommon. This is at least partially due to traditional teaching and protocols that have emphasized use of tourniquets exclusively as a last-ditch maneuver to control bleeding. The philosophy behind this approach was that more frequent tourniquet use was unnecessary and would potentially lead to severe complications such as nerve injury, muscle injury, compartment syndrome, or loss of limb. However, studies have not demonstrated that such complications have regularly occurred in patients who have been treated with tourniquets for bleeding control.

Mortality from isolated, poorly controlled extremity injury bleeding in the civilian population appears to be relatively rare.[1] In military situations in Viet Nam and Somalia, however, it has been suggested that some soldiers have died in action as a result of bleeding from extremity wounds that could have been controlled with the early use of a tourniquet. In the early phases of the current Global War on Terror, hemorrhage from extremity wounds was again identified as a leading cause of potentially preventable death in combat.[2] These data led to development of a policy that all US military personnel in the combat theatre must carry tourniquets and be trained in their use.[3,4] In January 2009, Colonel John Kragh and colleagues from the US Army Institute for Surgical Research published a report in which they examined emergency tourniquet use in patients arriving at the Combat Support Hospital in Baghdad, Iraq. They concluded that tourniquet use for patients with severe hemorrhage from extremity wounds was lifesaving when applied prior to the development of shock and that prehospital tourniquet application was more effective in saving lives than was later application in the emergency department.[5] A second study from the same group of authors examined the risk of complications after field application of tourniquets. They concluded that complications related to the use of the tourniquets were infrequent even with tourniquet times in excess of 2 hours.[6]

Some authors claim that using extremity tourniquets is a less effective technique for hemorrhage control than using a compressive dressing combined with deep gauze packing of a wound. The studies these authors reference, however, employed largely makeshift tourniquet designs and prehospital providers who were familiar with direct wound exploration. These scenarios will not likely be encountered by modern civilian EMS providers.[7,8] Concerns about systemic ischemia-reperfusion injury associated with tourniquet release were also cited, although clinical evidence that this injury is clinically significant is still lacking.

Another concern occasionally voiced with the early application of a tourniquet is that it will cause muscle damage in the involved limb, making use of alternative techniques to achieve hemorrhage control more desirable. Animal studies examining the effect of tourniquet application in a limb confirm that damage to function in certain critical muscle types can result from the tourniquet alone. These same studies, however, clearly demonstrate that such damage is substantially magnified when the tourniquet has been applied *after* substantial hemorrhage has already occurred.[9]

In the civilian setting, certain other problems may occur. If tourniquets are applied improperly, injury to underlying structures may result. This risk seems unlikely, however, given the military experience in which most tourniquets were self-applied or applied by other soldiers who were not trained EMS providers. With adequate training and use of tourniquets designed for extremity hemorrhage control, safe and effective civilian field tourniquet use by trained EMS personnel should be feasible. A second potential problem is that hospitals may not be aware of the presence of a tourniquet or of the potential for exsanguinating hemorrhage upon release of the tourniquet, which results in secondary complications at the receiving centers. This argument seems lacking also as it suggests that complications resulting from poor communication between EMS field providers and hospital care personnel are somehow worse in the tourniquet scenario than they would be in much more common scenarios. For example, if a paramedic treats a patient for first-time onset of chest pain with nitroglycerin with successful resolution of pain and then fails to advise the hospital that he did so or that the patient had severe pain on presentation, the patient could experience severe myocardial injury as a result of the delay in implementing more definitive treatment of the underlying condition. Such a risk of complication speaks strongly for educating EMS personnel about the importance of good communications and reporting upon arrival in the emergency department. It does not mean that use of nitroglycerin in the field to control chest pain is contraindicated.

Teaching control of hemorrhage from extremity wounds in the civilian sector has traditionally emphasized direct pressure followed by application of pressure at arterial pressure points proximal to the point of injury. Application of tourniquets has been reserved for situations in which the former modalities are ineffective. Recent experiences with management of severe extremity wounds in combat have suggested, however, that earlier application of tourniquets may result in a decrease in mortality. While the studies available have directly addressed the combat situation and resulted in development of protocols that call for primary tourniquet application immediately after diagnosis of extremity wound hemorrhage, civilian protocols have been slower to evolve. The information available, however, suggests that the benefits of early field tourniquet application outweigh the risks in the civilian environment also and that revising protocols for use of tourniquets in the civilian setting has the potential to save lives just as it has done for the military in Iraq and Afghanistan.

EMS systems should proceed with development of protocols for early application of tourniquets in the face of severe extremity hemorrhage. Providers should not be taught to rely on direct pressure for more than a short time to achieve bleeding control, and application of indirect pressure should be eliminated as a treatment step in favor of much earlier tourniquet application in the face of any recalcitrant bleeding. EMS systems should also make certain that providers are equipped with tourniquets that are easy to apply and effective once used and that they are appropriately trained in their use.

Andrew N. Pollak, MD
Associate Professor and Head, Division of Orthopaedic Traumatology, University of Maryland School of Medicine
Associate Director of Trauma, R Adams Cowley Shock Trauma Center
Medical Director, Baltimore County Fire Department
Special Deputy United States Marshal
Series Editor, Orange Book Series

References

1. Dorlac WC, DeBakey ME, Holcomb JB, et al. Mortality from isolated civilian penetrating extremity injury. *J Trauma*. 2005; 59:217–222.
2. Holcomb JB, McMullin NR, Pearse L, et al. Causes of death in US special operations forces in the global war on terrorism 2001–2004. *Ann Surg*. 2007; 245:986–991.
3. Walters TJ, Mabry RL. Issues related to the use of tourniquets on the battlefield. *Mil Med*. 2005; 170:770–775.
4. Walters TJ, Wenke JC, Kauvar DS, et al. Effectiveness of self-applied tourniquets in human volunteers. *Prehosp Emerg Care*. 2005; 9:416–422.
5. Kragh JF, Walters TJ, Baer DG, et al. Survival with emergency tourniquet use to stop bleeding in major limb trauma. *Annals of Surgery*. 2009; 249(1).
6. Kragh JF, Walters TJ, Baer DG, et al. Practical use of emergency tourniquets to stop bleeding in major limb trauma. *J Trauma*. 2008; 64:S38–S50.
7. Mellesmo S, Pillgram-Larsen J. Primary care of amputation injuries. *JEUR*. 1995; 8:131–135.
8. Hussum H. Effects of early pre-hospital life support to war injured: The Battle of Jalalabad, Afghanistan. *Prehosp Disast Med*. 1999; 14:75–80.
9. Walters TJ, Kragh JF, Kauvar DS, Baer DG. The combined influence of hemorrhage and tourniquet application on the recovery of muscle function in rats. *J Orthop Trauma*. 2008; 22:47–51.

bruising and irritation of the nerves in that area. Ecchymosis may not appear until 24–48 hours after the injury. In more severe sprains and strains, a patient will often report an audible snap or pop.

After inspection, gentle palpation and examination of the injured area may help to narrow the diagnostic possibilities. Identification of muscle defects, indentation, or bulging may indicate complete rupture that could require surgical repair. If a patient can move a joint, that can help rule out dislocation and rupture and suggests a sprain or strain. For example, in a quadriceps injury you can have a patient lie on their back and ask them to raise their leg off the ground. If there is a complete patella tendon or quadriceps rupture, the patient will not be able to hold the leg straight with the knee extended. This test is known as a straight leg raising test **FIGURE 7-13** .

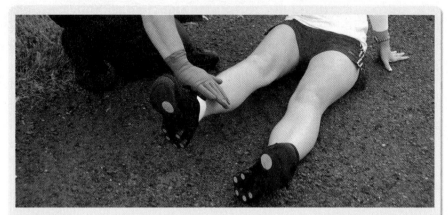

FIGURE 7-13 The straight leg raising test is used to check the quadriceps or patella tendon stability.

Vascular Injuries

Vascular injury in an extremity is often the result of penetrating injury **FIGURE 7-14** . Penetrating extremity injury can occur from industrial accidents or lacerations from broken glass. Explosive-type injuries, which can combine blunt and penetrating injuries, are also becoming more common, and providers are likely to encounter such injuries at some point in their careers.

High-speed motor vehicle collisions, often with fractures or dislocations, are a major cause of blunt trauma, but are not the only cause. Falls, assaults, and crush injuries can all result in vascular trauma and are made worse by any fractured long bones or dislocated joints. Certain injuries, however, are more likely to cause vascular injury than other injuries, for example a Colles fracture of the wrist.

The arteries and veins in the extremities have some natural protection from stretching and bending, which helps protect them from blunt injury. The **tunica adventitia** (arterial media), the outer layer of the blood vessel, protects the patient from stretch-type injuries and minor puncture wounds and can limit the chance of hemorrhage. When an arterial vessel is cut, vascular spasm and low systemic blood pressure help induce clotting at the injury site. This reaction allows better vital organ perfusion than occurs with ongoing hemorrhage.

Based on examination, vascular injuries can be divided into hard signs and soft signs. Hard signs include pulsatile bleeding, expanding hematoma, thrill or bruit, and evidence of ischemia (pallor, paresthesia, paralysis, pain, pulselessness, and poikilothermia [loss of temperature]). These obvious signs almost always indicate an underlying

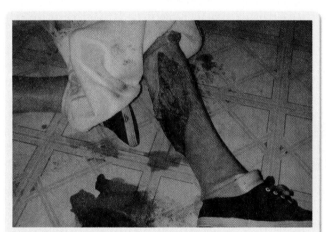

FIGURE 7-14 Vascular injuries are often the result of penetrating trauma.

arterial injury and are indications for immediate surgical intervention.

Soft signs include moderate hemorrhage occurring at the site of injury, stable hematoma, proximity to a penetrating wound, peripheral nerve deficit, and associated fracture or dislocation. Other equivocal or soft signs of arterial injury are persistent shock, an injury near an artery, and an injury to a nerve accompanying an artery.

A cool and pulseless extremity may be the result of low systemic blood pressure, but pulse abnormalities may indicate underlying vascular injury. Other indicators of extremity vascular injury include neurologic deficit, delayed capillary refill, and bone abnormalities.

TIP

Compare extremities side to side to determine whether signs of an injury are isolated to the extremity.

Assessment and Management

A rapid assessment may be the single most important part of saving a life when multisystem trauma is involved. The initial/primary assessment begins with the initial scene size-up and identification of the mechanism of injury and any potential immediate life threats. If there are no immediate threats to patient survival, the next step is to assess the rest of the body quickly and efficiently for pain and deformity that may indicate musculoskeletal trauma. When assessing an injured patient, do not be distracted by visually impressive injuries. It is essential to locate the life threats to the patient before focusing on limb-threatening injuries.

In cases of musculoskeletal injuries, patients may be classified based on the presence or absence of associated injuries:

- Life- or limb-threatening injury or condition, including life- or limb-threatening musculoskeletal trauma
- Life-threatening injuries and only simple musculoskeletal trauma
- Limb-threatening musculoskeletal trauma and no other life-threatening injuries
- Isolated, non–life- or non–limb-threatening injuries

Life-threatening injury takes priority over limb threats; however, the limbs should be protected by stabilizing the entire body on a long backboard before immediate transportation to a trauma center **FIGURE 7-15** **PROCEDURE 17** . If the patient has a significant mechanism of injury, complete a rapid trauma/secondary assessment and perform a detailed physical exam en route to the emergency department (ED). If the initial/primary assessment indicates the patient has no immediately life-threatening condition and only localized musculoskeletal trauma, continue with a focused history, physical exam, and stabilization prior to transport. The priorities throughout the assessment and management of musculoskeletal injuries should include identifying the injuries, preventing further harm or damage to the injured structures and surrounding tissues, supporting the injured area, and administering pain medication when necessary.

History of Present Injury

Obtain information about the incident that led to the injury from the patient and any bystanders. In particular, determine the condition of the patient immediately before the incident, the details of the incident, and the patient's position after the incident. Have the patient give a subjective description of the injury: How did this happen? Did you hear a pop? Do you have pain? Have you done anything to alleviate the pain? Are you able to move the extremity?

Medical/Surgical History

Obtain the patient's medical history using the standard SAMPLE format. During the previous medical history, the provider should ascertain tetanus immunization status. This history should also identify any preexisting musculoskeletal disorders and help the provider learn more about the injury. Knowledge of a previous injury, surgery, or arthritis that may alter the exam are some examples of information relevant to the injury.

Examination

When examining the patient, obtain a baseline set of vital signs. The focus can then shift to evaluating the injured extremity. Fractures are not always obvious, and diagnosis is often by clinical history, mechanism of injury, and thorough physical exam. Physical exam should follow the look, feel, and move model. Always begin with inspection of the skin for abrasions, discoloration, or abnormality that may indicate injury. One of the simplest ways to assess an extremity is to compare one side with the other, noting any discrepancy in length, position, or skin color. This holds true for any body part or joint and for all aspects of the exam, including palpation and range of motion. As you observe and palpate the soft tissue from head to toe, assess the patient for limitations, such as inability to move a joint.

While performing the exam, be sure to cover the six Ps of musculoskeletal assessment: pain, paralysis, __paresthesia__ (numbness or tingling), pulselessness, pallor (pale or delayed capillary refill in children), and pressure under the skin from swelling.

Pain Assessment

A person experiences acute pain when peripheral pain receptors (__nociceptors__) convert painful stimuli into electrical impulses that are transmitted via the peripheral nerve fibers to the spinal cord. The signal ascends along the spinal cord to the pain-sensing region of the brain.

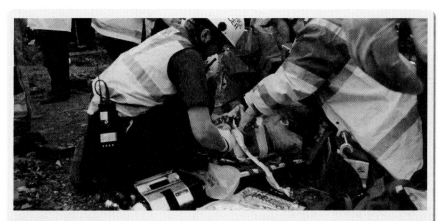

FIGURE 7-15 In the presence of life-threatening injury, extremity injuries can be minimized by securing the patient to a long backboard.

When a tissue is injured, various chemical mediators are released that facilitate the conduction of the painful stimulus to the brain. The brain stimulates endorphins in an attempt to decrease the pain.

When assessing a patient's pain, remember the OPQRST mnemonic: Onset of the pain; provoking or palliating factors; quality of the pain (such as sharp, pressure, cramplike); region of the pain, including its primary location and areas where pain radiates or refers; severity of the pain; and the time (duration) that the patient has been experiencing pain. It is also useful to have the patient quantify the severity of the pain by using a scale of 0 to 10 or visual images such as faces that appear to be happy or in pain.

Inspection

When inspecting an injured extremity, always evaluate the joint above and the joint below the site of injury because indirect forces may have affected these sites as well. If the patient can move the extremity, compare the range of motion (ROM) of the injured side with the uninjured side. While inspecting a patient's injuries, look for the following signs FIGURE 7-16 :

- Deformity, including asymmetry, angulation, shortening, and rotation
- Skin changes, including contusions, abrasions, avulsions, punctures, burns, lacerations, and bone ends
- Swelling
- Muscle spasms
- Muscle wasting
- Abnormal limb positioning
- Increased or decreased range of motion with patient motion
- Color changes, including pallor and cyanosis
- Bleeding, including estimating the amount of blood loss and the level of shock (see Chapter 4)

Palpation

Palpation of an injured extremity should include the injury site and the regions above and below it. Identify regions of point tenderness. Note that although point tenderness is one of the best indicators of an injury, it may be absent in patients who are intoxicated or who have an injury to the spinal cord. The upper and lower extremity exam should include palpation of the entire length of each arm or leg to identify any sites of injury. The most efficient way to accomplish this is to place your hands around the extremity and lightly squeeze FIGURE 7-17 . Repeat this procedure every few centimeters until you reach the end of the extremity. This type of exam will locate gross injury while a more specific exam may be required once you locate an area of tenderness.

When palpating an injured site, attempt to identify instability, deformity, abnormal joint or bone continuity, and displaced bones. Feel for crepitus, which is commonly found at the site of a fracture. Palpate distal pulses on all extremities, with special attention to comparing the strength of the pulses in the injured extremity with those in a normal one. When evaluating the upper extremities, always examine the cervical spine and shoulder because complaints within the arm may be caused by a more proximal disorder. Likewise, always conduct an exam of the pelvis and hip if the patient complains of pain in the leg.

On occasion, an arterial injury may be identified while palpating an extremity. Signs of an arterial injury include a pulsatile expanding hematoma, diminished distal pulses, a palpable thrill (vibration) over the site of injury that correlates with the patient's heartbeat, and difficult-to-control bleeding.

Motor Function and Sensory Exam

It is essential to assess a patient's distal pulse, as well as motor and sensory function, in cases of musculoskeletal injury. Perform a motor function exam whenever a patient has an injury to an extremity, provided the patient does not also have a life-threatening injury. When assessing motor function, consider the preinjury level of function. In some cases, weakness or motor deficits may be due to prior injuries or medical problems. For this reason, you should perform a careful review of the patient's history whenever a patient complains of being weak or unable to move an extremity.

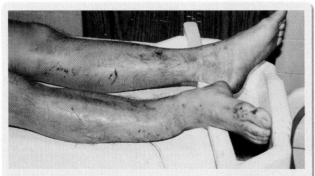

FIGURE 7-16 Inspect extremities by comparing opposite sides for symmetry.

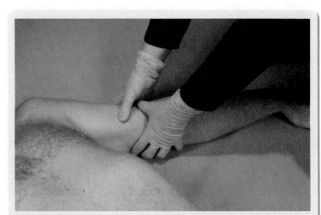

FIGURE 7-17 Encircle the extremity and palpate from the body outward to check for injury.

To evaluate the upper extremities, have the patient sit upright, shrug their shoulders, and then extend the upper arm outward. Continue by flexing the lower arm at the elbow and then extending it again. The patient should flex and extend at the wrist as well. Perform the test on both sides of the body simultaneously so that each extremity can be compared to the other. Use of the old child's game of "rock, paper, scissors" can help evaluate distal motor and nerve function in the upper extremity by testing the radial, medial, and ulnar nerves **FIGURE 7-18**. A more traditional method is to have patients put their thumbs up, make the OK sign, and spread the fingers.

If the lower extremity is to be examined, have the patient raise his or her upper legs toward the chest. The patient can then extend and flex at the knee and ankle. Lower extremity exams will not be able to be performed bilaterally without losing balance, so compare them visually. While performing a motor exam, carry out each test with and without resistance (injury permitting) because some patients may be too weak to overcome any outside resistance.

Perform a sensory exam on all patients who have an injury to an extremity, keeping in mind the dermatome areas (Chapter 6). The sensory exam and history should attempt to identify any preexisting deficits in function or other disorders, including diabetes and nerve disorders that may cause changes in sensation. It is important to assess not only for the presence or absence of sensation, but also for the quality and symmetry of sensation.

To perform a sensory exam, first ask the patient if he or she feels any abnormal sensations, such as numbness, tingling, or burning. Next, conduct a gross sensory exam by lightly touching the injured extremity and the unaffected side simultaneously; have the patient report whether the two sides feel the same or different. Compare both proximal and distal sites to determine specific sites of injury. In some cases, a patient may complain of an abnormally severe sen-sation of pain when just lightly touched. Such hyperesthesia may be a sign of an injury to the spinal cord.

Complications Due to Extremity Trauma

Volume Deficit

As with any injury, musculoskeletal injuries can come with many complications. These complications are divided into two groups: local and systemic. Hemorrhage from a rupture in the vascular system can be very dangerous and even life threatening if not controlled. Most external hemorrhaging will be readily seen and easily controlled with direct pressure, pressure dressings, elevation, and use of pressure points. Internal hemorrhaging, however, cannot easily be seen and must be found through assessment. This includes examining the patient for hypovolemic shock and hypotension. Fluid loss also occurs from interstitial fluid shifts seen as swelling around an injury. This swelling is a protective mechanism used by the body to limit further injury to the area. Fluid loss is most significant with long bone fractures when the loss is due to both bleeding and swelling. The larger the bone, the more potential for loss **TABLE 7-2**.

Compartment Syndrome and Crush Syndrome

Compartment syndrome is another possible complication of extremity injury and can be catastrophic if not diagnosed **FIGURE 7-19**. Muscles of the extremities, along with their neurovascular supply, are grouped with one another in muscle compartments. These muscle compartments are enclosed by a tough fascia that has little elastic property. Compartment syndrome is the increased tissue pressure from edema and/or hemorrhage within one of these muscle compartments that gradually compromises vascular perfusion, escalating to ischemia of the tissues and nerves. Ischemia can lead to necrosis of muscle and nerves in as few as 4 to 8 hours. The diagnosis is initially based on clinical suspicion. Crush injuries and fractures, especially in the forearm and tibia, are particularly susceptible. Delayed treatment can lead to fibrotic scar tissue, muscular contracture, and permanent dysfunction of the involved nerves and muscle. In severe cases, amputation may be indicated following hospital care.

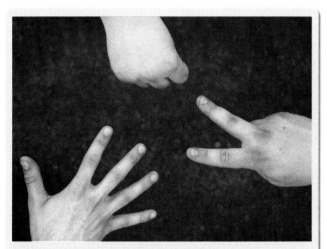

FIGURE 7-18 The child's game of "rock, paper, scissors" can be used to evaluate the distal nerves of the hand.

TABLE 7-2 Potential Fluid Loss from Fracture Sites	
Fracture Site	**Potential Fluid Loss (in mL)**
Pelvis	1,500–3,000
Femur	1,000–1,500
Humerus	250–500
Tibia or fibula	250–500
Ankle	250–500
Elbow	250–500
Radius or ulna	150–250

Signs and symptoms of compartment syndrome include pain that is out of proportion to obvious injury, edema that creates palpable firmness and tension of the compartment, and decreased sensation. The hallmark of examination is extreme pain with passive stretching of the muscle compartment. For example, extension of the fingers will stretch the volar forearm and plantar flexion of the ankle will stretch the anterior compartment of the lower leg. Pulses will remain palpable because the pressure rarely exceeds systolic blood pressure. Lack of pulse indicates arterial injury and not compartment syndrome. Never use circumferential splints or tight wraps acutely because they do not allow for expansion of tissue and subsequent swelling. Ice and elevation can help reduce swelling in early treatment, but surgical intervention is often required.

<u>Crush syndrome</u> is even more threatening than compartment syndrome and is the result of a severe crushing injury, particularly one involving large muscle masses. Extremities that get pinned following a motor vehicle collision or by falling debris are examples `FIGURE 7-20`. Crush syndrome is characterized by extensive soft-tissue damage with excessive blood and fluid loss. It can lead to life-threatening hypovolemic shock and renal failure that is brought on by significant hematuria and myoglobinuria. Potassium and calcium are also released from the damaged muscle cells. When the pressure is released from the body, blood that has been in stasis in the injured area is flushed into the circulatory system, causing the system to become overloaded.

Treatment is often geared at hemodilution with normal saline prior to extrication of the patient to assist the kidneys in filtering the toxic by-products. Lactated Ringer's or Hartmann's solution is not indicated because excess amounts of potassium and calcium have already been placed into the bloodstream. Sodium bicarbonate is often used to alkalize the urine, allowing the kidneys to clear the toxins from the body. If hyperkalemia is indicated by peaked T waves on the ECG, treatment should be to lower the intravascular levels. Albuterol (salbutamol), dextrose, and insulin are often used in combination. Local protocols should be used to determine treatment.

Thromboembolism

Any musculoskeletal injuries can also cause a blood clot (<u>thrombus</u>) in a vein, which can then break off, only to lodge elsewhere in the vein and cause a blockage of blood flow. This is then termed a <u>thromboembolism</u> and is life threatening if the clot goes to the lungs or (less commonly) brain. The most threatening blood clots occur in the deep veins (deep venous thrombosis [DVT]) between the hip and the knee. Blood clots can sometimes be found on physical exam and present as a tender, firm

mass or cord. Other signs of a DVT include tenderness to the calf, increased warmth in the affected leg, redness or bluish coloring, low-grade fever, tachycardia, and pain when the toes are pulled toward the head. Although anticoagulants are the mainstay of treatment, early warm compresses in the field may be helpful.

General Interventions

The overall goal in the management of a musculoskeletal injury is to identify the type and extent of the injury and to create a biologic environment that maximizes the normal healing process of the injured structure. This process begins in the field with a thorough assessment of the patient and proper immobilization of injuries to prevent further harm.

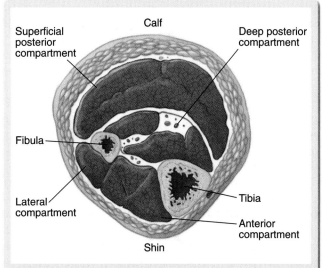

FIGURE 7-19 Compartment syndrome occurs when pressure in a muscle compartment stops blood flow through the compartment.

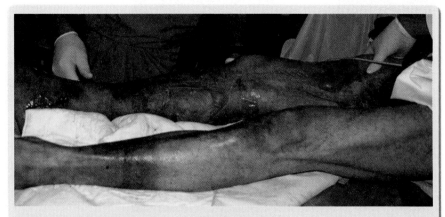

FIGURE 7-20 Patients who suffer injury where an extremity has been entrapped for a long period of time are at risk for crush syndrome.

Pain Control

A patient who has sustained a musculoskeletal injury may experience pain for a number of reasons. Pain may be caused by a fracture or continued movement of an unstable fracture, muscle spasm, soft-tissue injury, nerve injury, or muscle ischemia. Orthopaedic injuries are often extremely painful, so the goal of prehospital pain control should be to diminish the patient's pain to a tolerable level as early as is safe and feasible.

A number of interventions may be performed in the field to control pain from musculoskeletal injury. The first step is to assess the level of pain. Establish a baseline level of pain and reassess it after each intervention to determine the effectiveness of the treatment being provided. Simple methods for controlling pain include splinting, resting and elevating the injured part, and applying ice or heat packs.

Cold packs may be useful for treating patients during the initial 48 hours following an injury. They are thought to act by reducing pain and swelling. Cooling the injured area theoretically causes vasoconstriction of the blood vessels in the region and decreases the release of inflammatory mediators. As a result, swelling and inflammation are reduced when ice packs are used during the acute stage of an injury. The actual efficacy of this modality in reducing swelling has been debated, but there is abundant anecdotal evidence that cooling provides some level of symptomatic relief.

Conversely, heat therapy should not be used during the initial 48 to 72 hours following an injury because it may actually increase pain and swelling during this period. Once the acute phase of the injury ends and the damaged blood vessels become clotted, heat is useful for increasing blood flow to the region to decrease stiffness and to promote healing. As a consequence, heat packs may be beneficial for patients who report they sustained an injury several days before contacting emergency services.

When simple procedures do not effectively control a patient's pain, the administration of an analgesic or antispasmodic agent is indicated. Analgesics used in the field include narcotics, such as fentanyl and morphine, and non-narcotic options such as nitrous oxide or NSAIDs. Antispasmodic agents include diazepam and lorazepam. The anesthesia induction agent ketamine (Ketanest) has been used to assist in pain relief but can offer better responses when used with an opiate or benzodiazepine. These agents should be reserved for patients in hemodynamically stable condition who have an isolated musculoskeletal injury. It is important to obtain vital signs before and after administering any medication for pain and spasm and to monitor the patient's respiratory status for signs of respiratory depres-

sion. After pain medication is administered, reassess the patient's pain to ensure that pain relief is adequate.

Administering pain medication before splinting may allow the extremity to be immobilized more effectively. It is painful to have an injured extremity held in the proper position for splinting. Pain medication may make it possible for the patient to tolerate that position longer and allow the splint to be applied properly.

Splinting

Splinting is intended to provide support to and prevent motion of the broken bones. Correctly splinting an injured extremity not only decreases the pain a patient experiences, but also reduces the risk of further damage to muscles, nerves, blood vessels, and skin. In addition, splinting helps control bleeding by allowing clots to form where vessels were damaged. When a patient with multiple orthopaedic injuries must be transported immediately, you will not have time to splint each fracture one by one. The best way to stabilize multiple fractures when the patient's overall condition is critical is to use a long backboard and straps. This will serve two purposes:

1. It will protect against a spinal injury.
2. It will reduce the movement of injured extremities by securing them to the board.

Splinting is one of the most crucial skills to learn when caring for patients with musculoskeletal injuries. Failure to splint an injured extremity properly leads to unnecessary discomfort and the possibility of further injury or harm. Allowing a closed fracture in the distal tibia to become an open fracture owing to mishandling or improper splinting will result in the need for surgery and a hospital stay and may increase the patient's rehabilitation time. Keep the following points in mind when applying a splint:

- The injured area must be adequately visualized before splinting. Remove clothing as necessary so you can inspect the area thoroughly.
- Assess and record distal pulse, motor, and sensation (PMS) functions before and after splinting.
- Cover all wounds with a dry, sterile dressing before applying the splint. Do not attempt to push exposed bone ends back under the skin.
- Do not move the patient before splinting unless an immediate hazard exists.
- For fractures, the splint must immobilize the bone ends and the two adjacent joints. For dislocations, the splint must extend along the entire length of the bone above and the entire length of the bone below the dislocated joint.
- Pad the splint well to prevent local pressure and to provide optimal motion restriction.
- If a long bone fracture is severely angulated, gently apply longitudinal traction (tension) to attempt to realign the bone and improve circulation.
- If the patient complains of severe pain or offers resistance to movement, splint in the position of deformity and carefully monitor the distal neurovascular status (PMS).

TIP

Pain relief medications carried by services vary by region. It is important to check your local protocols for medications and dosing before administering pain medication to a patient.

- Splint firmly, but not so tightly as to occlude the distal circulation.
- If possible, do not cover fingers and toes with the splint to allow for monitoring of skin.

Any device used to immobilize a fracture or dislocation is considered a splint **FIGURE 7-21**. Commercially available splints include rigid splints, inflatable or vacuum splints, and traction splints. Lack of a commercially made splint should never prevent proper immobilization of an injured patient; multiple casualties may tax the resources of even the best-equipped ambulance, requiring improvisation.

A rigid splint is any inflexible device that can be attached to a limb to maintain stability—a padded board, a piece of heavy cardboard, or an aluminum splint molded to fit the extremity **PROCEDURE 31**. More elaborate rigid splints are designed to fit around two or three sides of an extremity quickly and be secured with straps or cravats. Some rigid splints are made of a radiolucent material that allows radiographs to be obtained without removal of the splint. Whatever its construction, the splint must be generously padded to ensure even pressure along the extremity and long enough to be secured well above and below the fracture site.

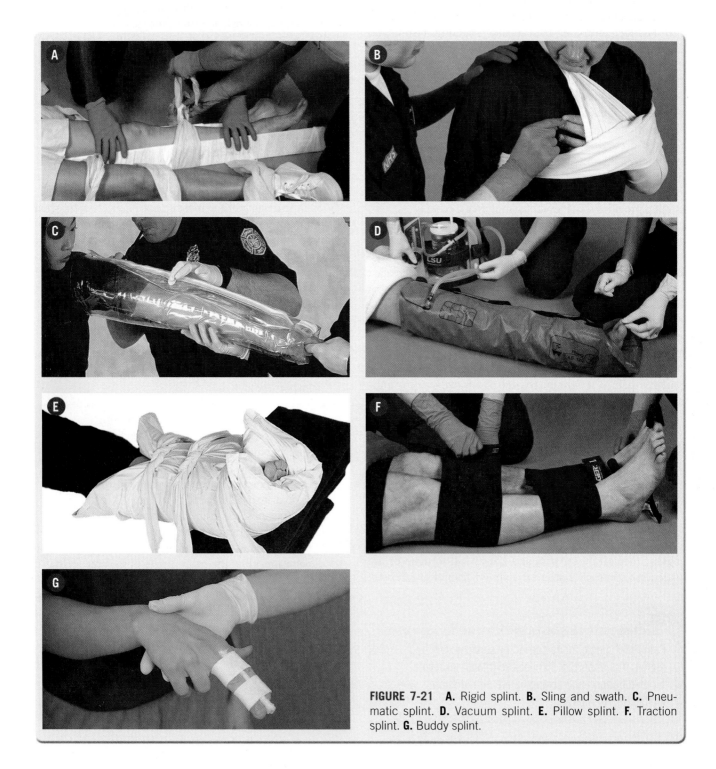

FIGURE 7-21 **A.** Rigid splint. **B.** Sling and swath. **C.** Pneumatic splint. **D.** Vacuum splint. **E.** Pillow splint. **F.** Traction splint. **G.** Buddy splint.

An arm sling may be fashioned from a triangular bandage or you can use a commercial device to immobilize injuries that involve the shoulder or as an adjunct to a rigid splint of the upper extremity. The sling holds the injured part against the chest wall and takes some of the weight off the injured area. To apply a sling, place the extremity in a comfortable position across the chest. Secure the sling so the hand is carried higher than the elbow and the fingers are visible for checking peripheral circulation.

An arm that is splinted with a sling can be further immobilized by adding a swath. Create a swath by using one or more triangular bandages to secure the arm firmly to the chest wall. This technique is particularly useful for injuries to the clavicle and for anterior dislocations of the shoulder. Do not use a sling if the patient has a neck injury.

Pneumatic splints (also known as air splints or inflatable splints) are useful for immobilizing fractures involving the lower leg or forearm **PROCEDURE 33**. They are not effective for angulated fractures or for fractures that involve a joint because they will forcefully attempt to straighten the fracture or joint. Likewise, air splints should not be used on open fractures in which the bone ends are exposed.

Air splints offer one distinct advantage over other splints: They can help slow bleeding and minimize swelling by applying pressure over fracture sites to decrease small-vessel bleeding. For injuries involving the pelvis or femur, the pneumatic antishock garment (PASG) may be used as an air splint and can potentially tamponade bleeding from larger vessels **PROCEDURE 36**. If a PASG is used for this purpose, it is necessary to use high pressure in the device (ie, 106 mm Hg or until the pop-off valves for the compartments blow off). Refer to your local protocols for use of the PASG/MAST (military anti-shock trousers) as a splint.

PRO/CON

Usage of the PASG/MAST garment is controversial and should be used only when adhering to local protocol. Extended transport times may benefit from the use of a PASG/MAST. With shorter transport times, required care may be delayed because hospital staff are forced to remove the garment in a slow, controlled manner.

You must watch air splints carefully to ensure they do not lose pressure or become overinflated. Overinflation is particularly likely when the splint is applied in a cold area and the patient is subsequently moved to a warmer area because the air inside the splint will expand as it gets warmer. Air splints will also expand when going to a higher altitude if the patient compartment is unpressurized, a factor that must be considered when patients are transported by air ambulance.

A vacuum splint consists of a sealed pad that is filled with air and thousands of small plastic beads **PROCEDURE 34**. A suction pump attached to the pad is then used to evacuate the air from inside the splint. The resulting vacuum inside the splint compresses the beads in such a way that the whole splint becomes rigid, much like a plaster cast that has been molded to conform to the contours of the patient.

There are multiple sizes of vacuum splints, including a mattress and smaller splints for the extremities. Because these splints form to fit the extremity, they can be used to splint angulated extremities in the position found. The splint is quite bulky, so it not only takes up a lot of storage room in the vehicle, but also can be difficult to work with in cramped quarters. Furthermore, like all vacuum splints, it requires a mechanical suction pump, yet another piece of equipment to grab.

A pillow is an effective means to immobilize an injured foot or ankle. To create a pillow splint, simply mold an ordinary pillow around the affected foot and ankle in a position of comfort, and then secure the pillow in place with several straps. Pillows can also be molded around an injured knee or elbow and are invaluable for padding backboards when they are used to immobilize patients with dislocated hips. Pillow splints are especially useful with pediatric patients because children are familiar with pillows and the splinting is less stressful.

Following a femur fracture, the strong muscles of the thigh begin to spasm in an effort to splint the fracture anatomically. This often leads to significant pain and deformity. Traction splints provide constant counterforce on these muscles, thereby preventing the broken bone ends from overriding as a result of unopposed muscle contraction **PROCEDURE 32**. In addition, these splints help maintain alignment of the fracture pieces and provide effective immobilization of the fracture site. As a result, patients are likely to experience less pain.

Traction splints also reduce blood loss. Normally, the thigh is shaped like a cylinder. In a femur fracture, the thigh is shortened and becomes spherical. The volume of a sphere can be substantially greater than that of a cylinder, so a person with an untreated femur fracture can accumulate more blood in the thigh than a person whose thigh is pulled out to length by a traction splint.

Traction splints are indicated for the treatment of most femur fractures. They should not be used, however, when the patient has an additional fracture below the knee on the same extremity. When the hitch is secure, the traction splint will apply gentle longitudinal traction using enough force to realign the extremity.

Buddy splinting can be used to splint injuries that involve the fingers or toes. With this technique, an adjacent uninjured finger or toe serves as a splint to the injured one. To buddy splint, tape the injured digit to an uninjured one. Place a gauze pad between the digits that are taped together and ensure that the tape does not pass over joints.

Injuries of the Upper Extremities

Shoulder Fracture

The shoulder girdle is a common area of injury. The shoulder joint allows the greatest range of motion of all the joints, but to do so it sacrifices stability. Unlike the hip joint, which has a deep, stable socket, the shoulder has a very shallow but mobile ball-and-socket joint. Acute injuries include fracture, dislocation, separation, and tendon ruptures.

Fractures of the shoulder girdle include clavicle, scapula, and humeral head or neck fractures. Clavicle fractures are very common and 80% of them happen at the middle third. History of injury is usually a fall on the shoulder or a high-impact blow directly to it. Patients will often be unable to lift their arm because of the pain caused at the fracture site.

Fractures of the humeral head and neck are also common and caused by a fall onto an outstretched arm. They are most common in elderly women due to osteoporosis. Fractures that occur in trauma are often avulsion type, secondary to dislocation. Avulsion fractures occur when a small teardrop-shaped piece of bone is torn from the larger bone by the connecting ligament. These injuries are very painful and pain can be elicited with the slightest movement of the arm. The patient will likely present with swelling, ecchymosis, and an obvious deformity of the skin.

Management of Shoulder Fracture

Check the distal extremity for pulses and sensation, the lack of which could indicate axillary artery or nerve damage, respectively. Treatment is rarely surgical, and most fractures are treated with a simple sling and swath depending on severity and pain. Indication for surgery is tenting of the skin (by bone ends) or significant displacement. Manage pain as indicated, although immobilization is often successful in minimizing pain.

Shoulder Dislocation

The shoulder is one of the most complex joints of the human body and allows the greatest range of motion. This greater capability of movement also brings a much higher possibility of dislocation or separation. Shoulders can dislocate when a strong force, such as a traumatic injury, abnormally stretches the ligaments and tendons, causing the ball-shaped end of the humerus to pop out of its socket `FIGURE 7-22`. It may or may not be associated with fracture. Anterior dislocations are far more common than posterior dislocations. Posterior dislocations are extremely rare and very painful. Possible causes of a posterior shoulder disloca-

tion include electrocution and severe seizures. In an anterior dislocation, the head of the humerus comes to rest anterior to the glenoid fossa. Shoulder dislocations can be caused by a fall, a throwing motion, or a punching motion.

A patient with a shoulder dislocation will likely have a history of a "pop" or sensation of movement of the joint. Other indications include pain or tenderness at the joint and inability to lift the arm.

Management of Shoulder Dislocation

Patients with a shoulder dislocation should be immobilized in a sling and swath. Ice can be applied to the shoulder to minimize the swelling. Additional pain medications are often required. In some instances, reduction of the shoulder may be required if local protocol permits, the mechanism presents no suspicion of fracture, and the time for transport will be delayed for more than several hours. Before reduction, perform a neurovascular exam of the shoulder, paying special attention to the axillary nerve. This can be tested by having the patient attempt an isometric contraction of the deltoid and assessing sensation over the lateral deltoid.

After giving analgesics and muscle relaxants, reduction can be performed by one of many valid techniques. One is gravity-assisted reduction, which is done with the patient lying prone with the affected arm hanging off the table. Ten to 15 pounds (4.5 to 7 kg) of weight is then hung around the patient's wrist. For a right-sided dislocation, place your right thumb on the posterior aspect of the acromion and your fingers on the humeral head, applying pressure toward the patient's back. For another technique, have the patient lie supine and place a rolled sheet around their chest with the tails of the sheet on the opposite side of the affected shoulder. One person stands at the level of the patient's waist and pulls gentle traction while another person pulls countertraction with the sheet. You should see and feel the shoulder relocate. Again, many variations are possible.

Shoulder Separation

Shoulder separation is a different injury from a fracture or a dislocation and involves a disruption of the acromioclavicular joint. These injuries commonly occur from a fall onto the superior lateral aspect of the shoulder. They are common injuries in athletics or falls off a bicycle. They can vary greatly in severity and are graded into six types, type I being the least separated and type VI the most. Tenderness at the acromioclavicular joint, pain with elevation of the arm, and deformity of the distal clavicle superior to the acromion all indicate shoulder separation.

Management of Shoulder Separation

Immediate management in the field is a sling, analgesics, and ice. The less severe type I and II separations can then continue to be treated in a sling for about a week. All others should be evaluated for surgical repair.

Scapula Fracture

Scapula fractures are not common and occur only after a high direct impact trauma, typically from motorcycle accidents or falls from a significant height. Scapula frac-

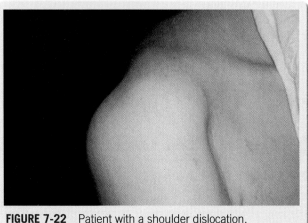

FIGURE 7-22 Patient with a shoulder dislocation.

tures are often missed due to the high rate of associated life-threatening injuries that are treated before a thorough assessment can be completed. Patients experience tenderness to gentle palpation of the posterior shoulder and present with swelling, ecchymosis, and possible abrasions.

Management of Scapula Fracture

Life-threatening injury often associated with scapula fracture can include head and spinal cord injury, pneumothorax from rib fractures, and pulmonary contusion. Scapula fracture patients naturally splint the shoulder by keeping the arm held tight to their side. As with shoulder fracture, sling immobilization followed by early motion restriction is usually sufficient with an isolated fracture.

Humerus Fracture

Fractures of the humeral shaft can be found following motor vehicle collisions or falls on an outstretched arm. These are one of the easier fractures to diagnose because movement of the arm will usually cause obvious movement and deformity at the fracture site. These injuries should be carefully examined because they are often associated with radial nerve injury.

Pain or tenderness at the fracture site, inability to extend the wrist or hand, and numbness or tingling at the back of the hand all indicate a humerus fracture. The patient will also present with deformity, swelling, or ecchymosis.

Management of Humerus Fracture

Fractures of the humeral shaft are also commonly open and at risk for development of infection. Look carefully for any associated breaks in the skin. Always check for radial pulse and examine the shoulder and elbow as well. Immobilize the fracture with a rigid splint, then sling and swath the arm to the body in preparation for transport. Even when there is significant initial displacement, these fractures can almost always be reduced and treated with a stabilizing brace around the arm. In older adults, humerus fractures can include the area immediately above the elbow and actually extend into the elbow. In these situations, the neurovascular structures around the elbow are also at risk for injury. Careful examination of distal pulses is necessary to ensure adequate perfusion of the hand. If perfusion is compromised and the elbow is malaligned, consider gently realigning the limb to help restore adequate circulation.

Elbow Fracture

Elbow fractures are a little more complex and variable than humerus fractures but are relatively less common. The elbow is formed by the articulation of the distal humerus with the proximal ulna and radius. Fractures of the elbow usually involve the epicondyles of the distal humerus, the <u>olecranon</u> (the rounded posterior projection we commonly call the "elbow"), or the <u>radial head</u> (the proximal articulating end of the radius).

A patient with an elbow fracture will present with deformity, ecchymosis, or crepitus. The patient will also experience pain at the site that increases with motion and significant effusion that is usually obvious and palpable. Pain with <u>supination</u> (rotation with the palm upward) or <u>pronation</u> (rotation with the palm downward) of the hand is an indication of radial head injury.

Management of Elbow Fracture

The ulnar nerve passes from the medial cord of the brachial plexus to the little finger in the hand with little to no protection from muscle or bone. Because of its subcutaneous location near the elbow on the medial side, it is the most frequently injured nerve in patients with elbow injuries and should be carefully assessed after elbow trauma. This assessment can be accomplished by checking sensation at the little finger. Check the radial pulse and capillary refill because elbow fractures can occlude the brachial artery. The elbow does not tolerate injury very well and is very susceptible to persistent pain and stiffness. Therefore, the goal of treatment is to achieve a stable reduction that will allow for early motion. Nondisplaced fractures can be treated with a sling or posterior splint. Almost all displaced fractures will require open reduction and internal fixation. Manage pain according to local protocols.

Elbow Dislocation

<u>Radial head subluxation</u>, also known as nursemaid's elbow (or pulled elbow), is the most common injury to the upper extremity in infants and children. Subluxation of the radial head is a minor injury in infants ages 6 months to 6 years old and typically results from a quick pull on a child's arm. The ligaments of young children are weak and underdeveloped, thus when longitudinal traction is placed on an extended pronated arm, one of the ligaments around it may slip out of place. The left arm is more commonly involved, presuming most caregivers are right handed, and girls are more often affected than boys. Typically this child presents in no distress, with the affected arm semi-flexed, adducted, and pronated. These injuries often go unnoticed initially until the parents realize the child is not using the arm. Reduction of the subluxated radial head is a quick and easy procedure that requires no anesthesia but should be attempted only after a thorough history and physical exam.

Adult elbow dislocations typically occur from a fall on an outstretched hand. The large majority are posterior dislocations where the ulna's olecranon is displaced posterior to the distal humerus. Concomitant olecranon and radial head fractures may occur along with brachial artery, median nerve, and ulnar nerve injuries. Complete a thorough neurovascular exam in these cases.

Management of Elbow Dislocation

Elbow dislocations should be reduced as soon as possible but require sedation or general anesthesia to do so. The reduction is done with the arm in slight flexion and with steady, downward traction on the forearm. When reduction is achieved, a "cluck" is typically felt. The neurovascular exam should be conducted again, followed by splinting the arm in 70° to 90° of flexion and some pronation.

Forearm Fracture

Forearm fractures of the radius and ulna are not very common and usually come from a direct trauma. They will typically occur when a patient has raised their arm in protection from an ensuing blow. In more severe trauma, if one of the bones is broken, be suspicious that both bones are broken or that an associated dislocation of the second bone is present. Forearm fractures of the ulna alone are sometimes called a *nightstick* fracture because they were often caused in defense of a swinging nightstick or baton. Distal radius or wrist fractures are far more common and the most common fracture in adults. These injuries are almost always caused by a fall onto an outstretched hand and less frequently by compressive impaction, such as jamming the wrist while holding the steering wheel. There are several types, but the most common are the Colles fracture, where the distal radius fragment is tilted posteriorly or dorsal, and the **Smith fracture**, where the distal fragment is tilted anteriorly or volar (FIGURE 7-23). This area is rich with blood vessels and nerves, so use caution when splinting these injuries.

Swelling, along with tenderness and ecchymosis at the fracture site, are typical indicators of a forearm fracture. A history of injury, deformity, and wrist pain make these fractures apparent. Posttraumatic wrist arthritis can occur in the joint after a distal radius fracture, due to possible cartilage damage, or because of wear and tear from a misaligned joint after the injury is healed. Pediatric fractures caused by the same typical history are less obvious because the fracture goes through the distal radius growth plate, resulting in pain but little to no deformity. These fractures are then often misdiagnosed as sprains and not properly immobilized.

Management of Forearm Fracture

Forearm fractures have to be splinted so that both distal and proximal joints are secured (FIGURE 7-24). When splinting the forearm, it is important to check pulse, sensation, and motor function before and after splinting to ensure the treatment did not cause further damage. Along with inspection for swelling, deformity, and discoloration, also check for sensation and circulation in the hand. Management of nondisplaced or minimally displaced wrist fractures varies from a simple cock-up wrist splint to short or long arm casting. Ice can also help in reducing inflammation at the site in the acute setting. Pharmaceutical treatment may be required for pain management. Significant displacement or comminution will require open reduction and internal fixation followed by cast immobilization.

Wrist Fracture

Wrist fractures that involve the actual carpal bones are far less common than long bone fractures (FIGURE 7-25). There are eight small bones lined up in two rows that make up the bones of the hand or carpal bones. The scaphoid, or carpal navicular, bone is most susceptible to fracture from a fall on the outstretched hand and therefore is the most commonly fractured. The scaphoid spans the two rows of carpal bones and sits between the radius and the thumb

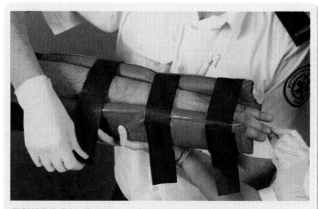

FIGURE 7-24   Splinting of a forearm fracture.

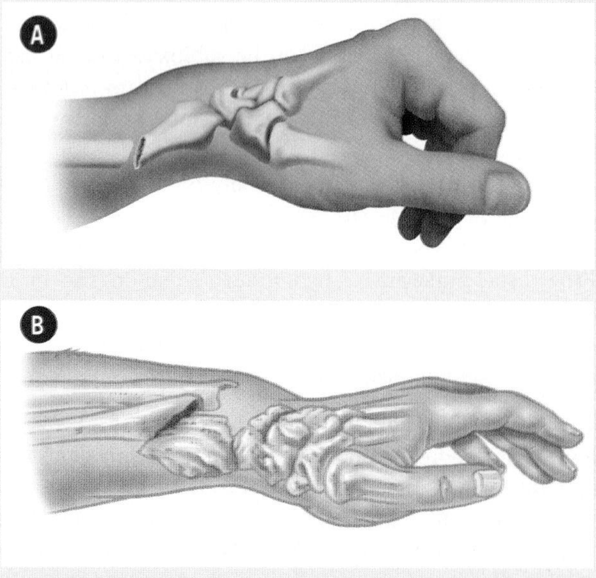

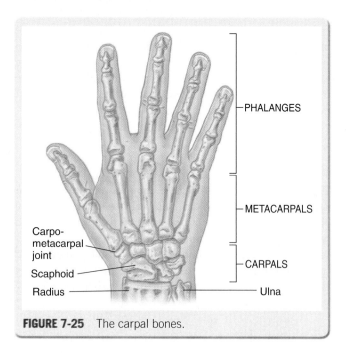

Carpo-metacarpal joint

Scaphoid

Radius

PHALANGES

METACARPALS

CARPALS

Ulna

FIGURE 7-25   The carpal bones.

FIGURE 7-23   Two common forearm fractures include the Colles fracture (**A**) and Smith fracture (**B**).

phalanges. Scaphoid fractures are important because they are often missed, leading to delayed treatment. This delay, along with naturally poor blood supply, puts this fracture at high risk for delayed union or nonunion. Diagnosis is not always easy because there is no obvious deformity and initial radiographs may not reveal a fracture. On examination, extension and abduction of the thumb will create a dimple between the tendons at the base of the thumb's metacarpal, forming an anatomic landmark called the snuff box. Palpate the area with a pinching type pressure applied to both the palmar and dorsal surfaces. Tenderness and swelling here indicates a wrist fracture.

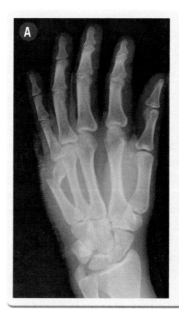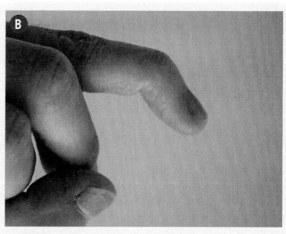

FIGURE 7-26 Common fractures of the hand include boxer's fracture (**A**) and mallet fracture (**B**).

Management of Wrist Fracture

Initially immobilize acute scaphoid fractures with a rigid splint. Apply ice to minimize swelling. Manage pain per local protocols.

Hand Fracture

Common hand fractures include metacarpal fractures and distal phalanx fractures **FIGURE 7-26**. The most common fracture is a <u>boxer's fracture</u>, which is a metacarpal neck fracture of the little finger. As the name implies, this fracture is usually caused by a closed fist striking an object. Another fracture common to fist fights is the <u>Bennett fracture</u> of the base of the thumb. <u>Mallet finger</u> is commonly caused by an athletic injury that occurs when the most distal joint of the finger is forcefully hyperflexed. This causes the extensor tendon to be avulsed traumatically from the distal phalanx to which it attaches. The result is a flexion deformity of the distal phalanx, which the patient cannot actively extend. Mallet finger is sometimes called a baseball fracture because it is seen when a player slides into the base head first and jams his finger on the base. It is also seen in basketball or football players who routinely jam fingers.

Indicators of a hand fracture include history, tenderness, and swelling. A boxer's fracture can be identified by a depressed knuckle on the little finger and overlapping of the little finger by the ring finger when making a fist. Deformity is the hallmark of mallet finger.

Management of Hand Fracture

Mallet finger should be splinted in neutral or even hyperextension immediately. The splint should stay on day and night until the fracture is healed. Ice can help reduce pain and swelling in the acute phase following an injury. If not splinted properly, or if left untreated, fractures of the hand that present with the deformity may need surgery to correct function and appearance.

Finger Dislocation

Dislocations of the fingers are usually obvious and largely occur at the proximal interphalangeal (PIP) joint. The patient will have a history of trauma with acute onset of pain and dorsal displacement of the distal finger. Patients will often instinctively pull the finger and reduce the dislocation themselves before medical evaluation; otherwise, there will be obvious deformity to indicate a dislocation. You should also expect to find swelling and tenderness of the finger. Associated volar fracture of the middle proximal phalanges is usually present.

Management of Finger Dislocation

A finger that has been dislocated should be splinted, as if it were fractured, with a rigid splint or by buddy taping. Apply ice for pain and swelling during the acute phase of the injury.

Injuries of the Lower Extremities

Pelvic Fracture

The pelvis consists of the ilium, ischium, and pubis bone, which form an anatomic ring with the sacrum. Disruption of this ring typically requires significant energy; because of the forces involved, pelvic fractures frequently involve organs and blood vessels contained within the pelvis, including the bladder, femoral arteries, and femoral veins. Due to the proximity of these large vessels, massive amounts of blood loss can occur within the pelvis with no external visible signs. The pelvis can hold 2–3 liters of undetected blood loss, which is about half of the adult blood volume.

A <u>pelvic fracture</u> is the disruption of the bony structure of the pelvis. In the elderly, the most common cause of pelvic fracture is a fall from a standing position; however, the most severe fractures involve significant forces, such as a motor vehicle collision or fall from a height.

There are four main classifications of pelvic fractures: lateral compression, anterior-posterior compression, vertical shear, and combined mechanical. **Lateral compression fractures** are transverse fractures of the pubis bone, along with associated sacral compression on the side of impact, or iliac wing fracture on the side of impact. **Anterior-posterior compression fractures (straddle fractures)** are associated with a slight widening of the pubic symphysis along with a fracture at the sacroiliac joint, whereby the pelvis is separated both front and back. **Vertical shear** is an actual displacement of both the anterior and posterior pelvic ring due to a high-energy impact. The **combined mechanical** is a combination of any of the above pelvic fractures, also due to high-energy impact, and is often caused by a motor vehicle collision or fall from a height.

Indicators of pelvic fracture include pain in the pelvis, groin, or hips; hematomas or contusions to the pelvic region; obvious external bleeding; hypotension without obvious external bleeding; unstable fracture of the pelvis; and pain with compression of the iliac crest.

Management of Pelvic Fracture

Any suspected pelvic fracture will need to be stabilized immediately in the field due to the high potential for underlying tissue and organ damage. Open pelvic fractures are very rare and must be considered a life-threatening injury. This is a very high-energy type of injury.

There are several ways to stabilize a pelvic fracture. The use of a commercial device, called a **pelvic girdle**, provides very good immobilization and is easily applied. The PASG can also be used to provide support to an unstable fracture with hypotension. The vest-type shortboard is another option that can be applied to one side of the pelvis. The device is centered laterally on the injured side, with the head of the device pointed toward the feet. The chest straps are then tightened around the waist and pelvis to secure it. The patient can also be placed on a simple long backboard or scoop stretcher, bolstered with pillows or padding and secured with straps PROCEDURE 20 .

Hip Fracture

The hip joint is a ball-and-socket joint that comprises the femoral head (ball) and the acetabulum (socket) of the pelvis. A broken hip is a common injury, especially among the elderly with osteoporosis. Hip fractures in the elderly are most commonly caused by a seemingly insignificant fall. In younger patients with stronger bones, hip fractures occur from more high-energy events. Hip fractures are usually placed in two categories: femoral neck or intertrochanter. The **femoral neck fracture** is when the femoral head is broken at its neck from the femoral shaft. The **intertrochanter fracture** occurs just below the neck of the femur. Typically, the patient has a history of a fall with inability to walk.

Shortening of the injured leg and external rotation of the foot indicate a potential hip fracture. A patient may also present with pain and tenderness, an inability to place weight on the leg, and crepitus with movement.

Management of Hip Fracture

Management of hip fractures should include gentle realignment of the limb and splinting. Supporting the injured extremity in the position found should be reserved for injuries where gentle realignment is unsuccessful or impossible FIGURE 7-27 . This may be accomplished by placing pillows or blankets under the affected extremity and securing them in place. In younger patients and in those with high-energy injuries, the use of a traction splint may be required to reduce the amount of bleeding. In this case, treat the patient as you would any other trauma patient: Fully immobilize the patient, monitor for shock, and transport to a trauma center.

Definitive treatment of a hip fracture almost always requires surgery. If possible, the bone is repaired with plates, rods, or screws. Sometimes, however, the hip must be replaced. Difficulty in determining the exact location of the fracture in the field causes concerns with the use of a traction device for these injuries. These injuries are best handled similar to a pelvic fracture and splinted with a rigid device or girdle-type device. Definitive treatment is almost always surgical fixation.

Hip Dislocation

Hip dislocation is very rare in adults because of the deep and secure ball-and-socket hip joint. When dislocations do occur, it is from a very high-impact injury such as a motor vehicle collision. Ninety percent of hip dislocations are posterior. The femoral head gets pushed out of the joint posterior to the acetabulum. The resulting deformity is a shortened, flexed, and internally rotated limb. The sciatic nerve may be injured during this trauma and the patient may complain of numbness or tingling throughout the limb. These dislocations are a true emergency and need to be reduced as soon as possible to prevent osteonecrosis of the femoral head, which occurs 10% of the time, perhaps because of a traumatic disruption of the

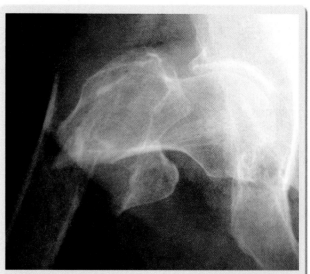

FIGURE 7-27 Hip fractures should be gently realigned and splinted.

femoral head blood supply. Unfortunately, reduction is often delayed while plain radiographs are obtained to rule out loose fragments and femoral head fracture. After reduction, patients will use crutches or another walking aid and advance weight bearing as tolerated until pain free.

Patients with hip dislocations may experience shortening of the affected leg, internal rotation of the foot, and pain in straightening the leg. Other signs to look for include deformity, local pain, and swelling.

Management of Hip Dislocation

Hip dislocations require support to minimize movement. Use blankets and pillows to buttress the patient when immobilizing them on a long backboard or rigid supporting device. Pain medication may be useful when trying to immobilize and move the patient. Use local protocols for pain management.

Femur Fracture

Because of the significant amount of surrounding muscle mass, it takes a great deal of force, directly or indirectly, to fracture the shaft of the femur. Once the fracture has occurred, it is usually the contracting force of the musculature that causes the shaft to displace, bringing increased pain and damage to the surrounding soft tissue. This is why a traction splint is applied. It is not uncommon for femur fractures to be open fractures, and the prehospital provider should conduct a careful inspection for one. A swollen or deformed thigh, a shortened extremity, and ecchymosis or deep bruising are all indicators of a femur fracture.

Management of Femur Fracture

Due to the rich blood supply and the vast tissue area of the thigh, large amounts of blood can be lost before any signs of hypovolemia will be evident after a femur fracture. Always evaluate the vascular status of the limb distal to the fracture. Because this injury is caused from a high-impact force, it is associated with multisystem injuries. Examination of the patient should therefore include assessment for life threats. Treatment for the mid-shaft femur fracture should include pain management, bleeding control if necessary, and application of a traction splint.

Knee Fracture

The knee is a hinge joint formed by the distal femur and the proximal tibia. It is protected anteriorly by the patella, or kneecap. The knee also includes several ligaments and cartilage that play a part in the function and stability of this joint. Because the knee supports almost the entire body weight, this joint becomes highly susceptible to injury during sports. The critically important anterior cruciate ligament (ACL) holds the anteromedial tibia to the posterior femur and prevents the femur from being pushed too far anterior relative to the tibia when the foot is planted. The ACL is often torn during high-energy twisting injuries. The posterior cruciate ligament (PCL) connects the anterior femur to the medial tibia and prevents posterior displacement of the femur and is typically injured only from blunt force trauma. The medial collateral ligament (MCL) prevents the medial side of the knee from being hinged open, and the lateral collateral ligament (LCL) protects the lateral side from being forced open. The **meniscus**, the shock-absorbing cartilage between the femur and tibia, protects the bone ends from rubbing together and effectively deepens the socket in which the femur articulates. It is common to tear one or more of these parts while playing contact sports and those that place a great deal of pressure on the knee, especially twisting-type pressure like sudden change of direction.

Trauma may cause two types of knee fractures FIGURE 7-28 . One is the **tibial plateau fracture**, which occurs

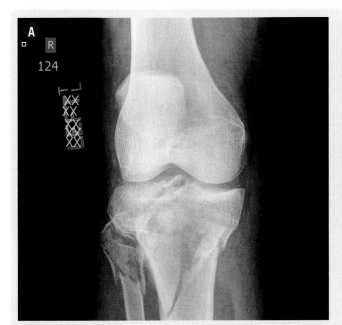
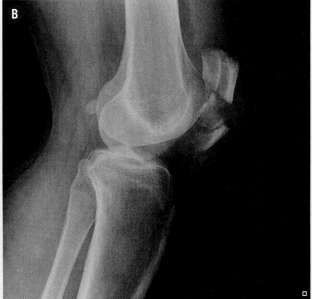

FIGURE 7-28   Knee fractures include (**A**) tibial plateau fractures and (**B**) patella fractures.

when a patient falls from a significant height like a roof or high ladder. The fracture occurs when the victim lands on their feet and the distal femur crushes the tibial head. These fractures are very painful and usually require surgical reduction. Even with surgery, the tibial plateau is difficult to reconstruct perfectly and the irregular surface will often lead to early arthritis. The other common knee fracture is the **patella fracture**, which is caused by direct trauma to the kneecap. These patients will have significantly painful knee effusions, swelling, deformity, inability to move the joint, and decreased distal sensation due to swelling near the nerves.

Management of Knee Fracture

Because knee fractures occur from high-energy trauma, they are often associated with other injuries. Prehospital providers should conduct functional assessment of the peroneal and posterior tibial nerves, along with distal pulses. The peroneal nerve has sensory receptors on the dorsal surface of the foot and is tested by asking the patient to lift their toes upward. Posterior tibial nerve function should be tested by checking sensation on the bottom of the foot and having the patient push their toes downward. All knee injuries must be splinted in the position in which they are found because of the large number of nerves and blood vessels running in proximity to the joint. Any manipulation of the injury may cause further damage to the surrounding structures.

Knee Dislocation

Knee dislocation is a rare condition but may include additional injury to the vascular and nervous structures that run through the joint. This dislocation occurs between the distal femur and the tibia. Many dislocations may spontaneously relocate, whereas dislocations in the context of multisystem trauma are often overlooked. Gross deformity, swelling and severe pain are all clues to knee dislocations. Decreased pulses at the dorsalis pedis or posterior tibial arteries should alert the provider to potential damage to the popliteal artery. Peroneal nerve damage will present with decreased sensation between the first and second toes and difficulty dorsiflexing the foot.

Patella dislocations of the knee are more common than knee dislocations. The patella is suspended in the anterior portion of the knee by ligamentous attachments that form the synovial capsule. These injuries are more common in women but also affect male athletes. The quadriceps muscle usually tightens to provide stabilization to the joint and almost always pulls the patella lateral to the knee. Women are more susceptible to this injury for two reasons: the greater ligamentous laxity females have over males and women have wider hips that cause the patella to be pulled or tilted slightly more lateral. Pain, swelling, and a decreased range of motion are signs of a patella dislocation. The sensation of a "pop" and visible deformity of the knee also indicate that a patient may have a patella dislocation.

Management of Knee Dislocation

A tibiofemoral dislocation is a limb-threatening injury often associated with vascular injury. Careful assessment for distal neurologic and vascular compromise is needed. When reduc-

tion is required in the prehospital phase due to absent blood flow, it is best done by extending the knee and applying forward pressure on the proximal tibia. Definitive treatment requires reconstructive surgery of the involved ligaments.

Management of Patella Dislocation

Patella dislocations are easily reduced with extension of the knee and medializing pressure to the patella. The knee should then be protected in a knee immobilizer for a few days, followed by a patella stabilizing brace.

Lower Leg Fracture

The lower leg is formed by the fibula on the lateral side and the tibia on the medial side. The tibia is the larger of the two and bears about 80% of the weight. Fractures of the tibia are more common. Fractures of the fibula are more likely to occur in connection with a tibial fracture.

There are three main areas of the tibia that can be affected by fracture: tibial shaft fractures, tibial plateau fractures, and plafond fractures which occur at the distal end of the tibia. Midshaft tibia fractures are the most common type of tibial fracture and typically require a very forceful direct blow. These fractures are often the result of motor vehicle collisions, falls, and sports injury. Assessment should attempt to determine the location of the fracture, whether the fracture is displaced, and whether there is associated injury to the soft tissue surrounding the bone. Plateau fractures, also called fender or bumper fractures due to their association with automobile impacts, occur just below the knee joint and usually involve the cartilage. Swelling usually accompanies the fracture and can cause decreases in distal blood flow. These fractures increase the chance of developing arthritis. Knee ligament and meniscal tears are common with plateau fractures. Surgery is often the choice for repair of the fracture due to the misalignment of the surface as it articulates with the femur. Plafond fractures, sometimes called tibial pilon fractures, involve the ankle joint. Plafond fractures are usually the result of axial loading and can occur with low energy (from skiing) or high energy (motor vehicle collision). As with plateau fractures, these too often involve the cartilage of the joint and can lead to arthritis. Because there is little tissue surrounding the distal tibia, swelling is often a problem.

Lower leg fractures are often open fractures because there is very little soft tissue covering the anterior tibia. Bleeding is a major concern with open fractures because the sharp bone ends may lacerate the large blood vessels during their displacement. Deformity, focal pain, and swelling all indicate potential lower leg fracture. The patient also may not be able to bear weight on the affected leg. Compartment syndrome is a concern with lower extremity injury because there is little soft tissue to accommodate the swelling.

Management of Lower Leg Fracture

In open fractures of the lower leg, bleeding can be extensive and hard to control. Tourniquet usage can be life saving in these instances. Appropriate management of the lower leg fracture involves applying a rigid splint to include both upper and lower joints, pain management, and ice to reduce

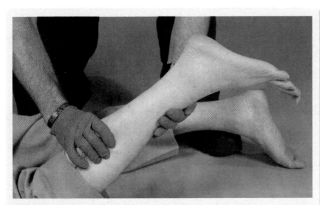

FIGURE 7-29   The Thompson test is used to test for rupture of the Achilles tendon.

inflammation. Apply sterile dressings to any open fractures to reduce risk of infection. These injuries are at significant risk of compartment syndrome and therefore serial examination should be conducted for increasing swelling and tension of the skin. As always, distal nerves and circulation should be examined.

Achilles Tendon Rupture

The Achilles tendon is a strong, fibrous cord that attaches the muscles in the back of the leg (gastrocnemius and soleus) to the heel (calcaneus). Overstretching this tendon can cause it to tear or rupture. It is most common in middle-aged men who are active with sports like basketball and tennis because the quick stop-and-go can put abrupt strain on the tendon. It may also occur from a sharp traumatic blow. This rupture usually occurs just above the heel, but can happen anywhere along the tendon.

A patient with an Achilles tendon rupture may present with a history of a sudden snap followed by immediate pain and swelling near the heel. Patients will commonly describe the sudden pain as "a gunshot," "snakebite," or direct hit from a ball. Pain with weight bearing and difficulty walking are common, and there is often a palpable defect in the tendon, typically 5–7 cm above the insertion into the calcaneus.

Management of Achilles Tendon Rupture

To determine a complete versus partial rupture, have the patient lie on his or her stomach (prone), with the knee flexed to 90°, and squeeze the calf of their leg. This will normally cause plantar flexion of the foot. If there is no such flexion, the Achilles tendon is ruptured and it is termed a positive Thompson test (or Simmon's test) **FIGURE 7-29**. Achilles tendon rupture should be splinted in equinus. Pull the toes downward to decrease the pressure on the tendon and

secure without putting pressure on the Achilles tendon with straps or cravats.

Ankle Injury

The ankle joint is formed by the distal ends of the tibia and fibula of the lower leg and the talus bone of the foot. The ankle joint allows for the extension, flexion, inversion, and eversion motion of the foot. The bony prominence of the inner ankle is called the medial malleolus, which is formed by the end of the distal tibia. The outer bony prominence is called the lateral malleolus, formed by the distal fibula. Ankle injuries are common to sports-related incidents, motor vehicle accidents, and falls. It is not uncommon to find open fractures to the ankle area.

There are several types of ankle fractures. Stable ankle fractures are one-sided fractures of the medial or lateral malleolus. Unstable fractures include fracture of both malleoli (bimalleolar), fracture of the lateral malleolus with rupture of the medial ankle ligament (bimalleolar equivalent), or trimalleolar fracture involving both the medial and lateral malleolus and the posterior distal tibia.

Indications of an ankle injury include pain, tenderness, swelling, and ecchymosis. Open fractures are common and abnormal rotation of the foot may be present.

Management of Ankle Injury

Vacuum splints or a rolled-up pillow work very well for stabilizing an ankle fracture. Pain management is appropriate. Check distal capillary refill and temperature of the toes frequently. Medial malleolus, bimalleolar, and trimalleolar fractures will typically need open reduction with internal fixation for complete repair.

Foot Injury

The calcaneus is the bone in the back of the foot, commonly referred to as the heel. This bone helps support the foot and allows for a normal walking motion. Calcaneus fractures are almost always the result of high-energy injuries like motor vehicle collisions or falls from a significant height. Calcaneus fractures cause severe pain and swelling to the back of the foot, along with an inability to bear weight. Check capillary refill because swelling can make pulses difficult to detect. Palpate the lumbar spine as well because the mechanism of injury to cause a calcaneus fracture can also cause a compression fracture of the spine.

Management of Foot Injury

Foot injuries should be splinted in the position found with a well-padded posterior splint from the toe to the upper calf. Do not withhold pain medication because these injuries can be very painful. Also elevate the foot to decrease swelling from venous pressure and apply ice.

CHAPTER RESOURCES

CASE STUDY ANSWERS

1 What are the priorities for assessment of this patient?

Treatment, as for all trauma patients, must be geared to life-threatening injury first. Your patient has significant bleeding from the right thigh that must be controlled. If you can do nothing more than maintain the ABCs, immobilize the patient, and transport to an appropriate center, you have done your job. When the bleeding has been controlled, additional assessment and treatment should be completed. A detailed assessment of the leg should include musculoskeletal deformity and distal neurovascular checks.

2 If direct pressure to the wound on the leg did not control the bleeding, what other options are available?

In cases of severe life-threatening bleeding, a tourniquet should be the first line of treatment. When a tourniquet is unavailable or does not fit above the wound, direct pressure with a dressing capable of covering the wound should be attempted. If the dressing soaks through, an additional dressing should be added to the top of the first one. If pressure does not control the bleeding, pressure to the artery above the site of bleeding may decrease the pressure, allowing a clot to begin forming. Clotting agents may also be an alternative if local protocols allow. If a large blood vessel has been severed, clamping the vessel with a hemostat may provide direct control of the bleeding. Blind clamping within a wound in an attempt to stop bleeding should be avoided because this often produces additional damage to the wound.

3 Would realignment and splinting of the leg be appropriate?

Following bleeding control, the leg should be assessed for additional injury and distal neurovascular status. Alignment of the extremity into normal anatomic position can decrease bleeding and restore neurovascular flow. Splinting assists in controlling bleeding by minimizing the space for blood to collect and by decreasing any additional injury that may occur following movement of the sharp bone ends from a fracture.

4 Describe your assessment for a lower extremity and an upper extremity.

Begin the assessment of the leg by checking the structure. Palpate the entire length looking for deformity or signs of localized injury. Check for distal pulses and capillary refill. Neurologic assessment should include both movement and sensation. In the leg this includes the ability for dorsiflexion (moving the toes upward) and plantar flexion (moving the toes downward away from the body) of the foot. Sensation should be assessed on both the dorsal (top) and plantar (bottom) surfaces of the foot. If the injury does not limit movement, have the patient move the extremity to check range of motion (ROM) passively and then with light resistance.

The arms include the same general steps: checking the structure and assessing distal pulses, neurologic function, and ROM. There are three nerves that create function and sensation in the hand that should be assessed: the radial (thumb), medial (top of the middle fingers of the hand), and ulnar (little finger) nerves.

Trauma in Motion

1. What types of splints are available for use at your service? Are you proficient in their use?
2. Isolated musculoskeletal injury does not often qualify for transport to a trauma center. What hospitals have the capability to handle these injuries in your area? Do you have protocols to allow you to transport patients to these facilities?
3. Pain is often a major factor in treating musculoskeletal injuries. What are your local protocols for pain management?
4. If an extremity is entrapped following an accident (of any type) and will not be freed in a timely manner and the patient has additional life-threatening injury, do you have a protocol that would allow personnel to do a field amputation or to bring additional personnel to the scene for the procedure?

References and Resources

American Academy of Orthopaedic Surgeons. *Emergency Care and Transportation of the Sick and Injured.* 9th ed. Sudbury, MA: Jones and Bartlett; 2005.

American Academy of Orthopaedic Surgeons. *Nancy Caroline's Emergency Care in the Streets.* 6th ed. Sudbury, Mass: Jones and Bartlett; 2007.

American College of Surgeons Committee on Trauma. *Advanced Trauma Life Support for Doctors.* 7th ed. Chicago: American College of Surgeons; 2004.

Doyle JR, ed. *Hand and Wrist.* Philadelphia: Lippincott Williams & Wilkins; 2006.

Elling B, Elling K, Rothenberg M. *Anatomy and Physiology: Paramedic.* Sudbury, MA: Jones and Bartlett; 2004.

Feliciano DV, Mattox KL, Moore EE. *Trauma.* 6th ed. New York: McGraw-Hill Medical; 2008.

Greene WB, ed. *Essentials of Musculoskeletal Care.* 2nd ed. Rosemont, IL: American Academy of Orthopaedic Surgeons; 2001.

Hoppenfeld S, ed. *Orthopedic Dictionary.* Philadelphia: J.B. Lippincott; 1994.

Hoppenfeld S. *Physical Examination of the Spine and Extremities.* New York: Appleton-Century-Crofts; 1976.

Korbeek JB, Turki SA, Ali J, et al. Advanced trauma life support, 8th edition, the evidence for change. *J Trauma Inj Infect Crit Care.* 2008; 64(6):1638–1650.

Melamed E, Blumenfeld A, Kalmovich B, et al. Prehospital care of orthopedic injuries. *Prehospital Disaster Med.* 2007; 22(1):22–25.

Richey S. Tourniquets for control of traumatic hemorrhage: a review of the literature. *World J Emerg Surg.* 2007; 2:28. Available at: www.wjes.org/content/2/1/28. Accessed January 14, 2008.

Schultz RJ. *The Language of Fractures.* 2nd ed. Baltimore: Williams & Wilkins; 1990.

Wilkins EW, Jr. *Emergency Medicine Scientific Foundations and Current Practice.* 3rd ed. Baltimore: Williams and Wilkins; 1989.

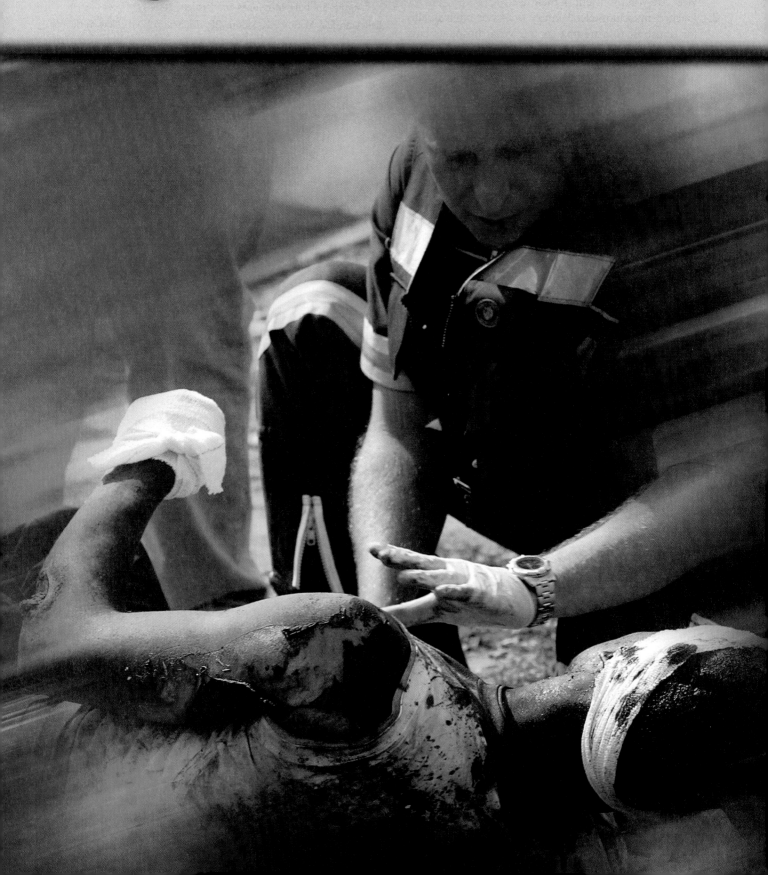

8 Burn Trauma

CASE STUDY

You are dispatched to a burn victim with the fire department. Details are sketchy as you respond to the side of a roadway in a part of town known for violence. As the fire department arrives they report a victim who was beaten and set on fire. Police are en route to the scene and arrive just before you. You notice a large crowd has grown around a man lying on the ground screaming in pain. The smell of burned flesh is in the air as you arrive at the patient's side.

Bystanders who have gathered around the victim begin to disclose the events leading up to this injury. They say a group of five men were beating and kicking the victim when one splashed the victim with fluid and then set him on fire. They state they ran over and chased the five men away and threw the victim to the ground and rolled him to put out the flames. The patient is anxious and crying out in pain. His clothes are still smoking and he is bleeding profusely from the head as you begin your assessment.

The initial/primary assessment shows a small amount of blood in the mouth but no soot or singed hair in the airway. Breathing is fast at 36 breaths/min and breath sounds are equal. The patient has a wound on the left side of his head that has a steady flow of blood coming from it. He has burns on his hands, upper chest, and back. His pulse is 130 beats/min and blood pressure is 90/60 mm Hg. You decide to move this patient to the hospital rapidly and to provide additional care en route.

1 What scene safety issues are present?

2 Approximately how much surface area is affected by the burn?

3 What is the first step in prehospital burn care?

4 Describe the priorities for assessment and initial care of your patient.

5 What is the cause of his shock?

Introduction

Burns are a devastating injury that occur with some frequency. More than a million people in the United States are burned each year. Forty-five thousand patients require in-hospital care annually for burns. Of the 45,000, about half are admitted to specialized burn treatment centers and half to other hospitals; 3% to 5% are considered to have life-threatening injuries.

In the United Kingdom, 250,000 people are burned each year, of which 175,000 visit the accident and emergency department with burn injuries and around 13,000 are admitted to the hospital. Across the United Kingdom, about 30% of children and 40% of adults suffering burns requiring admission to the hospital are admitted to nonspecialist units. Approximately 1,000 patients per year are admitted with severe burns requiring fluid resuscitation, about half of whom are children younger than 16 years old.

Burns are also a major problem in the developing world. Over 2 million burn injuries are thought to occur each year in India (population 500 million), but this may be a substantial underestimate. Mortality in the developing world is much higher than in the developed world. For example, Nepal has about 1,700 burn deaths per year for a population of 20 million, giving it a death rate 17 times that of Britain.

The incidence of burn injuries and deaths has decreased since the advent of stricter building regulation codes, safer construction techniques, and the use of smoke detectors. Children younger than 5 years old and the elderly are at a particularly high risk to die in fires. Deaths and serious injuries also occur from electrical, chemical, and radiation burns.

Just as building regulation code enforcement and smoke detectors have decreased fire-related deaths, our ability to treat large burns effectively has steadily improved. Before the medical advances of the 20th century, death was almost inevitable when more than one third of the body was burned, no matter how superficially. Now, however, better understanding of burn shock, advances in the use of fluid therapy and antibiotics, improved ability to excise dead tissue, and the use of biologic dressings to aid early wound closure have vastly improved burn care.

Although you probably will not see moderate and severe burns on a daily basis, you will certainly encounter some serious thermal injuries during your career. You may even encounter serious electrical, chemical, and radiation events as well. The appropriate recognition of the severity of such injuries can dramatically enhance the care received by the burned patient. Although emergency medical services (EMS) providers are often most concerned with the immediate life threats caused by burn injuries, their early actions can also impact the long-term morbidity and even the psychological impact of this devastating traumatic pathology.

To comprehend the patient treatments indicated for thermal injuries, we must first review the structure of the skin, which is the primary organ affected by burn injuries.

Anatomy and Function of the Skin

The skin, also known as the <u>integument</u>, is the body's largest organ. It plays a crucial role in maintaining <u>homeostasis</u>, or balance, within the body. The skin, which varies in thickness from 1 mm on the eyelid to 1 cm at the heel, is durable, flexible, and usually able to repair itself.

The primary functions of the skin are as a barricade against the outside world, a thermoregulatory organ, a fluid barrier, and a sensory organ. Significant damage to the skin may render the body vulnerable to bacterial invasion, temperature instability, and major disturbances of fluid balance, which is exactly what happens when burn trauma damages large portions of the integument.

Layers of the Skin

The skin is composed of two principal layers: the <u>epidermis</u> and the <u>dermis</u> **FIGURE 8-1**. The epidermis, or outermost layer, is the body's first line of defense—the principal barrier against water, dust, microorganisms, and mechanical stress. Underlying the epidermis is a tough, highly elastic layer of connective tissue called the dermis. The dermis is a

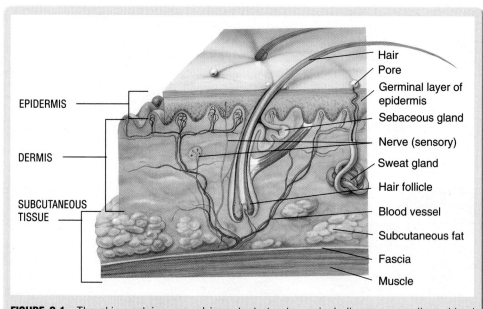

FIGURE 8-1 The skin contains several important structures, including nerve endings, blood vessels, sweat glands, hair follicles, and sebaceous glands.

complex material composed chiefly of <u>collagen</u> fibers, <u>elastin</u>, and a <u>mucopolysaccharide gel</u>. Collagen is a fibrous protein with a very high tensile strength, so it gives the skin a high resistance to breakage under mechanical stress. Elastin, as the name implies, imparts elasticity to the skin, allowing the skin to return to its usual contours. The mucopolysaccharide gel gives the skin resistance to compression. These tissues are all susceptible to destruction by heat or chemicals.

Enclosed within the dermis are several specialized skin structures:

- *Nerve endings*, which mediate the senses of touch, temperature, pressure, and pain.
- *Blood vessels*, which—like blood vessels elsewhere in the body—carry oxygen and nutrients to the skin and remove the carbon dioxide and metabolic waste products. Cutaneous blood vessels also serve a crucial role in regulating body temperature by regulating the volume of blood that flows from the body's warm core to its cooler surface.
- *Sweat glands*, which produce sweat and discharge it through ducts passing to the surface of the skin. Evaporation of water from the skin's surface is one of the body's major mechanisms for shedding excess heat. People who survive large-area full-thickness burns have often lost many of their sweat glands and are highly susceptible to heat stress.
- <u>Hair follicles</u> are structures that produce hair and enclose the hair roots. Each follicle contains a single hair. Full-thickness scalds sometimes destroy the follicles, and hair will fall out or be painlessly and easily pulled out of the scalded skin.
- The <u>sebaceous gland</u> at the neck of each hair follicle produces an oily substance called sebum. The precise function of sebum is not well understood, although it has been suggested that sebum keeps the skin supple so it does not crack.

The layer of tissue beneath the dermis is, by definition, the subcutaneous layer, and it consists mainly of adipose tissue (fat). Subcutaneous fat serves as insulating material to protect underlying tissues from extremes of heat and cold. It also provides a substantial cushion for underlying structures, while serving as an energy reserve for the body.

Finally, beneath the subcutaneous layer are the muscles, tendons, bones, and vital organs. Muscles have thick, fibrous capsules that are prone to hypoxia and anaerobic metabolism in a burn state. Bones are living, changing tissue that can be severely affected by burn injury. Lastly, the proper function of these vital organs is sensitive and easily destroyed by thermal, chemical, and electrical injury.

The Eye

The eye is particularly susceptible to thermal, ultraviolet, and chemical injury. Chemicals and heat denature the cellular proteins and cause secondary vascular ischemic damage. The cornea is most commonly injured because it is the part of the eye most susceptible to exposure. The tear ducts and eye-

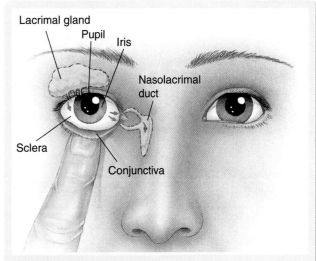

FIGURE 8-2   Tears act as lubricants and keep the front of the eye protected.

lids combine to lubricate the surface of the eyes constantly **FIGURE 8-2** . Unfortunately, intense heat, light, or chemical reactions on the surface of the eye can quickly burn the thin membrane or skin covering the surface of the eye.

Ocular damage is a common result of alkali (base) injury: The higher the pH of the substance, the more severe the damage to the eye. When a patient gets a substance like lime in the eyes, the damage is worsened by repeatedly rubbing the eyes. Initiate copious irrigation; the patient will also require follow-up treatment in the emergency department (ED).

Providers are typically quick to address chemical burns to the eyes, but may overlook thermal burns to the eyes in the complex scenario of a patient suffering burns from a house fire or motor vehicle crash. Ultraviolet eye burns present in skiers (snow blindness), people using tanning beds, or welders. Ocular burns represent as much as 20% of the eye trauma presenting to emergency departments in the United States. They are a common occupational injury. In the United States, 15% to 20% of patients with thermal burns of the face have sustained some degree of ocular burn.

Pathophysiology

<u>Burns</u> are diffuse soft-tissue injuries created by destructive energy transfer via radiation, thermal energy, or electrical energy. Thermal burns can occur when skin is exposed to temperatures higher than 111°F (44°C). A typical home heating system can deliver hot water out of a tap at temperatures between 130° and 140°F (55° to 60°C). At these temperatures, children will suffer superficial burns in only 7 seconds and full-thickness burns in 90 seconds. In general, the severity of a thermal injury correlates directly with temperature, concentration, and the duration of exposure. For example, solids generally have higher heat content than gases, so exposure to a hot solid (such as the rack inside an oven) typically causes a more significant burn than exposure

to hot gases (such as those coming out of an oven). Burns are a progressive process: The greater the heat energy, the deeper the wound.

Exposure time is another important factor. Thermal injury can occur to unresponsive or paralyzed patients from seemingly innocuous heat sources such as heating pads, transcutaneous oxygen sensors, and heat lamps left unattended for long periods.

Thermal Burns

A thermal burn is caused by heat energy that can be transmitted in a variety of ways in addition to fire. Thermal burns are all caused by heat (as opposed to electricity, chemicals, or radiation), but different situations can cause thermal burns and pose a safety hazard to responding providers.

Flame Burns

Most commonly, thermal burns are caused by open flame. Fires are chaotic and dangerous events, and patients involved in fires have often suffered other trauma in addition to their burns. Flame burns are very often deep burns, especially if a person's clothing catches fire **FIGURE 8-3**. They also are associated with inhalation injuries.

Scald Burns

Hot liquids produce scald injuries. Scalds are most commonly seen in children or disabled adults. They often cover large surface areas because spilled hot liquids will flow over any exposed body parts that are beneath them.

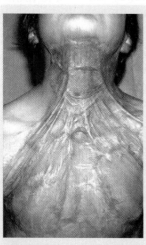

FIGURE 8-3 Flame burns are often very deep burns.

Hot liquids can soak into clothing and will continue to burn until the clothing is removed. Some hot liquids, such as oil or grease, will adhere to the skin and are more resistant to flushing with cool water, causing particularly deep scald injuries. Scald injuries generally are not as deep as those caused by open flame (although boiling grease or boiling oil can produce deep burns). They are sometimes associated with child abuse

FIGURE 8-4 . Many scalds could be avoided if people would practice a few well-known methods of prevention. Consider the information presented in **TABLE 8-1** , keeping in mind that your role as a provider includes public education about these important injury prevention issues.

Contact Burns

Contact with hot objects, such as a cooking stove burner, produces contact burns. Ordinarily, reflexes protect a person from prolonged exposure to a very hot object, so contact burns are not usually deep unless the patient was somehow prevented from drawing away from the hot object (eg, unconscious, intoxicated/impaired, disabled). Burns in children, older people, or people with

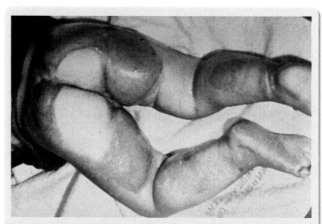

FIGURE 8-4 Scald burns, like the doughnut burn pictured here, may indicate child abuse.

TABLE 8-1	Scald Burn Exposure Times
Water Temperature	Time Required for a Full-Thickness Burn to Occur
155°F (68°C)	1 second
148°F (64°C)	2 seconds
140°F (60°C)	5 seconds
133°F (56°C)	15 seconds
127°F (52°C)	1 minute
124°F (51°C)	3 minutes
120°F (48°C)	5 minutes
100°F (37°C)	Safe temperature for bathing

Adapted from Moritz AR, Henriques FC Jr. *Am J Pathol.* 1947; 23:695–720.

disabilities may be cause for a raised suspicion for abuse. Burns with formed shapes or unusual patterns, or burns in atypical places such as genitalia, buttocks, and thighs, are often consistent with a history of abuse **FIGURE 8-5**. Detecting nonaccidental injuries is important because up to 30% of children who are repeatedly abused die as a result of the abuse.

Steam Burns

A steam burn can produce a topical (scald) burn. Steam (gaseous water) is also notorious for causing airway burns. Inhalation of other hot gases may cause **supraglottic** (upper airway) trauma but rarely leads to burns in the lower airway. Steam is unique because the minute particles of hot water *can* cause significant injury as they are carried into the lower airways.

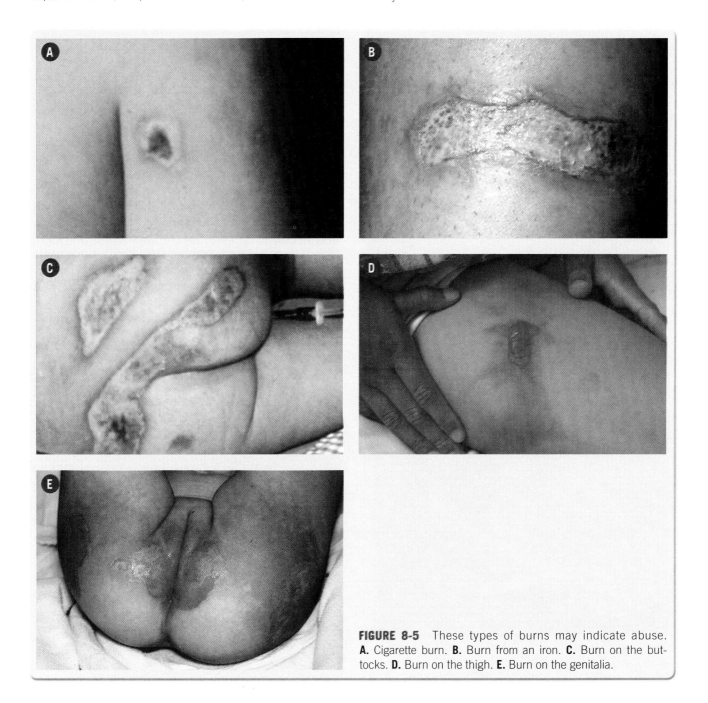

FIGURE 8-5 These types of burns may indicate abuse. **A.** Cigarette burn. **B.** Burn from an iron. **C.** Burn on the buttocks. **D.** Burn on the thigh. **E.** Burn on the genitalia.

Flash Burns

A relatively rare source of thermal burns is the flash produced by some form of explosion, which may briefly expose a person to very intense heat **FIGURE 8-6** . Lightning strikes can also cause flash burns. For more information on lightning strikes, please see Chapter 9: *Environmental Trauma*.

Burn Shock

Burn shock occurs because of fluid loss across the damaged skin and because of a series of volume shifts within the body itself. Capillaries become leaky, so intravascular volume oozes out of the circulation into the interstitial spaces. Meanwhile, cells of normal tissues take in increased amounts of salt and water from the fluid around them.

It is important to note that burn shock involves the entire body, not just the area burned. You may have experienced a sunburn over a reasonably large surface area (eg, your entire back is about 18% of your body surface area [BSA]). In addition to the discomfort from the burn, you may have experienced chills, nausea, and just feeling sick. This is secondary to the fluid shifts and electrolyte disturbances that are occurring in your body because of the burn. This is, in fact, a mild form of burn shock. Just as in other forms of shock, the changes that occur will limit the effective distribution of oxygen and glucose to the tissues, and limit the ability of the circulation to take away waste products from both healthy and damaged tissues. It is very important, therefore, that adequate fluid resuscitation of the burn patient occur at an early stage to prevent the devastating consequences of burn shock.

The burn shock process generally occurs 6 to 8 hours after the burn incident. You will not typically witness this in the field. Therefore, if an acutely burned patient is in shock in the prehospital phase, look for another injury as the source of shock. People caught in fires fall through floors, jump out of windows, and have things fall on them. There are ample opportunities for traumatic injuries on fire and explosion scenes, so you must be diligent in your assessment. At the same time, it is possible for you first to encounter a burn patient many hours after their injury, when the signs of burn shock are obvious.

Airway Burns

Inhalation burns can cause rapid and serious airway compromise. Advanced airway equipment, such as an endotracheal tube to secure the airway, should be readily accessible when treating any burn patient. Heat acts as an irritant to both the lungs and the airway. Airway edema, cough, nasal hair singeing, laryngeal edema, laryngospasm, and bronchospasm may result from heat inhalation. Patients may experience pulmonary damage from direct thermal injury or later from toxic inhalation injury. Lower airway damage is more often associated with the inhalation of steam or hot particulate matter, whereas upper airway damage is more often associated with the inhalation of superheated gases.

Smoke Inhalation

The process of combustion produces a variety of toxic gases. The less efficient the combustion, the more toxic gases (like carbon monoxide) may be involved. When furnaces, kerosene heaters, and other heating devices are in poor repair, or they are inadequately ventilated, they may emit unsafe levels of these toxic gases. Internal combustion engines may emit many of the same gases and should always have their exhaust vented to the outside. A common cause of carbon monoxide exposure is running a small engine in an enclosed space like a garage or basement.

When more complex materials (like plastic, PVC pipes, furniture foam fillings, and synthetic carpets) burn, more toxic and dangerous chemicals may be released. House fires and car fires may emit benzofurans, bicyclo compounds, carbon monoxide, cyanides, hydrochloric acid, and free radicals as their many synthetic components burn **FIGURE 8-7** . Regardless of the chemical composition of the smoke, it is best to stay low, thus limiting the chance of smoke inhalation **FIGURE 8-8** .

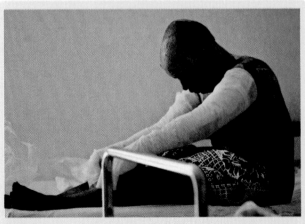

FIGURE 8-6 Flash burns may be minor compared with the additional trauma inflicted by the explosion.

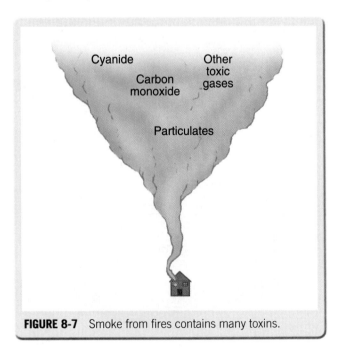

FIGURE 8-7 Smoke from fires contains many toxins.

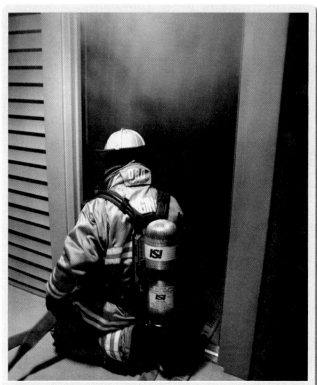

FIGURE 8-8 Staying low limits the chance of injury from smoke inhalation.

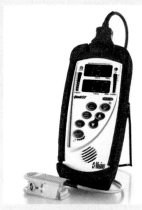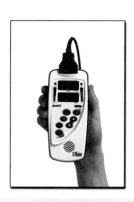

FIGURE 8-9 Pulse CO-oximeter devices can measure oxygen saturation as well as carbon monoxide levels.

Carbon Monoxide Intoxication

<u>Carbon monoxide (CO)</u> is an odorless, colorless, and tasteless gas produced by incomplete combustion of fuels. These fuels range from oil, natural gas, petroleum/gasoline, and diesel to wood and charcoal. CO builds up where there is poor ventilation, particularly in an enclosed area. CO is a common gas found in and around structural fires. Providers must be alert for the signs and symptoms of CO poisoning when treating burn patients rescued from enclosed areas.

CO has a 200–250 times greater affinity for hemoglobin (Hb) than oxygen does, making even small concentrations of it dangerous. The primary negative effect of carbon monoxide is that it binds to hemoglobin, forming carboxyhemoglobin (COHb). Once attached to Hb, CO does not easily detach, taking a critical number of Hb molecules out of action for the transportation of oxygen to tissues.

From living in an urban/industrialized society, most of us have a 1%–2% carbon monoxide level all of the time. Smokers might have a 3%–4% level. Symptoms of carbon monoxide intoxication, such as nausea, discoordination, and sleepiness, may occur at saturation levels of around 20%. Death can occur at 50%. Keep in mind that the "normal" 97% pulse oximetry reading may actually be 95% oxygen and 2% carbon monoxide. Patients with toxic, or even fatal, levels of carbon monoxide poisoning will show normal or high pulse oximetry values because

a typical pulse oximeter cannot recognize the difference between an oxygen molecule (O_2) attached to Hb, and a carbon monoxide molecule (CO) attached to Hb. Specialized pulse CO-oximeters are now readily available that can measure the level of COHb in the blood **FIGURE 8-9**. Some fire departments and ambulances now carry these devices, and providers can make use of them at fire scenes.

Unfortunately, carbon monoxide is a common molecule. It is formed from incomplete combustion of hydrocarbons, so it is present in vehicle exhaust, house fires, inefficient space heaters, small engines, wood fireplaces, or malfunctioning heating systems in homes. Patients exposed to high levels of carbon monoxide are in immediate danger from hypoxia, but are also susceptible to long-term consequences such as cognitive defects, memory loss, and movement disorders.

TIP

Effects of CO

As a point of interest, CO has other toxic effects on the body. CO interferes with the cytochrome oxidase mechanism in each cell (the same as cyanide does), making it difficult for cells to use any oxygen that is delivered. This is a less pronounced effect than Hb binding, but can contribute to mortality in the severely CO-intoxicated patient. This effect may lead to the cherry red color provider lore tells us patients exposed to carbon monoxide have. Although this is somewhat true, most experienced practitioners agree that an obvious red hue to the skin is not evident until the patient has a very high, perhaps fatal, dose. Never rule out carbon monoxide toxicity just because you don't see cherry red skin.

Cyanide Treatment in Fire Victims

WHETHER TO TREAT FIRE VICTIMS for cyanide poisoning has been an issue of controversy for two decades. Justification for such treatment is straightforward. About 75% of fire-related fatalities result from smoke inhalation, not burns, and hydrogen cyanide is among the most toxic components commonly found in smoke. On the other hand, evidence of the clinical benefits of such treatment remains sparse and uncertain.

Smoke is a complex mixture of toxic compounds.[1,2] Its actual composition changes from fire to fire and over time, reflecting the materials being burned, the temperature of the fire, the adequacy of oxygen, and the completeness of combustion. Hydrogen cyanide is routinely found in smoke generated by burning of nitrogen-containing compounds. Examples include natural (wool, silk, cotton, and wood) and synthetic (acrylic, nylon, and plastic) materials. Case reports and autopsy studies have documented elevated cyanide levels in victims of closed-space fires, with levels often greater than those regarded as "toxic" (ie, $> 39 \mu g/L$) or "lethal" (ie, $>100 \mu g/L$).[3] Such findings argue that cyanide toxicity should be a routine concern in smoke inhalation victims.

Acting on such concerns, however, has not been easy. Until recently, the only cyanide antidote available in the United States was the "cyanide kit" comprised of amyl nitrite, sodium nitrite, and sodium thiosulfate. That combination poses hazards to smoke inhalation victims.[4] Nitrite oxidizes hemoglobin to methemoglobin, a dysfunctional molecule that does not transport oxygen. In smoke victims with an oxygen-carrying capacity compromised by formation of carboxyhemoglobin, nitrite-induced methemoglobin further reduces oxygen transport to tissues and worsens hypoxia.

Some experts suggest that sodium thiosulfate be given alone to treat smoke inhalation victims, thereby avoiding the risks of methemoglobin formation.[5] Thiosulfate acts as a sulfur donor, facilitating the enzymatic conversion of toxic cyanide to harmless thiocyanate which is readily excreted. A few anecdotal reports describe treatment of victims with sodium thiosulfate (8–15 g IV), but no controlled trials have been undertaken. Based on animal studies, some have argued that the onset of thiosulfate effects is too slow to be useful for the treatment of acute life-threatening poisonings.

More recently, hydroxocobalamin, a natural form of vitamin B_{12}, has been approved by the US FDA for treatment of known or suspected cyanide poisoning with a recommended dose of 5 to 10 mg IV.[6] Its effectiveness has been well established in animal studies and it has been widely adopted.[2,6,7] There are few serious side effects of this agent; most reports describe only transient elevations of blood pressure, skin discoloration, and possible allergic reactions. In principle, its use for suspected cyanide poisoning seems to pose probable benefits and few risks.

On the other hand, however, its actual efficacy for fire victims remains unclear. The uncertain benefits of hydroxocobalamin for smoke inhalation reflect the substantial challenges to performing controlled trials in emergency settings. It has also been difficult to differentiate the benefits of cyanide antidotes from those resulting from other resuscitation efforts. Finally, most smoke victims found in cardiac arrest do not survive despite antidotes; in two series from the Paris Fire Brigade (where hydroxocobalamin is used routinely), 49 of 53 (93.5%) of smoke-related cardiac arrest victims died within 8 days.[2,7] Thus, determining the benefits of antidotal treatment will require a large, multicenter random-control trial which itself may raise important ethical concerns.

In summary, there is strong toxicologic evidence that cyanide inhalation contributes to the morbidity and mortality of smoke inhalation, especially in residential and closed-space fires. A cyanide antidote that seemingly poses few risks of side effects is now available and it appears to be useful in these cases. Nevertheless, the clinical benefits of intervention remain unclear.

Jonathan Borak, MD, DABT
Clinical Professor of Epidemiology and Medicine
Yale School of Medicine

References

1. Alarie Y. Toxicity of fire smoke. *Crit Rev Toxicol.* 2002; 32:259–289.

2. Fortin JL, Giocanti JP, Ruttimann M. Prehospital administration of hydroxocobalamin for smoke inhalation-associated cyanide poisoning: 8 years of experience in the Paris Fire Brigade. *Clin Toxicol (Phila).* 2006; 44(Suppl 1):37–44.

3. Baud FJ, Barriot P, Toffis V, et al. Elevated blood cyanide concentrations in victims of smoke inhalation. *N Engl J Med.* 1991; 325:1761–1766.

4. Hall AH, Kulig KW, Rumack BH. Suspected cyanide poisoning in smoke inhalation: Complications of sodium nitrate therapy. *J Toxicol Clin Exp.* 1989; 9:3–9.

5. Hall AH, Dart R, Bogdan G. Sodium thiosulfate or hydroxocobalamin for the empiric treatment of cyanide poisoning? *Ann Emerg Med.* 2007; 49:806–813.

6. Erdman AR. Is hydroxocobalamin safe and effective for smoke inhalation? Searching for guidance in the haze. *Ann Emerg Med.* 2007; 49:814–816.

7. Borron SW, Baud FJ, Barriot P, et al. Prospective study of hydroxocobalamin for acute cyanide poisoning in smoke inhalation. *Ann Emerg Med.* 2007; 49:794–801.

Chemical Burns

Chemical burns occur when the skin comes in contact with strong acids, alkalis/bases, or other corrosive materials **TABLE 8-2**. The burn will progress as long as the corrosive substance remains in contact with the skin. Thus, the cornerstone of therapy is safe and rapid removal of the chemical from contact with the patient's body.

Injuries from Chemical Burns

Skin destruction is determined by the chemical's concentration and the duration of contact. Systemic toxicity is determined by the degree of absorption. Immediately removing the patient's clothing will often remove the majority of the chemical from skin contact. Most chemicals are most efficiently removed by washing with copious amounts of low-pressure cool water (such as in a shower, sink, or eye-wash station) **FIGURE 8-10**.

TABLE 8-2	Acid/Alkaline Burns and Related Injuries	
Chemical Type	**Examples**	**Injury**
Acids	Battery acid, hydrochloric acid	Coagulative necrosis
Alkalis	Sodium hydroxide (bleach), drain cleaner, oven cleaner, lye	Liquefactive necrosis

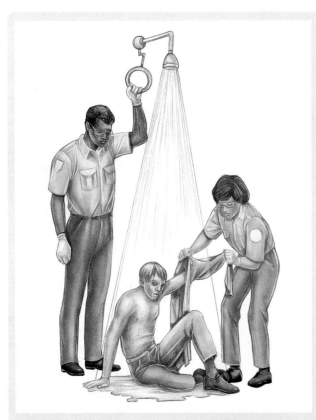

FIGURE 8-10 Chemicals must be removed from the skin as soon as possible to limit the burning process.

TIP

Acid Versus Alkaline Burns

Acid burns produce a <u>coagulative necrosis</u>, where burned tissue forms a tough layer of scar tissue. Alkaline (base) burns produce a <u>liquefactive necrosis</u>, in which burned tissue liquefies and becomes "soapy," allowing the base to burn deeper. This is why, in general, alkaline burns can be worse than acid burns.

Some chemicals react violently with water, which obviously precludes irrigation. Such chemicals are usually powders, so it is reasonable to brush off as much dry powder as possible before irrigation of the chemical.

Chemical Burns to the Eye

Improper handling can cause a variety of chemicals to splash into the eye, causing burns. Household bleach, chlorine for swimming pools, and splashed battery acid are common serious ocular burns. Chemical burns of the eye are also a common occupational injury, which could obviously be prevented by wearing safety glasses whenever pouring or working with any type of acidic or alkaline chemical **FIGURE 8-11**. Clouds of toxic chemicals, as may be released from pressurized containers of chlorine gas or ammonia, can also cause ocular burns. Providers should routinely wear eye protection when there is increased risk to their eyes at a scene.

Electricity-Related Injuries

One out of every five construction deaths is caused by electrical contact. National Institute for Occupational Safety and Health (NIOSH) statistics indicate that electrocution is the fifth leading cause of death in the workplace, with more than 400 deaths per year in the United States. Domestic injuries, on the other hand, are most likely to involve children **FIGURE 8-12**.

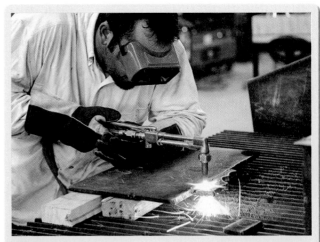

FIGURE 8-11 Common causes of eye burns include industrial incidents.

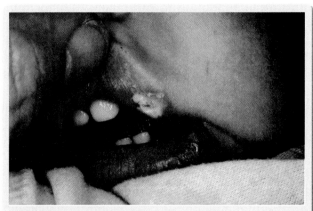

FIGURE 8-12 Children may sustain electrical burns from chewing on electrical cords.

Electrical burns can produce devastating internal injury with little external evidence. The degree of tissue injury in an electrical burn is related to the resistance of various body tissues, the intensity of current that passes through the victim, and the duration of contact.

As electric current travels from the contact site into the body, it is converted to heat, which follows the current flow, causing extensive damage to the tissues in its path. When the voltage is low (ie, under 1,000 volts, as in household sources), current follows the path of least resistance, generally along blood vessels, nerves, and muscles, which results in minor contact burns and cardiorespiratory complication. When the voltage is high (greater than 1,000 volts, as that from high-tension lines and industrial sites), the electric current takes the shortest available path. In either case, the greater the current flow, the greater the heat generated. These injuries are associated with massive tissue loss, with a high incidence of limb amputation.

Alternating current is considerably more dangerous than direct current because the alternations cause repetitive (tetanic) muscle contractions, which may "freeze" the victim to the conductor until the current source is turned off. Furthermore, alternating current is more likely than direct current to induce ventricular fibrillation. The direction of current flow is also significant. Current moving from one hand to the other is particularly dangerous because current may then flow across or near the heart; a current of only 0.1 ampere to the heart can provoke ventricular fibrillation.

Electricity-Related Burns

Electricity can cause three types of burns **FIGURE 8-13**. The most common is the type I burn, or contact burn, a true electric injury in which the current is most intense at the entrance and exit sites. At those points, you may see a char-

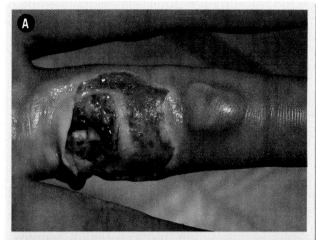
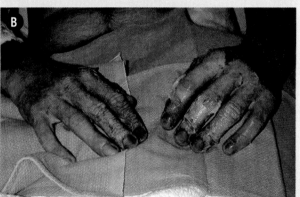
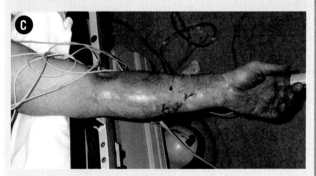

FIGURE 8-13 The three types of burns caused by electricity are (**A**) contact burns (type I), (**B**) flash burns (type II), and (**C**) flame burns (type III).

acteristic bull's-eye lesion, with a central, charred zone of full-thickness burns; a middle zone of cold, gray, dry tissue; and an outer, red zone of coagulation necrosis **FIGURE 8-14**. The contact burn, although usually not in itself very serious, is an important marker because it can signal devastating injury inside the body.

The type II burn, or flash burn, is really an electrothermal injury and is caused by the arcing of electric current. If a person passes close enough to a source of high voltage current, they will reach a point where the resistance of the air between the current source and themselves is sufficiently low that current arcs through the air from the current source to the passerby. An arc of that sort has a temperature

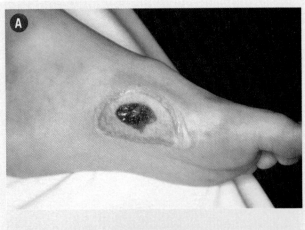

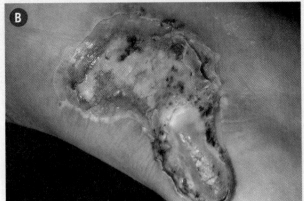

FIGURE 8-14 Electrical burns have entrance (**A**) and exit (**B**) wounds, characterized by bull's-eye lesions.

A whole host of neurologic complications have been reported in connection with electric injury, including seizures, delirium, confusion, coma, and temporary quadriplegia. Destruction of muscle tissue (rhabdomyolysis) occurs with deeper burns. Damage to muscle releases the contents of the muscle cells into the plasma. These cell contents include enzymes (creatinine kinase), myoglobin, and electrolytes such as potassium and phosphates. Damage to the kidneys is common after electric injury and resembles the syndrome seen after a crush injury, which is due to the breakdown products of damaged muscle (myoglobin) being liberated into the circulation.

Severe tetanic muscle spasms can lead to fractures and dislocations, which are often overlooked because of preoccupation with the electric injury itself. Posterior dislocation of the shoulder and fracture of the scapula—both otherwise rather rare injuries—have been reported in a number of cases of electrocution. And don't forget the cervical spine, especially in an electrical worker (lineman) who has fallen from a utility pole.

All of these potential injuries conspire to make the victim of an electrical contact a very complex assessment challenge. Never let obvious injuries distract you from a complete assessment including the neurologic, respiratory, cardiac, and musculoskeletal systems.

TIP

Electrical Cautions

- Seemingly "dead" wires can jump back to life because of automatically resetting breakers.
- The ground can become electrified by downed high-voltage wires.
- Take small steps—the electrical gradient can increase as you get closer to the source.
- Be wary if the hairs on your arm stand up on their own.
- Assume railroad tracks convey electrical current until proven otherwise.
- Look for dead animals on the ground.

anywhere from 5,400°F to 36,000°F (3,000° to 20,000°C)—high enough to produce significant charring. Victims standing near an object that was struck by lightning may get "splashed" and have areas of burns that resemble a fine red rash.

The type III electric burn, or flame burn, is another thermal injury; it occurs when electricity ignites a person's clothing or surroundings.

Nonburn Injuries from Electricity

Burns can be only one of the problems of a patient who has come in contact with an electric source—and not necessarily the most serious one. The two most common causes of death from electric injury are asphyxia and cardiac arrest. Asphyxia can occur when prolonged contact with alternating current induces tetanic contractions of the respiratory muscles; asphyxia can also be the result of current passing through the respiratory center in the brain and knocking out the impulse to breathe.

Cardiac arrest can occur either secondarily, from hypoxia, or as a direct result of the electric shock. As noted earlier, currents as small as 0.1 ampere can trigger ventricular fibrillation if they pass directly through the heart, which is particularly likely when current travels across the body from hand to hand or from upper to lower limb. In cases where cardiac arrest does not occur, cardiac damage can nonetheless be manifested in various rhythm changes seen on the electrocardiogram (ECG).

As soon as the electric hazard has been neutralized and made safe, proceed to the ABCs. Open the airway using the jaw-thrust maneuver, bearing in mind the possibility of cervical spine injury. Start cardiopulmonary resuscitation (CPR) as indicated. If the patient is not in cardiac arrest, but has received a significant electrical burn, cardiac monitoring is indicated for 24 to 36 hours after the injury.

Radiation Burns

Acute radiation exposure has become more than a theoretical issue as use of radioactive materials increases in industry and medicine. You must understand radiation exposure to function effectively in the prehospital arena. Since 1946, there have been more than 400 radiation accidents involving significant radiation exposure to more than 3,000 people worldwide. Potential threats include incidents related to the

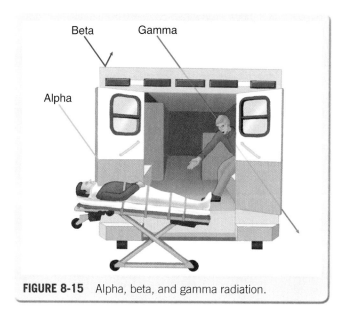

FIGURE 8-15   Alpha, beta, and gamma radiation.

use and transportation of radioactive isotopes or intentionally released radioactivity in terrorist attacks. To be effective, you must first suspect radiation and attempt to determine whether ongoing exposure exists. Increasingly, individual providers in some services and some special response units are equipped with pager-sized radiation detectors. Such detection also can be provided by other public safety services.

There are three types of ionizing radiation: alpha, beta, and gamma **FIGURE 8-15**. Alpha particles have little penetrating energy and are easily stopped by the skin. Beta particles have greater penetrating power and can travel much farther in air than alpha particles. They can penetrate the skin but can be blocked by simple protective clothing designed for this purpose. The threat from gamma radiation is directly proportional to its wavelength. This type of radiation is very penetrating and easily passes through the body and solid materials.

Radiation dosage is measured in joules per kilogram (J/kg); 1 J/kg is also known as 1 gray (Gy). Small amounts

of everyday background radiation are measured in rad; the amount of radiation released in a major incident can be measured in gray (100 rad = 1 Gy). Mild radiation sickness can be expected with exposures of 1 to 2 Gy (100–200 rad), moderate sickness at 2 to 4 Gy, and severe sickness at 4 to 6 Gy. Exposure to more than 8 Gy is immediately fatal.

The vast majority of ionizing radiation accidents involve gamma radiation or x-rays. People who have suffered a radiation exposure generally pose no risk to the people around them. However, in some types of incidents—particularly those involving explosions—patients can be contaminated with radioactive particulate matter. It is speculated that after a nuclear explosion, most patients will have sustained some type of trauma in addition to the radiation exposure.

It is important to limit any particulate contamination if the patient has been involved in an incident other than simple irradiation (explosions, aerosolization of material, etc). At the scene, clothes should be removed and patients should be decontaminated using soap and water. Open wounds should be irrigated. Washing should be gentle to avoid abrading the skin. The head and scalp should be irrigated the same way. Be sure to decontaminate the bottoms of the feet, because this is a commonly missed area. The receiving emergency department should be notified as soon as practical so they can prepare a special reception.

Acute Radiation Syndrome

Acute radiation syndrome causes hematologic, central nervous system, and gastrointestinal changes. Many of these changes occur over time and so will not be apparent during contact with providers. Patients who are rendered unconscious by radiation or who manifest vomiting within 10 minutes of exposure have a 100% chance of mortality. Those who manifest vomiting in less than an hour have severe exposure and a 20% to 70% mortality rate. Many people with moderate exposure will vomit within 1 to 2 hours and have a 0% to 50% mortality rate **TABLE 8-3**.

TABLE 8-3	Effects of Acute Radiation Exposure and Expected Mortality			
Assessment	**Lethal Exposure (> 8 Gy)**	**Severe Exposure (4–6 Gy)**	**Moderate Exposure (2–4 Gy)**	**Mild Exposure (1–2 Gy)**
Vomiting	Most will vomit in < 10 min	Most will vomit in < 1 h	Many will vomit in 1–2 h	Half will vomit after 2 h
Diarrhea	Most will have severe diarrhea in < 1 h	10% will have some diarrhea in 3–8 h	None	None
Unconsciousness	Some will be unconscious for seconds to minutes; in massive exposure (> 50 Gy), all will lose consciousness.	None	None	None
Fatigue	Yes	Yes	Yes	Yes
Headache	Severe	Moderate	Mild	Slight
Fever	High fever in < 1 h	Moderate fever in 4–24 h	Mild fever	No fever
Expected mortality	100% will die in 1–2 wk	20%–70% will die in 4–8 wk	0%–50% may die in 6–8 wk	Typically, all will survive

Adapted from IAEA and WHO. *Safety Reports Series No. 2: Diagnosis and Treatment of Radiation Injuries.* International Atomic Energy Agency, 1998.

Clearly, the onset of vomiting soon after exposure is a predictor of poor outcomes. Consider this fact when triaging patients or considering the risks of entering a high-radiation environment to attempt rescue.

Radiation Contact Burns

A person who briefly handles a radioactive source can sustain a local soft-tissue injury without a lot of total body irradiation. This scenario might arise, for example, in a collision involving a vehicle transporting radioactive material or after the detonation of a "dirty bomb." The injury could resemble anything from superficial sunburn to a chemical burn. Although chemical burns usually become apparent almost immediately after exposure, radiation burns could appear hours or even days after exposure.

General Assessment of Burns

Burned patients can fool you. We expect our critically injured patients to act sick. Most severely injured and dying cardiac and trauma patients are hypotensive and unresponsive, or in such distress that we can tell they are critical before we ever get close to them. On the other hand, patients suffering from isolated severe burn injury sometimes walk up to you on a scene. Their chief complaint may be "I'm terribly cold," and the severity of their injuries may not become apparent to you until you have completed your assessment and realized that they fit the criteria for transfer to a burn center.

Burn injuries sometimes happen in remote locations, and patients may be found hours after their traumatic burn event, where they may present with an entirely different spectrum of problems than we are typically used to dealing with. Burned patients often have additional traumatic injuries from falling debris, explosions, or injuries sustained while they were trying to get away from the source of the burn **FIGURE 8-16**. Serious burn patients may need to be transferred from tertiary facilities to larger burn centers, and you may be required to

deal with advanced issues like **escharotomies** and advanced fluid management during the secondary transport.

Scene Size-up

As always, begin with scene safety and body substance isolation (BSI) **FIGURE 8-17**. Do not proceed to the patient's side if the scene is not safe. Be wary of entering closed spaces if there is evidence of a recent fire—the heat may be intense and there may be a large residue of fumes. Never enter a burning building unless you are trained and wearing the appropriate protective gear. Make sure there is no continuing danger to you or the patient(s). Keep a high index of suspicion for the presence of toxic gases: CO, cyanide, and hydrogen sulfide. Cyanide can kill within 15 seconds of exposure. Look for placards indicating hazardous materials. Never enter an area that potentially has hazardous materials. Always follow direct instructions from the senior fire officer at the scene in relation to aspects of health and safety.

There are two aspects to maintaining scene safety. The first is staging yourself and others in a place that is safe to render patient care and that is outside of the hot zone. This allows you to stay far enough removed from the situation to keep a wider focus.

The second concern is to extinguish the flame. Always extinguish the fire before providing medical care. Extinguish overt flames using copious irrigation or covering with a heavy wool or cotton blanket that can smother the flames.

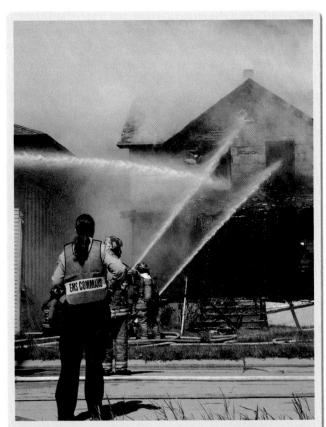

FIGURE 8-17 Checking for scene safety requires due diligence at every scene.

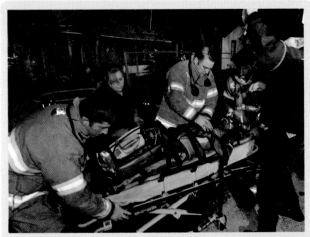

FIGURE 8-16 Burned patients often sustain additional traumatic injuries while trying to get away from the source of the burn.

Wet Versus Dry Dressings

Burns that cover greater than approximately 10% body surface area should be covered with dry clean dressings. Water-soaked dressings will encourage evaporation and cooling of the skin under the dressing. This can provide some pain relief; however, the damaged skin has become unable to limit the amount of temperature lost by the body. If larger burns are allowed to cool too much, the patient may become hypothermic. An exception to this rule is the gel burn bandages that insulate the skin from excessive heat loss by cooling down only to normal body temperature. These products have thermal properties that do not let the patient cool too quickly. It is advisable on all dressings to rewrap the patient with protective blankets to avoid wind chill.

That may seem obvious, but it is remarkable how many patients still arrive by ambulance at hospital emergency departments with clothes smoldering.

Initial/Primary Assessment

As mentioned earlier, patients who have been burned may have sustained other trauma. Consider and examine other mechanisms associated with the burn: Did the patient jump from a high window to escape flames? Do they have musculoskeletal trauma from tetanic spasms after an electrical burn? Were they trapped in an enclosed space? Did the patient lose consciousness? All of these questions affect the initial response to the patient and their ultimate care. Evaluate the need for additional resources and request them early on if necessary.

As you approach the burn trauma patient, simple clues can help identify how serious the injuries are and how quickly you need to assess and treat. If your patient greets you with a hoarse voice or is reported to have been in an enclosed space, you should be concerned about their airway. Similarly, if the patient has singed facial hair, eyebrows, nasal hair, or moustache, your general impression might be that the patient has a potential airway and/or breathing problem.

Evaluate Mental Status

Patients who have suffered from a burn injury can have a varied mental status response. All patients who present as combative must be deemed hypoxic until proven otherwise. Because burns are extremely painful injuries, the patient may present awake but not responsive, or be hysterical and inconsolable. Even patients with excessive burns will most likely be awake and attempting to communicate. Isolated burns do not cause unconsciousness (although toxic inhalations can). Unresponsive burn patients must be carefully assessed to search for sources of other lethal injuries.

TABLE 8-4 Clues to Airway Compromise in the Burned Patient

Standing and/or screaming while on fire
Burns in an enclosed space
Soot in the sputum
Hoarse voice
Singed eyebrows or nasal hairs
Burns of the face or in the mouth or nose

Ensure an Open Airway

As in any other seriously ill or injured patient, the airway comes first. In the burned patient, the airway may be in particular jeopardy; the same heat and flames that caused the external burn may have produced potentially life-threatening damage to the airway **TABLE 8-4**. Laryngeal edema can develop with alarming speed in burn patients, especially in infants and children where a small amount of edema can occlude their small airways. Early endotracheal intubation—before the airway has closed off—will be lifesaving in such cases and should be performed by the most experienced provider on your team. To intervene early, however, you need to spot the problem early.

Assess for Adequate Breathing

The vast majority of deaths from fires are not from burns, but from pulmonary injury due to the inhalation of toxic gases. Direct pulmonary injury may occur from the inhalation of very hot steam, which can conduct heat all the way down into the smaller airways and produce damage at the bronchiolar and alveolar level. At the same time, carbon monoxide and other toxic products of combustion can displace oxygen from both the alveolar air and the blood hemoglobin. Carbon monoxide binds to receptor sites on hemoglobin about 200 times more easily than oxygen, so the patient's hemoglobin is well saturated with the wrong chemical. For this reason, pulse oximetry readings may be inaccurate. Listen to lung sounds, paying special attention to stridor, which may predict upper airway compromise.

Ensure Adequate Circulation

During the first 24 to 48 hours of a patient's burn care, a great deal of emphasis is placed on fluid resuscitation by the ED and the burn center to prevent burn shock. Burn shock is caused by fluid shifts that typically occur 6 to 8 hours after the burn. This fluid shift may not be complete until 24–48 hours after the burn. Severely burned patients will ultimately require large volumes of fluid, but they don't need it during the first minutes of prehospital care unless their burn injury occurred some time ago. While prehospital IV access is an important route for analgesia and fluid, most patients will ultimately require central venous access, and most prehospital intravenous (IV) lines will be removed owing to tissue swelling and infection risk. If the patient is *not* grossly hypotensive (ie, detectable peripheral pulse), do not delay transport by making multiple attempts at vascular access.

Patients with other trauma may require immediate vascular access just like any other trauma patient. It is preferable, however, to avoid starting IV lines through burned tissue to decrease the chance of infection during the patient's recovery. Burned patients may challenge your vascular access skills. Options for intraosseous access may provide you with more choices than intravenous options. Access locations can include the tibia, femur, iliac crest, humerus, or sternum.

Burn Severity

The burn wound is identified by degree of injury. The injury may be described by three pathologic progressions or zones. Skin nearest to the heat source suffers the most profound cellular changes. The central area of the skin, which suffers the most damage, is called the **zone of coagulation**. The peripheral area surrounding the zone of coagulation has decreased blood flow and inflammation. This area can undergo necrosis within 24 to 48 hours after the injury, particularly if perfusion is compromised due to burn shock. This is known as the **zone of stasis**. Lastly, the area that is least affected by the thermal injury is the **zone of hyperemia**, in which cells will recover in 7 to 10 days. These three zones are important for providers because treatments rendered in the prehospital environment involve understanding these basic principles **FIGURE 8-18**.

Burn Location

One factor used to determine whether a burn is critical enough to require a burn specialty center is the location of the burn on the body. Most burns are determined to be critical by the depth and size of the burn. However, burns on particular parts of the body are critical regardless of the overall size of the burn. Burns must still be partial thickness or worse to be considered critical. Superficial burns are not counted when occurring alone.

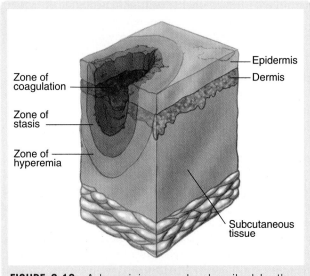

FIGURE 8-18 A burn injury can be described by three different zones. **A.** Zone of coagulation. **B.** Zone of stasis. **C.** Zone of hyperemia.

Burns to the face, eyes, ears, hands, feet, perineum, genitals, or major joints that may result in cosmetic or functional disability should be transferred to a burn specialty center when available. These burns often leave the victim physically, psychologically, and socially scarred if they do not receive careful debridement and cleansing of the wounds, definitive reconstructive surgery, proper follow-up wound care, and complete rehabilitation to assist the victim in returning to pre-injury function.

Burn Depth

Keep in mind that you are performing a rapid initial assessment with the goal of determining what level of care the patient requires (burn center, trauma center, local hospital), and also getting an idea of size and severity to pass on to the receiving facility. The nature of the patient's burns will evolve over the next 24 hours, and estimations of their size and severity will change, so there is little to be gained from a comprehensive and time-consuming evaluation of every inch of the patient's body in the field. That being said, you would obviously like to have a reasonably accurate estimation of the scope of the patient's injuries.

The first step in burn management is to assess the burns quickly. Consider the presence or absence of pain, swelling, skin color, capillary refill, moisture, and blisters; the appearance of wound edges; presence of foreign bodies, debris, contaminants, and bleeding; and circulatory adequacy. Assess for concomitant soft-tissue injury. Determination of burn depth is a subjective assessment dependent on provider judgment.

The traditional labels given to burns were first, second, and third degree. Most centers expanded that concept, and discussed fourth-, fifth-, and sixth-degree burns, as tissue destruction went into the deeper tissues, muscle, and bone. It is probably more appropriate for prehospital providers to limit their assessment to superficial, partial-, and/or full-thickness burns **FIGURE 8-19** to simplify the process and avoid confusion and miscommunication.

Sometimes called a first-degree burn, a **superficial burn** involves the epidermis only. The skin is red and when touched the color will blanch and refill. Blisters are not usually present. Patients will experience pain as the nerve endings are exposed to the air. This burn will heal spontaneously in 3 to 7 days. One common example of a superficial burn is a sunburn.

A **partial-thickness burn**, which is sometimes called second degree, involves the epidermis and varying degrees of the dermis. This category can be subdivided into superficial partial-thickness and deep partial-thickness burns.

A superficial partial-thickness burn is one in which the skin color is red and when touched the color will blanch and refill. Usually there are blisters or moisture present. Patients will experience extreme pain. Hair follicles remain intact. The burn will heal spontaneously, but may scar or have changed appearance.

A deep partial-thickness burn extends into the dermis, damaging hair follicles and sweat and sebaceous glands. Hot liquids, steam, or grease are usually to blame for these

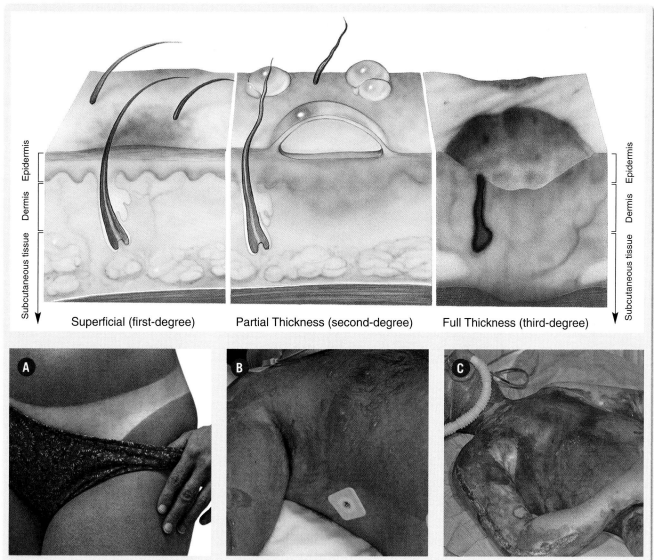

FIGURE 8-19 Classification of burns. **A.** Superficial (first-degree) burns involve only the epidermis. **B.** Partial-thickness (second-degree) burns involve some of the dermis but do not destroy the entire thickness of the skin. The skin is mottled, white to red, and often blistered. **C.** Full-thickness burns extend through all layers of the skin and may involve subcutaneous tissue and muscle. The skin is dry, leathery, and often white or charred.

injuries. In the prehospital setting, the difference between deep partial thickness and full thickness may be difficult to determine at this early stage.

Full-thickness burns, sometimes called third-degree burns, involve destruction of both layers of the skin, including the basement membrane of dermis, which produces new skin cells. The skin color is white and pale, or brown, or charred in appearance. The skin is dry and sometimes described as "leathery." There is no capillary refill because the capillaries are destroyed. Sensory nerves are destroyed so there is typically no pain in the full-thickness section. Patients usually have mixed depths of burns so they often will still experience significant pain in the areas surrounding the full-thickness burns. Treatment of this burn will require skin grafting because the dermis has been destroyed.

Burn Surface Area

Once the thickness of the burn has been determined, the provider must approximate the total body surface area (TBSA) burned. TBSA is based on all burned surfaces from reddened to partial- and full-thickness burns. The typical approach to calculating TBSA is using the Rule of Nines **FIGURE 8-20**, which is based on fractionalizing the body into 9% segments. The provider adds the portions of the body for a total of the percentage of the body affected by the burn injury. Because our proportions change as we grow, there is a different Rule of Nines for infants, children, and adults.

Another mechanism of assessing the TBSA is the Rule of Palms. This assessment utilizes the size of the patient's palm to represent about 1% of the patient's body surface area. This calculation is helpful when the extent of the burn is less than 10% TBSA or it is an irregularly shaped burn.

The Lund and Browder chart (FIGURE 8-21) is an even more specific and more accurate method used to estimate burn area, and its modifications take into account the proportional differences in adults and children. It recognizes that the proportion of body surface covering specific body parts changes with age (for example, the head and neck of an infant constitute 20% TBSA compared with 9% in an adult).

The provider must balance the need for accuracy against the time required to complete the assessment. The prehospital estimation of burn area is used to get the patient to the correct place for treatment. The emergency department estimation of burned area may be used to initiate fluid therapy. The burn center's estimation of injured area will undoubtedly need to be more accurate and specific. In any case, reassessment is vital after an hour to assess changes from the prehospital assessment.

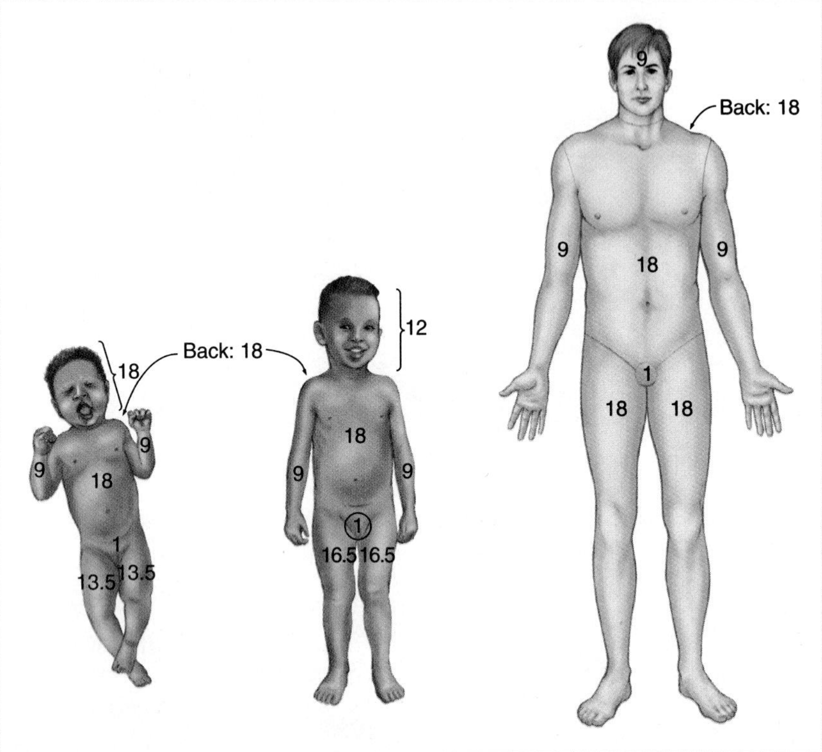

Rapid Trauma/Secondary Assessment

Once you have evaluated the ABCs and treated any conditions noted, then proceed through the steps of physical assessment in the usual sequence, starting with the patient's general appearance, then complete a set of vital signs. Obtaining vital signs may be challenging if the patient has extensive burns over the arms. It is still important to try to document accurate vital signs because the management of shock, airway compromise, and pain control will all depend to some extent upon them.

FIGURE 8-20 The Rule of Nines is a quick way to estimate the amount of surface area that has been burned. It divides the adult body into sections, each representing approximately 9% of the total body surface area. The proportions differ for children and infants.

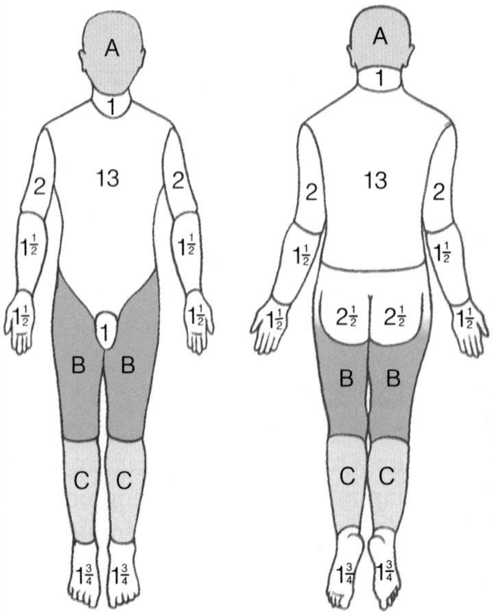

Relative percentages of body surface area affected by growth

Age (years)	A ($\frac{1}{2}$ of head)	B ($\frac{1}{2}$ of one thigh)	C ($\frac{1}{2}$ of one leg)
0	$9\frac{1}{2}$	$2\frac{3}{4}$	$2\frac{1}{2}$
1	$8\frac{1}{2}$	$3\frac{1}{4}$	$2\frac{1}{2}$
5	$6\frac{1}{2}$	4	$2\frac{3}{4}$
10	$5\frac{1}{2}$	$4\frac{1}{4}$	3
15	$4\frac{1}{2}$	$4\frac{1}{2}$	$3\frac{1}{4}$
Adult	$3\frac{1}{2}$	$4\frac{3}{4}$	3

Region	%
Head	
Neck	
Ant. Trunk	
Post. Trunk	
Right arm	
Left arm	
Buttocks	
Genitalia	
Right leg	
Left leg	
Total burn	

FIGURE 8-21 The Lund and Browder chart.

Source: Adapted from Lund CC, Browder NC. *Surg Gyn Obst.* 1944; 79:352–358.

When you have finished your brief inspection of the patient's skin, you have only just begun the head-to-toe exam. The purpose of doing the head-to-toe exam is to make sure there are no other injuries that have higher priority for treatment. Often the burn itself may obscure such injuries, so you need to pay attention to the circumstances of the burn and the possible mechanisms of injury. Look for injuries to the eyes, and cover injured eyes with moist, sterile pads or a water-gel face dressing. Check the neck, chest, and extremities for circumferential burns. Progressive edema beneath a circumferential burn—especially when the burned skin has become leathery and unyielding (as in a full-thickness burn)—may act as a tourniquet. In the neck, a circumferential burn may obstruct the airway; in the chest, it may restrict the respiratory excursion; and in an extremity, it may cut off the circulation and put the extremity in jeopardy. Patients with circumferential burns must therefore reach a medical facility quickly because it may be necessary to make an incision (called an escharotomy) into the burned area to allow blood flow in the limb, chest, or neck. An escharotomy is a surgical procedure that cuts the thickened and damaged external skin to allow the pressure in the tissue below to decompress and blood flow to continue through the constricted area. Measure and document the distal pulses in burned extremities.

If possible, attempt to get a brief history from the patient. Patients with preexisting pathologies, such as chronic obstructive pulmonary disease (COPD) or heart disease, may be triaged as critical burns even if their burn injury or area is small. As in any other trauma, allergies, medications, and other pertinent past medical history may affect the patient's care plan.

Detailed Physical Exam and Reassessment

If the patient is considered to have a significant mechanism of injury (MOI), then the provider should perform a detailed physical exam relative to the time criticality of the assessment, as well as the continued reassessment, while en route to the ED or burn center. The specific steps to these are not significantly different than for any other trauma patient. Reassessment of vital signs to establish trends is done every 5 minutes for time-critical patients and every 15 minutes for the lower priority (stable) patient.

> **TIP**
>
> A quick tool to assist the provider in assessing burns is the mnemonic OLDEST.
>
> **O** Other injuries (c-spine, etc.)
> **L** Location of burn injury
> **D** Depth of burn
> **E** Exposure time
> **S** Surface area estimation
> **T** Temperature (eg, was coffee freshly brewed or standing for a minute or two)

Assessment Considerations for Specific Burn Types

Assessment of Airway Burns

Initial/primary assessment of the burn patient must include a careful examination of the external and internal airway. Look at the mouth, lips, and nares for swelling or blistering. Review the interior of the mouth and nasal passages for soot, reddening, swelling, or obstruction. Examine the tongue and oral pharynx for signs of burns, thick secretions, or soot. Suction any secretions and remove any obstructions that can be cleared.

Listen for stridor, the noisy breathing heard from air passing through swollen air passages in the upper airway. If the patient is conscious, ask them a question and listen to how they speak. A harsh or raspy voice can indicate burns or swelling of the vocal cords. Finally listen to lung sounds for wheezing or rhonchi indicating swelling or obstructions from smoke inhalation or deeper burns. When signs of airway burns are noted, continuous care and reassessment are indicated. Airway burns can become life threatening in minutes. Immediate transport is indicated to a hospital with a suitably set up ED. Securing an advanced airway should be attempted by the most skilled provider available because additional swelling from the attempt may worsen the condition.

Assessment of Chemical Burns

The scene of a chemical burn is by definition a hazardous materials scene. Personal safety must be assessed before the provider or additional personnel enter the scene without personal protective equipment (PPE). When possible, have the patient moved to a well-ventilated area for further assessment. Most chemical exposures require flooding the skin with copious amounts of water. Do not position yourself in the runoff from the patient. Strip the patient while irrigating the patient, looking for burns in the folds of skin and along areas where the chemical can collect, such as the shirt collar, along the beltline, and in socks, shoes, and gloves.

After the patient has been decontaminated, assess the patient's breath for odd smells indicating the patient inhaled additional chemicals. Assess the airway as noted above. Although personal modesty is to be considered, all areas of the body exposed or potentially exposed must be examined for burns, including along the folds of the skin under the breasts, under the scrotum, and around the buttocks.

Assessment of Electrical Burns

The first priority at the scene of an electric injury is to protect yourself and bystanders from becoming the next victims. Do not rush in and attempt to dislodge the patient from the current source, even if you intend to use a rope, wooden pole, or any other object. High voltage will still have the capacity to jump the relatively short distance. Clearly, relatively low domestic voltage from lamps and the like are not such an area of caution. Do not go anywhere near a high-tension line. There is only one safe way to deal with a live high-tension wire, and that is to call the electric company. Wait until a qualified person has shut off the power before you approach the patient, who in reality will mostly likely be close to death if not already dead.

Make careful note of the patient's state of consciousness and record his or her vital signs. Try to determine the path the current has taken through the body by looking for an entrance wound and an exit wound and by carefully palpating the skin and soft tissues. When deep tissues have been seriously damaged by heat, the surrounding muscle swells and becomes rock hard. Thus, if you find a rigid abdomen or rigid extremity, there is a high probability of serious internal injury. Be alert for fractures or dislocations, and check the distal pulses on all four extremities.

Assessment of Radiation Burns

First and foremost, the assessment of a patient who may have been exposed to radiation involves a scene size-up to determine that the scene is safe for rescuers. In some cases, it may be appropriate to contact the hazardous materials response team so they may determine the appropriate precautions, including exposure-limiting suits, and the most appropriate ED for the patient's treatment. Not all EDs are set up to handle a patient who has been exposed to radiation, so learn the capabilities of your hospitals before an incident occurs. If in any doubt, contact your local ED via dispatch and establish their up-to-date capability. In general, EDs do not like surprise visits of radiation burns. EMS agencies that operate in an area where there is a nuclear power plant or other research facility typically have additional training offered by the facility and regularly practice responding to radiation-related emergencies.

Once the scene is deemed safe, you may proceed with your initial assessment of the patient. Unfortunately, patients who have sustained a significant radiation exposure and a major burn are unlikely to survive, even with major resources expended to keep them alive. You should also

consult with the ED via dispatch in these complicated cases. In the field, it is difficult to determine the extent of the patient's internal injuries because radiation can "cook from the inside out."

Management of Burns

Burn care can be divided into five phases. Although prehospital providers will be most involved in the first phase, it is important to appreciate the magnitude of care that a severe, or even moderate, burn patient must receive. Early actions of the prehospital provider may dramatically affect the long-term outcome for the patient. Providers may also find themselves transporting patients to specialty or rehab facilities at later stages of their care. The five phases of burn care are outlined in **TABLE 8-5**.

Note that, unlike many emergencies you will encounter, burn patient care is measured in weeks, not hours. Burns are devastating multisystem traumatic injuries that will dramatically alter your patient's life. It is valuable for providers to comprehend not only the massive physical trauma caused by burns, but also the emotional, psychological, and financial burdens caused by these horrific traumatic events. Once appreciated, it is easy to understand the importance of teaching injury prevention strategies to those we serve.

General Management

Management of the burned patient begins with the steps taken during the scene size-up and initial/primary assessment to extinguish the fire and ensure adequate ABCs. Only when the active burning is extinguished and the ABCs are under control should you turn your attention to the burn itself. It is important to have all resuscitative equipment ready for use when treating the burn patient. This includes advanced airway equipment and heart monitors.

TABLE 8-5	Five Phases of Burn Care	
Phase	**Time Frame**	**Treatment Objectives**
At emergency scene	First 30 minutes	Stop the burning, airway, pain relief, wound dressing, and rapid transport
Initial evaluation and resuscitation	First 72 hours	To achieve accurate fluid resuscitation and perform a thorough evaluation
Initial wound excision and biologic closure	Days 1 through 7	To identify and remove all full-thickness wounds and obtain biologic closure
Definitive wound closure	Day 7 through week 6	To replace temporary covers with definitive ones and close small complex wounds
Rehabilitation, reconstruction, and reintegration	Entire hospitalization	To maintain range of motion and reduce edema, and to strengthen and prepare for return to the community

Keep the following equipment and materials handy for burn management:

- Foil blanket
- Woven blanket
- Large sterile burn sheet
- Face mask dressing
- Hand and finger dressings
- Sterile gauze bandages of various sizes
- Conforming gauze roll bandages
- Tape rolls
- 1,000-mL sterile water bottles
- Eye wash
- Scissors (shears)
- Ring cutter
- Some kits may include gel dressings, which have TBSA in percentage on the back of the wrappings

It is important to determine accurately the extent of the burn injury to facilitate proper treatment and transportation of the burn patient. All the patient's clothes must be removed to assess accurately the extent of the burn injury and to make sure all hot materials have been removed. Do not try to remove clothing that is adhered to the patient's skin. It is important to maintain warmth during this process because there is an alteration in the normal thermal regulation process. Anticipate shivering and loss of body temperature in all burns exceeding 20% of the total body surface area. Evaporative heat losses can be enormous. For this reason it is imperative to monitor the patient's temperature. Avoiding wind chill is ideal and can be helped by providing a blanket.

The following three areas should be assessed:

- Depth of the burns
- Total body surface area burned (calculate partial and full thickness only)
- Need to transfer to a burn specialty center with consideration to running time

Immediate Management

Stop the Burning When a person burns their hand on a hot oven rack at 375°F (190°C), they will usually stick their hand under cool running water for a few seconds. Is that long enough to cool the tissues and stop the burning? It often takes a few minutes under cool running water to completely cool the burned area and achieve some pain relief. That being the case with a minor burn in the home, providers should be aware that a quick spray from a fire hose will not completely stop the burning in a patient whose clothing was on fire a few moments before. The burned areas need to be cooled to 98.6°F (37°C).

Watchbands, zippers, and rings not only can retain enough heat to continue burning the patient, they can melt your gloves and burn you as well! Take extra care to be certain that metal on the patient's person has been cooled appropriately.

If the hands are burned, they will swell considerably and rings will become tourniquets if not removed early. If bits of smoldering cloth adhere to the skin, do not pull them

TIP

The following steps list the approach to the burn patient:

1. Ensure scene safety and body substance isolation.
2. Put out the fire.
3. Safeguard the airway: Be alert for clues to an airway in jeopardy. Consider the need for spinal immobilization if the burn is associated with trauma. Intubate early if clinically necessary; defer to the hospital if reasonable to do so.
4. Help the patient breathe: Give high-flow, high-percentage oxygen to reduce CO concentrations via nonrebreathing mask. Consider a nebulized beta-agonist if respiratory distress is present.
5. Ensure the circulation: Start intravenous or intraosseous fluids, but don't extend your on-scene time to do so.
6. Give narcotics (or other agents as directed by your protocols) IV for pain management.
7. Perform the rapid trauma/secondary assessment:
   a. Find out the circumstances of the burn.
   b. Check vital signs often.
8. Be alert for the following:
   a. Injuries sustained in falls (fractures, spine injury)
   b. Circumferential burns
   c. Absence of distal pulses
9. Treat the burns.
   a. Do not use remedies such as creams or lotions on the burn.
   b. In the prehospital setting, and in the first stages of the ED, burns of less than 10% should have cool, wet dressings applied until the burning process stops. Otherwise, cover with clean, dry dressings.
   c. Elevate burned extremities; remove constricting jewelry.
10. Transfer the patient to an appropriate treatment facility.
11. Maintain the patient's temperature; do not allow them to cool too rapidly.

off the skin; cut them away. Pulling fabrics from the skin may cause additional tissue trauma and bleeding, which will worsen the situation. Let the burn center or hospital deal with items that are melted to the flesh.

In addition to extinguishing flames, the skin should be cooled. Never use ice on a burn. Cool partial-thickness burns of less than 10% body surface area or full-thickness

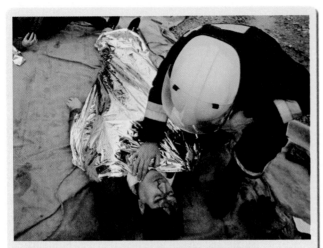

FIGURE 8-22 Maintain the burn patient's warmth.

burns of less than 2% body surface area with irrigating solution (normal saline) in the first 10 to 15 minutes after the burn. Cooling larger surface areas will contribute to hypothermia, especially with wind chill factors.

Maintain the Patient's Warmth This seems like a contradiction to the above because it is. The trick is to cool the burn without making the patient hypothermic. Remember, people with large area burns have lost their primary mechanism for thermoregulation. Keep the burn patient covered and move them into the ambulance as soon as possible to minimize hypothermic stress **FIGURE 8-22**.

Do Not Forget Other Injuries If the patient is at risk for spinal trauma from a fall or explosion, that trauma needs to be addressed the same way as it would in any other trauma patient. The same is true for gross bleeding or other traumatic injuries. Burns can also exacerbate a patient's underlying medical conditions. COPD, asthma, and cardiac conditions may all need attention. Follow the same priorities for these emergencies as you would for any other time-critical patient.

Airway Management

Bear in mind that intubation of an awake, scared patient in the field is particularly challenging, and considerable damage can be inflicted on the airway if the patient is struggling. If intubation does become necessary under such circumstances, consider the consequences of failure before using paralytics or muscle relaxants to intubate (Chapter 3). Have all the equipment set up at your side so that intubation, once begun, can proceed rapidly and smoothly. Select and use the largest tube in relation to the lumen of the available airway. Burn patients' secretions are sometimes thick and sooty, so be sure to have a suction unit with large catheters available. Progressive airway swelling will make it difficult to reintubate or change the endotracheal (ET) tube at the hospital. Even if there is no evidence of airway

involvement, early intubation should also be considered in any fire victim who is stuporous or comatose, but it is preferable that it be performed in the more controlled environment of the hospital, where additional drugs and devices are available if the airway is difficult to achieve.

Many burn patients will ultimately require intubation, even though they were talking to you and in no distress in the field. Although it is obviously preferable to have such patients intubated in a controlled environment with a full complement of anesthesia agents, there will be a few patients who absolutely require an emergency airway in the field. Burn patients fall into four general categories for airway management:

1. *The patient with the acutely decompensating airway that requires field intubation.* This will include those burn patients who are in cardiac or respiratory arrest and conscious patients whose airways are swelling up before your eyes. These are chaotic and difficult situations where you need to have planned for the possibility that you cannot intubate. Supraglottic swelling or complete obstruction can occur in some burn scenarios, and surgical airways or rescue devices may be necessary if intubation is not possible and bag-mask ventilation fails or is inadequate.

2. *The patient with the deteriorating airway from burns and toxic inhalations.* This is also a very difficult scenario. It is obviously better for the patient to defer this airway to hospital teams with anesthesia, surgery, specialized equipment, and a fully stocked pharmacy. The patient will often be conscious and may become combative with attempts to place them supine, let alone to intubate them. "Awake" techniques, such as nasal intubation, are dramatically more complicated in victims of upper airway burns, and should be avoided. Attempt to intubate this patient only if left with no other choice. If their airway continues to swell and will become impossible to intubate if you wait for arrival at the hospital, you will have little choice but to attempt intubation. Where applicable, try to consult medical direction for advice in this situation.

3. *The patient whose airway is currently patent, but who has a history consistent with risk factors for eventual airway compromise.* Cool, humidified saline or a beta-agonist from a nebulizer is appropriate for this patient. If this equipment is not available, consider using an aerosol nebulizer with saline **FIGURE 8-23**. This patient will probably not require acute interventions in the field, but make sure you pass on their history to the hospital. Many of these patients may ultimately undergo elective intubation.

4. *The patient with no signs of, or risk factors for, airway compromise, and who is in no distress.* It is reasonable to provide supplemental oxygen to burned patients, even if they are not in distress. Remember

that carbon monoxide can make oxygen saturation readings inaccurate. It is safe to oxygenate until you are very comfortable with the situation surrounding the burn and have completed a full assessment.

Fluid Resuscitation

The two reasons to establish an intravenous (IV) or an intraosseous (IO) line are to administer fluids and to administer pain medications. An IV/IO should be established as early as possible in any patient who has been severely burned. Do not delay transport to do so, but try to get a large-bore IV catheter into an antecubital vein, or an IO into the tibia and hang lactated Ringer's or Hartmann's solution. Normal saline can be substituted if local protocols prohibit lactated Ringer's. You can use a superficially burned extremity if you cannot find another site—an IV in a burned upper extremity is still preferable to an IV in a lower extremity.

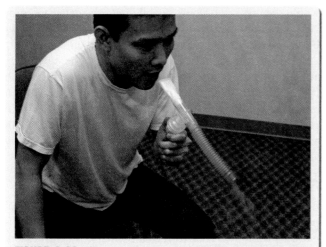

FIGURE 8-23 For a patient with a history consistent with risk factors for eventual airway compromise, provide oxygen using a nebulizer.

Approximate the amount of fluid the burned patient will need by using the Parkland formula (TABLE 8-6), which states that during the first 24 hours, the burned patient will need:

$$4 \text{ mL} \times \text{kg body weight} \times \% \text{ of body surface burned}$$
$$= \text{total mL of fluid needed}$$

Half of that amount needs to be given during the first 8 hours. For example, if a 70-kg man has sustained burns to 30% of his body, his fluid needs over the first 8 hours will be:

$$4 \text{ mL} \times 70 \text{ kg} \times 30\% \div 2 = 2{,}100 \text{ mL to be infused in 8 hours}$$

Half of the 4,200 mL (2,100 mL) needs to be administered in the first 8 hours.

As aggressive as the Parkland formula may seem, current trends actually lean toward delivering *more* fluid than the Parkland formula indicates. In instances of high-tension electrical injuries, substantially more fluid is required. At the same time, keep in mind that you do not need to attempt to deliver the entire initial amount in the field. It is *not* helpful to administer *too much* fluid in the field. Most serious burn patients will ultimately need central venous access, and prehospital IV lines will most often be lost as the patient begins to swell peripherally. Do not focus all of your prehospital, on-scene attention on vascular access and fluid delivery.

Pain Management

Beyond oxygenation, cooling the burn to stop damage, and maintenance of core temperature for the patient, it is important to provide aggressive pain management. Even minor burns are painful and need analgesia. The provider should assess the patient's pain before administering medication. Burn patients may require high doses of pain medications to achieve relief. Their metabolism rates are accelerated, requiring higher than normal doses of pain medicines.

TABLE 8-6	Parkland Formula Chart								
% Burn	10 kg	20 kg	30 kg	40 kg	50 kg	60 kg	70 kg	80 kg	90 kg	100 kg
10	25	50	75	100	125	150	175	200	225	250
20	50	100	150	200	250	300	350	400	450	500
30	75	150	225	300	375	450	525	600	675	750
40	100	200	300	400	500	600	700	800	900	1,000
50	125	250	375	500	625	750	875	1,000	1,125	1,250
60	150	300	450	600	750	900	1,050	1,200	1,350	1,500
70	175	350	525	700	875	1,050	1,225	1,400	1,575	1,750
80	200	400	600	800	1,000	1,200	1,400	1,600	1,800	2,000
90	225	450	675	900	1,125	1,350	1,575	1,800	2,025	2,250
20 mL/kg	200	400	600	800	1,000	1,200	1,400	1,600	1,800	2,000

This table represents the fluid recommended in the *first hour* (1/8 of the initial 8-hour dose) by the Parkland formula. The final row represents the amount of a 20-mL/kg bolus.

Narcotic pain relief medications are often the first line of relief for these patients beyond cooling the burn. These medications often produce a decrease in blood pressure and a decrease in respiratory effort. Titration to adequate pain relief with careful monitoring of vital signs is necessary. Narcotics should be given only by IV or IO and in doses no larger than is needed for pain relief. Doses will need to be adjusted when coexisting trauma or preexisting medical conditions are present.

Pain relief may be enhanced by appropriate relief of anxiety. Agents such as diazepam or midazolam must be used with caution when combined with narcotic analgesics unless a provider with advanced airway skill is available to deal with the respiratory depression or hypotension that can result from synergism.

Nitrous oxide mixtures are useful and provide immediate oxygen. Nitrous oxide must not be continued together with narcotics and sedatives because the effect of these three types of drugs together is essentially a general anesthetic. Reassessment of pain should be completed using the same scale (for example, 0 to 10) every 5 minutes. Seek advice from the ED or medical command via dispatch regarding increasing pain medication and dosages that are beyond normally accepted dosage. Non-narcotic analgesics can be valuable in certain scenarios.

Management of Superficial Burns

Although superficial burns can be very painful, they rarely pose a threat to life unless they involve nearly the whole surface of the body. If you reach the patient with superficial burns within the first hour of the injury, immerse the burned area in cool water or apply cold compresses to the burn **FIGURE 8-24**. Burned hands or feet may be soaked directly in cool water, while towels soaked in cool water may be applied to burns of the face or trunk.

The object of the exercise is twofold: to stop the burning process and to provide relief of pain. Commercial products are available to do both those things and also to

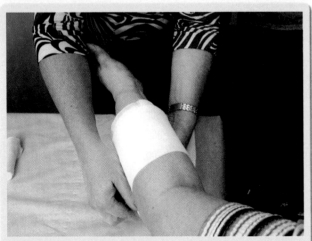

FIGURE 8-24 Moisten dressings of superficial burns to stop burning and reduce pain.

provide a good burn dressing. However, in cooling the burn, take care not to overcool the whole patient; that is, do not let the patient become chilled. A dry sheet or blanket applied over the wet dressings will help prevent systemic heat loss, especially in inclement weather conditions **PROCEDURE 28**.

Whatever you put on the burn, do not use salves, ointments, creams, sprays, or any similar materials on any type of burn. They will just have to be scrubbed off in the emergency department, causing the patient further pain. No additional treatment should be necessary in the field for the uncomplicated (no other injury) superficial burn. Simply transport the patient in a comfortable position to the hospital.

Management of Partial-Thickness Burns

Treatment of partial-thickness burns in the field is very similar to that of superficial burns. Again, cool the burned area in cool water or apply a wet or water-based gel dressing within the first hour. Doing so will diminish edema and provide significant pain relief. Burned extremities should also be elevated, again to minimize edema formation.

Do not attempt to rupture blisters over the burn; they are the best burn dressing in the short term. Establish IV fluids with lactated Ringer's or Hartmann's solution or normal saline, as dictated by local protocol. Pain in partial-thickness burns may be very severe. Complete a pain assessment and administer pain medication as allowed by your protocols.

Management of Full-Thickness Burns

Although full-thickness burns do not cause the same level of pain for the patient, most patients will have varying degrees of burns within the affected region of injury. For this reason, a pain assessment should be completed and pain medication should be administered as described above. There is little else you can do for a full-thickness burn in the field, but be sure to cover with a sterile dressing and monitor any areas of circumferential burns as noted above.

Management of Chemical Burns

As with any burn, rapidly stopping the burning process is central to early management. Flush the exposed area of the patient's body immediately with copious quantities of water to remove the offending chemicals. A few chemicals react violently with water, which obviously precludes irrigation. Such chemicals are usually powders, so it is reasonable to brush off as much dry powder as possible before irrigating any chemical exposure **FIGURE 8-25**. Skin destruction is determined by the concentration and duration of contact. Systemic toxicity is determined by the degree of absorption.

Immediately remove the patient's clothing, especially shoes and socks that may have become contaminated with the chemical agent, taking care not to get any of the hazardous chemicals on your own clothing or skin. This will often remove the majority of the chemical from skin contact. Most chemicals are most efficiently removed by washing with

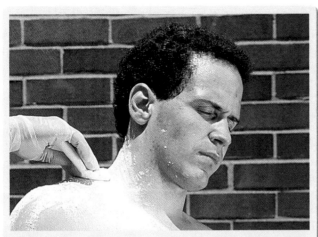

FIGURE 8-25 Dry chemicals may burn the patient further if you add water. Before flushing a dry chemical burn with water, brush off as much of the chemical as you can.

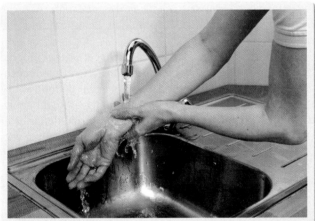

FIGURE 8-26 Have the patient wash areas that are along joints and between fingers and toes.

copious amounts of low-pressure water, as may be available in a shower, sink, or eye wash station. If the patient is in or near the home, the shower or a garden hose is ideal. Have the patient bend over when washing hair and head, to avoid having residual chemicals run over the rest of the patient's body. Chemicals collect in skin folds, where they remain in contact with the tissue, causing more severe damage. Care must be taken to wash the skin folds at joints, and between fingers and toes meticulously **FIGURE 8-26** .

In an industrial setting, use the decontamination shower or a hose. After a thorough initial flushing (usually at least 5 minutes), some chemicals may adhere to the skin and a mild detergent (dishwashing liquid) will aid in the washing. Remember to rinse and wash gently to avoid abrading the skin and causing increased injury or absorption of the chemical.

Do not waste time looking for specific antidotes; copious flushing with water is more effective and more immediately available. Furthermore, so-called neutralizing agents often work by combining with the chemical that caused

the burn in an <u>exothermic reaction</u> (ie, a reaction that produces heat). Thus, the very process of neutralizing the offending chemical may cause further burns to the patient.

Flushing should be continued for a minimum of 30 minutes; for chemical burns caused by strong alkalis (eg, oven and drain cleaners), 1 to 2 hours of flushing is recommended. It is obviously preferable that you begin transport as soon as is practical and continue the flushing en route. Specialist burn centers have specialized equipment to complete the flushing and cleaning process. When flushing is complete, cover the burned area with a sterile dressing or cover the whole patient with a sterile sheet.

Special Cases of Chemical Burns

In alkali burns caused by dry lime, mixing with water may produce a highly corrosive substance. For that reason, when a patient has been in contact with dry lime, first remove his or her clothing and brush as much lime as you can from his or her skin (wearing gloves). Then start flushing copiously with a garden hose or shower, and continue flushing for at least 30 minutes. The potential for overcooling is great; take care.

Sodium metals produce considerable heat when mixed with water and may explode. Although rarely practical, consider covering the burn with oil, which will stop the reaction by preventing the sodium from coming in contact with the atmosphere.

Hydrofluoric acid (HF) is used in drain cleaners in the home; industrially it is used for etching glass and plastic. The patient burned with HF will complain bitterly of pain, and the pain will not get any better even with continuous flushing—a sign that the process of tissue destruction is ongoing. Treatment of HF burns requires the injection of calcium chloride (CaCl) into the burn wound, a procedure that should be undertaken in the ED, not in the field. The patient with HF burns, therefore, should be moved to the hospital after an initial 5 to 10 minutes of flushing to remove surface chemical. A slurry of 10% CaCl and a water-soluble lubricant can be applied to small HF burns and may provide some pain relief.

Hot tar burns are, strictly speaking, thermal burns, not chemical burns, although they tend to be classified with chemical burns. The most important treatment in the prehospital phase is to immerse the affected area in cold water to dissipate the heat from the tar and speed up the hardening process. Once the tar has cooled, it will not do any further damage, and there is no need to try to remove it in the field.

If you do not know the identity of the chemical that caused the burn, assume it is not a special case. Flush the burn wound with water for at least 30 minutes as previously described.

Chemical Burns of the Eye

If chemicals have splashed into the patient's eyes, the eyes too must be flushed with copious amounts of water. The most efficient way to do so is simply to support the patient's head under a faucet, directing a steady stream of lukewarm

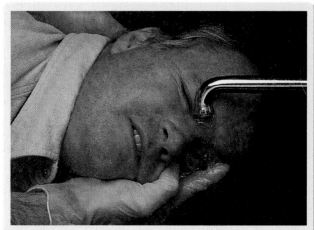

FIGURE 8-27 Flood the affected eye with a gentle stream of water. Hold the eyelids open, a challenging task because the patient's natural reflex is to close the eye or even keep the eye shut. Take care to prevent any of the chemical from getting into the other eye during the flushing.

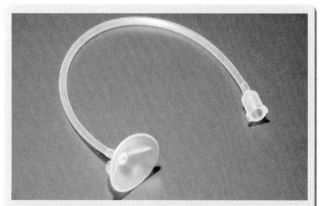

FIGURE 8-28 The Morgan Lens makes eye irrigation more comfortable, efficient, and effective.

tap water into the affected eye **FIGURE 8-27**. If the patient wears contact lenses and the stream of water does not flush them out, pause after a minute or two of irrigation to allow the patient to remove their own contact lenses. If the lenses remain in place, they will prevent water from reaching the cornea underneath. Be sure to irrigate well underneath the eyelids **PROCEDURE 30**.

Never use any chemical antidotes (eg, vinegar or baking soda) in the eyes. Irrigate with water only. After irrigating for a minimum of 30 minutes, patch the patient's eyes with lightly applied dressings and transport the patient to the hospital for evaluation.

Eye irrigation is extremely important in any situation where a chemical has gotten into the eye. It is uncomfortable and inefficient to attempt to irrigate an eye by prying it open and rinsing with a standard normal saline IV set. The Morgan Lens makes eye irrigation more comfortable, efficient, and effective **FIGURE 8-28**. Ocular anesthetic drops are preferable (if allowed by your local protocols), but care must be taken when the eye is numb to keep the patient from scratching or rubbing it **PROCEDURE 29**.

Management of Electrical Burns

The first priority at the scene of an electrical injury is to protect yourself and bystanders from becoming the next victims. Do *not* use a rope, wooden pole, or any other object to try to dislodge the patient from the current source. Do *not* try to cut the wire. Do *not* go anywhere near a high-voltage line.

Many parts of the electrical grid are protected by automatically resetting breakers. Should the wind blow a branch into wires, bridging the gap between two wires, it is desirable to have the breaker reset after a few moments to avoid power outages. As a consequence, a downed wire that "looks dead" can jump back to life, perhaps several times. There is only one safe way to deal with a downed high-tension wire: Call the electric company. Wait until a qualified person has shut off the power before you approach the patient. This can be a traumatic event for providers, who will feel helpless waiting for the power to be shut down while a possibly critical patient lies on the ground nearby. But remember—*providers can die in these situations*. You can help the greatest number of people by being cautious and safe in this circumstance.

Once the electric hazard has been neutralized, proceed to the ABCs. Open the airway using the jaw-thrust maneuver, keeping in mind the possibility of cervical spine injury. If the patient is in cardiac arrest, beginning CPR and applying an ECG monitor or the automated external defibrillator (AED) will, of course, have priority. There is usually a very good chance of successfully resuscitating the patient with an electric injury, but doing so might require prolonged CPR.

If the patient is not in cardiac arrest, arrhythmias remain a risk and cardiac monitoring is indicated for 24 hours after significant burns. Take the following steps when treating patients with electrical burns:

1. Administer high-flow oxygen.
2. Monitor the patient's cardiac rhythm.
3. Start at least one IV or IO and run in a lactated Ringer's, Hartmann's, or normal saline solution bolus to keep the kidneys flushed.
4. Contact the ED or base physician via dispatch for advice, which may include:
   a. If the patient has fallen, immobilize the cervical spine.
   b. Cover any surface burns with dry, sterile dressings.
   c. Splint any fractures.

Management of Radiation Burns

Patients with radiation burns might be contaminated with radioactive material, so they should be decontaminated before transport. The majority of contaminants can be removed simply by disrobing the patient.

Irrigate open wounds. Washing should be gentle to avoid further damage to the skin, which could result in additional internal radiation absorption. The head and scalp should be irrigated the same way. The ED should be notified as soon as practical if you are transporting a potentially contaminated patient. In contrast with other types of contamination, radioactive particulate matter probably poses a relatively small risk to the rescuer. Consider providing basic care to the patient before decontamination if you are wearing protective clothing.

Radiation injury follows the <u>inverse square law</u>: Exposure drops exponentially as distance is increased. Increasing your (and your patient's) distance from the source by even a few feet may dramatically decrease your exposure, so it is important to identify the radioactive source and the length of the patient's exposure to it. You must try to limit your duration of exposure, increase your distance from the source, and attempt to place shielding between yourself and sources of gamma radiation.

With contact radiation burns, decontaminate the wound as if it were a chemical burn to remove any radioactive particulate matter. You may then treat it as a burn.

Many radioactive isotopes are used in medicine and industry. Some of these isotopes can be absorbed or have their toxic effects blunted by another substance. Like their radioactive effects, the toxic effects of these isotopes vary. Antidotes may help bind an isotope, enhance its elimination from the body, or reduce the toxic effects on other organs **TABLE 8-7**. Such expert antidotal therapy should be considered only under the guidance of a knowledgeable doctor or specialist radiographer.

Potassium iodide is distributed to people who live near a nuclear power plant and may help protect the thyroid gland if taken within 6 hours of exposure. Contrary to popular belief, however, it is effective only for radionuclides released from fission products from nuclear power plants and would be of little value for exposure to medical radiation.

Management of Burns in Pediatric Patients

Escaping from a fire can be difficult for children. More than half of child fire fatalities and injuries are preschoolers. Recent research suggests that young children are not as effectively awakened by smoke detectors and are often disoriented immediately after waking. Young children are also more likely to suffer severe scald injuries. Children's thin skin and delicate respiratory structures are more easily damaged by thermal insults than in older children and adults.

In children, fluid resuscitation may be more challenging because they have an increased body surface-to-weight ratio. They may have a greater fluid requirement than adults. It is acceptable to start with the Parkland formula in children; however, local protocols may provide for standard pediatric dosing of fluids. In addition, because of poor glycogen stores, children might require dextrose-containing solutions earlier than adults. Certainly routine blood glucose monitoring should be done.

In children, it is vitally important to differentiate accidental burns from child abuse. Pay careful attention to the mechanism of injury, which should be relayed to the hospital staff at the ED.

TABLE 8-7 Antidotes to Selected Isotopes*

Isotope	Antidote
Cesium 137	Prussian blue adsorbs cesium in the GI tract and may enhance elimination.
Iodine 131	Potassium iodide blocks thyroid uptake.
Plutonium 239	DTPA or EDTA can be used as a chelator and for wounds. Aluminum hydroxide antacids may bind plutonium in the GI tract.
Radium 226	Provide immediate lavage with 10% magnesium sulfate followed by saline solution and magnesium purgatives. Ammonium chloride may increase fecal elimination.
Strontium 90	Aluminum hydroxide antacids may bind strontium in the GI tract. Aluminum phosphate can decrease its absorption by 85%. Ammonium chloride can acidify urine and enhance its secretion. Barium sulfate may reduce strontium absorption.
Tritium	Oral fluids will reduce biologic half-life from 12 to approximately 6 days.
Uranium	Sodium bicarbonate reduces nephrotoxicity.

*GI indicates gastrointestinal; DTPA, diethylenetriamine pentaacetic acid; and EDTA, ethylenediaminetetraacetic acid.

Reprinted from *Dis. Mon.*, vol. 49, J.B. Leikin, et al., A primer for nuclear terrorism, pp. 485–516, Copyright (2003), with permission from Elsevier. [http://www.sciencedirect.com/science/journal/00115029]

Management of Burns in Elderly Patients

In the United States, 1,200 older adults die from fire each year, making fires the sixth leading cause of death in this population group. Thirteen percent of older adults smoke, and smoking is the leading cause of fires that lead to death in the elderly. Elderly patients are particularly sensitive to respiratory insults. The leading sentinel event in home health care is fires caused by smoking while wearing supplemental oxygen. Cooking fires represent another distinct hazard to the elderly.

Older patients may also have poor glycogen stores, and their blood glucose levels should be checked to determine possible hypoglycemia. In addition, careful cardiac monitoring should occur. Although fluid resuscitation is important, elderly patients are more likely to develop pulmonary edema. The provider must routinely assess lung sounds for developing rales.

Transfer to a Specialty Burn Center

The American Burn Association has identified the following referral criteria. Patients suffering from any of the following burn injuries should be transferred to a specialty burn center:

- Partial-thickness burns of greater than 10% body surface area
- Burns that involve the face, hands, feet, genitalia, perineum, or major joints
- Full-thickness burns in any age group
- Electrical burns, including those from lightning
- Chemical burns
- Inhalation burns
- Burn injury with preexisting medical conditions that could complicate management, prolong recovery, or affect mortality
- Burns and concomitant trauma in which the burn injury poses the greatest risk of morbidity or mortality
- Burn injury that requires special social, emotional, long-term rehabilitation intervention

There are some differences between European and American guidelines that relate to both burn care and the capabilities of different burn centers. The European Practice Guidelines for Burn Care mirror the American Burn Association but also include:

- Any type of burn if any type of doubt about the treatment exists
- Diseases associated to burns such as toxic epidermal necrolysis, necrotizing fasciitis, staphylococcal scalded child syndrome, etc
- Burns over 10% TBSA for children
- Burns over 15% TBSA for the elderly

The American Burn Association also has published burn severity classifications **TABLE 8-8**. All critical burns should be transported to a specialty burn center.

Consequences of Burns

Burns are horrifying injuries. They leave scars on both the victims and rescuers, and they tax the system's resources. Sophisticated burn centers are available to treat these complex injuries, but the total number of burn center beds has decreased in recent years. These limited beds are often occupied by patients who require care for weeks or months. The surge capacity of burn units is limited, and an incident that generates multiple burn patients can tax this limited resource.

The Patient

As previously mentioned, burns are devastating injuries that may require months of recuperation. Burn patients must survive not only their traumatic burn injuries, but

TABLE 8-8	Burn Severity Classifications	
Minor burns	Superficial	Body surface area less than 50% (sunburns, etc)
	Partial thickness	Body surface area less than 15%
	Full thickness	Body surface area less than 2%
Moderate burns	Superficial	Body surface area greater than 50%
	Partial thickness	Body surface area less than 30%
	Full thickness	Body surface area less than 10%
Critical burns	Partial thickness	Body surface area greater than 30%
	Full thickness	Body surface area greater than 10%
	Inhalation injury	
	Partial- or full-thickness burn involving hands, feet, joints, face, or genitalia	

also end-organ dysfunction and the specter of infection. The psychological trauma inflicted by burns may be as bad as the physical trauma. After the acute phase, months or years of rehabilitation might be necessary to maximize the use of limbs and joints damaged by the burn and extensive immobility. Patients with major injuries average about 1 day of inpatient treatment for each percentage of TBSA burned. After initial treatment, extensive rehabilitation may be necessary to regain function. Serious burn survivors are left with a host of long-term consequences including problems with thermoregulation, fluid imbalance, and neurosensory deficits. Tremendous improvements in the care of critical burn patients have made long-term survival possible for many who would have died from their injuries a decade ago, but large surface area burns remain a critical care challenge on par with other forms of severe multisystem trauma.

The Provider

Caring for patients with severe burn emergencies can be one of the most horrifying tasks undertaken by a provider. Fire scenes are chaotic and dangerous places. Patients are often in severe pain. The smell of burned hair and flesh permeates your clothes and equipment. Sheets of skin may peel off the patient when you perform simple tasks like attempting to take vital signs or moving the patient. These calls are among the most traumatic events most providers will be called upon to cope with. Providers should consider psychological first aid after any major burn event.

CHAPTER RESOURCES

CASE STUDY ANSWERS

1 What scene safety issues are present?

Scenes of violence require constant vigilance to maintain scene safety. The fire that was present and the fluid that was used to start the fire are concerning as well. The developing crowd can also become an issue of safety if the crowd becomes difficult to control.

2 Approximately how much surface area is affected by the burn?

Using the Rule of Nines, the upper chest is 9% + the upper back 9% + hands 6% = 24%. This burn estimate may be high or low and should be adjusted based on the patient's actual presentation. Other methods could also be used to help estimate the burns.

3 What is the first step in prehospital burn care?

Stopping the burning process must be addressed immediately following scene safety. It is appropriate to wet the patient to stop the burning. Thermal transfer is a concern that can be managed after the burning process has stopped. Warming the patient with dry blankets and dressing wounds can be completed in the treatment phase of burn management.

4 Describe the priorities for assessment and initial care of your patient.

Immediate threats to life from thermal trauma revolve almost exclusively around the airway and breathing. The initial/primary assessment is completed with these in mind, however bleeding and early presentation of shock is more often a significant sign of traumatic injuries, not burns. Your patient has only minor trauma to the airway and while he is breathing fast, he is not having difficulty moving air in and out. Shock does appear to be present based on his appearance and vital signs. Treatment should be geared at stopping the burning and treating for shock.

5 What is the cause of his shock?

Your patient is most likely in shock due to the injury sustained from the assault prior to being set on fire. Look for additional signs of bleeding such as internal blunt trauma or unseen penetrating trauma. The fluid loss from burns has a delayed presentation as it takes time for the fluid to shift out of the damaged cells into the tissue.

Trauma in Motion

1. What are the local burn specialty hospitals in your area?
2. How will you transport to those facilities if they are far away?
3. What are the capabilities of your local hospitals for chemical exposures? Radiation exposures?
4. Does your agency have protocols for response to a chemical or radiation exposure? Have you reviewed them recently?

References and Resources

American Burn Association. Scalds: a burning issue. Burn Awareness Kit. 2000. Available at: www.ameriburn.org/Preven/ScaldInjuryEducator'sGuide.pdf. Accessed: February 21, 2009.

Centers for Disease Control and Prevention. Available at: www.cdc.gov/niosh/docs/2002-123/pdfs/02-123.pdf. Accessed: February 21, 2009.

Decker WJ, Garcia-Cantu A. Toxicology of fires—An emerging clinical concern. *Vet Hum Toxicol.* 1986; 28(5):431–433.

Electrocution. *Construction Safety.* 2000; 11(1). Available at: www.csao.org/uploadfiles/magazine/vol11no1/shock.htm. Accessed: February 21, 2009.

Moritz AR, Herriques FC Jr. Studies of thermal injuries: II the relative importance of time and surface temperature in the causation of cutaneous burns. *Am J Pathol.* 1947; 23:695–720.

Priani P, Quaintenne EJ. Ocular burns: etiology, diagnosis and treatment. *Arch Oftalmol B Aires.* 1966; 41:281–301.

Royal Society for the Prevention of Accidents. Accidents involving electricity. January 2007. Available at: www.rospa.co.uk/factsheets/electrical_accidents2007.pdf. Accessed: February 21, 2009.

Saffle JR. What's new in general surgery: burns and metabolism. *J Am Coll Surg.* 2003.

U.S. Fire Administration, National Fire Data Center. Older adults and fire. *Topical Research Series.* 2001; 1(5).

U.S. Fire Administration, National Fire Data Center. The fire risk to children. *Topical Research Series.* 2004; 4(8).

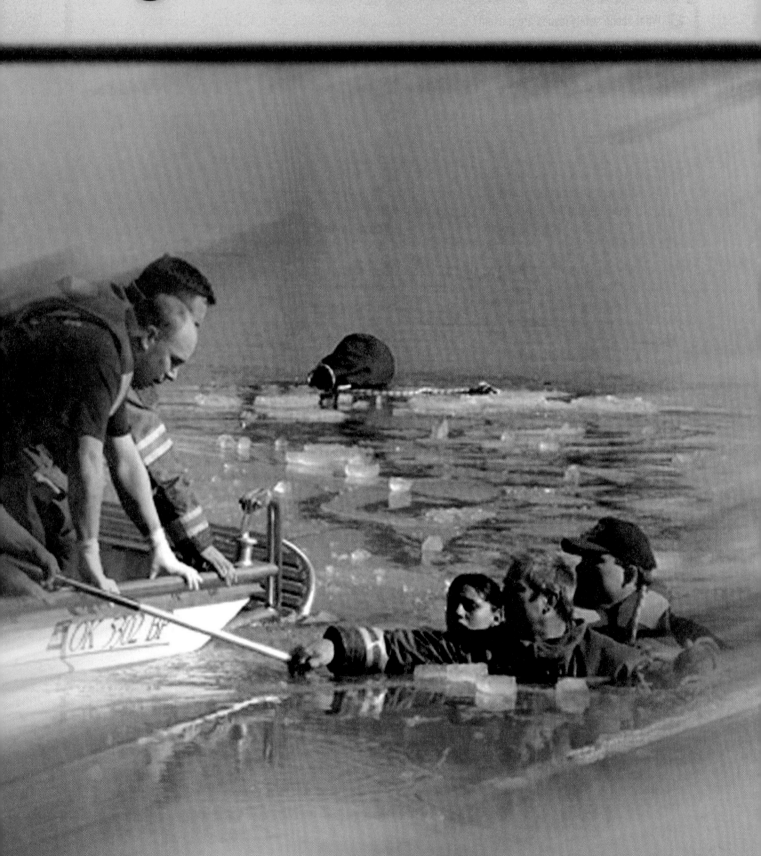

CASE STUDY

You have been dispatched with rescue to a woman who fell through the ice. While monitoring the radio en route to the pond, the fire/rescue team begins issuing an additional priority call for a fire fighter who has fallen through the ice while attempting a rescue. The temperature outside is 50°F (10°C) and the woman and fire fighter are 150′ (45 meters) from the shore in chest-deep water. Upon your arrival you find three victims in the water because another rescuer has jumped in to help.

The original patient is an 18-year-old woman who has reportedly been in the water for 20 minutes. When she is delivered to you she has had a blanket wrapped around her shoulders and is dressed only in light clothing because the day was unseasonably warm. The patient is anxious and having a hard time talking due to vigorous shivering but tells you she does not remember why she went onto the ice. Bystanders state she ran out after her hat blew off. The two rescuers who went into the water have walked off to their truck to warm up.

After moving the patient to the warm ambulance, your patient tells you she is on a beta blocker for a heart arrhythmia and does not take any other medicine. She tells you she did not get hurt when she fell into the water but she could not pull herself free. Her pulse is 84 beats/min, respirations are 14 breaths/min, and blood pressure is 90/60 mm Hg. Her skin is cold, pale, and mottled. Her wet clothes are removed and she is wrapped in warm blankets. She continues to shiver uncontrollably and has little control over fine motor skills as you prepare for transport. She has no visible trauma.

1 How could scene safety have been improved?

2 How does being immersed in water affect body temperature?

3 Will the patient's body temperature continue to be affected if she remains in her wet clothing?

4 Does this patient's medical history affect her ability to control her temperature?

5 Does this patient require aggressive warming?

Introduction

Environmental emergencies can occur in isolation, but many will be clustered around an abnormal weather pattern or event. Unseasonably cold or hot periods will often cause high demands on emergency medical service (EMS) systems. These demands can be increased by large gatherings of people, such as a concert, fair, or sporting event. An integral part of being a good health care provider is focusing on the entire patient. An exploration of environmental emergencies will provide a better understanding of how these pathologies affect your patients. More importantly, it will give you patient care tools to help improve survival and decrease morbidity.

Temperature may not be the primary injury; however, it can adversely affect the outcome of trauma patients. When an injury occurs in a hot or cold environment, patients can be at risk because they are trapped in the situation with no way to protect themselves. Patients also are at risk of decreasing body temperature when they are exposed for the trauma assessment in these environments. Providers should take care to minimize these situations to protect the patient from further harm.

Thermoregulation

Temperatures and Measurements

When discussing environmental emergencies, Celsius temperature readings are typically used. The conversion from Fahrenheit to Celsius is °F − 32 ÷ 9 × 5.

Converting 72°F to Celsius:
72°F − 32 = 40
40 ÷ 9 = 4.44
4.44 × 5 = 22.2°C

A simpler method is to memorize key Celsius points and then estimate the numbers between those points. The key points to remember are found in **TABLE 9-1**.

FIGURE 9-1 demonstrates the comparisons between Celsius and Fahrenheit systems. One of the fundamental questions to ask is where, and with which instrument, you should take the temperature of the patient. Treatment plans when managing environmental emergencies are often based on core body temperatures.

TABLE 9-1   Key Celsius to Fahrenheit Points

°C	°F	Example
0	32	Freezing
10	50	Cold tap water
22	72	Room temperature
37	98	Normal body temperature
40	104	High fever
100	212	Boiling water

Every instrument to measure temperature has an error factor. The goal is to understand the various types of technologies and their limitations in accurately reading body temperature. Different types of temperature reading technologies have different styles and clinical issues. Glass thermometers are very low-tech and require little maintenance. They can be used orally, rectally, or axillary but can take up to 3 minutes to get an accurate reading and can break. Electronic probe-style thermometers have been shown to spread disease if not cleaned properly. Infrared systems are accurate but work best in controlled settings. They need to be acclimated to the surrounding temperature or they can be inaccurate. Electronic thermometers obviously need batteries. Plastic strip thermometers used on the skin can take 2–3 minutes and can be affected by atmospheric temperature and skin perfusion. If no thermometer is available, you can get a general idea of the patient's temperature by feeling the skin under the patient's clothes.

TABLE 9-2 provides information on the places temperatures can be measured and the accuracy of each. For conscious patients, oral temperatures are accurate provided they are done according to the device's recommendations. In unconscious patients, rectal, tympanic, and temporal artery readings all have value.

Heat Exchange

Heat exchange refers to the movement of heat from one source to another. **Heat production** deals with the speed at which the body is burning fuels. Both exchange and production have impacts on a patient's temperature and how easily it is maintained. Let's look in more detail at the exchange side of the equation.

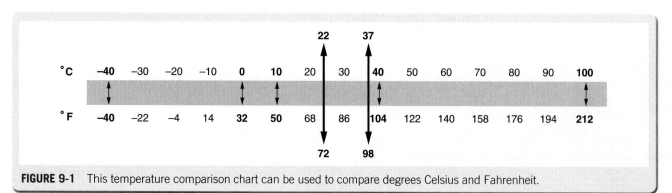

FIGURE 9-1   This temperature comparison chart can be used to compare degrees Celsius and Fahrenheit.

TABLE 9-2 Temperature Locations and Recommendations

Location	Results	Recommendations
Oral	Near core temperature ($-0.5°C$) Affected by mouth breathing, fluids in the mouth, smoking, and mouth movement	Use for conscious patients. Coach the patient to keep the mouth closed. Electronic devices are more accurate than glass.
Axillary	Near core temperature ($-1.0°C$) Affected by sweating and blood flow	Use as a backup method. May be useful in infants.
Rectal	Near core temperature Affected by depth of probe, contents of bowel, and blood flow Uncomfortable for patient (and provider)	When used, it is a reliable indication of near core temperature.
Tympanic	Core temperature Very technique sensitive Ear wax can interfere with accurate reading. Must have probe resting on tympanic membrane	This method is effective on conscious and unconscious patients.
Temporal artery	Core temperature May be affected by sweating May be more accurate on children than on adults	This method is effective on conscious and unconscious patients.

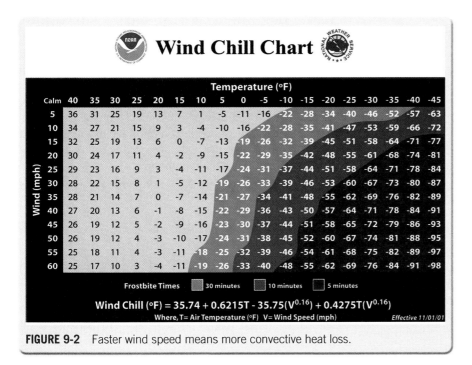

FIGURE 9-2 Faster wind speed means more convective heat loss.

Energy tends to move from areas of high concentration to areas of low concentration. There are various means by which this heat can be transferred:

- Conduction
- Convection
- Radiation
- Evaporation (respiration)

Conduction is the transfer of heat from a source of relatively high heat to one of lower heat through physical contact. As you sit on a chair, you are heating the chair directly. Technically, you heat your clothing, which becomes warmer.

Your warm clothes then heat the chair. The limiting factor with this method is the density of the objects involved.

The denser the substances in contact, the more efficiently the heat transfers. When a person is standing, clothed, in a temperate environment, the amount of conductive heat loss is low. If you change the air temperature or make the environment denser, conduction can have a profound impact. Water is denser than air and conducts heat 25 times more efficiently than air.

The next factor that affects care relates to the temperature gradient. The greater the temperature difference between two substances, the greater the heat will flow downhill. It is important to recognize the implications of conductivity and density.

Convection heat transfer involves the movement of a liquid or air over a surface. Convection is a key element in how quickly a person cools when exposed to cold temperatures. Under nonemergency conditions, it is estimated that almost 40% of all heat loss from an unclothed person is from convection.

For people who live in colder areas, wind chill is a common forecast during winter months. Wind chill calculates the effects of moving air over the body. The greater the wind speed, the greater the convective heat loss **FIGURE 9-2**.

Everything within the universe has some degree of heat. Anything that has heat will emit electromagnetic radiation. **Radiation** is the transfer of heat through electromagnetic waves. All living organisms emit infrared radiation. This radiation of heat can be seen when looking through an infrared scope to locate victims in smoke-filled rooms or by the infrared camera systems used on police helicopters to follow criminal suspects. Although invisible to the naked eye, infrared emission occurs regardless of the pigment of the skin or color of the clothing. Heat transfer from radiation accounts for about 45% of net heat loss.

The final mechanism for transferring heat is **evaporation**. Evaporation involves the loss of heat through the transition of water from a liquid state to a gas. As the air moves over a wet surface, some water molecules are picked up and incorporated into the gas. Primarily, the water involved within this transition is sweat and moisture within the respiratory tract. Evaporation accounts for approximately 15% of heat transfer within a neutral temperature environment (30% if sweating).

This mechanism is greatly affected by a variety of conditions. As the relative humidity climbs, the ambient air becomes so saturated with water that sweating becomes ineffective. Another factor is the speed at which the air is moving over the moist area. Greater speed equals greater evaporative heat exchange from the skin. This speed can come in the form of wind speed or respiratory rate.

Air is a poor conductor of heat. The more layers of clothing present, the more air is trapped between those layers, providing a barrier to the effects of cold weather. Blankets work the same way **FIGURE 9-3**. Blankets are nothing more than thermal reflectors and air trapping units. If you place a blanket on a cold floor, you will not have a warm floor. Blankets reflect your body heat and at the same time provide a layer of air between you and the cold environment. That is why the best blankets are fluffy and full: lots of fibers loosely bound means lots of places for air to be trapped.

Heat Production

Life is a series of chemical reactions; therefore, life is heat. The speed at which your cells are burning fuel is referred to as your **metabolic rate**. The **basal metabolic rate (BMR)** (the number of kilocalories [Kcal] created by the body per hour) is how medicine measures this process. The thyroid gland is responsible for controlling the BMR, which is the set point of the body's engine speed. The faster your cells are working, the more fuel they use and therefore the more heat they generate. Your BMR can change based on the demands placed on the system.

STATS

The average American consumes approximately 2,000–2,200 Kcals/day. Men and women who are stationed in the Antarctic face extremes in temperature. Depending on the work being done, Antarctic scientists may need 6,000 Kcals/day or more just to maintain body weight.

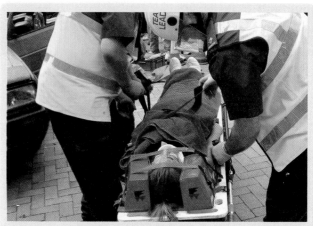

FIGURE 9-3 Blankets can provide a barrier to temperature loss in cold weather.

When you work outside during a hot summer day, your body produces sweat in an attempt to stay cool. This dehydration through sweat creates a sense of thirst so your body will replenish the lost fluids. However, individuals will experience loss of appetite during a very hot day. The body is trying to decrease its heat production. When the environment is warm, the body's BMR does not need to be as high to maintain the same core temperature.

Cold climates present other challenges to maintaining core temperature. Shivering is essentially muscles quivering. As they move, they must burn fuels, thus liberating needed heat. Any work that the body does will generate heat. This activity helps to stave off hypothermia.

Heat can be produced by other nontypical methods. Fevers are used by the body's immune system to create an internal environment that is unsuitable for the growth of invading organisms. For this reason, fevers are generally viewed as a beneficial symptom of disease.

Medications can also change a person's temperature. One class of medications that does this is **sympathomimetics**. Epinephrine, norepinephrine, cocaine, and methamphetamines all place the patient at risk of hyperthermia. These sympathomimetic medications increase the patient's BMR. This increase, if unchecked, can lead to increased heat generation and hyperthermia.

Other medications can alter the patient's ability to maintain a normal temperature. Aspirin, acetaminophen, and ibuprofen all work to block the patient from generating additional heat during an infection. Although these medications do not lower body temperature, they can impact core temperature during a time of cold stress.

Additionally, there are other medications that will alter the body's ability to manage excess heat, making patients more prone to heat-related illnesses. These medications can prevent sweating and even distort a patient's perceptions of environmental temperature. A partial list of medications that affect heat is found in **TABLE 9-3**.

TABLE 9-3 Medications That Can Affect Heat Regulation	
Drug Types	Drug Names
Anticholinergics	benztropine (Cogentin)
	atropine
Antihistamines	diphenhydramine (Benadryl)
Tricyclic antidepressants	amitryptiline (Elavil)
	imipramine (Tofranil)
Antipsychotics	
Phenothiazines	chlorpromazine (Thorazine)
	fluphenazine (Prolixin)
Butyrophenones	haloperidol (Haldol)
	clozapine (Clozaril)
Atypical antipsychotics	risperidone (Risperdal)
	olanzapine (Zyprexa)
Diuretics	hydrochlorthiazide (HCTZ)
	furosemide (Lasix)
Lithium	chlordiazepoxide (Librium)
	lithium carbonate (Eskalith, Lithobid)
Beta-blockers	sotalol (Betapace)
	propranolol (Inderal)
	metoprolol (Lopressor)
	esmolol (Brevibloc)
Ethanol	alcoholic beverages
Stimulants	cocaine
	amphetamine
	methamphetamine
	ecstasy (MDMA)

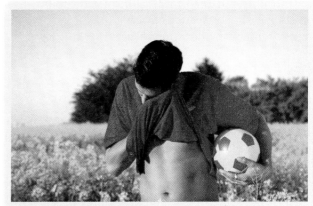

FIGURE 9-4   When the skin detects heat or cold, it sends signals to the brain.

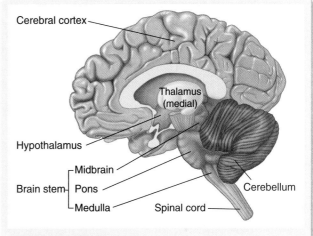

FIGURE 9-5   The hypothalamus works with the midbrain and pons to regulate the body's temperature.

Physiologic Effects of Temperature Change

As temperature deviations occur, the body fights to maintain control. The organ that is most sensitive to temperature changes is the brain. The brain receives information from the entire skin surface about the degree of cold or heat FIGURE 9-4 . Additionally, the body has internal thermometers within the abdominal cavity, spinal cord, hypothalamus, and brain stem. Together these internal and external sensors provide enough information for the brain to maintain an internal temperature within 2°C.

The main portion of the brain responsible for temperature monitoring and correction is the hypothalamus. The hypothalamus interconnects with other areas within the brain stem to affect changes designed to return temperature deviations to normal FIGURE 9-5 .

The brain is able to regulate the body's temperature using three main actions:

1. Vascular control
2. Shivering and sweating
3. Behavioral responses

Vascular control represents the first of these major control methods FIGURE 9-6 . During periods of thermal stress, the brain can cause blood to be shunted either into the periphery or to the core. If heat needs to be released from the body, **vasodilation** occurs. More of the warm blood is exposed to the surface of the skin, allowing more effective radiation and convective heat loss. When this occurs, the skin becomes flushed and hot, and peripheral pulses are easily felt.

When the body is cold, **vasoconstriction** shunts warm blood away from the periphery. This prevents the exposure of warm blood to the coldness surrounding the body. The results are cool, pale skin with decreased peripheral pulses. Vasoconstriction can be so effective that the temperature of the skin can closely approximate the temperature of the environment.

Shivering and sweating are the second major control methods initiated by the hypothalamus. **Shivering** is the rhythmic, involuntary movement of muscles. This muscular activity generates heat through burning of fuels needed by the moving muscle cells.

Sweating, on the other hand, assists in heat dissipation. Sweating is controlled by the sympathetic nervous system. The entire skin can sweat. Some areas have a higher density of sweat glands: the forehead, the neck, anterior and posterior portions of the trunk, and dorsal surfaces of the hand and forearms. Sweating increases the effectiveness of evaporative heat loss by providing more moisture to carry away heat.

The third major way the brain helps maintain thermal balance is through behavioral responses. As the internal temperature climbs, you become uncomfortable. You tend to shed clothing. This improves airflow over the skin, thereby increasing heat loss. The average person will reduce work during the heat of the day and have increased thirst. These conscious behaviors assist in preventing hyperthermia.

During times of decreased temperature, you will seek additional layers of clothing to help insulate your body. This obviously decreases heat loss. You spend more time indoors and crave a warm environment. You perceive temperature changes similarly to sensations of pain. The body tries to eliminate this uncomfortable stimulation.

Children, the elderly, and neurologically and psychologically altered patients have difficulty using these actions to change their temperature. Some lack the ability to alter their vascular system to retain temperature (very young children cannot use vasoconstriction to alter temperature), some do not have the ability to shiver or sweat (the changes in the skin of the elderly decrease the sweat response), and some do not sense the change in temperature (seen in patients following a stroke, spinal cord injury, degenerative neurologic diseases, or psychological conditions). This lack of actions makes these groups more prone to injury from temperature changes.

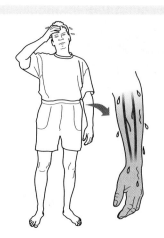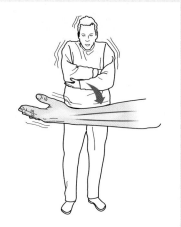

Hot Environment
- Hypothalamus stimulated
- Blood vessels dilate, maximizing heat loss from skin
- Body sweats, causing evaporation and cooling

Body temperature *decreases*

Cold Environment
- Hypothalamus stimulated
- Blood vessels constrict, minimizing heat loss from skin
- Muscles shiver, generating heat

Body temperature *increases*

FIGURE 9-6 The hypothalamus is the "master thermostat" for the body, sensing a temperature change and then using the body systems to regulate it.

is generally thought to be around 49°C (120°F). At this temperature, cell damage is extreme and cell death nearly instantaneous.

Incidence

Heat emergencies occur more often during summer months. Heat waves are responsible for many of the heat-related deaths and illnesses around the world. Patients also suffer from heat emergencies during times of moderate temperatures. These emergencies occur to laborers, patients with preexisting medical conditions, patients with mental illness, the very young or older patients, and those who are poorly acclimated. When circumstances are present in which patients cannot compensate effectively, even moderate heat can pose a problem.

STATS

The human body is home to around 2.6 million sweat glands.

Heat Emergencies

The body uses changes in metabolism, shivering and sweating, modifying vascular diameter, and behavioral responses to maintain a core temperature of between 36° and 38°C (96.8° and 100.4°F). The maximum upper limit for humans

STATS

According to the US Centers for Disease Control and Prevention (CDC), a total of 3,442 deaths resulting from exposure to extreme heat were reported in the United States from 1999 through 2003. Of that number, 40% were in people over the age of 65. Cardiovascular disease was listed as the underlying cause of death in over half. In the United Kingdom over 60% of patients who died from heat exposure had a previous history of cardiac or respiratory disease.

Pathophysiology

Patients suffer from hyperthermia in conditions of increased environmental heat and/or when they have a decreased ability to shed heat. It is important to note that fevers are not included in this grouping.

As core temperature rises, cellular injury can occur. This damage may take hours to become evident as the body attempts to compensate. Cells need to work ever harder to maintain their internal chemistry. This increased work requires more and more fuel. Eventually, supply and demand for fuel become unbalanced and cellular damage begins.

In an effort to prevent cellular damage, a complex series of compensatory mechanisms are used to maintain core temperature at normal levels. Vasodilation moves heated blood to the skin for cooling. This improves the dissipation of heat but can have the negative effect of decreasing available blood for the heart to pump (preload). Combine this with the loss of actual volume through sweating, and the potential for hypotension becomes real.

To prevent this potential crisis, epinephrine and norepinephrine are released. This causes an increase in heart rate and force of contraction (beta-1 adrenergic effects) in an attempt to maintain blood pressure. This is one of the reasons for bounding peripheral pulses in early heat emergencies. Vasoconstrictive forces from epinephrine and norepinephrine (alpha adrenergic effects) are balanced with the vasodilation forces of the hypothalamus. The net effect is blood vessels that remain dilated, but not overly so.

If the heat continues, the **renin-angiotensin-aldosterone system (RAAS)** is activated, causing vasoconstriction and decreased urine production. The RAAS increases systemic vascular resistance and works to increase fluid retention by the kidneys by increasing sodium reabsorption and stimulating the release of antidiuretic hormone (ADH). Blood flow to the intestines and kidneys will decrease to allow for sufficient core blood volume. The loss of liquid through sweating further reduces the volume and composition of the blood.

As the blood becomes thicker, the patient has a strong urge to drink **FIGURE 9-7**. If the replacement fluid is electrolyte balanced, in sufficient quantity, and the gastrointestinal system can absorb it effectively, the patient will be able to maintain this compensation without a drop in blood pressure.

As the cells burn more fuels, increased levels of metabolic byproducts are present. This can create metabolic acidosis. To compensate for the increased acid load within the blood, the respiratory rate is increased.

This is the critical tipping point. How healthy is the patient? What medications are being taken? How acclimated is the patient? How well hydrated was he or she before the heat stress? The answers to all of these questions will help predict how quickly the patient will move from heat stress to heat illness.

If the heat is excessive or unrelenting, or if the body's reserves are inadequate to the task, decompensation can occur. Cells begin to suffer damage. The body works to repair the damage to the cells. In a similar manner to fighting an infection, inflammation begins. This inflammatory response can lead to capillary leakage, microhemorrhage, and **disseminated intravascular coagulopathy (DIC)**.

DIC is essentially a coagulation system supply and demand problem. As more and more hemorrhages occur, more and more clots are needed. In turn, more resources are needed to make these clots. The result is that the demand for clots exceeds the ability to create them. Clots are formed incorrectly, inappropriately, or not at all. Essentially, patients bleed to death and clot to death simultaneously. Hemorrhage and infarctions are the hallmarks of this coagulation disturbance **FIGURE 9-8**.

Increased capillary permeability is one of the final steps in the patient's battle to survive. As permeability increases, the amount of precious fluid within the blood is allowed to exit the blood vessels and enter the interstitial space. Peripheral edema and reduced circulating volume are the results. With limited volume for the heart to move, blood pressure begins to fall. Perfusion to the skin decreases. Effective cooling stops and the core temperature rises rapidly. Cerebral perfusion is impaired. Very soon, hypoxia and death will occur.

The speed at which the patient travels through this process is, like most diseases, very difficult to predict. Acclimation of the person is an important consideration. As one's body becomes more adept at managing increased environmental heat or increased physical activity, cells are not as stressed. Acclimatized laborers and trained athletes have been able to maintain core temperature of 40°C (104°F) without significant injury.

General Management Guidelines

Heat emergencies can present as a minor illness or a serious condition. Heat edema is a relatively benign condition, whereas heat stroke is life threatening. Many patients will display findings that may confuse and confound the provider. The best approach for the management of any heat emergency, regardless of how minor it may appear, is to ensure that the patient is not suffering from heat stroke.

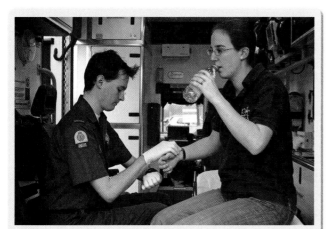

FIGURE 9-7   Patients will often experience extreme thirst as sweating decreases the fluid in the body.

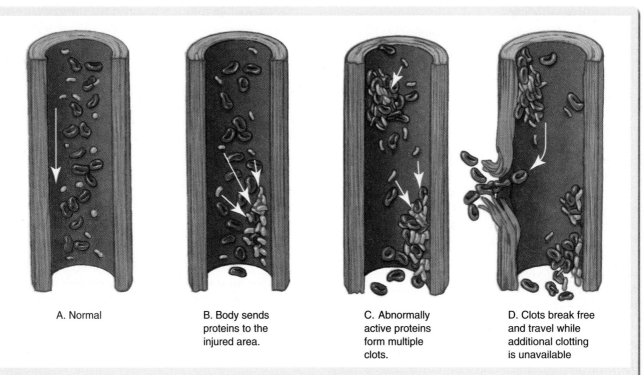

A. Normal

B. Body sends proteins to the injured area.

C. Abnormally active proteins form multiple clots.

D. Clots break free and travel while additional clotting is unavailable

FIGURE 9-8 Disseminated intravascular coagulopathy (DIC) occurs when the patient's normal repair system is overloaded.

Patients should be removed from hot environments as soon as possible. Do not underestimate the benefits of shade. When facing a heat emergency, shade is certainly better than direct sunlight. Either move the patient or improvise to protect the patient from the sun. Perform a good, detailed assessment. While this is occurring, excess clothing should be removed and the need for active cooling assessed. If the patient has an altered level of consciousness, assessment of core temperature is indicated. A detailed assessment with particular focus on history of present illness, past medical history, medications, and level of consciousness will help to determine the degree of heat emergency.

If you are preparing an oral rehydration solution for your patient, there are several choices. A solution containing carbohydrates is absorbed through the GI system up to 30% faster than free water. Free water is water that also has little or no electrolyte complement. Bottled water and tap water are examples. **TABLE 9-4** lists solutions that can be used for rehydration. Note that all water used within these recipes is to be disinfected and clean. Encourage the patient to take about 1 L per hour of the rehydration solution. A good measurement of effectiveness is the ability of the patient to urinate at least every 2–3 hours.

Specific Hyperthermia Emergencies
Heat Edema
Heat edema is a condition in which vasodilation and pooling of fluids in the interstitial space cause swelling in the hands and feet. It often occurs when people are standing for long periods of time in a hot environment. This condition is self-limiting and rarely poses any real threat to the patient's general health.

TABLE 9-4	Oral Rehydration Solutions
Solution	**Comments**
1 L water 1 tsp salt 2–3 Tbsp honey or sugar	This solution lacks bicarbonate and potassium.
3 cups water 8 oz fruit juice, such as orange juice or apple juice 1 tsp salt	This solution lacks potassium.
Half-strength sports solution, such as Gatorade	Full-strength solutions can cause stomach cramps.
1 L water 3/8 tsp salt 1/4 tsp salt substitute 1/2 tsp baking soda (bicarbonate) 2–3 Tbsp sugar or honey	World Health Organization's oral rehydration solution

Patients should be removed from the hot environment. The affected extremity(s) should be placed in a comfortable position above the level of the heart to assist with venous drainage. In this case, diuretics can make the patient's condition worse by further complicating potential volume and electrolyte loss.

Heat Cramps
When individuals are involved in strenuous activity during periods of high environmental heat, **heat cramps** can occur as patients try to replace lost volume with free water

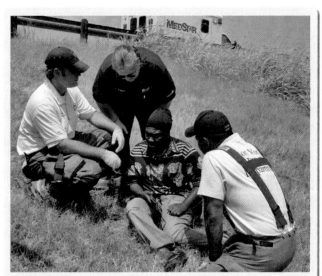

FIGURE 9-9 A patient with heat cramps should be moved to a cool area to complete the assessment.

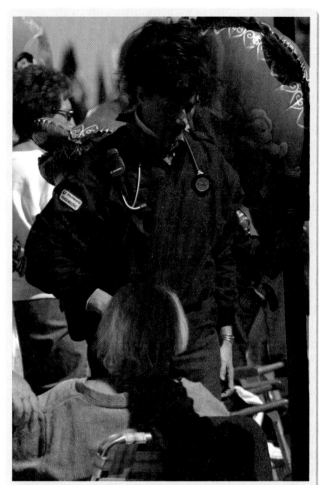

FIGURE 9-10 Heat syncope is transient and will often present as resolved upon provider arrival.

FIGURE 9-9 . Because one of the major components of sweat is sodium, people who drink only free water during times of extreme sweating run the risk of developing **hyponatremia**, or low sodium levels. Sodium is one of the electrolytes required for muscle contraction. When sodium levels become depleted, muscles can suffer from continuous contraction.

Heat cramps often occur hours after the activity is completed. These spasms are painful but should not pose any life-threatening emergency. The contractions of the muscles are localized to the muscles that were involved in the activity. As one portion of the affected muscle contracts another relaxes, so it appears as if the contractions are wandering over the area. Core temperatures may be normal or slightly elevated.

Treatment for heat cramps involves replacement of the lost sodium, with a goal of returning electrolyte balance, along with rest. Patients should be given oral rehydration solutions. If the patient is unable to drink, intravenous fluids including normal saline solution can be administered; however, if the patient is so incapacitated that he or she is unable to drink, a closer assessment of the patient is in order. This patient may be suffering from a more severe form of heat emergency.

Heat Syncope

As discussed earlier, vasodilation is one of the compensatory mechanisms to manage heat stress. As the vascular container increases in size, the amount of blood volume available to the heart to pump (preload) can diminish. Patients who have not been keeping up with fluid replenishment, those with preexisting cardiac conditions, and those who have not been well acclimated are more prone to **heat syncope**.

The classic setting for this event is a person who has just entered a hot environment and is standing for a long period of time. Standing in one position allows for pooling of blood within the lower extremities. Combine this

with a dilated vascular container, and a temporary state of decreased cerebral perfusion is possible. Patients will often complain of restlessness, nausea, sighing, or dysphoria (not feeling well) just before they pass out.

Heat syncope is a transient event that is self-resolving. Once the patient has lost consciousness and has assumed a position in which blood pressure demands have decreased, consciousness should spontaneously return. One of the most important considerations is not so much that the patient went unconscious, but what the patient struck during the fall FIGURE 9-10 .

Treatment for this patient is mainly supportive. Assessment should be accomplished as normal. Assess the risk for cervical injuries. If needed, apply spinal immobilization. Assess and manage any injuries that occurred during the fall. Lacerations needing sutures are not uncommon in these patients. Patients should be given oral rehydration solutions if tolerated.

A wide array of factors can cause patients to have syncopal episodes. A heat emergency is only one. A detailed assessment with special focus on past medical history, medications, and history of present illness is in order. Providers should apply a cardiac monitor and check blood glucose to rule out medical causes of the syncope.

Heat syncope is typically present without an increase in core temperature. It results from a misdistribution of volume. This is not a true volume loss. If the patient does not awaken rapidly after the syncopal episode, you should consider that a more serious condition. Check the core temperature to ensure that heat stroke is not present.

Acclimatization is an important factor with this condition. Heat syncope peaks on the first day when exposed to a hot environment. By day five, this syndrome is rarely seen, demonstrating the beneficial effects of acclimatization. If a provider is required to work during a heat wave, remember that he or she is susceptible to heat syncope in the first few days. Rest and plenty of electrolyte replacement solutions are vital in maintaining the ability to serve the public.

Heat Exhaustion

The most common form of heat emergency encountered by providers, **heat exhaustion**, represents the beginning of a continuum of heat-related emergencies with mild exhaustion at one end and heat stroke at the other.

In heat exhaustion, water and salt levels within the body have been depleted. Patients typically present with headache, fatigue, weakness, dizziness, orthostatic hypotension, nausea, vomiting, and muscle cramps. Tachycardia and dehydration are also present. Because this condition is at the beginning of compensatory failure, patients often present with profuse sweating. Classic skin conditions are flushed, hot, and moist. More important than the presence or absence of sweating, however, is the effect of heat on the level of consciousness (LOC). Heat exhaustion patients should be able to maintain a normal LOC.

Heat exhaustion usually takes several days to occur. This condition results from a continued strain of the compensatory mechanisms as they work to maintain core temperatures within normal limits. Patients with this condition may experience irritability and anxiety but should not suffer from generalized decreases in level of consciousness. Assessment of the core temperature is important. In heat exhaustion, core temperatures are rarely above 40°C (104°F).

Treatment for this condition is directed at extrication from the hot environment and replacement of lost body fluids. Clothing should be removed as the assessment process is continuing. Assess vital signs and core temperature. In cases where patients are able to take oral fluids and their vital signs are stable, administer oral rehydration solutions. These patients should improve quickly and should expect a full recovery.

When patients are more unstable with orthostatic vital signs or are unable to take oral fluids, it may be necessary to administer intravenous fluids. IV fluid administration of normal saline should be given at a rate based on the patient's vital signs. A conservative approach is to administer 250 mL boluses and then reassess. Saline boluses can dramatically improve vital signs. Indications of effectiveness are the following:

- Decreased tachycardia
- Decreased nausea and vomiting
- Negative orthostatic tilt test

It is important to note that in this environment of fluid loss and electrolyte abnormalities, excess administration of normal saline can cause cerebral edema from the overload of sodium in the blood.

Because determination of this condition can be difficult, the prudent provider needs to assess very closely for heat stroke. If the patient has a decreased level of consciousness or does not improve quickly with cooling and fluid replacement, assume heat stroke and aggressively begin to cool the patient.

Heat Stroke

Heat stroke is a true medical emergency. When medical treatment is delayed, mortality from this condition can be as high as 80%. The cardinal signs of heat stroke are core temperatures above 40°C (104°F) with alterations in central nervous system function. Failure to recognize and rapidly treat this form of hyperthermia can result in permanent disability or patient death.

Heat stroke has two separate and somewhat different forms. In **classic heat stroke**, core temperature rises due to exhaustion of the compensatory mechanisms. In **exertional heat stroke**, compensatory mechanisms are overwhelmed by more heat than they can manage. These two different causes will be effectively demonstrated in patient assessment findings and history of present illness differences.

Classic heat stroke is a condition that occurs over several days. Patients who are least able to manage heat stress are at risk. Particularly in poorer areas, where there may be an inability to maintain hydration, people will seek a cooler location; the very young, the elderly, and those with previous medical problems are at highest risk. This condition often occurs during periods of increased heat, such as a heat wave.

Heat stroke has a gradual presentation, with the more severe signs and symptoms occurring longer into the heat exposure.

Exertional heat stroke has a different presentation; and, a different patient population is at risk. In this condition, young, healthy individuals who are involved in strenuous physical activity are the typical patient. Military personnel, fire fighters, construction workers, and athletes are the patients most often affected by exertional heat stroke.

These relatively healthy individuals can place themselves at greater risk. Factors such as obesity, baseline dehydration, sleep deprivation, fatigue, poor physical fitness, recent viral infection, and decreased acclimatization can impact the body's ability to compensate effectively for heat stress. Patients who are using sympathomimetics, such as cocaine or amphetamines, increase the risk of heat stroke.

Exertional heat stroke has a more sudden presentation than classic heat stroke, occurring over hours with a rapid cascade of signs and symptoms including those presented in **TABLE 9-5**.

In addition to the effects of heat on the nervous system, exertional heat stroke patients will often have **rhabdomyolysis**, the breakdown of muscle fibers releasing the contents into the bloodstream. As muscle cells are being stressed by the combination of work and heat, they begin to

TABLE 9-5 Comparison of Signs and Symptoms of Severe Classic Heat Stroke and Exertional Heat Stroke

Body System	Signs and Symptoms	
	Classic Heat Stroke	**Exertional Heat Stroke**
Central nervous	Irritability	Irritability
	Delusions	Headache
	Irrational behavior	Dizziness
	Hallucinations	Weakness
	Seizures	Delirium
	Cerebellar dysfunction	Seizures
	Cranial nerve dysfunction	Syncope
		Coma
	Coma	
Cardiovascular	Bounding peripheral pulses early	Bounding peripheral pulses early
	Absent peripheral pulses later	Absent peripheral pulses later
	Hypotension	Hypotension
	Tachycardia	Tachycardia
	Widened pulse pressure	Widened pulse pressure
Respiratory	Hyperventilation	Dyspnea
Renal	Oliguria	Oliguria
	Anuria	Anuria
		Dark urine
Gastrointestinal	Nausea	Nausea
	Vomiting	Vomiting
		Abdominal muscle cramps
		Diarrhea
Integumentary	Anhidrosis (lack of sweating)	Sweating
		Hot
	Hot	Flushed
	Flushed	
Musculoskeletal	N/A	Severe muscle cramping

TIP

Heat stroke patients need to be viewed similarly to other major trauma patients. The provider must decide how to get this patient to a hospital efficiently. The major trauma patient needs care the provider is unable to provide: surgery. The heat stroke patient is in a similar situation in regards to cooling. These patients need rapid controlled cooling, which most EMS units will be unable to provide.

die. The cell membranes rupture and __myoglobin__ (oxygen-transporting protein), potassium, and other cellular contents are released. Rhabdomyolysis will result in decreased urine production, hyperkalemia, and metabolic acidosis.

Treatment for heat stroke, regardless of whether classic or exertional, is directed at rapid recognition and rapid dropping of core temperature. It cannot be stressed enough: *Failure to drop core temperature will result in increased mortality and morbidity*. Once patient contact is established, remove the patient from the hot environment as quickly as possible. This may be as simple as getting out of the patient's house or moving into a shaded area.

As you assess the patient, remove the clothing and begin cooling. Manage the ABCs. The airway should be secured by the most appropriate method. Some patients will require endotracheal intubation, others may need only airway monitoring. Level of consciousness will guide you to the correct airway intervention.

Capnography can be a valuable assessment tool with heat stroke patients. Cellular hyperactivity will result in increased carbon dioxide generation. This hypermetabolic state can be measured accurately using capnography. Beyond using the waveform to assist the provider in ensuring proper endotracheal placement, it can be helpful in monitoring the effectiveness of cooling. As core temperatures drop, cellular metabolism will follow. This should translate to a decrease in expired CO_2 levels over time.

Heat stroke patients will need high-flow oxygen. The accelerated cellular activity will consume oxygen at a rate much higher than normal. Even if pulse oximetry readings are near normal, ensure that heat stroke patients receive high-flow O_2 either by advanced airway or by nonrebreathing mask.

Providers should begin cooling by removing the patient's clothing. Place washcloths over the groin and breasts for privacy. The patient needs to be soaked and maintained wet during transport. The goal is to maximize radiational and convective cooling. For convective cooling to work, skin must be exposed to airflow; therefore, modesty will need to be compromised. Turn on the ventilation system within the ambulance to amplify airflow over the patient.

Access to large quantities of water may be difficult to come by during a call. If available, simple tap water through a garden hose will be very effective. Consider using irrigation saline or sterile water as a coolant. If water resources are limited, soaked sheets can be used. Place one layer of soaked sheets over the patient; the sheets may need to be rewet en route to the hospital to help the evaporative process. More aggressive cooling can be accomplished by placing ice packs in areas of major blood flow such as the axilla and groin if local protocols permit. Although bags of IV fluids can be cut, these should be used as a last resort. The IV solutions may be needed for blood pressure management.

Very aggressive cooling is needed in these patients. As cooling continues, body temperature should be monitored. Assessment and reassessment of core temperature will assist the provider in controlled cooling. Cooling should be halted when the core temperature reaches 39°C (102.2°F) or when shivering is noted.

ALS-level care for the heat emergency is predominantly supportive. IV/IO access is needed for volume support and medication access. If the patient is hypotensive, provide fluids to expand the vascular compartment. Administer 1–2 L of normal saline over 1 hour. Be cautious with fluid administration. Large quantities of IV fluids can cause cerebral and pulmonary edema. (Providers should follow local protocols because they may quantify the amount and type of fluid to be administered.)

The use of vasopressors should be avoided. Dopamine at high doses and epinephrine will cause vasoconstriction. This may increase core temperature by preventing peripheral blood flow. Blood pressure that does not respond to IV fluids should be augmented with dobutamine (where available).

Although it may seem to be a good idea, internal methods of cooling are not as effective as external methods in cooling heat stroke patients. Cooled IV fluids, gastric lavage with cold fluids, and cooled ventilations do not drop core temperatures nearly as effectively as ice water baths.

Providing continuous monitoring of the ECG is required. Arrhythmias may be present due to electrolyte imbalances. Assess and monitor the T wave shape and progression. Flattened T waves are an indication of hypokalemia.

Contact the hospital as soon as possible so they can prepare for continued cooling methods within the emergency department. The fastest method to decrease core temperature is ice water immersion. Within the hospital, this method is economical and easy to implement. Patients are placed in a basin filled with water and ice. This method is capable of reducing core temperatures as quickly as 0.13°C/minute. This can result in dropping the temperature to near normal levels in 10–40 minutes.

A summary of information for heat emergencies can be found in **TABLE 9-6**.

Cold Emergencies

When the body loses more heat than it produces or gains, **hypothermia** occurs. Cold emergencies can be localized to an extremity or can be a general decrease in overall core temperature. An elderly man who falls, fractures his hip, and remains on the floor of his home for several hours or days until he is discovered is at risk for hypothermia.

Incidence

Cold emergencies occur in colder climates; however, patients are able to suffer from hypothermia even in the warmest environments. In the United States, more cases of hypothermia tend to occur within the urban setting because patients can have circumstances that make them ill prepared to keep warm. Homelessness, drug use, and alcoholism all play major roles in preventing patients from finding and maintaining a warm environment. For similar reasons, the mentally ill also are at risk. Older age is another risk factor for hypothermia, and people older than 80 years account for the highest number of cold deaths every year in the United Kingdom, according to the Office of National Statistics.

TABLE 9-6   Common Heat-Related Syndromes

Syndrome	Signs and Symptoms	Treatment
Heat edema	Swelling of the extremities, hands, and/or feet	Elevate affected area above the level of the heart. Avoid diuretics.
Heat syncope	Sudden loss of consciousness with spontaneous return after patient assumes horizontal posture	Assess for trauma from fall. Rehydrate by either oral or intravenous routes.
Heat cramps	Painful muscle cramps, typically in the legs and shoulders, occurring hours after exertion	Allow patient to rest. Administer oral rehydration solution.
Heat exhaustion	Core temperature less than 40°C, tachycardia, hypotension, orthostatic hypotension	Remove patient from heat and allow to rest. Rehydrate by either oral or intravenous routes.
Classic heat stroke	Core temperature over 40°C; CNS dysfunction; hot, flushed, and dry skin	This is a life-threatening situation. Aggressively cool the patient. Monitor the core temperature. Support vital signs.
Exertional heat stroke	Core temperature over 40°C; CNS dysfunction; hot, flushed, and wet skin	This is a life-threatening situation. Aggressively cool the patient. Monitor the core temperature. Support vital signs.

STATS

Approximately 800 Americans and 140 Canadians die from hypothermia each year. The very young and very old are at the greatest risk. Mild hypothermia patients tend to have fewer fatalities, whereas patients with severe decreases in core temperatures (below 30°C [86°F]) can have mortality rates above 20%.

When discussing nonurban incidents of hypothermia, a second group appears. These are the individuals who are enjoying the outdoors. Hunters, skiers, climbers, boaters, swimmers, and those whose jobs require them to work outside all have an increased risk.

Pathophysiology

The effects of generalized hypothermia can be quite profound on most of the body systems. The central nervous system is one of the first systems to demonstrate derangement. As temperatures drop, judgment, memory, speech, and eventually consciousness will be impaired. In mild hypothermia, the patient will begin with <u>ataxia</u> (lack of muscular coordination), slurred speech, and loss of fine motor skills. This presentation can be easily confused with cerebral vascular accidents (CVAs).

As the core temperature continues to drop, difficulty thinking and judgment problems are present. It is not uncommon for the patient to begin to take off protective clothing under the misguided assumption that they are hot. This action will only accelerate the cooling process. Eventually, core temperature will be too low for neuron activity and the patient will slip into unresponsiveness.

One of the more interesting aspects of hypothermia on the nervous system is its protective effects. As the temperature drops, metabolism within the neurons decreases. The cells now need less oxygen to survive. This provides an environment where complete restoration of nervous system function is possible.

The cardiovascular system is dramatically affected by hypothermia. As the body is cooled, the initial response will be tachycardia and vasoconstriction. These effects will increase the workload on the heart. As core temperature continues to drop, myocardial cell function is impaired. This will modify the repolarization aspect of myocardial function. The result is conduction delays, which are displayed in a variety of ways. PR interval, QRS duration, and QT interval are all prolonged. The T wave becomes flattened. A characteristic of hypothermia is the J wave or Osborne wave. This wave, initially seen in leads II and V6, is indicative of delayed repolarization. It can be seen as a wave immediately following the end stroke of the QRS and before the flattened T wave **FIGURE 9-11**. The size of the J wave is related inversely to the temperature of the patient.

Arrhythmias become more common as coordination among sections of the heart becomes more disjointed. Other ECG changes caused by hypothermia include bradyarrythmias, consisting of sinus bradycardia, junctional rhythm, or atrial fibrillation with a slow ventricular response.

Bradycardia is one of the cardinal effects of hypothermia. When assessing the moderate to severe hypothermic patient, one should expect to find bradycardia. If the patient's core temperature is below 30°C (86°F) and bradycardia is not seen, a repeat assessment is warranted. There is a distinct possibility of some level of trauma, hypovolemia, drug overdose, and/or hypoglycemia present in concert with the hypothermia. A continued decline in core temperature will result in extreme bradycardia, leading to asystole. This rhythm is commonly seen in patients with profound hypothermia.

The increased cold slows down the speed of the sodium/potassium pump. This is demonstrated in the prolongation in the QT interval. The myocardial cells remain in depolarization longer than normal; therefore, the relative refractory phase is also prolonged. This is an important issue because myocardial cells are prone to random firing. Rough handling can accidentally cause an R on T event, which can lead to ventricular fibrillation.

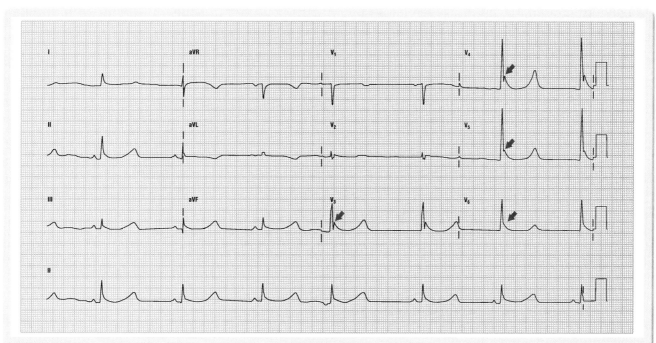

FIGURE 9-11 The J waves on this ECG are indicated with arrows.
From *12-Lead ECG: The Art of Interpretation,* courtesy of Tomas B. Garcia, MD.

The respiratory system responds in a similar manner to the cardiovascular system. Initial **tachypnea** (fast respiratory rate) is followed by **bradypnea** (slow respiratory rate). As alveoli are cooled, the movement of gases across the semipermeable membrane is impaired. Fluids can build up within the alveoli, causing decreased oxygen diffusion. The saving grace is that as the body cools, the amount of oxygen needed by cells decreases.

Additional changes within the respiratory system include a decrease in the pliability of the chest wall. It becomes more difficult to move the chest, so the patient may need to work harder to move air. As resuscitation efforts are in progress, providers may note that the compliance of the respiratory system seems stiff. Patients will also have an increase in respiratory secretions that tend to be thicker than normal.

Peripheral blood flow is diminished in an attempt to keep the warm blood within the central circulation. As peripheral blood flow is decreased, central blood flow is increased. This results in increased renal perfusion. The **glomerulus** (the main filter in the nephron of the kidneys), being very blood-flow dependent, responds to this increased flow by creating more dilute urine. Hypothermia patients will initially begin to produce more urine than normal. Consequently, this effect places them at risk for dehydration due to **polyuria** (excessive passage of urine).

Coagulation is also impaired by the cold. Blood at temperatures below 34°C (93.2°F) has significant difficulty manufacturing clots. The result is that areas of the body that need clots either have none or have clots that are weak and fragile. The polyuria will result in decreased circulating plasma, thus increasing the thickness or viscosity of the blood. The patient is now at risk for random clot formation due to the slower, thicker blood. This results in a situation similar to DIC. **FIGURE 9-12** shows the effects of decreasing temperature on the human body.

The four main factors associated with a predisposition to hypothermia are **TABLE 9-7**:

- Decreased heat production
- Impaired thermoregulation
- Increased heat loss
- Comorbid factors

General Management Guidelines

Cold emergencies can present as an isolated injury or a serious medical condition. **Frostnip**, for example, affects a relatively small area, whereas hypothermia can be life threatening. Assess the environment to help determine the possibility of hypothermia, because it can happen even when a patient is indoors.

Patients should be isolated from the cold environment as soon as possible. Move to a warm environment to perform a good, detailed assessment. While this is occurring, wet clothing should be removed and the need for active warming assessed. If the patient has an altered level of consciousness, assessment of core temperature is indicated.

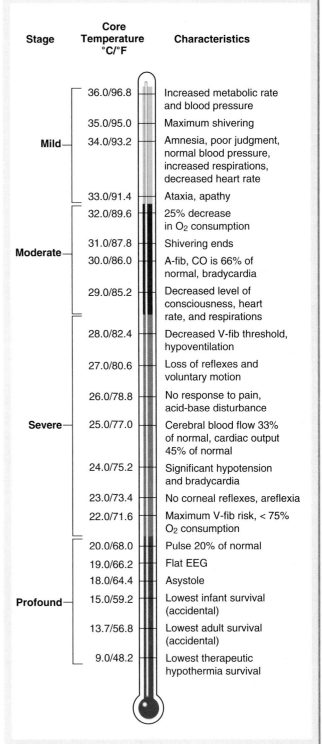

FIGURE 9-12 Physiologic effects of decreasing core temperature.

TABLE 9-7	Predisposing Factors to Hypothermia		
Decreased Heat Production	**Impaired Thermoregulation**	**Increased Heat Loss**	**Comorbid Factors**
• Age extremes • Diabetic ketoacidosis • Hypothyroidism • Hypoglycemia • Immobility • Impaired shivering • Malnutrition	• Brain tumor • CNS trauma • CVA • Diabetes • Multiple sclerosis • Parkinson's disease • Spinal cord injury	• Burns • Heat stroke treatment • Immersion accidents • Medication-induced vasodilation • Overdose • Psoriasis	• Cardiopulmonary disease • Infections • Multisystem trauma • Recurrent hypothermia • Shock (any type) • Sickle-cell disease • Vascular disease

Specific Hypothermia Emergencies

Cold emergencies can be divided into four specific pathologies. The three most common forms of cold emergencies, in which the temperature drop is limited to a relatively small section of the body, are trench foot, frostnip, and frostbite. The fourth is generalized hypothermia.

Trench Foot

Trench foot is a condition in which the feet are exposed to long-term and/or repeated insults of hypothermia. The feet are never actually frozen. A typical presentation is the patient who has been walking in wet, cold environments for several days without the ability to warm and dry the feet. The military have seen this condition over several wars as soldiers, pinned down by the enemy, were unable to appropriately warm and care for their feet. It is not too far a stretch to imagine a hiker lost for days in the cold suffering from trench foot.

The main culprit with trench foot is **ischemia** (inadequate blood flow to the cells). The cold causes peripheral vasoconstriction, which decreases blood supply to the tissues of the feet. Environmental temperatures often associated with trench foot are a range from 0° to 15°C (32° to 59°F). If the boots worn are tight fitting, circulation is diminished before the effects of cold begin. These two factors create a prime environment for cellular ischemia.

Immediately after the exposure to the cold, the feet will appear pale and blanched and will be cold to the touch **FIGURE 9-13**. Patients will report sensations of cold and numbness in the affected areas, or complete anesthesia may be present. Attempts at walking can result in severe injury and unbalanced gait due to decreased sensation in the feet.

Once warming has begun, the feet may swell and become reddened. The skin may appear dry and then the pain will be severe. The exact presentation will depend on the degree of damage to the tissues. The pain is described as burning, aching, and excruciating. As the days and weeks of recovery continue, the effects of the cellular damage become more evident.

Patients are often plagued by pain, decreased function, extreme cold sensitivity, increased sweating on the soles of the feet, and chronic fungal infections. If the ischemia is

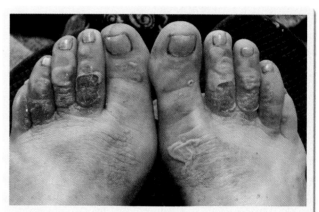

FIGURE 9-13 Scaling of skin occurs with trench foot.

severe, areas of the foot may have suffered necrosis. Partial foot amputation is not uncommon in this type of patient.

Treatment in the field for this condition is supportive. Shoes and socks should be removed and the foot gently dried. Warm the foot using passive measures. Place dry dressings over the foot and toes and provide blankets for warmth. Do not massage the feet or apply hot packs directly to the feet.

Pain management is very difficult. Narcotics and nonsteroidal anti-inflammatory agents tend to be ineffective at providing relief. If the patient needs to be evacuated from a wilderness area, walking may not be an option due to extreme pain or the risk of further injury.

TIP

Prevention is the key to managing trench foot. If you are in an environment that is cold and wet, you need to ensure that your feet are kept warm and dry. Get into a routine of visually inspecting your feet to ensure there is no injury. Signs to look for include slow capillary refill or pale or cold areas on the feet. These are the signs of decreased blood supply. Focusing on prevention will decrease the chance of injury and potential amputation.

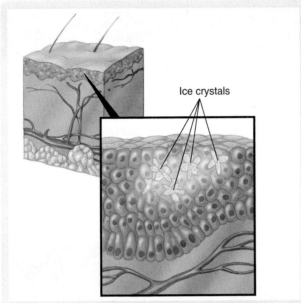

FIGURE 9-14 Rubbing the tissue in an attempt to warm it can cause the ice within the cells to rip open the cells, creating damage.

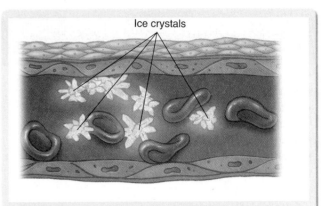

FIGURE 9-15 Frozen crystals within the blood plasma cause damage throughout the circulatory system.

Frostnip

Frostnip is a condition of superficial and reversible partial freezing of tissues within the body. Ice crystals are formed but there is little, if any, tissue damage. The main presentation for frostnip is pain and discomfort within the affected regions. Exposed portions of the body are most susceptible.

To manage a patient with frostnip, first remove the patient from the cold environment and assess for generalized hypothermia. Passive rewarming with blankets should be initiated. Do not rub the affected area. Rubbing can move the ice crystals, causing cellular damage **FIGURE 9-14**. There is no need to apply hot packs or other heated items to the affected area. This condition is so mild that it is often argued that it does not merit being classified as a cold emergency. With little or no destruction of tissues, patients make a full recovery.

Frostbite

<u>Frostbite</u> injury is caused by the freezing of tissue. The most vulnerable areas of the body are the nose, fingers, hands, toes, feet, and male genitalia due to their distal location.

The key factor involved in the pathology of this condition is blood flow. As an area of the body detects the cold, vasoconstriction occurs. The intent is to decrease the heat loss of the body. Unfortunately, this process also sacrifices the areas that are now vasoconstricted. The decreased blood flow places a smaller amount of liquid within the blood vessels. This decreased volume freezes rather easily.

Without the underlying heat to protect the area, temperatures locally begin to drop. The speed of the temperature drop will help dictate the outcome of cells. If temperatures drop very quickly, over seconds to minutes, intracellular ice crystals will form. These crystals are often fatal to the cell membrane and ultimately the cell itself. If temperatures decrease more slowly, extracellular ice crystals form. Although not immediately threatening to the cell, these crystals also have deleterious effects. Once formed, a potentially lethal imbalance occurs between the intra- and extracellular environments. Water is pulled out of the cell, causing shrinkage. This movement leads to a toxic buildup of electrolytes within the cell. The combination of decreased intracellular water and increased electrolytes is not compatible for cellular function.

Although cellular damage and destruction are profound, they do not tell the entire story. As the tissue is frozen, the cells move into a state of inactivity. Many of the cells will survive the freezing process relatively unharmed. It is during the thawing that the majority of damage occurs. As temperatures rise, blood flow attempts to reinitiate within the frozen area. Arterioles, venules, and capillaries are now filled with partially frozen blood. The movement of this liquid with its ice crystals causes injury to the walls of those structures **FIGURE 9-15**. Occurring at the same time are showers of microemboli. These result in clogging blood supply to the now awakening cells. The net result is a situation where cells that survived the freeze are starved to death due to lack of blood supply.

Presentation of frostbite is dependent on the depth of freezing to the tissue. Numbness, pain, **paresthesia** (temporary or permanent loss of sensation to an area, often associated with a pins-and-needles feeling), skin color changes, blister formation, and changes in tissue consistency are some of the signs associated with frostbite. Many of these signs and symptoms may not be present until the exposed area is thawed. Once frozen, patients may have little sensation. During the frozen period, the only clinical sign will be extreme pallor of the affected region.

First-degree frostbite is also called frostnip (discussed earlier in this chapter) and occurs in people who live in very cold climates or engage in outdoor activity in winter. It involves the top layer of skin (epidermis) and presents as numbed skin that has turned white in color. The skin may feel stiff to the touch, but the tissue underneath is still warm and soft. Blistering, infection, or scarring seldom occurs if frostnip is treated promptly.

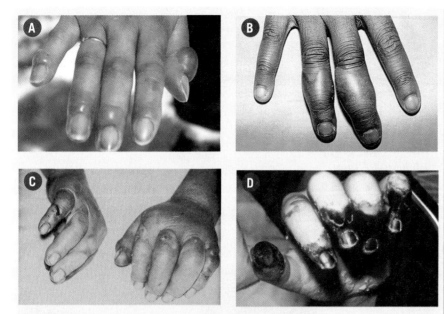

FIGURE 9-16 **A**. First-degree frostbite (frostnip). **B**. Second-degree frostbite. **C**. Third-degree frostbite. **D**. Fourth-degree frostbite.

Second-degree frostbite is superficial frostbite and presents as white or blue skin that feels hard and frozen. Blisters usually form within 24 hours of injury and are filled with clear or milky fluid. The tissue underneath is still intact but medical treatment is required to prevent further damage.

Deep, or third-degree, frostbite appears as white, blotchy, and/or blue skin. The underlying skin tissue is damaged and feels hard and cold to touch. Blood-filled blisters form thick, black scabs over a matter of weeks. Proper medical treatment by personnel trained to deal with severe frostbite is required to help prevent severe or permanent injury. Amputation may be required to prevent severe infection.

Fourth-degree frostbite is where full-thickness damage affects muscles, tendons, and bone, with resultant tissue loss. See FIGURE 9-16 for the clinical presentation of frostbite based on the visual appearance of injury.

Initial treatment for these patients is to ensure that generalized hypothermia is not present. If an environment is present that can cause frostbite, it is certainly cold enough to cause a global core temperature decrease. If the patient has a decrease in core temperature, that will take priority over the care of local injuries.

Correct treatment for frostbite is essential to any hopes of salvaging tissue. Rewarming of the frozen body part should be done only when there is very little risk of refreezing. If a hiker is found in the wilderness with clear frostbite to his or her feet, no rewarming should be attempted until he or she is in the ambulance. All patients need to be removed from the cold as soon as possible.

Once in a warm environment, remove restrictive clothing, watches, rings, and other jewelry. Due to the potential hazards to tissue caused by the removal of rings and other

jewelry, if the item cannot be easily removed, cut it off. Forceful removal can shatter frozen tissue, ending any chance of recovery in that area. Do not massage the area, because this will cause movement of the ice crystals, potentially augmenting tissue damage.

Place the affected area in dry dressings. Pad the areas, such as between fingers and toes, to help protect tissues from grating together. Ensure that the patient is in a warm environment with blankets, but do not apply any direct heat to the affected area. If in the wilderness, it is not recommended to warm the affected area near a fire. Freezing, thawing, refreezing, and then rethawing is perilous to cells.

Blisters should not be ruptured. If they spontaneously rupture, place a dressing over the area. If transportation is delayed or impossible for many hours or days, administer ibuprofen 400 mg by mouth every 12 hours to help decrease the creation of microemboli.

If the patient is unable to reach a hospital within 2 hours, rewarming should be started. The recommendations are for rewarming to be rapid and controlled. The affected area should be immersed in water warmed to 40° to 42°C (104° to 107.6°F). The water temperature must be ensured. Using hot water from a tap is not recommended.

Hot water heaters are often set at 49° to 54°C (120° to 130°F), which will result in cellular damage due to excess heat. If the conditions for rewarming cannot be guaranteed, rewarming should not be initiated. Continue a controlled rewarming until the tissue is pliable and the most distal portion of the tissue involved has returned to normal color (about 15–30 minutes). Transportation to a local hospital remains important and should not be delayed to rewarm a patient.

Patients should not be allowed to consume anything that can produce vasoconstriction. For example, caffeine and tobacco will only worsen the situation by decreasing blood supply to areas during the rewarming process. IV therapy can be initiated and pain medication administered, particularly during the rewarming process, because frostbite can be painful.

Care in the hospital is directed at warming tissue and limiting potential damage. Antibiotics, ibuprofen, and surgical care are used to limit infection, limit microemboli, and improve chances of functional use of affected tissue.

Generalized Hypothermia

In generalized hypothermia, the core temperature is decreased. As described in this section, the effects of cold on the body systems create an overall slowdown in functioning. Without intervention, the body essentially slows to death.

Presentation of the hypothermic patient is dependent on the degree of hypothermia. What is important with these patients is to look at the entire assessment and not focus on one or two details. In isolation, many of these signs and symptoms can be caused by an overdose, metabolic disease, trauma, CVA, or the like. The diligent provider will complete a full head-to-toe assessment, integrating all of the findings to get a clearer picture of the patient presentation.

The signs and symptoms of generalized hypothermia by body system are:

- **Neurologic:** Decreased corneal reflexes, decreased level of consciousness, amnesia, areflexia, ataxia, dysarthria, and irritability
- **Cardiovascular:** Arrhythmia, bradycardia, hypotension, initial tachycardia, J waves, jugular venous distension, pallor, and peripheral vasoconstriction
- **Respiratory:** Abnormal lung sounds, apnea, **bronchorrhea** (excessive mucus production), hypoventilation, and initial tachypnea
- **Renal:** Oliguria/anuria and polyuria
- **Gastrointestinal:** Abdominal distension and constipation
- **Integumentary:** Cyanosis, ecchymosis, edema, frostbite, frostnip, and **icterus** (jaundice)
- **Musculoskeletal:** Increased muscle tone, pseudo-rigor mortis, and shivering
- **Psychiatric:** Depression, flat affect/apathy, impaired judgment, neuroses, psychosis

Arguably more important than the assessment in these patients is the history of present illness. As with many patients, the history and mechanism of injury can reveal key factors that assist in discovering the correct field impression. Gather information related to the following:

- Environmental temperature
- Length of exposure to environment
- Type of dress
- Heat sources available/used
- Degree of mobility or immobility
- Access to food and water
- Past medical history and medications predisposing to hypothermia
- Alcohol or recreational drug use
- Associated trauma

Immersion injuries result from prolonged exposure to cold water, usually 12 hours or longer at temperatures of 10°–21°C (50°–70°F) or for shorter periods at or near 0°C (32°F). It is customary to refer to incidents of near drowning as *immersion* or *submersion*. In submersion incidents, the head goes below the water and the main problems are asphyxia and hypoxia. With immersion, the head remains

TABLE 9-8	Water Temperature and Effects	
Water Temperature	Time Frame for Exhaustion or Unconsciousness	Expected Survival Time
21°–27°C (70°–80°F)	3–12 hours	3 hours–indefinitely
16°–21°C (60°–70°F)	2–7 hours	2–4 hours
10°–16°C (50°–60°F)	1–2 hours	1–6 hours
4°–10°C (40°–50°F)	30–60 minutes	1–3 hours
0°–4°C (32.5°–40°F)	15–30 minutes	30–90 minutes
<0°C (32°F)	Under 15 minutes	Under 15–45 minutes

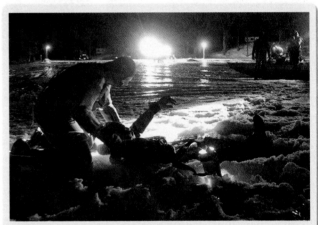

FIGURE 9-17 The mammalian diving reflex is credited with increased survival rates from lengthy resuscitations following submersion injuries.

above the water and the problem will be hypothermia. Trauma is often a major complicating factor in an immersion incident and can often happen secondarily to water recreation incidents such as boating or personal watercraft usage or falling through the ice during winter recreation. **TABLE 9-8** shows the effects and dramatic survival times for people in cold water.

Many authors have suggested that a primitive mammalian diving reflex may be responsible for survival after extended immersion in cold water **FIGURE 9-17**. The mechanism for this reflex is reflex inhibition of the respiratory center (apnea), bradycardia, and vasoconstriction of the nonessential skin capillary beds triggered by the sensory stimulus of cold water touching the face. These responses preserve the circulation to the heart and brain and conserve oxygen, thereby prolonging survival. The sudden temperature drop also helps depress cellular metabolism significantly, limiting the harmful effects of hypoxia and metabolic acidosis.

Treatment for these patients begins with scene safety. It is imperative that providers ensure to a reasonable degree that it is safe for them to enter this scene. If a search or rescue is initiated, ensure that you have adequate training and communication, and stay with your team.

After the patient is found, ABCs need to be assessed and stabilized. Preventing further cooling is as important as establishing an airway. Although patients have been successfully resuscitated even after severe decreases in core temperature, you should not view these patients as somehow in suspended animation, waiting to be reawakened. Hypothermia patients are critical and unstable and need to be cared for with calm urgency.

Examine the patient's clothing very closely. Is it wet? If so, it must be removed as soon as possible. Remember that a wet piece of clothing will disperse heat much faster from the body than a dry one. All care must be done gently. Avoid jostling or roughly handling the patient. Patients with severe hypothermia are at risk of sudden onset ventricular fibrillation.

As with other patients, management of the airway is based on the patient's level of consciousness and his or her ability to protect the airway. Patients need to be preoxygenated to help prevent ventricular fibrillation (V-fib). Intubation should not be avoided for the fear of precipitating V-fib. The key is gentle, smooth, controlled intubation.

Ventilation of the severely hypothermic patient will be complicated by stiff, somewhat unyielding muscles. Compliance will be low because cold chest muscles will not move freely. This will make identification of a pneumothorax difficult. The provider should have suction available and be prepared to manage secretions that are increased in both quantity and thickness.

The cold body does not respond to the standard interventions providers would initiate in other cardiac arrest patients. Defibrillation, external pacing, and medication administration are generally ineffective until the core temperature reaches levels that are above critical. As a rule, these interventions will be deferred until the patient's core temperature is above 30°C (86°F). Case studies have not provided definitive information on whether defibrillation should be attempted in the severely hypothermic patient or the number of defibrillation attempts that should be made. If pulseless ventricular tachycardia (V-tach) or V-fib is present, however, the ECC and the ERC recommend the patient receive defibrillation with one shock immediately followed by resumption of CPR. If the patient does not respond to one shock, further defibrillation attempts should be deferred until the patient has been warmed to a range of 30°–32°C (86°–89.6°F).

Remember that bradycardia is an expected finding in hypothermic patients. This slow heart rate can often be effective in maintaining adequate tissue perfusion for cold cells whose need for oxygen is dramatically decreased. Do not attempt to increase heart rates below 60 based solely on a heart rate; base your interventions on all available assessment information.

The hypothermic liver is unable to metabolize medications well. For this reason, medications should be withheld in patients who have a core temperature below 30°C (86°F).

Using the same logic, IV solutions should be limited to dextrose 5% or normal saline. Lactated Ringer's solution (or Hartmann's solution) should be avoided due to the inability of the cold liver to metabolize this solution. If the patient is in moderate hypothermia, medications should be spaced over longer intervals and/or dosages decreased to prevent toxic medication buildup.

A treatment algorithm can be helpful in organizing care for the patient with hypothermia. As you can see in **FIGURE 9-18**, one of the key elements with this algorithm is the need to know the patient's core temperature. Estimation of core temperature in the prehospital setting can obviously be problematic. Use history of present illness and mechanism of injury to assist.

You will note that the algorithm discusses various rewarming techniques. In the field you will obviously be limited in what you can accomplish. Ensure you follow local treatment protocols.

Passive external rewarming uses the patient's own body heat. Efforts should be made to prevent any increased heat loss into the environment.

Active external rewarming involves applying heat directly to the skin. Specialized blanket systems that pump heated air directly onto the patient can effectively increase core temperature. Hot water bottles or hot packs can be applied to the neck and axilla where major blood vessels are closest to the skin. Ensure that the patient is not burned by the application of heat by any of these methods.

Active internal rewarming involves directing the heat into the core and essentially warming the body from the inside. Prehospital care will typically be limited to heated ventilation and warmed IV fluids. In the hospital, catheters can be placed within the gastrointestinal tract, bladder, chest, and abdomen. Warmed fluids are then infused, allowing the temperature to equilibrate, and then the fluid is removed. Check your local protocols for specific skills to be performed in your area.

With **extracorporeal rewarming**, the patient's blood can be removed from the body, heated, and then returned. Cardiopulmonary bypass involves artificial oxygenation and circulation of the blood. Arteriovenous and venovenous systems involve placement of catheters within blood vessels. Blood is then directed out of the body, heated, and returned via another catheter into a vein.

One reason for the various methods of rewarming is to prevent **afterdrop**. In this situation, cold blood sequestered in the peripheral areas of the body is moved into the core. Warming of the periphery creates vasodilation. This in turn allows cold blood into a warmer core, thus decreasing the core temperature.

Care for the patient with generalized hypothermia can be summarized as follows:

1. Ensure scene safety by preventing rescuer hypothermia.
2. Complete a thorough assessment, including core temperature.
3. Check the ABCs and stop the cooling process.

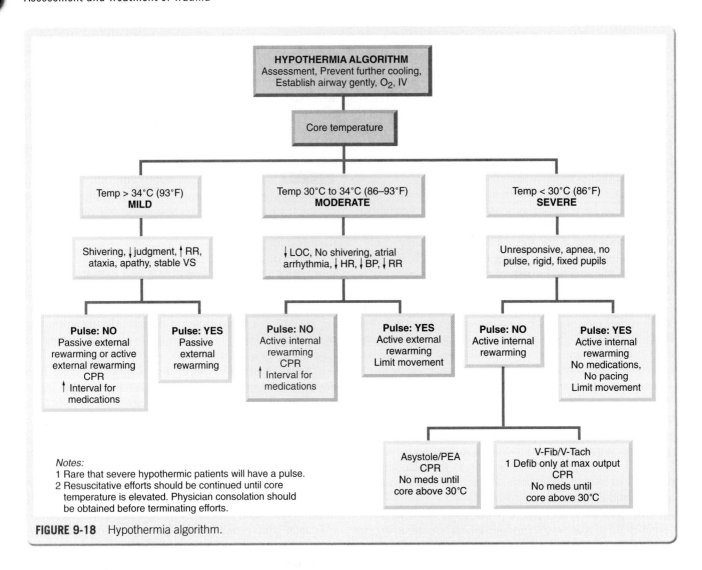

FIGURE 9-18 Hypothermia algorithm.

4. Begin rewarming based on degree of hypothermia.
5. Manage associated injuries and illnesses.
6. For most hypothermia arrest patients, provide CPR, one defibrillation (as needed), and no medications until core temperature is elevated.
7. Continue resuscitation until the patient is evaluated by a physician.

Lightning Emergencies

The awesome power of lightning is a truly remarkable environmental phenomenon. Myths about lightning are prevalent. Many people believe that being struck by lightning means instant death. Some imagine that people struck will burst into flames and be completely consumed by fire. Others think that victims are vaporized with little remains as evidence of the event.

Most patients who are struck by lightning survive. Burns, although certainly possible, are often not present. Patients tend to have the energy from the strike travel around the periphery of their body and not through their core. Patients do not truly absorb the force of the strike; they merely conduct it to ground. Do not forget, however, that a lightning strike is a very serious injury and many people struck by lightning do die or suffer permanent disabilities.

Incidence and Injury Patterns

Lightning strikes are a common event around the world, with nearly 1.2 billion lightning events occuring each year. Over 3 million flashes of lightning occur worldwide every day (about 30 flashes per second). The United States has over 20 million cloud-to-ground strikes per year. Lightning strikes are more common near the global equator. Central Africa has the most frequent lightning strikes, whereas the Pacific islands are rarely struck.

It is estimated that in the average year between 50 and 300 people are killed by lightning. In Australia, lightning accounts for 5 to 10 deaths and over 100 injuries annually. What is truly remarkable is that, worldwide, between four and five times the number of people killed by lightning are merely injured. Injuries can range from very minor to severely disabling, but the majority of people who have the misfortune of being involved are not killed.

Because most lightning is caused by thunderstorm activity, it is not surprising to learn that the summer months are most often associated with lighting. Areas that have year-round warmer climates can experience lightning frequently during any month. More than half of the strikes occur between 3 and 6 PM. This also is consistent with thunderstorms, which often gather their energy from heated air. Men comprise 84% of those involved in strikes. This does not mean that men are more potent lightning rods than women; rather, men are involved more often because more men work outside or are engaged in sports activities. This places men in potential lightning situations more often than women. Of all lightning events, 91% involve only one person. This information helps to create an injury pattern.

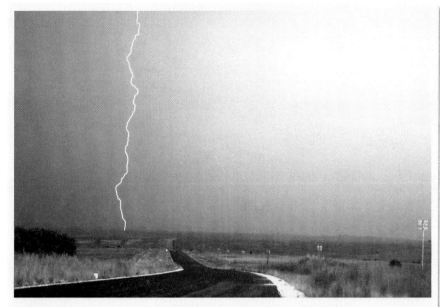

FIGURE 9-19 Lightning strikes are among the deadliest weather-related injury mechanisms.

Physics of Lightning

During warm days, air is heated by the sun. Thunderstorms are caused by rapidly rising warm, moist air. As this air rises, it condenses within the ever colder upper atmosphere. The moisture within the air can condense to form ice crystals. These begin to fall to the earth. Warm updrafts then begin to collide with cold downdrafts. The rapid movement of such large amounts of air, dust, moisture, ice, and rain causes a change in electrical potential between the sky and the earth below. Typically, the earth has a negative charge, but as the thundercloud approaches, the bottom of the cloud becomes more negative than the earth, thus imparting the ground with a relative positive charge. As the electrical difference between cloud and ground increase, a lightning strike may occur **FIGURE 9-19**. This process is similar to what is experienced with static electricity.

A bolt of lightning is relatively small in diameter, measuring only about 2–3 cm (1″). Around the main bolt is a sheath of ionized, super-heated plasma measuring about 3–20 m (10–66′). The temperature at the point of connection is estimated to measure between 8,000° and 50,000°C (14,432° to 90,032°F). The temperature of the surface of the sun is only 6,000°C (10,832°F). Why is there such tremendous heat? This heat is generated by the enormous amount of power involved. A single stroke of lightning can generate 30 million volts and 50,000 amperes.

Effects of Lightning on the Human Body

The most important facet related to lightning strikes is how they differ from generator-produced energy. In a classic electrical injury, a person grabs a charged wire, and the power from the line travels into the person's arm, making their forearm muscles contract. This prevents the person from letting go, so the energy is able to flow through the body. The power seeks ground and exits typically through a foot or leg. Total contact time is measured in seconds. The main problem in this setting is <u>voltage</u>, or amount of power.

Lightning, which has many times more volts and amperes than typical generator-produced energy, travels around the body and not through it. Lightning is a unidirectional, massive current impulse that is not direct or alternating current. Contact time with the energy of this event is measured in milliseconds. The main problem is not voltage, but <u>current</u>. Current is the flow of power over time.

The science related to understanding exactly how a lightning strike affects the human body is limited. What is postulated is that as the bolt of lighting strikes the person, the current contacts the skin and is transmitted externally. Very quickly the skin is damaged **FIGURE 9-20**. A flashover effect occurs where the energy is now moved along the outside of the body. This flashover may result in vaporization of moisture on the skin. Clothing may also be blasted apart as the current travels around the patient.

This initial leaking of current from the skin internally is limited. What is known is that portions of the body that are already electrically active are susceptible to this current impulse. The brain, heart, spinal cord, muscles, and arteries all have large interconnections or compositions of nerves. In these structures, a short circuit occurs.

The brain, subjected to this touch of power, overloads. Central and peripheral nervous systems collapse. Patients can be rendered unconscious and apneic with no brainstem activity. Muscles can contract and arteries can vasospasm. Asystole is the most common arrhythmia seen with significant lightning strikes.

Similar to a computer that needs rebooting, the brain attempts to restart itself. As the brain is working to reorganize chaos, the heart begins to fire. Occasionally, the brain will lag behind the heart in reestablishing normal activity.

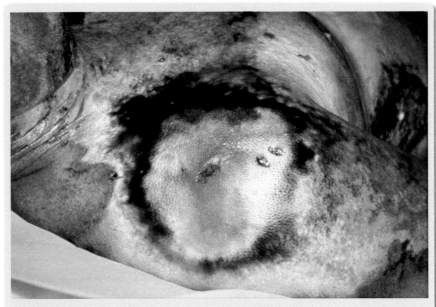

FIGURE 9-20 The skin is the organ most often injured in a lightning strike victim.

The heart establishes a normal rhythm, but quite quickly it will deteriorate due to lack of available oxygen because the respiratory centers are not operating. The patient dies a second time.

Signs and symptoms associated with lightning strikes can be seen in the nervous and cardiovascular systems. Injuries to the nervous system include:

- Loss of consciousness
- Confusion
- Amnesia
- Acute pain
- Numbness
- Neurocognitive deficits
- Peripheral nerve damage
- Spinal cord injury
- Epidural and/or subdural hematoma
- Cerebral edema
- Transient blindness
- Unreactive or unequal pupils
- Corneal edema
- Intraocular hemorrhage
- Tympanic membrane perforation
- Deafness

Cardiovascular symptoms include:

- QT prolongation
- ST segment changes
- Premature ventricular contractions (PVCs)
- Tachycardia
- Bradycardia
- Asystole (most common lethal rhythm)
- Ventricular fibrillation
- Severe vasospasm resulting in pulseless extremity

As the energy travels through the nervous system, damage can occur. Seizures are one of the most obvious effects. The massive current impulse causes cells within the brain to fire. Organized activity erodes and is replaced by random cell firing. Couple this grand mal (tonic-clonic) seizure with respiratory arrest, and brain cells will be depleted of oxygen and glucose a short time after the strike.

Another phenomenon that can occur affects the extremities. Patients may have cold, pale, pulseless, paralyzed limbs. This can be clinically confusing. The spinal cord and peripheral nerves may be damaged in such a way that prevents signals from the cerebral cortex from reaching the extremities. These peripheral nerves also provide signals to the blood vessels, so severe vasospasm can occur. This combination can lead care providers to assume the patient is in shock. This effect is caused by nerve impairment and not loss of blood volume.

During this massive discharge, muscles can contract violently and patients can suffer minor to severe musculoskeletal trauma. Falls from the strike may cause fractures or dislocations. In addition, the shockwave caused by the violent heating/expansion and subsequent rapid cooling/compression of the air can propel patients up to 10 m (30′).

Presentation of Injuries

Patients who have been struck can be categorized into minor, moderate, or severe injuries. Although the majority of patients suffering lightning strikes will survive, severe and greatly disabling injuries can be incurred. **TABLE 9-9** outlines the common presentations based on the degree of acuity.

Further discussion of the types of burn patterns is warranted. There are six types of burn patterns typically found in lightning strike patients. Each has its own cause and unique pattern rarely found in other pathologies. Treatment of burns is discussed in Chapter 8.

- **Linear burns:** As the flashover effect occurs, moisture is vaporized. Wherever there are concentrations of moisture, one can experience burns. Areas commonly associated with linear burns are the axilla, under the breasts, and over the top of the sternum.
- **Keraunographic marks:** Fern-like patterns appearing on the skin indicate keraunographic marks, also called feathering, lightning prints, or Lichtenberg's figures or flowers. These are not true burns because

TABLE 9-9	Common Lightning Injuries	
Degree of Acuity	**Common Presentation**	**Progression of Presentation**
Minor	Antegrade amnesia, confusion, temporary loss of consciousness, temporary deafness, tinnitus, blindness, dysesthesias within extremities, neurocognitive deficits, aphasia, and mild hypertension	Usually transient; patients can have lifelong deficits.
Moderate	Disorientation, combativeness, coma, lower extremity dysfunction, cardiopulmonary standstill with spontaneous recovery, seizures, and partial-thickness burns	Patients are prone to sleep disorders, fine motor deficits, weakness, and nervous system dysfunctions.
Severe	Cardiac arrest	Good recovery is possible with prompt CPR. Poor survival if CPR is delayed.

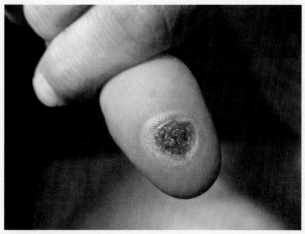

FIGURE 9-21 Punctuated burns present as small, circular burn marks.

there is no skin damage. They are thought to be caused by capillary damage and subsequent leaking of red blood cells underneath the skin. This injury resembles the effect of placing a feather over the skin, shining a bright light on the feather, and having the resulting shadow imprinted on the skin.

- **Punctuated burns:** Punctuated burns are small, circular burn marks over dry skin. They resemble cigarette burns **FIGURE 9-21**.
- **Classic thermal burns:** These occur if the patient's clothing catches fire. They appear as other burns that are seen from thermal injury.
- **Contact burns:** These result from the heating of metal objects (eg, glasses, jewelry, belt buckles, and zippers) on the person or on the person's clothing.
- **Flash burns:** These are caused by the excessive heat of the flashover, resulting in a brownish, discolored partial-thickness burn.

The nervous system is particularly prone to damage. Antegrade amnesia, or memory loss from the time of the strike, is a common finding. Neurocognitive deficits may also be seen. These deficits are very subtle and it takes a keen assessment eye to discover them. Patients are typically

able to hold entire casual conversations without evidence of deficit to the provider. Testing the patient's memory skills may reveal more valuable information. Tell the patient your name and then see if they can remember your name later. Instruct the patient to remember a series of seven random numbers. Later during the transportation, ask the patient to repeat the number list accurately.

Talk in detail about the patient's past, likes and dislikes, job activities, sports facts, and so on. This more in-depth conversation may yield gaps in the patient's ability to recall and process information. Ensure that your conversation involves the patient's past memory as well as new memories.

As with other assessments of memory, guide the conversation to areas with which you are familiar. This will provide you with a foundation to determine if the patient's responses are accurate. Also, do not be afraid to ask the patient how it feels to concentrate on a subject. The patient may report that it is difficult to recall certain facts or that his or her mind seems to be wandering.

Patients can suffer from a wide array of symptoms. A stroke-like presentation is possible. The centers of the brain involved in speech and object recognition can be impaired. Patients can experience **aphasia** (the inability to communicate through speech, writing, or signs because of brain dysfunction), **agnosia** (the inability to comprehend auditory, visual, or sensational stimuli, even though the eyes, ears, and other sensory organs are intact), or **apraxia** (the inability to perform purposeful movements when the motor and sensory organs are not directly impaired). In combination with a paralyzed limb, providers may draw the incorrect conclusion that a stroke has occurred. The key to correct management is a detailed, complete assessment.

Although some of these subtle nervous system effects may take days or months to manifest, they are important to note. Patients can experience severe personality and cognitive impairments. Short-term memory can be damaged, although prestrike memory is usually intact and stable. The ability to concentrate on tasks, problem-solving skills, and multitasking is often impaired. This brain damage can lead to social isolation, job loss, and depression.

Management of Lightning Injuries

Care for the patient who has been struck by lightning begins with the mantra of emergency care: Is the scene safe? Lightning has no memory; it certainly can strike twice in the same location. Tall buildings are struck often. See the next section on lightning safety for recommendations on how to be safe during a thunderstorm.

Once it is determined safe to enter a scene, care should begin with triage. There is a significant change in philosophy when caring for lightning strike patients as compared to other mass casualty traumatic events. Patients involved in a multiple car accident, when discovered dead, are passed over so care can be rendered to the living. But in lighting strikes, patients who are pulseless and apneic should be cared for first. This **reverse triage** approach is based on the concept that patients may be dead simply because of a disconnection between the nervous and cardiovascular systems. In addition, patients who are alive have already reconnected these two body systems and typically need only supportive care.

It is important to note that although many of these patients who are in cardiac arrest are in good physical health and are relatively young, there is no supporting data that suggests increased survival after prolonged CPR. As with other normothermic patients, chance of recovery after 20–30 minutes of resuscitation is very poor. Unusual heroics in attempting to resuscitate these patients are not warranted.

Cardiac arrest management is accomplished using the same algorithms as those for nonlightning injuries. As with other arrest victims, it is important to focus on what has caused cardiac arrest. Lightning strike patients suffer cardiac arrest initially from an electrical overload to the heart causing asystole. Respiratory arrest occurs at the same time. If the heart restarts before the respiratory center can provide sufficient oxygen, cardiac arrest will reoccur, this time due to tissue hypoxia.

The other reasonable causes for cardiac arrest in a lightning strike may revolve around the force of the blast. Though rare, hypovolemia due to blunt trauma, fractures, or chest or abdominal injuries is possible. Examine the jugular veins while performing effective compressions. Jugular venous distension (JVD) is a normal finding during CPR, but flat jugular veins may indicate severe blood loss. In cases where a hypovolemic cause for cardiac arrest is suspected, IV fluids should be administered.

For patients suffering from minor to moderate injuries, assessment stands at the core of effective patient care. Patients involved should have all clothing removed to ensure an accurate and detailed examination. After the patient has received an initial/primary and rapid trauma/secondary assessment, use the information in **TABLE 9-10** to guide your detailed assessment.

TABLE 9-10	Detailed Assessment Focus Point
Body System	**Detailed Assessment**
Nervous system	Monitor for changes in level of consciousness—either increasing or decreasing. Determine orientation to person, place, time, and event.
	Assess patient affect. Is the patient calm, confused, cooperative, anxious, irritable, angry, crying? What is the patient's mood?
	Listen closely to speech. Assess clarity and appropriate use of words and sentence structure.
	Perform a cranial nerve test.
	Test memory skills. Ask the patient to remember a series of seven numbers. Ask them to remember your name, the name of the ambulance, or something similar.
	Perform a pupil and visual acuity test.
	Perform a hearing test bilaterally. Speak into one ear and then the other.
	Assess motor skills. Have the patient follow commands to move arms and legs, squeeze hands, tap each finger on thumb, and so on.
Cardiovascular system	Apply the ECG monitor and perform a 12 lead. Continuous cardiac monitoring is recommended for all patients due to dysrhythmia and ST changes.
	Monitor vital signs with close attention to blood pressure.
Respiratory	Assess respiratory pattern.
	Note use of accessory muscles and/or retractions.
	Assess lung sounds.
Genitourinary	Assess for incontinence.
Extremities	Closely evaluate bilateral peripheral pulses. Assess for equality.
	Assess skin color and temperature for evidence of severe vasoconstriction.

Standard care for a lightning strike is directed at support. If the patient begins to seize, an antiseizure medication such as diazepam may be indicated. Hypovolemic shock due to blast trauma should be approached as with other traumatic injuries. Neurocognitive deficits should be documented and a very supportive, caring environment maintained. Regardless of whether the patient has injuries, being struck by lightning is a terrifying experience.

Below is an outline of care for lighting strike patients:

1. Reverse triage.
2. Spinal immobilization when required.
3. Oxygen—base delivery method on stability of patient.
4. Standard care for any burns. Usually burns are so superficial they will require little care.

5. Close assessment and reassessment of nervous system.
6. During cardiac arrest, follow standard advanced cardiac life support (ACLS) guidelines.
7. IV access to keep vein open. Patients may be prone to intracranial edema.
8. Administration of fluids to patients with evidence of hypovolemia.
9. Cardiac monitoring. Treat arrhythmias following ACLS guidelines.
10. 12-lead ECG when possible.
11. Seizure management following standard seizure protocol.
12. Encourage all patients to be transported for evaluation in the emergency department.
13. Take seizure precautions. Pad railings on ambulance cot. Do not restrain patient.
14. Provide emotional support.

Lightning Safety

It is important to understand that you can make wise decisions to help reduce your risk of being struck by lightning. One of the most effective ways to limit your risk is to have information and a plan. Because most lightning is associated with thunderstorms, Internet weather sites are a valuable resource that can provide local and regional Doppler radar, allowing you to estimate the speed, direction, and intensity of storms. Recently, lightning strike data have been added to help people determine the danger level of a storm.

Know where shelters are in the area you are entering and how to get there quickly. Your ambulance will provide some level of safety. When out in the storm, even without online information, you can still decrease your chances of becoming a victim.

Lightning travels at nearly the speed of light. This is fast enough to go around the world approximately eight times in one second. It is so fast that it will appear to be instantaneous to the naked eye. Sound, however, travels much slower at approximately 1.6 kilometers (1 mile) in 5 seconds. To estimate where the storm is, count the seconds between the flash of lightning and the sound of thunder.

For every 5 seconds between lightning flash and thunder, the lightning strike occurred an additional 1 mile away. You are in the danger zone and should seek shelter whenever the storm is within 5–6 miles, or you hear the thunder 25 to 30 seconds or less after seeing the flash of light.

Seek shelter in a substantial structure or all-metal vehicle. Avoid convertibles or vehicles with soft tops. Outbuildings like sheds, bus shelters, and golf shelters are not considered safe. Tents, especially those with metal support rods, may actually increase your risk of being struck. If planning a gathering, having a group of vehicles nearby as a shelter is certainly a good idea.

If no buildings or shelters are available, seek a location where you are not the tallest object. Avoid metal objects such as towers, power lines, fences, pipelines, and ski lifts. Do not seek shelter out in a field or clearing. This makes you the tallest object.

TIP

When you hear thunder within 25 to 30 seconds or less following a flash of lightning, you are in the danger zone and should seek shelter. Remember the 30 and 30 rule. If you hear the thunder within 30 seconds of seeing the flash, seek shelter. Wait at least 30 minutes after the last lightning is seen before resuming normal activities.

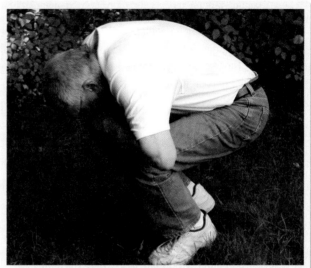

FIGURE 9-22 If you are in an open area and at risk for a lightning strike, assume the lightning position.

If you are caught in the open, you should assume the **lightning position** FIGURE 9-22. Get into a squatting, seated, cross-legged position or a kneeling position. These positions are maintainable for several minutes for the average person. Sitting in this position will decrease the amount of surface area exposed to the ground while decreasing the overall height of the person. People should not gather together, but try to place at least several yards distance between each other. Clustering individuals provides a larger target with potentially more than one victim injured.

If you need to call for help, cell phones are considered to be safe to operate during thunderstorms. Although landlines are susceptible to energy transmission down the phone line and therefore into the user of the phone, cell phones, which receive their signal via electromagnetic radiation, cannot transmit lightning energy.

In summary, death from lightning strikes is rare. Scene safety and appropriate planning are essential to preventing providers from becoming victims. Care for victims begins with rapid CPR, as needed, using a reverse triage approach. Care for individuals not in cardiac arrest is mainly supportive, with excellent assessment skills needed to find subtle injuries. Lightning victims may have peculiar patterns of burns and injuries that should help lead the provider to the correct field impression. Finally, emotional support for patients who have been struck is essential.

CHAPTER RESOURCES

CASE STUDY ANSWERS

1 How could scene safety have been improved?

Preplanning and training could have helped the first responders recognize and prepare for safe action in the unstable environment. The on-scene plan should have included a plan for how to rescue a rescuer if it should become necessary. The insecure and dynamic nature of EMS places providers at risk for many hazards at a trauma scene, making scene safety a priority at every incident.

2 How does being immersed in water affect body temperature?

The density of water surrounding the body will allow heat to transfer 25 times more efficiently than through air. The temperature gradient is yet another factor when considering thermal transfer. This patient will become colder quicker in the water than if she were in the cold air.

3 Will the patient's body temperature continue to be affected if she remains in her wet clothing?

Wet clothing allows moisture to evaporate away from the body, taking heat with it. Much like sweating allows the body to cool, wet clothing wicks heat away from the body. It is important to remove wet clothing and dry the patient to decrease additional heat loss by the patient.

4 Does this patient's medical history affect her ability to control her temperature?

This patient has a history of cardiac arrhythmia that is controlled by a beta blocker. This medication can block the body's ability to compensate for rapid heat loss and alter the assessment findings. Many medical conditions and medications can interfere with the body's response to cold.

5 Does this patient require aggressive warming?

This patient appears to be in mild hypothermia as represented by the shivering, loss of fine motor control, and amnesia. The most prudent care would require only passive warming in a warm environment after removing the wet clothes.

Trauma in Motion

1. Does your agency have a plan to deal with a large gathering if a heat or cold event were to exist? How do you fit into that plan?

2. What steps could you take to prepare yourself to perform your job safely if several days of hot weather were expected? What would you do for cold?

3. How does heavy safety gear affect the body's ability to regulate temperature? Are additional precautions required?

4. Does your system track weather changes that can affect health concerns in your town, such as people who are homeless or low income who might require heat or cooling during temperature extremes?

5. In every environment there is the ability to become too hot or too cold given an emergency situation. Nontraditional causes for thermal emergencies might include working in a factory where heat is part of the production process or being stuck in water or cool liquid for an extended time. List three ways a patient might experience a hypothermic emergency in your town. List three ways heat may be the cause of an emergency.

References and Resources

American Heart Association. Hypothermia. *Circ.* 2005; IV-136–IV-138.

Auerbach P. *Wilderness Medicine.* 5th ed. St Louis: Mosby; 2007.

Auerbach P, Donner H, Weiss E. *Field Guide to Wilderness Medicine.* 3rd ed. St Louis: Mosby; 2008.

Bouchama A, Dehbi M, Chaves-Carballo E. Cooling and hemodynamic management of heatstroke: practical recommendations. *Crit Care.* 2007; 11:R54. Available at: http://ccforum.com/content/11/3/R54. Accessed December 6, 2007.

Casa D, McDermott B, Lee E, et al. Cold Water Immersion: The Gold Standard for Exertional Heatstroke Treatment. *Exerc Sport Sci Rev.* 2007; 35(3):141–149.

Commonwealth of Australia, Bureau of Meteorology. Severe thunderstorms: facts, warnings and protection. Available at: www.bom.gov.au/info/thunder/. Accessed July 15, 2008.

Cooper M. Lightning injuries. *eMedicine.* Available at: http://emedicine.medscape.com/article/770642-overview. Accessed October 26, 2005.

Edlich R. Burns, lightning injuries. *eMedicine.* Available at: http://emedicine.medscape.com/article/1278040-overview. Accessed September 5, 2007.

Gatewood M, Zane R. Lightning injuries. *Emerg Med Clin North Am.* 2004; 22(2):369–403.

Glazer J. Management of heatstroke and heat exhaustion. *Am Fam Physician.* 2005; 71(11):2133–2140.

Hadad E, Rav-Acha M, Heled Y, et al. Heat stroke—a review of cooling methods. *Sports Med.* 2004; 34(8):501–511.

Joint Royal Colleges Ambulance Liaison Committee. Trauma emergencies, the immersion incident. *UK Ambulance Service Clinical Practice Guidelines.* October 2006. Available at: http://www2.warwick.ac.uk/fac/med/research/hsri/emergencycare/jrcalc_2006/guidelines/the_immersion_incident_2006.pdf. Accessed July 15, 2008.

Kithi R. Manifestations of lightning deaths and injuries. *National Lightning Safety Institute.* Available at: www.lightningsafety.com/nlsi_lls/deaths_injuries01.html. Accessed December 2007.

Lugo-Amador N, Rothenhaus T, Moyer P. Heat-related illness. *Emerg Med Clin North Am.* 2004; 22(2):315–327.

National Weather Service. NWS windchill index. Available at: www.nws.noaa.gov/om/windchill/index.shtml. Accessed November 27, 2006.

Plasqui G, Kester A, Westerterp K. Seasonal variation in sleeping metabolic rate, thyroid activity and leptin. *Am J Physiol Endocrinol Metab.* 2003; 285:E338–E343.

Statistics Canada. Home page. Available at: www.statcan.ca/start.html. Accessed July 15, 2008.

Ulrich A, Rathlev N. Hypothermia and localized cold injuries. *Emerg Med Clin North Am.* 2004; 22(2):281–298.

US Search and Rescue Task Force. Cold water survival. Available at: www.ussartf.org/cold_water_survival.htm. Accessed December 6, 2007.

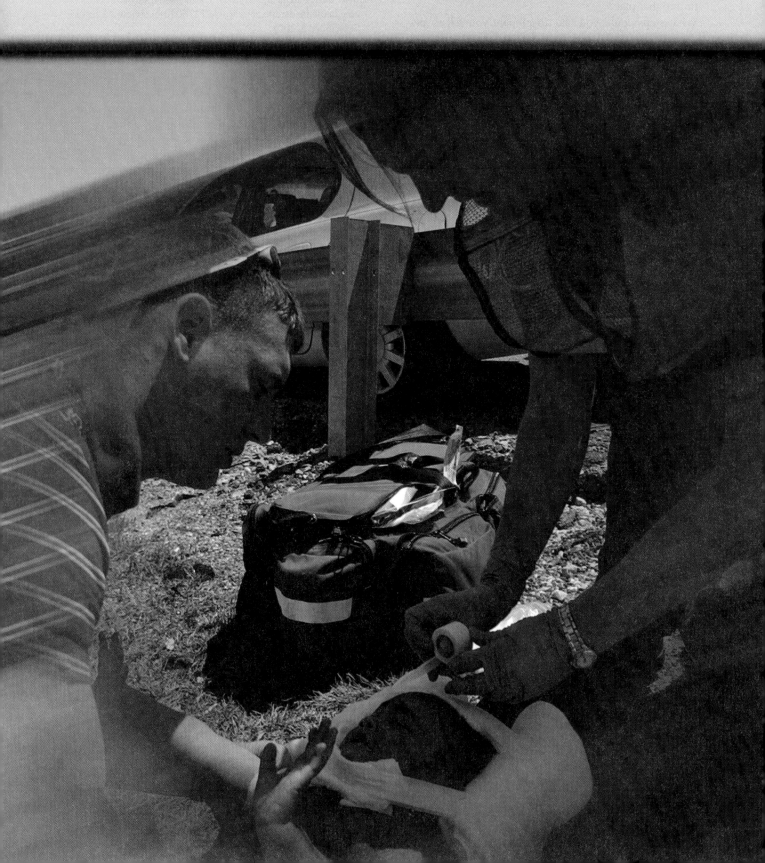

You are dispatched to the scene of a motor vehicle collision for a child with injuries. Updates from the scene report a 2-year-old girl who is awake and crying. Your stress level drops slightly as you begin to mentally prepare to care for a young child. Upon arriving at the scene you notice a midsize car with significant damage to the rear passenger door. There is a child seat in the rear seat that has been pushed further into the car by the collision.

You are directed onto the shoulder of the roadway where a woman is holding a screaming child. The woman introduces herself as the child's mother and begs you to help her child. The child does not stop crying, even when her mother tries to soothe her. You notice the child is holding herself upright in mom's arms but she does not appear to be paying attention to her mother or to your arrival. You also notice a hematoma starting to develop above her right ear.

The child has a good, strong cry and appears to take a good strong breath in between cries. You feel for a radial pulse and find a weak, rapid pulse; the child's hand is cool to the touch. You immediately begin a rapid trauma/secondary assessment that reveals pain in the lower right ribs. The pulse is 140 beats/min, blood pressure is 82/40 mm Hg, and respirations are 36 breaths/min as best as you can count with her crying. Pulse oximetry is 98% and she is moving all of her extremities well. You immobilize the child and begin transport to the hospital with the mother on board.

1 How can the child's appearance assist you in your assessment?

2 Are the child's signs and symptoms significant for shock, or are they signs of pain or anxiety?

3 You cannot find a cervical collar to fit the child. How should you immobilize the child's spine?

4 Should this child be transported to a trauma center?

5 How would your answers change if the patient were the driver's elderly mother?

Introduction

Trauma is the leading cause of death among children older than 1 year of age. Motor vehicle collisions cause the most deaths in this age group, followed by falls and submersions. Death from injury in people older than 65 years old accounts for one fourth of all trauma deaths in the United States and is one of the top 10 causes of death among elderly people worldwide. Approximately 6% to 8% of pregnant women will experience some type of trauma during pregnancy, usually during their third trimester. Major causes of trauma during pregnancy are motor vehicle collisions, falls, domestic abuse, and penetrating trauma such as gunshot wounds. An obese patient is more likely to die from blunt force trauma than his or her leaner counterpart.

As prehospital providers, we may not be able to change these events but we can take the necessary steps to gain the knowledge that may make a difference in the outcome.

Pediatric Trauma

Half of the children seen by emergency medical services (EMS) in the United States are acute injuries **FIGURE 10-1**. That ratio is one third in the United Kingdom. Injuries that young patients sustain vary across the pediatric age groups based on psychological and physiologic development. Prehospital providers must be able to modify their assessment and treatment skills based on the developmental level and social maturity unique to each pediatric age group. Fear and pain can make the assessment of children suffering from injuries difficult, and EMS providers must know how to contend with distraught and sometimes irrational parents or caregivers.

Differences in Anatomy and Physiology

At no time in the human lifespan will the body and mind change as drastically as during childhood. There are many unique features that affect children's assessment and treatment. A solid understanding of these anatomic and physiologic differences in the pediatric population will help the prehospital provider perform his or her duties with confidence and success.

Head

Young children have very large heads in comparison to their body mass. A large head means more surface area and increases the incidence of head injuries because when children fall they tend to land on their heads. Traumatic brain injury is the leading cause of death and significant disability in pediatric trauma. A large head can interfere with attempts at spinal immobilization because the larger occiput flexes the head forward when the child lies on a flat surface. This inequality between the patient's head and torso can be minimized by placing a pad under the torso effectively raising the torso and bringing the spine back into neutral alignment **FIGURE 10-2**. Failure to pay attention to this anatomic difference could lead to poor spinal immobilization and airway occlusion.

Airway

The neck and airway of pediatric patients have some significant differences from adults'. The pediatric tongue is proportionally much larger than in an adult and therefore presents an increased risk for airway obstruction. The pediatric trachea is smaller and narrower than in an adult, making it more susceptible to obstruction with positioning or secretions **FIGURE 10-3**. Newborns are obligate nasal breathers, so congestion may increase their level of respiratory distress because they are unable to breathe through their mouths. Pediatric patients have an increased amount of soft tissue

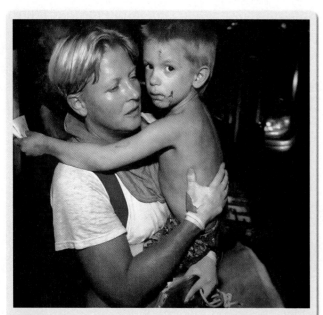

FIGURE 10-1 Injury is a large part of EMS calls involving children.

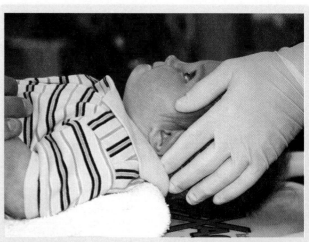

FIGURE 10-2 The child's head is larger in proportion to the body than an adult's and a pad under the torso can assist in spinal immobilization.

in their airways that may be susceptible to swelling from trauma, virus, or allergic reaction.

Finally, remember that the narrowest part of a young child's airway occurs at the cricoid cartilage rather than at the vocal cords as found in adults. This anatomic difference may influence your choice of airway management, especially the size of an endotracheal (ET) tube. Intubation requires working around a larger, more horseshoe-shaped epiglottis that is more vagally innervated than in an adult.

Spine

The vertebral column is developing as the child grows. Ligaments are more lax, which allows for increased mobility and the potential for cord injury, even in the absence of identifiable fractures and dislocations. This is a condition known as spinal cord injury without radiographic abnormalities (SCIWORA). This may present to EMS as a patient with neurologic injury of unknown origin.

Chest and Abdomen

The pediatric chest wall is more flexible than that of adults. Chest trauma is the third leading cause of serious injury in pediatric trauma. Children may have fewer rib fractures and flail chest events, but there is a significant increase in pulmonary and cardiac contusions due to the pliability of the chest. A young child's chest has considerably less muscle mass and subcutaneous fat and their rib cage is more com-

pliant. Infants and small children have fewer alveoli, so to enhance minute volume they need to breathe faster to compensate for decreased oxygenation. Compensated shock is likely to be accompanied by an increased respiratory rate and higher minute volume.

The term *belly breather* comes from the infant age group that is dependent on the use of the diaphragm as the primary muscle used during respirations. Injuries associated with the chest and abdomen will have a significant effect on a child's ability to breathe.

A child's ribs are more horizontal in shape and have much less musculature than an adult's. This forms a smaller proportion of the torso that is afforded the protection of the rib cage. The lack of developed musculature in the chest wall can also lead to a child tiring quickly when the body is forced to increase the respiratory rate or depth. Less developed abdominal muscles decrease the protection of internal organs and prehospital providers should expect more intra-abdominal injuries in the pediatric population than in adults. Abdominal injuries are the second leading cause of trauma in children (after head injuries).

Children are more prone to chest injuries than adults are, especially in the instance of a motor vehicle collision. When struck by a moving vehicle in a standing position, an adult will most likely sustain lower extremity injuries, whereas a child struck by the same vehicle is more likely to

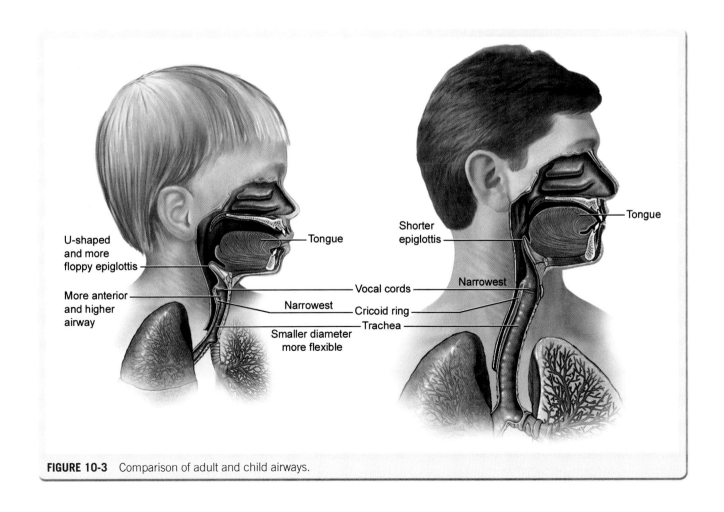

FIGURE 10-3 Comparison of adult and child airways.

have chest and abdomen injuries from the primary impact, and then head injuries from the secondary collision when thrown to the ground.

Children's intra-abdominal organs are larger in proportion than in an adult, which puts them at risk for injury during blunt trauma incidents. The pediatric body has not had time to develop, so there is less muscle tone and less fat protecting thoracic and abdominal organs. It is possible to have catastrophic injury in the abdominal cavity without major outward signs. The liver and spleen actually extend below the protective cover of the ribs, making them easy organs for injury.

Musculoskeletal

The growth plates of a child's bones are made of cartilage, are relatively weak, and can be damaged easily. These growth plates extend the length of long bones through the formation of new bone on the surface of the epiphyseal plates. In the epiphyseal plate, osteoclasts remove the cartilage and new deposits of calcium are left by osteoblasts, a process known as remodeling. When an injury occurs at the epiphyseal plate, unequal growth may occur, interrupting the remodeling process and making long-term disability possible. Most growth plates will cease the production of new growth by late adolescence. The bones of growing children are weaker than the ligaments, making fractures more common than sprains.

Compensation for Blood Loss

Children are legendary for their ability to compensate while in hypovolemic shock. Cardiac output is rate dependent in infants and young children. They have a relatively poor ability to increase stroke volume, which is reflected in rate response to physiologic stress and hypovolemia. Pediatric patients also compensate through vasoconstriction, similar to adults, but more pliable blood vessels allow the child greater control over the vascular bed. When a child suffers a dramatic insult that causes them to become hypovolemic, they may lose up to 25% of their blood volume prior to showing any outward sign of insult. Baroreceptors in the aortic arch and carotid sinus are stimulated by hypotension, and as a result the body stimulates an increase in heart rate, blood pressure, and cardiac output. A child's renin-angiotensin system will allow for reuptake of sodium and water. Chemoreceptors respond to sudden acidosis and result in both vasoconstriction and respiratory stimulation. Humoral responses within the circulatory system lead to a catecholamine release, stimulating contractility and vasoconstriction. And finally, autotransfusion within the circulatory system allows for reabsorption of interstitial fluid. Remember that when a child is in compensated shock, vital organ functions are maintained and the blood pressure remains normal.

Developmental Changes

Each age comes with its own stages of psychological development and characteristics. Unlike an adult who is usually calmed by the appearance of EMS following an injury, the young child may fear the new arrivals. There are several

TABLE 10-1 Pediatric Development Changes		
Development Stage	Age	Milestone
Neonate/infant	0–1 year	Sleeps, sits, babbles, crawls
Toddler	1–3 years	Language development, walks
Preschool-age	3–6 years	Verbal, interactive, understands
School-age	6–12 years	Analytical, abstract thought
Adolescent	13 years–adult	Experimentation, risk taking

milestones during development that affect the types of injuries a child may receive TABLE 10-1.

Infants have a limited number of behaviors during the first 2 months of life. Because they are completely dependent on caregivers for feeding, movement, and temperature control, child abuse should be suspected when they are injured. From 2 months to 1 year old, the child will learn to roll over, reach and grab items, and crawl around, making injuries from movement more possible. Infants prefer a warm environment and should be examined in a warm, quiet area.

Toddlers begin to walk, play with toys, and communicate with others. This new freedom, combined with the lack of fear of the universe around them, makes toddlers prone to injury. Bumps and bruises on the shins and knees may be a product of the normally clumsy attempts at walking. Burns from pulling a hot item onto them through curiosity can be explained. However, child abuse becomes more prevalent in this age group. Toddlers begin to develop separation anxiety, which may require a toe-to-head approach following the ABCs to assess further injury.

Preschool-age children develop the use of language but are still illogical thinkers. Many behaviors may be misinterpreted as punishment for bad actions. This group becomes more mobile and is transported more often in automobiles, making motor vehicle collisions a more common form of trauma.

School-age children are able to understand cause and effect. Their knowledge of how bodies work is sketchy and they have limited ability to judge the seriousness of injuries. Common fears for this group include separation from parents, loss of control, pain, and physical deformity. During the school years, children become more active in sports and motion activities (bicycling, skating, and running). Bicycling injuries with or without automobile collision are possible FIGURE 10-4.

Adolescents are very mobile but sometimes seem to lack common sense. These years are a time of experimentation and risk-taking behavior, leaving them prone to injury. New drivers account for the highest rate of motor vehicle

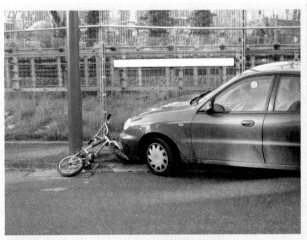

FIGURE 10-4 Bicycling injuries become more common in preschool and school-age children.

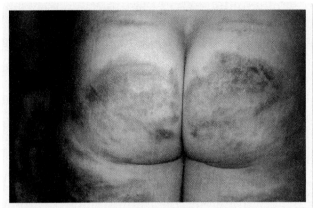

FIGURE 10-5 Child abuse is a possible cause of trauma to young patients.

TABLE 10-2 Top 10 Unintentional Injuries Seen in Children Under Age 15 Worldwide
Concussion/contusion of the brain
Open wound
Poisoning
Fracture of radius or ulna
Burns (< 20% total body surface area affected)
Fractured clavicle, scapula, or humerus
Internal injuries
Fractured femur
Fractured patella, tibia, or fibula
Fractured hand bones

injury of any age group. Their bodies have become more like an adult's but they are still developing socially and psychologically.

Injury Patterns

Blunt trauma is the mechanism of injury (MOI) observed in more than 90% of all pediatric trauma cases. Because children have less muscle and fat mass than adults do, they also have less protection. Injury patterns need to be assessed by MOI and anatomic region involved, which includes specific anatomic differences TABLE 10-2.

Bicycle injuries are frequent in the preschool and school-age group, especially with the child who is starting to learn how to operate a bicycle. The characteristic injury pattern involves hitting the handlebars during a fall, which can produce duodenal hematomas and/or pancreatic injuries. Prehospital providers must also consider head injuries in a child who is not wearing protective equipment, like a helmet.

Motor vehicle collisions present with a wide variety of injury patterns based on the child's age and position in the vehicle, and whether the child was using safety restraints or a correctly sized child seat. Restrained children may sustain chest and abdominal injuries from seatbelts. With seatbelt injuries, prehospital providers must also have a high index of suspicion for spinal trauma. One must also consider the pediatric patient's relative position and size when there is a deployment of air bags in a motor vehicle. Providers can see injuries to the head, neck, chest, spine, and abdomen from air bag deployment.

Car-versus-pedestrian collisions are likely to produce multisystem trauma, which is dependent on the speed of the vehicle, the child's height, and the height of the vehicle's bumper. The injuries produced will typically be chest, abdominal, and lower extremity injuries from the impact and head and neck injuries sustained when the child is thrown to the ground.

Falls are common in pediatric patients, and the injuries are consistent with physiologic and anatomic development. An infant, with a large head and undeveloped protective reflexes, could easily sustain a skull fracture and possibly an intracranial hemorrhage whereas an older child typically will sustain long bone fractures due to outstretched arms during a fall.

EMS providers need to be aware of the potential for child abuse when dealing with pediatric patients FIGURE 10-5. Abuse can be physical, emotional, sexual, or neglect. Children younger than 5 years are at the highest risk for abuse. Child maltreatment occurs in all ethnic and socioeconomic groups from the richest mansion to the poorest household. Be a child advocate, consider the possibility of child maltreatment, and if you suspect abuse, document your findings in detail, being sure to inform the emergency department staff. If you suspect any sort of abuse, it is your duty to report it in accordance with your local jurisdiction. Common signs of child abuse can be found in the CHILD ABUSE mnemonic in TABLE 10-3.

TABLE 10-3 CHILD ABUSE Mnemonic for Suspicion of Child Abuse

C	Consistency of the injury with the child's developmental age
H	History inconsistent with injury
I	Inappropriate parental concerns
L	Lack of supervision
D	Delay in seeking care
A	Affect (of the parent or caregiver and the child in relation to the caregiver)
B	Bruises of varying ages
U	Unusual injury patterns
S	Suspicious circumstances
E	Environmental clues

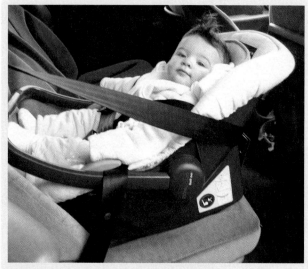

FIGURE 10-6 Infants under 10 kg (22 lb) should be in a rear-facing car seat.

Child Safety Seats

Because of young children's small stature and their underdeveloped musculoskeletal systems, seatbelts cannot provide a proper and safe means of restraining them in the event of a crash. Safety seats are designed for each age group, must fit appropriately, and must be used in any type of moving vehicle to provide the additional safety measures needed to protect the fragile pediatric population. In the first year following the new car seat law in Great Britain, the number of children under 12 injured in vehicle collisions dropped by more than 1,000.

Types of child safety restraints vary by age, manufacturer, and intended use. Many areas have adopted child seat legislation; check your local areas to see if car seats are legislated and the specifics of their use. Some guidelines are provided by the National Highway Traffic Safety Administration (NHTSA) and are very similar to the guidelines from the United Kingdom's Department for Transport. Infant seats are designed for children from birth until at least 9 kg (20 lb) and/or 1 year of age **FIGURE 10-6**. A weight of 20 lb becomes key because if an infant is forward facing and there is a deceleration injury, extremely strong gravitational forces affect the small bones in the neck and head. The resulting injuries from an infant who is too small in a forward-facing car seat may be cervical spine fracture (with spinal column elongation by up to 2″ [5 cm]) or closed head injury. Some car seat literature points out that a child may be changed from a rear-facing position to a forward-facing position when his or her feet touch the seat back or must be bent to get him or her into the seat.

Convertible safety seats will convert from rear-facing for infants to forward-facing for toddlers weighing at least 10 kg (22 lb). Children should remain in a forward-facing seat from 10 kg (22 lb) until they reach approximately 18 kg (40 lb) and 4 years of age **FIGURE 10-7**. At that time, children can move to a booster seat. Booster seats are designed for children older than 4 years old who have not grown tall enough to fit the adult restraint systems (57″ [1.5 m] tall, or usually by age 9 years) **FIGURE 10-8**. These seats are used

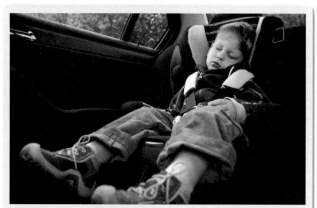

FIGURE 10-7 Children between 9 kg and 18 kg (20 lb and 40 lb) should ride in an approved child restraint device.

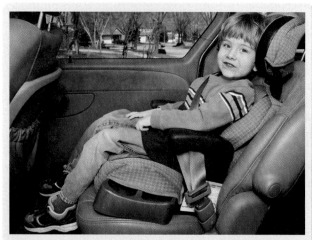

FIGURE 10-8 Place children in a booster seat until they become large enough to fit an adult seatbelt.

as a transition to safety belts by older kids who have clearly outgrown their convertible seat and are not quite ready for the vehicle belt system. Some automobile manufacturers have designed these seats hidden into the conventional interiors of some vehicles. When a child finally is old enough and large enough to be secured in an adult safety belt, they can be moved out of a booster seat. To size an adult safety belt properly, the lap belt should fit snugly and properly across the upper thighs and the shoulder strap should cross over the shoulder and across the chest, not over the child's abdomen.

The international consensus confirms that seatbelts save lives, and countries have fallen into line with mandating seatbelt usage. In Canada, the driver is responsible for ensuring that passengers younger than 16 years use their seatbelt. Over the age of 16, passengers are responsible for ensuring that they wear their own safety belt. England has similar car seat laws to the United States, and anyone older than 14 years is responsible for wearing a safety belt if one is available. (It is the driver's responsibility to ensure safety belt usage in passengers younger than 14 years.)

Alterations in Assessment

The scene size-up and initial/primary assessment in pediatric trauma patients use a similar approach to that of other trauma patients. Prehospital providers can use a hands-off approach when making a general impression, except in cases where there are serious problems with the ABCs and immediate hands-on intervention is necessary. In pediatrics, the pediatric assessment triangle (PAT), which is a "from-the-doorway" approach, can be used to make an important distinction between sick and not-sick pediatric patients **FIGURE 10-9**. The PAT approach includes three important and specific elements—the child's appearance, work of breathing, and circulation to the skin. It employs a rapid method of assessing a pediatric patient without using your hands and will answer three important and necessary questions:

1. Is the patient sick or not sick?
2. What is the most likely physiologic abnormality?
3. Does the child require emergency treatment?

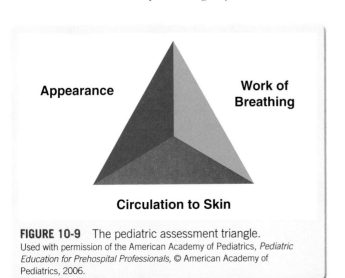

FIGURE 10-9 The pediatric assessment triangle.
Used with permission of the American Academy of Pediatrics, *Pediatric Education for Prehospital Professionals,* © American Academy of Pediatrics, 2006.

TABLE 10-4		Mnemonic to Assess Appearance
T	Tone	Muscle tone is a good indicator of how a child is doing. A child reduces movement to shunt energy to needed areas of the body.
I	Interactivity	A child should be naturally interactive with his or her caregivers. Children who do not interact are not well.
C	Consolability	Although a young child who is hurt is expected to cry, a child who cannot be consoled for even a short time is an indicator for a sick child.
L	Look or gaze	Children should look at movement around them. A child who does not look or watch the movement around them shows decreased mentation.
S	Speech or cry	Can the child speak or cry? Is it loud or soft? Movement of air through the vocal cords can demonstrate good air movement and an open airway.

Appearance reflects adequacy of ventilation, oxygenation, brain perfusion, body homeostasis, and central nervous system function. It can be assessed using the TICLS mnemonic **TABLE 10-4**. Work of breathing will assess the patient's oxygenation and ventilation status by looking for signs of increased breathing effort and abnormal airway sounds. Signs of increased work of breathing include intercostal or suprasternal, subcostal, or substernal retractions/recessions; nasal flaring; tripoding; and airway noises such as stridor, wheezing, or grunting. Finally, a circulatory assessment will determine cardiac output and core perfusion by looking at skin color. Pale or mottled color to the skin can indicate decreased perfusion to the skin, and cyanosis indicates a decrease in oxygenated blood reaching the skin. The individual parts of the PAT can be used alone or in tandem to help qualify the child's physiologic abnormality. For example, a child with an altered appearance may be having an endocrine/neurologic emergency. A child with an altered appearance and signs and symptoms of respiratory distress has a high potential for respiratory failure. A child with decreased circulation and altered mental status is most likely in shock; however, a decreased appearance always gives the provider a way to determine the child's need for immediate treatment.

The PAT method allows prehospital providers to form a general impression of the patient and to assess the patient's mental status further. Hands-on assessment of the ABCs allows providers to determine the priority of care and need for transport. Children at differing developmental stages may require alterations in assessment technique to get more accurate assessments. Toddlers may respond better to a toe-to-head approach in the secondary or detailed assessment. Adolescents require privacy during exposure of injuries and during history taking to allow accurate exchange of information. Obvious injury sites should be examined last in all age groups, when possible, to avoid causing pain and anxiety during the rest of the exam.

Child Restraint Safety

IN THE UNITED STATES, APPROXIMATELY 13% of all emergency medical service (EMS) calls are for pediatric patients, of whom slightly more than half are in the age range that requires some form of child safety restraint.[1] As the number of pediatric transports rises each year, questions have surfaced regarding the proper use of restraint of children in ambulances for prehospital transport. The problem is compounded by the fact that each state has its own restraint law, and EMS agencies vary in their definitions and practice regarding restraint of children in ambulances.[2] What is clear is the need for continued, comprehensive educational programs for parents, and uniform EMS policies for prehospital professionals, to restrain children consistently and appropriately for transport.

Multiple surveys and observational studies reveal an alarming trend of non- and misuse of child safety restraints (CSRs). The National Highway Traffic Safety Administration's survey of private vehicles reports 72.6% of CSRs were improperly used; factors included loose safety belt attachments, improper age- and weight-appropriate facing direction of CSR (forward-facing versus rear-facing), cracked car seat shells, torn harnesses, and use of after-market devices. Nearly 12% of children observed in this study did not have any type of CSR, the largest issue being the lack of booster seats for older children.[3]

Similarly, a voluntary survey of EMS personnel shows that adherence to guidelines varies. Over 25% of respondents reported that they "sometimes, almost always, or always" transported pediatric patients in a parent's lap "if the patient is stable." This is double the rate of non-restraint in private vehicles. Given that an estimated 4,500 ambulances per year in the U.S. are involved in crashes, it seems that young children are at a significant and disproportionate risk for in-transport injury.[4]

Three major factors impact the safety of ambulance transport of pediatric patients: child restraint, EMS provider restraint, and the overall judgment and performance of the ambulance driver.

If the infant or child is stable and weighs less than 40 pounds (approximately 18 kilograms), he or she should be secured in a child safety restraint (CSR). The CSR is best secured in an upright position against the stretcher that has also been placed in the upright position. Younger infants weighing up to 20 pounds should be secured in the rear-facing position to the stretcher. An alternative but less optimal method is to secure the CSR across the ambulance stretcher. It should be noted, however, that car seats and other CSRs are not designed for optimal lateral stability; securing a CSR across the stretcher requires vigilance in transport, in case of a collision or abrupt stop. If there is visible damage to the CSR after a motor vehicle collision or if a suitable CSR is not available, the infant or young child should be transported in the supine position.

Stable children over 40 pounds may be secured with age- or size-appropriate straps to the stretcher or gurney. Children should not be transported in the parent's arms in the stretcher. Unstable patients of any weight or those who require active interventions or a backboard may be transported in the supine position with special caution.[5]

An often overlooked aspect of ambulance safety is EMS provider restraint. Most providers do not wear seatbelts when caring for patients in the rear compartment, citing that this interferes with patient care.[4] Multiple studies using the Fatality Analysis Reporting System (FARS) database have shown that riding in the rear compartment of the ambulance during a crash substantially increases provider injury and mortality. Furthermore, an unrestrained passenger may act as a projectile in a collision, possibly injuring others as well as himself.[4] Ongoing efforts to improve provider restraint while allowing unencumbered access to the patient and ambulance equipment should be encouraged to reduce the risk of harm in a collision to provider, patient, and driver.

EMS responders are faced daily with injuries of varying degrees of acuity and questions involving expedition of transport. The natural anxiety in caring for sick children and pressures from the scene or bystanders may push prehospital professionals to transport very quickly. The decision to transport a patient with lights and/or sirens may be made, therefore, more by emotion than by medical necessity. It is important to note that the use of lights and sirens carries an inherent risk and is associated with a higher incidence of collisions and serious injury; in a review of the FARS data, 69% of ambulance crashes occurred with the use of lights and sirens, even on good roads and during daylight hours.[6] It is therefore vital to continue to reinforce the importance of weighing the risks against the potential benefits of "Code 3" lights and sirens transport on an individual basis and to consider this when deciding on methods of child restraint.

The Emergency Department and admitting service have a unique opportunity to intervene and educate parents in automotive child safety restraint.[7] Although restraint laws vary widely from state to state, The American Academy of Pediatrics has established guidelines for the restraint of children in private vehicles. The main determinants of type of restraint and facing direction (rear-facing or forward-facing) are the child's age, weight, height, and developmental status:

- **Booster seat:** A transition seat for older children who have outgrown convertible seats (over 40 lb), but are not tall enough to use an adult seatbelt. Available in high-back, low-back, or booster base only.
- **Car bed:** A device used for premature, low-birth weight babies, or children who cannot tolerate the upright sitting position, usually due to risk of airway occlusion.
- **Child safety seat/child safety restraint (CSR):** A general term for a crash-tested device designed for restraint of children in automotive collisions.
- **Convertible child safety seat:** A car seat that can be used as a rear-facing seat for infants or a forward-facing seat for toddlers.
- **Infant seat:** A smaller car seat appropriate to restrain infants.
- **Shell:** The molded plastic casing of the child restraint system, which may be reinforced with a metal frame.

Among the guidelines, a few points may be stressed regarding car seat safety:

- Follow the manufacturer's installation instructions without deviation.
- Do not replace or customize parts of your car seat.
- You must disable any air bags that may possibly come into contact with the car seat during a collision.
- Many parents graduate their children directly from car seat to seatbelt; booster seats are overlooked, but are an important part of child safety.

The National Highway Traffic Safety Administration (NHTSA) recently revised its recommendation regarding the use of car seats and other CSRs after a motor vehicle collision. NHTSA recommends that a CSR involved in a moderate or severe crash be replaced. CSRs involved in minor crashes do not necessarily need to be replaced if all of the following criteria are met:[8]

- The vehicle was in driving condition away from the crash site
- The vehicle door nearest the safety seat was undamaged
- There were no injuries to anyone in the vehicle
- The air bags were not deployed
- There is no visible damage to the safety seat

Motor vehicle collisions remain the leading cause of death of children ages 1 to 14.[9] Although use of restraints in the United States has improved in the past decade, a significant number of children are either poorly restrained or not at all. Through continued educational programs and restraint equipment improvement—both in the civilian and prehospital setting—unnecessary risk for children in transport may be reduced.

Timothy Horeczko, MD
Department of Emergency Medicine
Harbor–UCLA Medical Center
Torrance, California

Marianne Gausche-Hill, MD
Department of Emergency Medicine
Harbor–UCLA Medical Center
Torrance, California

References

1. Shah MN, Cushman JT, Davis CO, et al. The epidemiology of emergency medical services use by children: an analysis of the national hospital ambulatory medical care survey. *Prehosp Emerg Care*. 2008; 12(3):269–276.

2. National Highway Traffic Safety Administration. Counter-measures that work: a highway safety countermeasure guide for state highway safety offices, 4th ed. *NHTSA Report DOT HS 811 081*. Washington, DC. 2009; 2-1–2-38.

3. National Highway Traffic Safety Administration. Misuse of child restraints. *NHTSA Report DOT HS 809 671*. Washington, DC. 2004.

4. Johnson TD, Lindholm D, Dowd MD. Child and provider restraints in ambulances: knowledge, opinions, and behaviors of emergency medical service providers. *Acad Emerg Med*. 2006; 13:886–892.

5. American Academy of Pediatrics. Dieckmann, RA (ed). Transportation Considerations. In *Pediatric Education for Prehospital Professionals*, 2nd ed. Sudbury, MA: Jones and Bartlett Publishers. 2006; 273–281.

6. Seidel JS, Greenlaw J. Use of restraints in ambulances: a state survey. *Ped Emerg Care*. 1998;14(3).

7. National Highway Traffic Safety Administration. NHTSA Dictionary of Child Safety Seat Terms. Available at: www.nhtsa.dot.gov. Accessed February 16, 2009.

8. National Highway Traffic Safety Administration. Child Restraint After Minor Crashes. Available at: www.nhtsa.dot.gov. Accessed February 16, 2009.

9. National Safe Kids Campaign. Child passengers at risk in America: national study of restraint use. Washington, DC. 2002.

Management Specifics

Your management priorities with pediatric patients should be to manage life threats as they appear in order of importance: airway, breathing, and circulation. If you strongly suspect that the patient could have a life-threatening MOI, the patient should be spinal immobilized. Keep pediatric patients warm and use care when exposing the child to cold environments.

All trauma victims with suspected spinal injury require appropriate spinal stabilization. It is often difficult to find an appropriate-size cervical collar for infants or very young children. Do not attempt to place a collar that is too big on a small child; use towel rolls and tape them in a horseshoe pattern to immobilize around the head FIGURE 10-10 . Do not put towels around a pediatric patient's neck, because you may occlude the airway PROCEDURE 24 .

Remember, the goal in immobilization is to minimize the movement of the head and cervical spine. Apply the tape across the temples and forehead, but avoid tape over the chin or throat because it may impair ventilation. When additional tape is required, it can be placed across the maxilla, just under the nose. Choose a pediatric immobilizer (long backboard) with a recess for the child's large occiput or place a towel or small blanket under the shoulders and back. The towel should be an appropriate thickness to prevent neck flexion in infants and toddlers (usually about 1″ to 2″).

Trauma patients should be assessed for risk of developing shock from visible external bleeding or internal bleeding. Assess the child's circulation by checking the heart rate and quality, capillary refill, skin temperature, and blood pressure.

Hypovolemic shock could take quite awhile to present itself to EMS, because a child can lose up to 25% of their circulatory volume prior to presenting with signs and symptoms of shock. When a child can no longer compensate for a volume deficit, the cardiac output begins to fall, resulting in hypotension and inadequate perfusion of key organs. Once the child has begun to decompensate, the health care provider must act quickly to avoid irreversible shock and untimely death of the pediatric patient.

If the MOI is concerning and the child is tachycardic, assume the presence of compensated shock and initiate volume resuscitation with up to 20 mL/kg (5–10 mL/kg in the United Kingdom) of isotonic fluid (normal saline, lactated Ringer's, or Hartmann's solution). This fluid bolus can be repeated two more times if needed to support perfusion. It is important to remember not to overvolume resuscitate pediatric patients because too much fluid could be as dangerous to the pediatric patient as not enough. Local protocols may assist the provider in deciding when to provide fluid and how much to administer. Ideally, two peripheral IV lines should be started after initial assessment, stabilization, and the transport decision. When IV access is unavailable, the IO route should be used as long as there are no contraindications.

PRO/CON

Fluid replacement therapy in adults has become controversial in recent years, with pressure to give just enough fluid to keep the blood pressure at a minimum. In children, some systems have changed their protocols to give smaller fluid boluses with quicker reassessments and additional boluses if the patient's condition requires it.

Some traumas are load-and-go situations because of the severity of injuries and the patient's unstable condition. Examples include trauma involving an ominous MOI regardless of how the patient looks on scene, a child with an unstable or compromised airway, a child in shock, a child with difficulty breathing, and a child with a severe neurologic disability. For these patients, perform lifesaving procedures on scene or en route and transfer them quickly to an appropriate trauma center according to local trauma triage protocols FIGURE 10-11 .

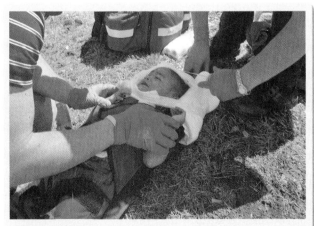

FIGURE 10-10 If an appropriate-size cervical collar is unavailable, the child should be padded and immobilized to the longboard.

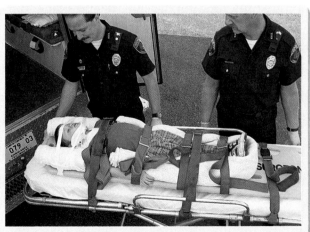

FIGURE 10-11 Significant MOI, regardless of how the child looks, is a load-and-go situation.

Elderly Trauma

Geriatrics is the branch of medicine that deals specifically with problems of the elderly. In 2003, people over the age of 65 years accounted for more than 12% of the US population and more than 15% of the UK population; by 2030, this percentage is expected to grow to 20%, largely driven by aging of the baby boomers (born in the period 1946–1964). Although the US numbers are not universal, populations in the rest of the world are facing similar growth rates, and by 2050 even underdeveloped countries will have a peak in their populations and one in three Europeans will be over the age of 65. Furthermore, the elderly population is itself growing older; indeed, the most rapidly growing segment of the world population is people 85 years or older. Currently, the aged population accounts for more than 34% of emergency medical responses **FIGURE 10-12**.

Age alone cannot define a geriatric patient. The bottom line about geriatrics and injury is the body's ability to withstand a traumatic event and mend itself. As a general rule, patients who have a condition regarded as normally afflicting the elderly (chronic obstructive pulmonary disease [COPD], congestive heart failure [CHF], hypertension, osteoporosis, etc) and patients who look like they are older than 65 years old as a result of difficult life experiences should be considered within the geriatric age grouping.

Differences in Anatomy and Physiology

Human development usually peaks in the late 20s and early 30s, at which time the body has its largest reserves in each of the body systems. Changes in the body's homeostatic compensatory mechanisms become less effective over time. Compensation for trauma-related deficits is successful when each of the systems is able to maximize its ability to function. Reduced cardiac reserves, decreased respiratory function, impaired renal activity, and ineffective vasoconstriction, by contrast, may lead to

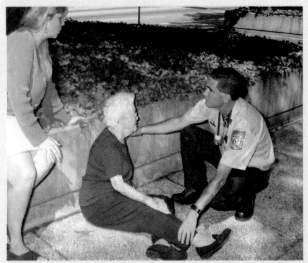

FIGURE 10-12 Older patients account for a disproportionate amount of EMS responses.

unsuccessful recovery from traumatic situations. Furthermore, an elderly person is more likely to sustain serious injury from trauma because stiffened blood vessels and fragile tissues tear more readily and brittle, demineralized bone is more vulnerable.

Respiratory System

A person's respiratory capacity undergoes significant reductions with age, largely due to decreases in the elasticity of the lungs and in the size and strength of the respiratory muscles. The chest wall becomes more rounded with increasing age, and calcification of costochondral cartilage tends to make the chest wall stiffer. In the lungs, the alveoli decrease in number but increase in size. These larger alveoli become less elastic and remain open at the end of an expiration, leaving air unused. As a result of these changes, the **vital capacity** (the amount of air that can be exhaled following a maximal inhalation) decreases, and the **residual volume** (the amount of air left in the lungs at the end of a maximal exhalation) increases. Thus, although the total amount of air in the lungs does not change with age, the proportion of that air actually used in gas exchange progressively declines.

Cardiovascular System

A variety of changes occur in the cardiovascular system as a person grows older. **Arteriosclerosis**—the stiffening of vessel walls—contributes to systolic hypertension in many older patients. These stiffened vessels make it harder for older patients to compensate for volume changes such as loss of blood. Vasoconstriction also assists in the formation of clots by clamping down the area. The sinoatrial (SA) node decreases in size over time making atrial arrhythmias more prevalent. In patients over the age of 80, atrial fibrillation is the rhythm most often experienced. The decrease in atrial movement of blood decreases the overall cardiac output and decreases the reserve compensatory ability of the older patient. The heart **hypertrophies** (enlarges) with age, probably in response to the chronically increased afterload imposed by stiffened blood vessels caused by arteriosclerosis. Over time, cardiac output declines, mostly as a result of a decreasing stroke volume.

Nervous System

Changes in the nervous system include a slowing of the sensory and motor nerve pathways, a decrease of the sensory organs, and a slowed response from the body's internal monitoring system. Thinking (cognitive) speed and postural stability are not affected by age and adverse changes should be considered abnormal at all ages. Falls in the elderly should be evaluated for the cause. Often the patient did not sense the object that caused a trip to occur (due to poor eyesight or decreased sensation in the feet) and then had a delayed motor response to try to stop the fall. (Wrists are often fractured due to slow responses telling the arms to reach out to stop the fall.)

As we age, our brains slowly shrink in volume and weight **FIGURE 10-13**. Instances of closed head injury become more common with geriatric patients, and providers should

Younger adult   **Older adult**

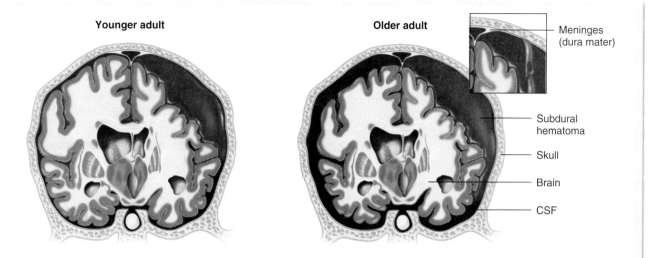

Meninges
(dura mater)

Subdural
hematoma

Skull

Brain

CSF

FIGURE 10-13   The aging brain decreases in size within the skull, causing a potential space between the brain and the dura mater. Any bleeding here can have delayed signs as the blood fills in the void first.

be aware of a coup-contrecoup injury resulting from falls and motor vehicle crashes. Bleeding occurs when the veins bridging the meninges to the brain are sheared in a sudden movement. Because there is more physical room in the skull, symptoms are often delayed as the blood fills the space before putting pressure on the brain.

Musculoskeletal System

Aging brings a widespread decrease in bone mass in men and women (**osteoporosis**). This process is accelerated in postmenopausal women. Bones become more brittle and tend to break more easily. Joints lose their flexibility and may be further immobilized by arthritic changes. In fact, more than half of all elderly people have some form of arthritis. Muscle mass decreases throughout the body, with an accompanying decrease in muscle strength.

Kyphosis, commonly referred to as humpback or hunchback, occurs as the muscles in the neck and upper body weaken and allow the head and shoulders to fall forward and the bones to become misshapen **FIGURE 10-14**. This curvature causes many issues in the elderly trauma patient. Neutral positioning for airway control or c-spine stabilization cannot be completed due to stiffness. Narrowing of the intervertebral disks and compression fractures of the vertebrae contribute to a decrease in height with age.

Renal System

The kidneys are responsible for maintaining the body's fluid and electrolyte balance and play important roles in maintaining the body's long-term acid-base balance and eliminating drugs from the body. Kidneys decline in weight as a person ages, which results in a loss of functioning nephron units. This translates into a smaller effective filtering surface. At the same time, renal blood flow decreases by as much as 50% as a person ages. Although the kidneys of an elderly person may be capable of dealing with day-to-day demands, they may not be able to meet unusual challenges, such as

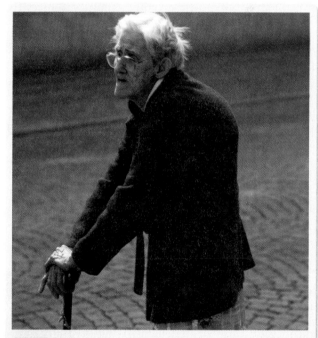

FIGURE 10-14   Kyphosis causes the elderly body to take on a different shape.

those imposed by injury. Aging kidneys respond sluggishly to sodium deficiency. Because of its lower glomerular filtration rate, the aging kidney is less able than its younger counterpart to excrete a large sodium load, making the patient vulnerable to acute volume overload.

Injury Patterns

Most trauma cases in the elderly involve falls or motor vehicle collisions. The incidence of falls, for example, increases with increasing age. Although most falls do *not* produce serious injury, elderly people account for 75% of all fall-related deaths. It is this statistic that should alert providers that a fall, even from a standing position, could present a significant MOI in the geriatric population. This increased mortality in geriatric patients is directly related to the patient's age, preexisting disease processes, and complications related to the trauma.

Falls are associated with a higher incidence of anxiety and depression, a loss of confidence, and **postfall syndrome**. Postfall syndrome occurs when an elderly patient has a significant fall that requires hospitalization and rehabilitation. After returning home, the patient develops a lack of confidence with movement and anxiety about potential falls and decreases his or her amount of activity. This decrease of activity leads to muscle wasting and leaves the patient at a higher risk of future falls. The largest predictor for a fall is the history of a previous fall.

Falls among elderly people are evenly divided between those resulting from extrinsic (external) causes, such as tripping on a loose rug or slipping on ice, and those resulting from intrinsic (internal) causes, such as a dizzy spell or a syncopal attack. The risk of falls increases in people with preexisting gait abnormalities (such as from neurologic or musculoskeletal impairment from previous injuries) and cognitive impairment (such as a previous CVA). Older patients with osteoporosis have lower density bones, so even a sudden, awkward turn may fracture a bone.

After falls, motor vehicle accidents are the second leading cause of accidental death among elderly people. Impaired vision, errors in judgment, and underlying medical conditions contribute to the higher risk **FIGURE 10-15**. Impairments in vision and hearing, along with diminished agility, also contribute to pedestrian deaths involving elderly people.

Burns are a significant risk of morbidity and mortality in elderly people because the skin is thinner and more fragile, the immune system is lessened, and the homeostatic balance is decreased. The risk of mortality is increased when there are preexisting medical conditions, defense mechanisms to protect against infection are weakened, and fluid replacement is complicated by renal compromise. The pain impulse moves through a slower peripheral nervous system, allowing the patient longer contact time with the hot surface before he or she reacts. Simply put, it takes longer for the geriatric population to react to pain stimuli. As a result, they tend to sustain more severe burns than would a younger patient given the same stimuli.

Head Injury

Head trauma or injury is a serious problem. The increased fragility of cerebral blood vessels, enlargement of the subdural space, and a decrease

in the supportive tissue of the meninges all contribute to make an elderly person more vulnerable than a younger person to intracranial bleeding, particularly subdural hematoma. In many cases, the hematoma develops slowly, during days or weeks. By the time the patient becomes symptomatic, the person or his or her caretakers may not remember the incident, or the family or caretakers may feel guilty about their own negligence in the incident. As a result, it may be difficult to obtain an accurate history of the initial trauma. The most important early symptom of a subdural hematoma is headache, which may be worse at night. Sometimes the headache occurs on the same side of the head as the blood clot. With increasing intracranial pressure, the state of consciousness becomes depressed, and the patient becomes increasingly drowsy.

Spinal Injuries

Elderly people are more vulnerable than their younger counterparts to spinal cord injury and cord compression, even after apparently minor trauma. Degenerative changes in the spine (**spondylosis**) cause arthritic "spurs" and narrowing of the vertebral canal; the nerve roots exiting from the cervical spine gradually become compressed, and pressure on the spinal cord increases.

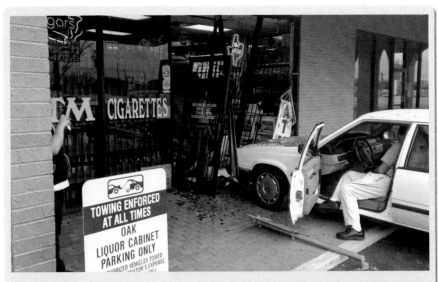

FIGURE 10-15 The elderly often attribute motor vehicle incidents to sensory deficits or medical conditions.

Chest Injuries

Injuries to the chest in elderly people are much more likely to produce a rib fracture and/or flail chest, owing to the brittleness of the ribs and overall stiffening of the chest wall. Be suspicious of a great vessel tear or an aortic arch rupture in any patient having severe chest pain following a sudden deceleration injury. Atherosclerosis can put the aorta at higher risk for tearing. These injuries are life-threatening and the patient should be transported into the trauma system quickly.

Abdominal Injuries

Abdominal trauma often produces liver injury, perhaps because the liver is less protected by abdominal musculature. The geriatric patient may delay complaints of abdominal injury simply because the nervous system in the elderly has decreased sensation in the abdomen.

Musculoskeletal Injuries

Orthopaedic injuries are a common result of falls in geriatric patients, with hip fractures the most common acute orthopaedic injury, followed in severity and frequency by fractures of the femur, pelvis, tibia, and upper extremities. The most important risk factor for hip fracture is osteoporosis: Approximately half of older women and one of eight older men will have an osteoporosis-related fracture (hip or other).

STATS

An estimated 15 to 20 million people in the United States older than 45 years have osteoporosis, and it leads to nearly 1.3 million fractures annually. In the United Kingdom, 20% of orthopaedic patients are those with osteoporosis.

Alterations in Assessment

Begin the assessment by looking at the mechanism of injury. When treating a patient who has fallen, a complete history is required. Although the patient often attributes the fall to an accidental cause ("I must have tripped over the rug"), meticulous questioning often reveals a period of dizziness or palpitations just before the fall, suggesting a different cause. Always look for signs or symptoms that an elderly patient may have experienced a medical problem before the trauma. A syncopal event while driving, for example, may result in a collision.

TIP

A complete fall history should answer the question, "mechanical or medical?" Mechanical causes include slips, trips, and falls. Medical causes include medication-induced issues, syncope, cardiac arrhythmias, or hypotension.

By the age of 65, most people are taking from three to seven different medications for medical conditions related to aging. Many of these medications can alter or contribute to the exam findings in the trauma exam. Blood thinners prevent the patient from clotting to stop bleeding, while medications for hypertension will prevent the patient from making a good effort at compensating for the blood loss. Some medications, like an antihyperglycemic or seizure medication, may give a clue to the events leading up to the traumatic event. It is very important to get a SAMPLE history early in the patient exam, because this information may be lost if the patient becomes unconscious.

Because vital signs, range of motion, and mental abilities change with age, it is often difficult to determine the patient's normal values without talking to relatives or caretakers. People who remain physically active well into their older years are better able to compensate for injury than a more sedentary individual. History taking for the elderly should include looking for the patient's normal values and how they relate to the signs and symptoms that are presenting.

Previous injuries leave scarring and decreased mobility in an extremity that can be confused with a current injury. An example would be a patient who suffered a broken lower leg as a child that when healed left the leg shortened and twisted slightly. Are the signs all from the previous injury or are they partially from the new? Conditions that are pre-existing may also become exacerbated by a new injury. A patient who has suffered a stroke in the past and who now has struck his head may develop new neurologic symptoms beyond the deficits left from the stroke or making them appear worse.

When assessing the ABCs, little changes with the older patient. Elderly patients may have dentures or dental bridges that may become an airway obstruction if loose. If assisted ventilation is required, use a bag mask gently, exerting just enough pressure to inflate the lungs so as to lessen the chance of creating a pneumothorax. When evaluating circulation, remember that what is a normal blood pressure in a younger person may mean hypotension in an older person. If possible, try to determine the patient's normal baseline blood pressure and circulatory status. The initial/primary assessment of disability (neurologic status) should include an evaluation of the pupils and the level of consciousness. Finally, be sure to expose the entire injured area, even if it means peeling away many layers of clothing. Conduct the physical exam as usual, staying particularly alert for signs of injuries to the head, cervical spine, ribs, abdomen, and long bones. Pain from fractures or peripheral injury may be difficult to assess if the patient has decreased pain perception.

Management Specifics

Aggressive suctioning of blood or secretions is required because of the older patient's weakened airway and gag reflexes. Remove dentures only if they are loose and are causing an obstruction. Dentures provide structure to the

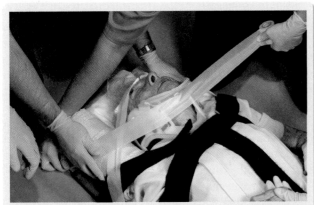

FIGURE 10-16 Padding is vital when placing an older patient on a long backboard.

face to allow bag-mask ventilations if needed. Administer supplemental oxygen early to assist the body in compensating for early states of trauma.

Use caution when fitting elderly patients with cervical collars, because the smallest collar may still be too large. This can be addressed in one of two ways. First, try a pediatric collar. The second option is a towel roll horseshoe. Because of kyphosis in the geriatric torso and cervical spine, this may be a more comfortable alternative to an ill fitting cervical collar **FIGURE 10-16**.

Additional treatment will depend on the patient's specific injuries, although there are a few general principles to keep in mind:

1. **IV catheters may need to be smaller**. Skin is more fragile and can rip during an IV insertion. A blood pressure cuff can make a good alternative to a thin tourniquet as long as the pressure allows arterial flow. Use small boluses and reassess the patient frequently by listening to lung sounds and looking for signs of pulmonary edema.

2. **Monitor cardiac rhythm throughout care of the patient and be alert for changes**. Previous or continuing cardiac disease predisposes a person to electrocardiogram (ECG) changes. A cardiac monitor will alert providers with visual and audible alarms quickly when changes occur.

3. **Take steps to preserve temperature in elderly trauma patients**. Regulation of temperature is slowed in elderly people, and the blood in cold patients does not clot as well.

4. **Frail elderly patients may not do very well with a traction splint for a femoral fracture**. If possible, place the patient on a well-padded backboard, buttress him or her well with pillows, and secure firmly in place.

5. **Immobilize the cervical spine before transporting the patient**. Pad the backboard generously because the skin of an older person may be damaged by the direct trauma of the pressure and the decrease in blood flow. Pad areas where the bone

is near the surface, from top to bottom, especially the occiput, scapula, spinous processes, elbows, sacrum, and heels. A pressure ulcer can develop in as little as 45 minutes and can complicate the original injury. Remember that the definition of *immobilization* is prevention of something from moving, and it may be accomplished in less conventional ways like using a vacu-mattress, an EMS cot, or other devices.

Pregnancy

Trauma is a serious complicating factor in pregnancy, partly because of the many physiologic changes that occur during pregnancy, but mostly because of the involvement of two patients—the woman and her fetus. Both patients are particularly vulnerable to trauma because of the unique features of pregnancy. Motor vehicle trauma accounts for up to two thirds of injuries in pregnancy but accounts for only one tenth of maternal deaths. In the United States, 324,000 women are abused each year by an intimate partner during their pregnancy, and it is reported that 30% of domestic violence in the US and the UK either starts or intensifies during pregnancy. Homicide is one of the leading causes of death for the pregnant patient. Nearly all pregnant homicide victims were killed by their current or ex-partners. Gunshot wounds account for almost one fourth of maternal deaths in the United States, while stab wounds account for 14% of maternal deaths. Nearly 70% of all penetrating abdominal wounds result in injury to the fetus.

During pregnancy, physiologic changes occur in nearly every organ system in the body **TABLE 10-5**. These changes can alter the signs and symptoms of trauma and the response to care. Even the types of trauma involved with a pregnant patient are different. Many of these changes can alter the normal response or create additional medical conditions that can threaten the health of both the woman and the fetus.

Differences in Anatomy and Physiology

The most significant physiologic changes occur in the uterus. Before a woman's first pregnancy, the uterus measures about 3″ (7.5 cm) long by 2″ (5 cm) wide and is approximately 1″ (2.5 cm) thick. As the uterus enlarges and the diaphragm becomes elevated, internal maternal organs begin to shift to make room. The measurement of the <u>fundus</u> (top portion of the uterus, opposite the cervix) can be used to estimate developmental dates **FIGURE 10-17**.

Respiratory System

During pregnancy, the respiratory system undergoes stresses as well. The uterus pushes the diaphragm up toward the abdominal cavity. To compensate for this change, the rib margins flare outward, which allows the respiratory system to maintain intrathoracic volume. The abdominal muscles tend to lose their tone during pregnancy, which allows respiration to be more diaphragmatic.

TABLE 10-5   Overview of Approximate Changes in the Body by Trimester

	Cardiovascular	Respiratory	Gastrointestinal	Urinary	Endocrine	Musculoskeletal
First trimester (weeks 1–13)	None	Increased minute volume	Prolonged emptying time	Increased filtering rate	Increased pituitary gland	None
Second trimester (weeks 14–27)	Increased cardiac output, slight decrease in blood pressure, increased heart rate		Increased appetite	Continues to increase	Glucose levels are lower at night	Joints become more lax
Third trimester (weeks 28–40)	ECG changes possible	Hypocapnea common	Intestine relocated to the upper part of the abdomen	Renal flow and filtering are 50%–60% higher than prepregnancy		Increased lordosis

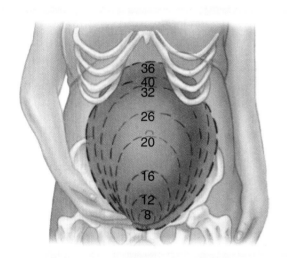

FIGURE 10-17 Approximation of gestational dates can be made using the height of the fundus from the pubic bone.

As maternal oxygen demand increases, the respiratory physiology changes to accommodate this need. The hormone **progesterone**, which is produced early in pregnancy by the corpus luteum and later by the placenta, decreases the threshold of the medullary respiratory center to carbon dioxide. It also acts on the bronchi, causing them to dilate, and regulates mucus production, causing an overall decrease in airway resistance. Oxygen consumption increases by about 20% and tidal volume increases gradually to about 40%, caused in part by hormone changes. The increase in tidal volume causes minute ventilation to increase by as much as 50% over prepregnancy values and $Paco_2$ to drop by about 5 mm Hg. The latter change is accompanied by a decrease in blood bicarbonate and a slight increase in plasma pH levels, which in turn affects acid-base balance. Thus, in the pregnant state, metabolic acidosis caused by increased metabolic demands is balanced by a respiratory alkalosis. The acid-base changes become quite marked during actual labor, but return to normal about 3 weeks

postpartum (after birth). At term, the displacement of the diaphragm by the fully enlarged uterus causes a decrease in expiratory reserve volume, functional residual capacity, and residual volume. Tidal volume and inspiratory reserve volume increase, causing the inspiratory capacity to increase.

Cardiovascular System

As the pregnancy progresses, the maternal metabolism undergoes phenomenal changes—most obviously, weight gain and alterations in physical structure. Weight gain is partly due to increased blood volume and increases in intracellular and extracellular fluid (6 to 7 lb, or 2.7 to 3.2 kg), uterine growth (3 lb, or 1.4 kg), placental growth (2 lb, or 0.9 kg), fetal growth (7 lb, or 3.2 kg), and increased breast tissue (2 to 3 lb, or 0.9 to 1.4 kg). Some weight gain is also attributable to increased proteins and fat deposits, with the average weight gain in pregnancy being 27 lb (12.3 kg).

As blood volume increases, so does the size of the pregnant woman's heart, by an average of 10% to 15% from prepregnancy levels. Cardiac output increases to about 40% more than before pregnancy, reaching its maximum capacity at about 22 weeks' gestation and then maintaining this level until term. A pregnant woman's heart rate gradually increases during pregnancy by an average of 15 to 20 beats/min by the end of the pregnancy. ECG changes that can occur during pregnancy include ectopic beats and supraventricular tachycardia, which is often considered normal.

As gestation increases, a woman's sensitivity to body positioning increases as well. Resting or lying supine can cause the uterus to impinge upon the inferior vena cava or common iliac veins, thereby decreasing venous return to the heart. Over time, if pressure is not relieved, cardiac output is decreased, blood pressure drops, and lower extremity edema results.

The pressures exerted on the circulatory system and the increased blood volume combine to produce venous distension of about 150% of prepregnancy levels. Blood return to the heart is reduced as the venous ends of the capillaries become dilated. Gravid women who are bedridden or who spend a great deal of time lying down are in particular danger of experiencing deep venous thrombosis, which can lead to pulmonary embolism. The slow return also causes delayed absorption of subcutaneously or intramuscularly injected medications. When a gravid patient goes into labor, the position she is in stresses the cardiovascular system as well.

Hemodynamics

The average woman has about 4 to 5 L of blood available as total circulating volume. Blood volume in the pregnant female increases gradually throughout gestation, such that there may be as much as a 40% to 50% overall increase at term. The level of increase depends on such factors as patient size, number of times **gravid** (total pregnancies, but not necessarily carried to term) and **para/parity** (pregnancies carried to more than 28 weeks' gestation, regardless of whether delivered dead or alive), and number of fetuses she is carrying. This increase in blood volume is necessary to meet the metabolic needs of the developing fetus, to adequately perfuse maternal organs—especially the uterus and kidneys—and to help compensate for blood loss during delivery.

A woman's white blood cell (WBC) count also increases during pregnancy, with an average of 4,300 to 4,500 mcL before pregnancy to as high as 12,000 mcL or more in the third trimester of pregnancy. Clotting factors are similarly increased, whereas fibrinolytic factors are depressed. These issues are important considerations if the provider has to deal with obstetric hemorrhage or thromboembolic disease.

Musculoskeletal System

The hormone relaxin, which is released during pregnancy, causes collagenous tissues to soften and produces a generalized relaxing of the ligamentous system, especially along the spine. This effect contributes to the characteristic **lordosis** (forward curvature of the lumbar spine which accentuates the buttocks) of later pregnancy and the increased flexion of the neck, both of which help the pregnant patient compensate for balance.

Injury Patterns

The anatomic changes during pregnancy have important implications for trauma. As the woman approaches term, her abdominal contents are compressed into the upper abdomen. The diaphragm is elevated by about 1.5″ (4 cm), so there is a higher incidence of abdominal injuries in association with chest trauma. Meanwhile, because the peritoneum is maximally stretched, significant abdominal trauma may occur without peritoneal signs. In the second and third trimesters of pregnancy, the uterus grows out from the pelvis and extends into the abdomen, making it more vulnerable to blunt and penetrating trauma. In motor vehicle crashes, for example, the improper use of a lap belt increases the likelihood of uterine damage because the looser lap belt compresses the uterus. Shoulder restraints, by contrast, decrease the chance of uterine injury. In penetrating injuries, the large uterus protects the other organs from injury. Because the uterus shields the other organs, pregnant women with penetrating wounds have excellent outcomes, although the fetus is often injured by the trauma.

As early as the second trimester of pregnancy, the bladder is displaced upward (superior) and forward (anterior) so that it lies outside the pelvic cavity. It is therefore at increased risk of injury, particularly from a deceleration injury caused by a lap seatbelt. Should you encounter a restrained pregnant patient in a motor vehicle collision, make a note of belt placement. If the patient is found with the belt placed over the abdomen or on top of the uterine dome, this positioning should dramatically increase your index of suspicion for internal injuries to the woman and fetus. The uterus also becomes more vulnerable to injury as it increases in size, and deceleration forces, such as those produced by vehicular trauma, may bring about abruption placenta or uterine rupture.

In patients with major injuries such as blunt vehicular deceleration, placenta abruption can occur in up to 67% of mothers with major injury but only 2%–4% with minor injuries. Associated with up to 100% fetal mortality and 10% maternal morbidity, to definitively diagnose abruption, two of the following criteria must be met: tense abdomen with flaccid fundus, maternal hypo- or hypertension, and ultrasound evidence of abruption.

Fetus and Trauma

The muscular wall of the uterus acts as a cushion for the fetus against the direct effects of blunt trauma, but fetal injury can occur as a result of rapid deceleration of circulation or may be secondary to impaired fetal circulation. The most common cause of fetal death from trauma is maternal death, but a woman will often survive an incident that proves fatal for the fetus. If the pregnant woman has sustained trauma and is bleeding massively, the maternal circulation will shunt blood away from fetal circulation to maintain maternal homeostasis—maternal circulation takes precedence over the requirements of the fetus. Therefore, any injury that involves significant maternal bleeding will threaten the life of the fetus. By the time the woman shows clinical signs of shock, fetal circulation will be so compromised that you can expect a fetal mortality rate of 70% to 80%.

The best indication of the status of the fetus after trauma is the fetal heart rate. A normal fetal heart rate is between 120 and 160 beats/min. A rate slower than 120 beats/min means fetal distress and signals a dire emergency. To measure the fetal heart rate, listen with the bell of the stethoscope over the pregnant woman's abdomen **FIGURE 10-18**. You may have to move the stethoscope around the abdomen until you can hear the fetal heart tones. Palpate the woman's pulse at the same time as you count the fetal heart rate. If the fetal heart rate is identical to the maternal pulse, you are probably listening to an echo of the maternal heartbeat and not the fetal heart, so change the position of your stethoscope and try again. It takes a lot of practice to hear fetal heart tones and requires quiet surroundings. Some modern ambulances may be equipped with Doppler stethoscopes, which make assessment of fetal heart sounds much easier.

Alterations in Assessment

As noted earlier, pregnancy is accompanied by a significant increase in vascular volume. Normal vascular volume increases by nearly 50% during the first 6 months of preg-

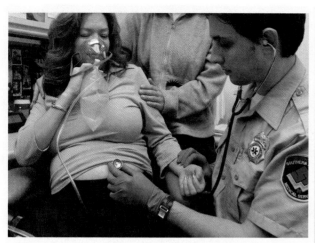

FIGURE 10-18 You may need to try different areas of the woman's abdomen to hear the fetal heart tones.

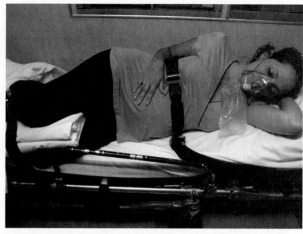

FIGURE 10-19 Patients in the third trimester of pregnancy should be transported with the right side elevated to avoid pressure on the vena cava.

nancy as a result of the pregnant woman having to perfuse her own circulation and that of the fetus. To meet this demand, normal cardiac output increases by about 40% as a result of the increasing pulse rate and stroke volume. The resting pulse rate increases by 15 to 20 beats/min over the rate in a nonpregnant patient, so the resting pulse may be as high as 100 beats/min by the end of the second trimester of pregnancy. This physiologic change makes it much more difficult to interpret tachycardia. Furthermore, because of the pregnant woman's vastly expanded blood volume, other signs of hypovolemia, such as a falling blood pressure, may not be evident until she has lost as much as 40% of her blood volume. Therefore you need to be aggressive in managing a pregnant woman with an MOI that indicates shock.

A relative redistribution of blood volume also occurs during pregnancy, with blood flow to the pelvic region increasing tenfold. If a pregnant woman sustains a pelvic fracture, her chances of bleeding to death are therefore significantly higher than those of a nonpregnant woman. A good deal of blood volume can be lost before signs and symptoms of shock develop because other mechanisms are compensating for the loss.

Regarding respiration, the pregnant woman has a higher basal metabolism and therefore an increased need for oxygen. At the same time, she has more carbon dioxide to eliminate—hers and that produced by fetal metabolism. She responds by increasing her tidal volume and, therefore, her minute volume. If she should need artificial ventilation, you will have to administer supplemental oxygen at a higher minute volume than usual. During pregnancy, digestion slows and bowel motility decreases, resulting in the stomach staying full longer. With the gravid uterus placing pressure on the stomach, the chances of aspiration are dramatically increased.

Management Specifics

Although trauma in a pregnant woman involves at least *two* patients, we can treat only one of them directly: the woman. In general, what is good for the woman will be good for the

fetus. For example, any effort to improve maternal perfusion will have a collateral effect of improving fetal circulation. Potential damage to the fetus cannot be adequately assessed in the field, however, only presumed or suspected. Although a decreased fetal heart rate signals an emergency situation, a normal fetal heart rate does not guarantee that all is well. Even minor deceleration forces can cause significant injury to the fetus. In general, the prehospital management of pregnant women with abdominal trauma is the same as for nonpregnant patients.

Airway, breathing, and circulation remain the highest priorities. However, because the large uterus can compress the vena cava (decreasing right atrial preload), a pregnant woman should be transported to the hospital on her left side unless a spinal injury is suspected **FIGURE 10-19**. If you must transport a patient in the supine position, elevate her right hip about 6″ (15 cm) to minimize the pressure on the vena cava.

Be aware that because of the physiologic changes that occur in a woman's body during pregnancy, the fetus may lack appropriate circulation even if the woman's vital signs appear normal. In other words, the fetus may be in shock before signs appear in the mother, so initiate early, aggressive fluid resuscitation.

Field treatment of a pregnant trauma patient is as follows:

1. **Ensure an adequate airway.** Regurgitation and aspiration are much more likely in a pregnant woman than in a patient who is not pregnant, so if the patient is unconscious, provide early endotracheal intubation to isolate the airway. Provide cricoid pressure until the airway is secured.
2. **Administer oxygen.** A pregnant woman's oxygen needs are 10% to 20% higher than normal, so provide 100% supplemental oxygen via nonrebreathing mask if the patient is conscious to achieve an oxygen saturation of 94%–100%.
3. **Assist ventilations as needed and provide a higher minute volume than usual.** Because the

uterus of a pregnant woman presses up against the diaphragm, she will be more difficult to ventilate. Once the patient is intubated, therefore, you may want to use a positive-pressure ventilator to ensure visible chest rise (representing an adequate tidal volume).

4. **Control external bleeding promptly**. Splint any fractures.

5. **Start one or two IV lines of normal saline**. Administer a bolus if signs and symptoms of hemodynamic compromise are present, with the goal of maintaining blood pressure. Remember that a larger volume of fluid is necessary for the pregnant patient.

6. **Notify the receiving hospital**. Alert them to the patient's status and your estimated time of arrival.

7. **Transport the woman in the lateral recumbent position**. If she is on a backboard, tilt the backboard 30° to the left by wedging pillows beneath it. This will cause the uterus to shift, taking the weight off the inferior vena cava and improving venous return to the heart. If cardiac arrest occurs, provide CPR and ALS as you would for a nonpregnant patient.

Trauma in the Obese Patient

Management of the injured morbidly obese patient has a number of peculiarities, including abnormal size, body composition, deranged physiology, and comorbid disease. Critically injured obese trauma patients are nearly seven times more likely to die than leaner patients with similar injuries.

Overweight and obesity are defined as abnormal or excessive fat accumulation that presents a risk to health. **Bariatrics** is the branch of medicine that deals with obesity and related health issues. A crude population measure of obesity is the body mass index (BMI), a person's weight (in kilograms) divided by the square of his or her height (in meters). A person with a BMI equal to or greater than 25 is considered overweight, with a BMI of 30 to 40 is considered obese, and 40 or greater is considered morbidly obese. The World Health Organization (WHO) projects that by 2015, approximately 2.3 billion adults will be overweight and more than 700 million will be obese. Motor vehicle safety standards have been developed in most countries to provide protection to individuals with a BMI equal to 24.3 kg/m² riding in a motor vehicle. Obesity is considered an independent risk factor and is autonomously associated with an increase in mortality. It is believed that the increases in comorbid factors are the cause for an increase in the overall mortality of obese patients. As prehospital providers, we must consider the potential for preexisting medical conditions when dealing with the treatment of obese individuals involved in a traumatic situation **FIGURE 10-20**.

Differences in Anatomy and Physiology

Anatomically, obese individuals differ from nonobese persons in several key areas, and obesity can alter the normal physiology of these patients. The airway will become altered by excessive soft tissues. Almost all pharyngeal structures increase in

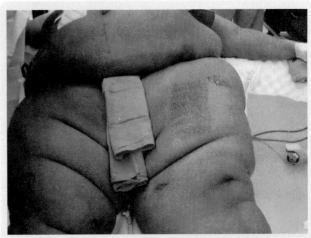

FIGURE 10-20 Obese patients present a unique problem for EMS.

size from increased adipose tissue. Because of the decreased pharyngeal space available between the fatty tissues of the upper airway, intubation and advanced airway care is more difficult. It is more difficult to landmark on a thick, obese neck. Cricoid pressure for airway control and landmarks for a cricothyrotomy may leave the provider with limited options for airway control. The laryngeal mask airway has been shown effective in managing the airway of an obese patient.

The respiratory system is most affected by morbid obesity. The weight of the chest wall and the impingement of a large abdomen on the diaphragm limit respiratory expansion in these patients. In addition, fatty deposits on the diaphragm and intercostal muscles impair the mechanics of breathing. These patients may normally suffer with chronic hypoxia and hypercarbia and may have little if any respiratory reserve. An increase in metabolic activity from the digestive system and at the cellular level will increase oxygen consumption and carbon dioxide production. Both of these factors (decreased lung capacity and greater oxygen demand) will increase an obese patient's work of breathing **FIGURE 10-21**. Morbid obesity can also lead to increased

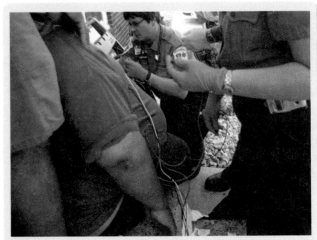

FIGURE 10-21 Large patients may have difficulty breathing while lying flat due to the weight on their chest.

episodes of obstructive sleep apnea, which will increase the potential for hypoxia, hypercapnia, and pulmonary and systemic hypertension. All of the physiologic changes should alert prehospital providers to become aggressive with the oxygen management of obese patients, even when the signs of respiratory compromise may not be evident.

The cardiovascular system has an increase in blood volume to fill the additional tissue on the body. The heart enlarges due to the increased pressures to pump blood around the larger body and pulmonary hypertension becomes the norm.

Injury Patterns

It appears that obese patients sustain different injury patterns than their leaner counterparts after blunt trauma. Obesity can play a major role in changes in injury pattern from nonobese patients, and some studies have shown that the sudden change in velocity and the type of collision (same-side impacts) may be a factor. Fewer head injuries, increased amounts of blunt chest injury, and more severe lower extremity injuries are seen in the obese patient. An increase in diaphragmatic injuries associated with near-sided motor vehicle collisions also has been reported.

Obese patients are more likely to sustain pulmonary contusions as well as pelvic, rib, and extremity fractures from blunt trauma such as a fall. Other reported injuries include distal femoral fractures along with an increased rate of cardiac, vascular, pulmonary, and wound complications. These typical complications, with the increase in comorbid factors, can be cause for an increase in mortality.

Alterations in Assessment

Assessment of obese patients often requires specialized equipment **FIGURE 10-22**. To obtain an accurate blood pressure reading, the bladder inside a blood pressure cuff must be able to encircle the arm. Inappropriately sized equipment can actually skew important patient data. For example, utilizing a blood pressure cuff that is too small falsely elevates a patient's blood pressure by as much as 10 points both systolic and diastolic. The reliability of ECG readings may be affected by incorrect lead placement due to difficulty locating anatomic landmarks or inconsistent voltages due to adipose tissue.

Prehospital providers should be aware of the more common types of injuries encountered and that the visual assessment of some of the injuries may be difficult due to the patient's size. You may find that patients stay in their homes due to decreased physical activity levels. Because the bariatric patient's respiratory and cardiac systems are already taxed by maintaining the patient without exertion, look for

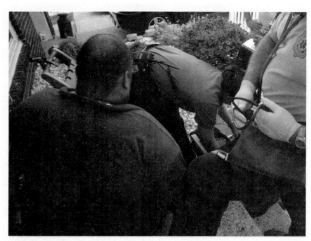

FIGURE 10-22   Assessing the obese patient requires the correct sized equipment.

exertional causes when treating a complaint of shortness of breath or chest pain.

Management Specifics

Patients with a body weight of greater than 350 lb (158 kg) are likely to require specialized tools, additional personnel, and treatment alterations. The management of traumatic injuries in the morbidly obese patient must include a plan for potential complications before the treatment plan can take effect. Providers must consider the technical limitations of the equipment being used as well as the limitations of the provider **FIGURE 10-23**. Consider the weight limitations of backboards, seated spinal immobilization devices, stretchers, appropriate size cervical collars, and the correct size blood pressure cuffs.

Specific management of obese patients must target early respiratory support and higher oxygen concentrations. The metabolic oxygen demand for obese patients has already been maximized to accommodate for the individual's size and the substantially decreased total lung capacity. When possible, morbidly obese patients should be transported in the Fowler's or upright position. Supine positioning may cause the patient increased respiratory compromise due to the weight of the chest and abdomen forcing the diaphragm upward and limiting the amount of inspired air with each breath. This may force the provider to decide whether aggressive airway care or spinal immobilization is the priority.

Common management considerations prehospital providers may encounter with bariatric patients include the following:

- There are extreme difficulties in bag-mask ventilations. Appropriate mask seal and head position are of paramount importance. Bag-mask ventilations should utilize the two-person technique to maintain mask seal on the face.
- Tracheal intubation problems are due to increased fat at the upper airway, a short neck, a high anteriorly placed larynx, and restricted cervical

TIP

Many obese trauma patients are encountered in their homes because they have difficulty moving themselves for long distances without exertional distress or injury.

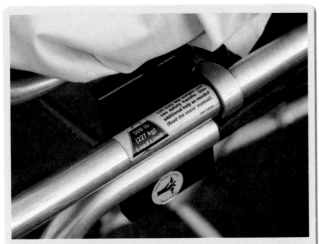

FIGURE 10-23 Consider the weight limitations on equipment when choosing an appropriate transport device.

spine movement. When possible, have the most experienced provider attempt the intubation, because multiple attempts will cause swelling in an already small airway. Use of a large laryngoscope blade is recommended.

- IM medications are not recommended and IV routes are preferred. Standard length IM needles are often too short to penetrate the muscle under the subcutaneous fat.
- Obesity leads to alterations in distribution, binding, and the elimination of drugs. Drug dosing may require alterations due to the increase of fatty tissue. Some medications use the total body weight (TBW) whereas others use an adjusted body weight (ABW) or indexed body weight (IBW). The difficulty is knowing which medication to base on which body weight calculation to avoid over- or underdosing the patient.
- Larger extremities make placement of IVs harder. Tourniquets are often too thin and a blood pressure cuff often does the job better. IO placement is an alternative to difficult IV sticks. Alternative sites for IVs are often overlooked. Scalp, abdominal, or breast veins may be considered when difficulty is encountered, if allowed by local protocols.
- Chest decompressions are difficult. A 2″ (10 cm) catheter may not reach the pleural space in 35% of the population. Consider the use of a commercially available decompression kit.

CHAPTER RESOURCES

CASE STUDY ANSWERS

1 How can the child's appearance assist you in your assessment?

The brain is the most oxygen-sensitive organ in the body and the first to show signs when it becomes hypoxic. Signs such as inconsolable crying, not looking around at her surroundings, and not interacting with her mother or you demonstrate decreased functioning of the brain.

2 Are the child's signs and symptoms significant for shock, or are they signs of pain or anxiety?

This child has an increased heart rate and cool skin and is crying inconsolably. These are all signs of shock. Pain and anxiety can also make the heart rate increase and the child may cry to try to communicate the problem. Although it is often difficult to differentiate the signs and symptoms of shock, using observations about the mechanism of injury and the signs and symptoms allow you to make the working diagnosis of shock.

CASE STUDY ANSWERS

3 You cannot find a cervical collar to fit the child. How should you immobilize the child's spine?

If a properly sized cervical collar that fits your young patient cannot be located, stabilize the neck manually until padding or an immobilizer is available. Secure the child's head from movement using the padding and tape or straps to keep her from moving. She will require tape or a strap over the forehead but no strap should be used under the chin without a collar to keep it from constricting the airway.

4 Should this child be transported to a trauma center?

Children with a mechanism of injury suggestive of trauma and any signs or symptoms that suggest the child is injured should be transported to a trauma center capable of dealing with pediatric patients.

5 How would your answers change if the patient were the driver's elderly mother?

Elderly patients have many correlations with young patients. They experience hypoxia more often than most patients, present differently from shock, and require alterations to make equipment fit them correctly. It is more difficult, however, to use the general appearance of the older patient to determine the physiological state of the patient, because altered appearance can be due to many other nontraumatic causes. If the older patient had these vital signs and mechanism of injury, they would be in shock. Also, because osteoporosis and kyphosis affect the position of the neck in everyday life, cervical collars may become hard to place without forcing the neck into a position of discomfort. If a cervical collar cannot be fitted to the patient, secure the patient to the long backboard and use padding to secure the head in place. Just like pediatric patients, elderly patients should be triaged to a trauma center if they present with injury and a mechanism of injury that suggests significant forces.

Trauma in Motion

1. Which facilities in your area are prepared to handle pediatric, geriatric, pregnant, or obese patients?
2. What specialty equipment do you carry to care for pediatric, geriatric, pregnant, or obese patients?
3. Are specialty transport vehicles or teams available in your area to assist in the transportation of pediatric, geriatric, pregnant, or obese patients?
4. What are your local protocols regarding vascular access and fluid replacement therapy in pediatric, geriatric, pregnant, or obese patients?

References and Resources

American Academy of Orthopaedic Surgeons, Pollak AN, ed. *Nancy Caroline's Emergency Care in the Streets.* 6th ed. Sudbury, MA: Jones and Bartlett; 2007.

Canadian Institute for Health Information. National Trauma Registry 2007 injury hospitalizations highlights report. In: *Focus: Pediatric Injury Hospitalizations in Canada, 2005–2006.* Ottawa, Canada; 2006.

Department for Transport. Child car seats. 2008. Available at: www.dft.gov.uk/think/focusareas/children/childincar. Accessed December 15, 2008.

Dieckmann RA, ed. *Pediatric Education for Prehospital Professionals.* 2nd ed. Sudbury, MA: Jones and Bartlett; 2006.

Gausche-Hill M, Henderson DP, Goodrich SM, et al. *Pediatric Airway Management for the Prehospital Professional.* Sudbury, MA: Jones and Bartlett; 2004.

Gazmararian JA, Petersen R, Spitz AM, et al. Violence and reproductive health; current knowledge and future research directions. *Maternal Child Health J.* 2000; 4(2):79–84.

Lewis, G (ed) 2007. The confidential enquiry into maternal and child health (CEMACH). Saving mothers' lives: reviewing maternal deaths to make motherhood safer: 2003–2005. The Seventh Report on Confidential Enquiries into Maternal Deaths in the United Kingdom. London: CEMACH.

Peden M, et al. World report on child injury prevention. Geneva, Switzerland: World Health Organization; 2008.

Revell M, Porter K, Greaves I. Fluid resuscitation in prehospital trauma care: a consensus view. *Emerg Med J.* 2002; 19:494–498.

Royal Society for Prevention of Accidents. Child car seats: the law. 2007. Available at: www.childcarseats.org.uk/law/index.htm. Accessed December 15, 2008.

Snyder DR, Christmas C, eds. *Geriatric Education for Emergency Medical Services.* Sudbury, MA: Jones and Bartlett; 2003.

United Nations. *World Population Prospects, The 2006 Revision, Executive Summary.* New York, NY: 2006. Available at: www.un.org/esa/population/publications/wpp2006/English.pdf. Accessed February 26, 2009.

World Health Organization. *The Injury Chart Book: A Graphical Overview of the Global Burden of Injuries.* Geneva, Switzerland: World Health Organization; 2002.

World Health Organization, Unicef. What you can do to keep kids safe from injury. 2008. Available at: www.who.int/violence_injury_prevention/child/injury/world_report/What_you_can_do_english.pdf. Accessed December 15, 2008.

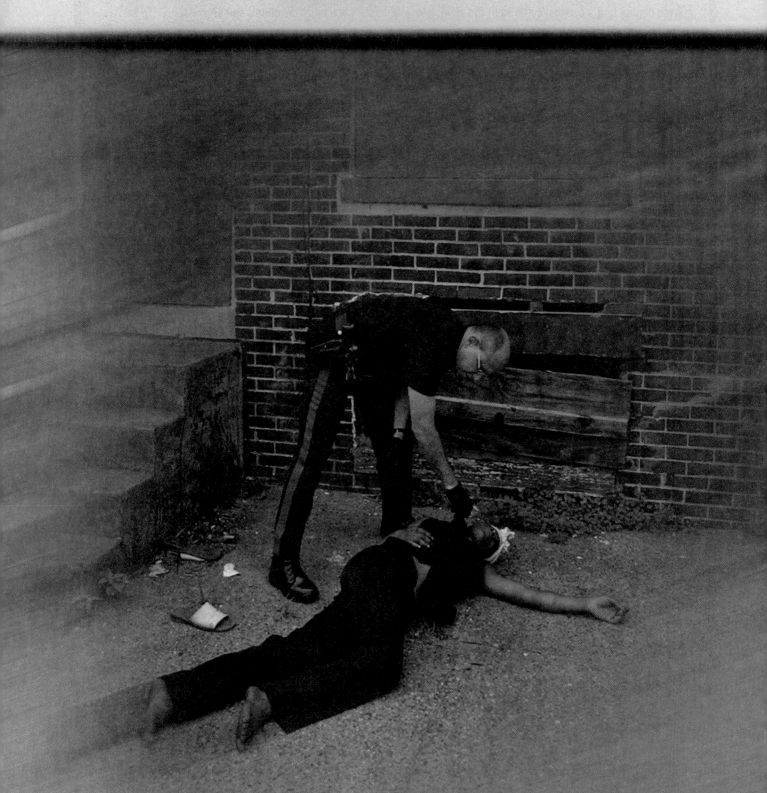

CASE STUDY

You have been requested by police to check an intoxicated female who appears to have been assaulted. Dispatch advises that police are on scene and the scene has been declared safe for you to enter. You arrive to find a middle-aged woman lying on the ground with a police officer trying to get information from the patient. You immediately notice that the patient has slurred speech and that there is an odor of alcohol surrounding the patient.

Further examination reveals a disoriented female with an abrasion on her forehead and a swollen and split lower lip. When asked about the injury the patient states she does not have an injury. She begins to pull away from you as you attempt to take her vital signs and tells you to go away. She has not been able to correctly answer anything other than her first name, and her speech has been getting more garbled as time has passed. She is refusing to allow you to touch her and she stumbles and falls several times.

As you attempt to restrain her from injuring herself any further, she becomes unconscious. Her breathing is nonlabored at 14 breaths/min with a pulse of 92 beats/min and a blood pressure of 122/78 mm Hg. It is a warm summer day and her skin is hot and sweaty. The examination of her pupils reveals that they are mid-point and slowly reactive to light. The abrasion to her forehead has no bleeding and the laceration to the lip appears to be several hours old. She has small abrasions to her hands and left knee from stumbling as she tried to get away from you.

1. This patient told you she did not want your help. Does she have the ability to refuse your care?

2. When this patient became unconscious, you began to treat her for possible injury or intoxication. What legal doctrine allowed you to care for her without her verbal permission?

3. This patient stumbled away from you during your attempt to assess her and sustained injury to her hands and knee. What elements would be required to claim malpractice?

4. You have completed your transportation of the patient to the hospital and are returning to your station when the dispatcher asks you to contact the police officer who is completing the report on the patient. He asks for information about the patient to fill in the details on his report. What information can you give to him?

Introduction

Many issues come into play when discussing the correct management, treatment, and triage of trauma patients. From early on in the history of medicine, patients have been afforded certain rights to make decisions about their medical care or lack thereof. Sometimes traumatic events can make it difficult to determine when a patient has the ability to make some of these life and death decisions.

Legal Issues Associated With Trauma Management

To function effectively in the emergency medical services (EMS) system, a provider must not only be capable of delivering the highest quality of medical care, but also must be prepared to address certain legal considerations that invariably arise. Trauma will often find the provider interacting with various law enforcement agencies because law enforcement personnel are often on scene at motor vehicle collisions, assaults, fires, and other trauma calls. These personnel may be conducting functions such as traffic control, scene safety, or criminal investigation. Furthermore, a provider may become involved in civil or criminal litigation as either a defendant or, more likely, as a witness for one of the parties.

Additionally, in the course of managing a trauma patient in the field, many legal issues will arise directly related to treatment and transportation. These issues may include consent or refusal of treatment, abandonment, turning over care to other providers, patient competence, and any Good Samaritan law that may be applicable. This chapter will review basic legal principles associated with the delivery of emergency care, allowing the EMS provider to deal with these issues effectively when they arise in the field.

In discussing legal issues, it is important to point out that laws frequently differ from state to state and country to country. In addition, local protocols and operating procedures may provide guidance or direction for the provider as to how issues discussed in this chapter should be handled. Accordingly, the legal principles presented here should not be considered legal advice. They are an overview of the general principles of law that commonly apply. For specific advice, the reader is strongly encouraged to seek guidance from legal counsel in the jurisdiction in which he or she is involved in EMS. In countries with a paramedic registrant body, such as the Health Professions Council in the United Kingdom, providers can review the standards set forth by that body.

Consent and Refusal of Treatment

It is a fundamental concept of health care that medical treatment may be provided only if the patient has expressed **consent**. This concept has evolved from the principle of autonomy that essentially gives each of us the right to make decisions about how we wish to be treated. Accordingly, a patient has a right to make a personal decision either to con-sent to or to refuse treatment. Consent can be considered a function of three significant factors: legal status, information, and decision-making capacity.

Legal Status

Does the patient have the legal right to make a health care decision? In some cases this issue will relate to the individual having reached the age of legal majority, because often a minor may not make decisions regarding health care. In the United States, most states allow minors who are considered emancipated to make decisions. Emancipation will vary among jurisdictions, but generally applies to minors who are married, members of the armed forces, or no longer being supported by their parents. Sometimes decisions for treatment may be legally made by a third party who is either a legal guardian or someone designated as a decision maker in a health care power of attorney or by court order.

In the United Kingdom, the term *emancipation* is not commonly used. The principle of *Gillick competence* (sometimes incorrectly referred to as *Fraser competence*; the Fraser guidelines relate solely to contraception), puts forward a principle for minors to give consent when they fulfill all of the requirements of capacity. This principle does not, however, allow minors to withhold consent if their parents wish an intervention to be carried out. In all cases, the best interests of the child should be the main consideration of health care providers.

Information

To make an informed decision regarding consent, a patient should have adequate information available to assist in the decision-making process. At the very least, the patient should be provided with the following information:

- The nature of the patient's suspected injury or illness
- An explanation of the treatment the provider feels is indicated and the benefits and risks associated with that treatment
- The possible consequences of refusing treatment

The nature of trauma care in the prehospital environment requires that consent be a far less formal process than what we typically see in a hospital admitting office where patients are asked to review and then sign a multipage consent document. Rarely does a patient sign a consent form in the field or the provider offer a detailed explanation of the treatment being suggested. We may simply tell a patient that we feel they may be suffering from internal injuries and we would like to start an IV so we will be able to administer fluid or medication if necessary. The patient may say yes, nod their head, or extend their arm to provide access to a vein. All of the foregoing may be considered forms of expressed consent and will generally suffice to authorize treatment. Indeed, consent to treat can sometimes be inferred from the mere fact that the patient called for an ambulance. Of course, in trauma situations the ambulance is often requested by another person such as a passing motorist or a police officer.

It is important to understand that consent to treatment may be withdrawn at any time and that consent may be selective. This means that a patient may consent to treatment and allow you to perform an assessment and apply a splint to their potentially fractured left ankle but then refuse to allow you to start an IV and administer an analgesic. This is not uncommon and is within the patient's rights.

Decision-Making Capacity

A valid consent or refusal may be given only by someone with the mental capacity to make a rational decision. We often refer to this as competence, but because competence is a legal concept that often requires judicial determination, the preferred term is <u>decision-making capacity</u>. Evaluating a patient for decision-making capacity can be quite simple, as in a case in which the patient is unconscious. At other times, however, the issue of capacity may be much more complex and involve a number of factors, including:

- Level of consciousness
- Ability to respond to questions
- Orientation to person, place, time, and event
- Influence of drugs or alcohol
- Influence of underlying mental disease
- Level of education
- Distracting injuries or pain
- Presence of shock or head injury
- Vital signs
- Preexisting mental capacity issues

TIP

In the United Kingdom, the Mental Capacity Act 2005 protects patients who have lost their capacity by putting in place mechanisms for a proxy to make medical decisions on the patient's behalf. The act is, however, more related to debilitating illness and end-of-life care as opposed to trauma.

The provider will have to assess each of these criteria and come to a rapid conclusion because patients who have suffered traumatic injuries often deteriorate quickly and therefore require prompt action. In many cases it may be helpful to contact online medical control (where applicable) to assist in determining decision-making capacity.

If the provider believes the trauma patient lacks decision-making capacity, it will be necessary to consider what further action should be taken. In some cases, where injuries are minor, treatment may be withheld until medical control or ambulance control is consulted and direction is given as to how to proceed or a family member or other authorized person arrives to give consent. In other cases it may be necessary to take immediate action to save the life of the patient. Trauma often involves circumstances where decision making cannot be delayed and the provider must act quickly. In cases where the provider must act promptly, it is often appropriate to proceed under the doctrine of <u>implied consent</u>. In certain circumstances, when the provider truly believes that life or limb is at stake, it may be necessary to

TIP

When the provider finds a situation that cannot be resolved, he or she can often call a physician for assistance. This is referred to as online medical control because the physician can offer assistance over the radio or phone as to how to proceed. Protocols or standing orders are available so providers can follow a doctor's order without having to seek direct contact. This is called off-line medical control because no radio or phone contact is required.

contact medical control and law enforcement and consider whether some form of civil custody and treatment over the objection of the patient is appropriate. Each jurisdiction has specific laws that control the manner in which this procedure should be handled.

Implied Consent

Implied consent, also known as the *emergency doctrine* or *doctrine of necessity*, is a legal doctrine that permits a health care provider to render emergency treatment under circumstances in which the patient is incapable of making a rational decision either to consent to or to refuse treatment. This may result from unconsciousness, severe shock, head injury, dementia, or the influence of drugs or alcohol. The legal basis for the application of implied consent is the assumption that the patient, if competent to do so, would desire and consent to treatment. These same principles may be applied in the case of a minor who is injured and requires treatment. In the absence of a parent or legal guardian, the EMS provider may assume that the parent or guardian, if available, would have wanted the child treated and would have provided consent.

It is important to note that the doctrine of implied consent should be used only in the case of serious injuries and not for minor conditions that do not require immediate treatment. In general, if time permits, it is wise to involve medical control in the decision to treat a patient using the doctrine of implied consent and to document any direction you receive from the physician.

Patient Refusal

Providers may encounter a trauma call where the patient refuses to be treated or transported. In many cases, the patient never requested an ambulance in the first place and the call may have been placed by a passerby who witnessed an accident and assumed an ambulance would be needed. Refusals in such cases are common. What is important to understand, however, is the fact that the standard for refusing care is the same as it is for granting consent to treat. In other words, the patient must be legally and mentally capable of making a decision and must have sufficient information about his or her medical status to make an informed

Treating Minors Unaccompanied by Parents

VIRTUALLY ALL HEALTH CARE WORKERS have some concerns about how the legal system impacts their jobs. They should be concerned. Decisions made by health care providers can significantly impact peoples' lives. The legal system will address poor decisions by health care workers in a number of ways. Patients may sue if they believe they have suffered an injury as the result of a negligent act. They may also sue if they feel their *autonomy* (right to make their own decisions) has not been respected.

Health care is one of the most highly regulated industries in our society. State and federal governments have enacted a myriad of statutes and administrative regulations governing all facets of patient care. Additionally, there is a rich body of "common law" emanating from over 200 years of court decisions. Some people refer to the "common law" as "judge-made law" because the rulings are not based on statutes, but rather on previous court decisions and societal norms. Understanding how all of these sources of law impact clinical decisions can seem daunting. Emergency providers have the additional pressure of time. Rarely is there an opportunity to obtain a formal legal opinion prior to taking action in a true emergency. Nevertheless, poor decisions made "under the gun" may result in legal consequences. To health care workers providing emergency care, this may seem like unfair second-guessing.

Injured minors present a special legal challenge to EMS providers. In your initial training, you likely learned that, because minors have no legal status, they can neither consent to nor refuse medical care. The rule of thumb is generally that consent must be obtained from a parent or legal guardian to provide care to minors. The term *emancipated minor* refers to those patients who are under the legal age in a given state but, because of other circumstances such as marriage, parenthood, pregnancy, and service in the armed forces, can be legally treated as adults.

EMS providers are often called to motor vehicle collisions involving teenagers who are not accompanied by parents or guardians. If these minors are injured badly enough to require medical attention, but they refuse care, what is the appropriate course of action for the EMS provider and what are the legal implications?

The most difficult and controversial situation may be cases in which minors refuse care. Such cases may arise when bystanders decide to call for emergency services at the scene of a collision. Many emergency care providers over think the legal issues involved in providing care to minors. You may wonder whether the patient is an emancipated minor and therefore able to consent or refuse care or whether you can legally allow a family friend to stand in for the legal guardians and refuse care in their place.

Some emergency care providers have erroneously reasoned that if a minor lacks the power to consent to care, he or she therefore is powerless to refuse. The flaw here is the false premise that minors lack the power to consent to their medical care. There is no blanket law denying a minor the right to consent to any medical care. State statutes exist that specifically empower minors to consent to medical care in a variety of settings, such as treatment of sexually transmitted infections, treatment of drug abuse, or psychiatric counseling. Some have erroneously deduced these specific consent statutes must be an exception to an underlying common law or statute, holding minors as powerless to consent to medical care. This is simply untrue. Generally, a mature minor may consent to his or her medical care.[1] Logically, this patient can therefore refuse care. However, any patient, adult or minor, should receive emergency medical care if there is an imminent risk of harm *and they lack the decisional capacity to refuse*.

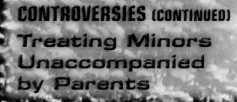
The greater the medical risk of foregoing care, the more willing an emergency care provider should be to provide necessary treatment to a minor under the doctrine of implied consent. In situations in which there is little or no risk, the provider should be more willing to accept the mature minor's refusal. For example, if EMS providers respond to a "fender bender" and the 16-year-old driver refuses transport to a hospital, I would honor his choice as long as there was no apparent injury. On the other hand, if the accident was more serious, and I was concerned about a life-threatening injury, I would transport the patient to the nearest trauma center despite his or her refusal of care. In all cases, reasonable efforts should be made to contact the parents or another responsible adult willing to assist in the final disposition.

The legal analysis relevant to the question of a minor's ability to consent to medical care can be complicated and involves not only state common law and statutes, but also federal statutes. However, if the emergency provider applies common sense and treats the minor with the respect and care he would want for his own child, the law will almost invariably support his decision.

Joseph P. Wood, MD, JD
Consultant and Vice-Chair
Department of Emergency Medicine
Mayo Clinic in Arizona
Phoenix, Arizona

Reference

1. Schlam L, Wood JP. Informed consent to the medical treatment of minors. *Health Matrix: Journal of Law-Medicine* 2000; 10(2):141–174.

decision. If all relevant criteria have been met, the patient is free to refuse care even if it does not appear rational to do so. Refusals to treat can easily result in potential liability, however, so it is wise to handle these situations cautiously.

Once the provider is satisfied that the patient has decision-making capacity, the patient should be advised about their medical status and the type of treatment indicated. If they continue to refuse treatment and transportation, every effort should be made to have the patient sign a release or similar local documentation. The document should be explained to the patient before it is signed and the signature should be witnessed by a third party. A law enforcement officer makes an excellent witness. If you are truly concerned that the patient may have injuries that could be serious and will require medical attention, the following steps should be considered before EMS departs from the scene:

1. Make every effort to emphasize the importance of treatment and transport to a hospital; make sure a clear explanation of the potential consequences of refusing treatment has been given to the patient.
2. Try having another person speak with the patient to see if they can convince the patient to be treated. A family member, friend, or police officer may be effective.
3. Contact medical control and let them know the circumstances. In certain cases it may be useful to have the patient speak directly with the physician.
4. Advise the patient to contact their own physician promptly.
5. Provide the patient with your emergency telephone number and advise them to call back immediately if they change their mind or if their condition becomes more serious.

Handing Over Care to Lower Level Personnel

In certain cases, a paramedic or other advanced life support (ALS) provider may feel it unnecessary to accompany a trauma patient to the hospital from the scene because the injuries are relatively minor, it does not appear that ALS care is needed, and a basic life support (BLS) team or Urgent Transfer crew would be sufficient during transport. The question that often arises is this: Does such a practice constitute abandonment of the patient? Many providers have been told they may be guilty of abandonment if they hand over patient care to someone who has a lower level of training. This is not a correct statement of the law. Under general principles of negligence, a health care provider should hand over patient care to another provider only if that provider has the credentials and training required to provide for the needs of that patient. In the hospital, a physician routinely hands over patient care to nurses, technicians, and mid-level providers such as a physician assistant. In the emergency setting, it is similarly appropriate for an ALS provider to hand over care to a BLS colleague if the transfer decision is handled properly **FIGURE 11-1**. When such a transfer of care takes place, the decision to do so should be made by the

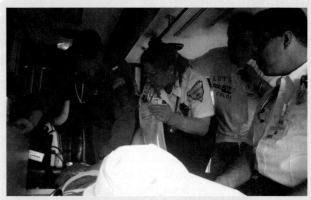

FIGURE 11-1 Paramedics are often able to transfer the care of a patient to a provider with a lesser level of training when protocols allow.

ALS provider on scene and not by BLS personnel. A number of factors should go into the decision-making process:

- Nature of the patient's injuries
- Age and past medical history of the patient, including medications
- Distance to the hospital
- Availability of ALS en route if the patient unexpectedly deteriorates
- How comfortable the BLS provider feels handling the patient and accepting responsibility for the patient

If, after considering these factors, both the ALS and BLS providers are comfortable, then the transfer of care may be appropriate. To ensure that these transfers are done appropriately, it is strongly advised that protocols be developed that outline the procedures to be followed. It is also important to be aware that other factors may have an impact on whether transfer of care is appropriate. For example, an EMS service may be contracted to guarantee that a paramedic will be on every emergency call. It is also possible that local protocols may require ALS on all calls. It is essential to understand these issues before making a decision to turn over care. The facts surrounding any transfer of care should be well-documented.

Abandonment

Abandonment may be defined as the termination of the provider-patient relationship without providing for the appropriate continuation of care. Some of the more common ways this may occur are as follows:

- Leaving a patient who requires treatment and transportation in the field without the consent of the patient
- Handing over patient care to another provider who lacks the level of training required by the patient
- Dropping off the patient in the emergency department without handing over care to a nurse or physician and providing a written and oral report regarding your findings and treatment **FIGURE 11-2**

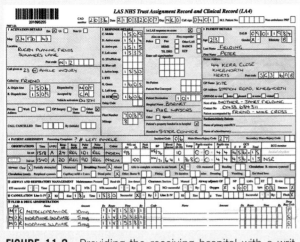

FIGURE 11-2 Providing the receiving hospital with a written and oral report limits the risk of being charged with abandonment.

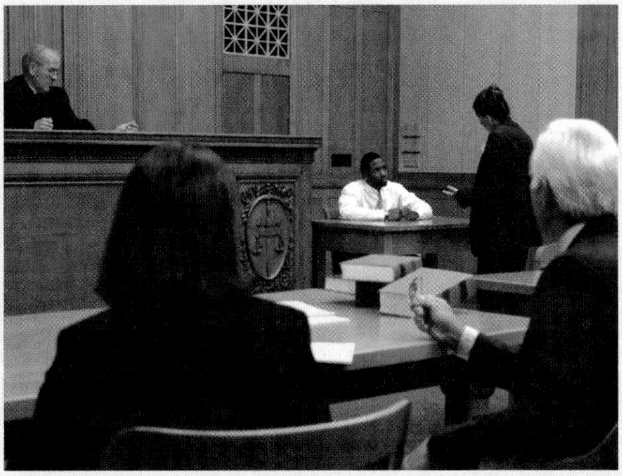

FIGURE 11-3 Paramedics can be taken to court for many reasons.

If a patient deteriorates or sustains any injury as a result of any of the foregoing, the provider may be liable for abandonment or negligence.

Good Samaritan Legislation

Many countries and jurisdictions, including every state in the United States, have passed Good Samaritan laws for the purpose of encouraging individuals, including health care providers, to assist at the scene of medical emergencies. There are countries where no such laws exist, for example in the United Kingdom, where there is generally felt to be a less litigious approach. Good Samaritan laws provide legal protection in the form of immunity under certain conditions. Most such laws protect average citizens as well as health care providers who render care at an emergency scene. Some laws cover only those who are volunteers but others also apply to paid health care professionals who are rendering emergent care in the course of their employment.

There are some common elements typically found in all Good Samaritan legislation:

- The person providing assistance must act within his or her scope of practice.
- Aid must be offered and rendered without any expectation of compensation of any kind.
- Immunity will not apply if the person acted with **gross negligence**.

In relation to Good Samaritan legislation, there is a difference between gross negligence and ordinary negligence. Most lawsuits are the result of **ordinary negligence**, which generally consists of errors in judgment, mistakes in treatment, and faulty handling of the patient **FIGURE 11-3**. Examples of ordinary negligence might include failure to recognize a tension pneumothorax, administration of an incorrect dose of medication, or dropping a patient while transferring him or her onto a stretcher.

Gross negligence consists of conduct that is reckless and bears no relationship to the accepted standard of care.

Acting beyond the scope of practice or engaging in conduct that exposes the patient to substantial harm would be considered gross negligence. Examples might include an attempt by an EMT-Basic to perform a surgical cricothyrotomy despite the fact that he has never been trained to perform this skill and the skill is outside his scope of practice as an EMT-B, or administration of a medication although advised not to do so by medical control (in the United States) or another authority. In such cases the Good Samaritan law would probably not protect the provider. Negligence can relate to acts of omission as well as commission. When a provider should provide a skill and does not, then a case of negligence can also be brought forward.

Elements of a Malpractice or Professional Negligence Claim

At this point it may be useful to review the elements of a lawsuit. Certain elements are necessary to prove for a plaintiff to prevail in a lawsuit and recover a judgment against the emergency medical service or provider:

- Duty to act
- Breach of that duty
- Injury or damages
- Proximate cause

If the plaintiff in a lawsuit is unable to prove each and every one of these elements, the suit will fail.

Duty to Act

Duty to act refers to the relationship that exists between the parties that requires the emergency medical service or paramedic to respond to a request for assistance. This may arise out of a contract, a statute, a mutual aid agreement, or some other legal relationship. In some cases, duty may arise out of custom and tradition if a volunteer ambulance service has provided emergency services for a period of time and thereby created an expectation on behalf of the residents of the town that they would respond when requested. Duty is generally very easy to establish. For example, when a patient calls to request an ambulance and you put your uniform on and respond to the call for help, you have adopted a duty to act.

Breach of Duty

A **breach of duty** results when the provider deviates from what would be considered a safe and competent standard of practice. In evaluating a claim against a provider, the provider's conduct will be compared to that which would be expected from a similarly trained provider under similar circumstances. The accepted standard is often established in court by the use of expert witnesses and reference to medical textbooks and local protocols. For example, during a response you determine that the patient requires a skill that is not in the protocols. If you provide that skill to the patient, then you have breached your duty. This breach of duty more often exists when the patient requires a skill but it is not completed by the provider.

Damages

The mere fact that a provider acted negligently is not sufficient to prevail in a lawsuit. The plaintiff must prove that actual damages or injuries were sustained. If a patient was administered an incorrect medication but suffered no adverse reaction, he or she could not prove damages, despite the fact that a clear error was committed. The patient must experience additional injury or a worsening of the condition to complete a suit of negligence.

Proximate Cause

The plaintiff must prove that the injuries he or she sustained were caused by the provider's negligence. In other words, there must be a direct relationship between the negligent conduct and the physical injury to the patient. The question asked in court is "Were it not for the negligence of the defendant, would these injuries have occurred?" The provider's action or lack of action must be tied directly to the damages sustained for negligence to have been committed.

Interacting With Law Enforcement Personnel

In the course of responding to trauma calls, the provider will often interact with law enforcement personnel who may be on scene for traffic or crowd control, crime scene investigation, or to make an arrest. In some cases, providers may rely on them for protection. It is therefore important to develop an effective working relationship despite the fact that the responsibilities of the provider might sometimes appear to be in conflict with those of the police officer on scene **FIGURE 11-4**. At all times, providers must remember that they have a primary responsibility to patient care and they should never allow themselves to assume the role of criminal investigator or detective. On the other hand, providers should cooperate with law enforcement to the extent possible and not interfere with an investigation or disrupt evidence on scene unless absolutely necessary to provide good patient care.

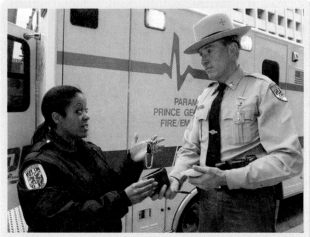

FIGURE 11-4 It is important to balance care of the patient and cooperation with law enforcement personnel.

While infrequent, conflicts may arise when a police officer directs a provider to remove an injured accident victim from the scene before the provider believes it is safe to do so to facilitate the flow of traffic, or refuses to allow treatment of an injured rape victim for fear of destroying evidence. Such circumstances create a real challenge for the provider and must be handled carefully.

The best way to avoid difficult issues on scene is to address them before they arise. The EMS agency should develop policies around these potential law enforcement interactions so the provider on scene will have some guidance as to how to proceed. It is also useful to meet regularly with local law enforcement agencies to develop an understanding of each others' roles and discuss possible ways of handling various issues that might arise.

The provider should always keep the following points in mind:

- Your primary responsibility is to your patient.
- Contact law enforcement when it is believed that a crime may have been committed or when provider safety is in danger. Never enter a scene unless you know it is safe to do so.
- At a possible crime scene, do not move, destroy, or tamper with anything unless it is necessary to do so to provide patient care. If you find it necessary to move or tamper with anything, let the police know what you have done.
- Do not allow a rape or sexual assault victim to use the bathroom or take a bath or shower until police arrive.
- Do not turn over patient care reports or other documentation to law enforcement personnel unless proper procedure is followed. Local laws and, where applicable, the Health Insurance Portability and Accountability Act (HIPAA) must be followed at all times. Such laws will vary greatly among

jurisdictions. In some areas, providers are required to turn over run reports on scene whereas in others a subpoena is required.

- Try to resolve conflicts on scene by carefully explaining your position to the law enforcement personnel on scene and attempting to solicit their cooperation.
- Document all contact with law enforcement carefully and in detail.

Mandatory Reporting

It is important to understand that many areas have laws that require health care providers to report certain events. Many of these mandatory reporting statutes involve events related to trauma, in particular industrial accidents. Although laws vary among areas, some examples of mandatory reporting include child, spousal, or elder abuse; gunshot and stab wounds; animal bites; sexual assault; and certain communicable diseases FIGURE 11-5.

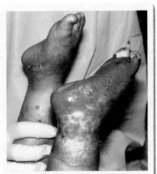

FIGURE 11-5 Certain types of trauma, including trauma from abuse, require mandatory reporting to governmental agencies.

The manner in which such reports must be made varies among jurisdictions, and the provider should become familiar with the laws of the area where he or she is employed. Consequences for failure to report may be either civil or criminal and could potentially affect the provider's license or certification.

Documentation

Every provider has been educated on the importance of documentation. Documentation of an emergency response might be used for many different reasons, including medical documentation of the care and treatment delivered by the provider, billing purposes, quality improvement reviews, medical and statistical research, as part of a criminal investigation, and as evidence in criminal or civil litigation.

REPORTING AGENCY | IDENTIFIER # 30176 | BLS ☐ ALS ■ | SERIAL # 292281 | INCIDENT # 213412A | CENSUS TRACT OR CODE 30176A | TODAY'S DATE 020206

PATIENT INFO

PATIENT'S LAST NAME Smith | FIRST John | M.I. A. | PHONE 555-1212 | INCIDENT LOCATION

ADDRESS 123 | STREET Ave. A | CITY Anywhere | STATE Wa | ZIP CODE 04132 | AGE 38 | BIRTH DATE 052767 | SEX M | PATIENT # 1 of 1

INSURANCE CODE | SOCIAL SECURITY OR MEDICAID # 123-45-6789 | GROUP INSURANCE # A23174 | PUBLIC ASSISTANCE ☐ YES ■ NO | PRIVATE PHYSICIAN N. Pain, M.D.

BILL TO OR NEAREST RELATIVE | LAST NAME Smith | FIRST John | MIDDLE INITIAL A. | PHONE NUMBER 555-1212

ADDRESS 123 | STREET Ave. A. | CITY Anywhere | STATE Wa. | ZIP CODE 04132

HOSPITAL CONTACTED University Hospital | TIME 0848 | PHYSICIAN CONTACTED Medical Control | TIME 0834 | OTHER N/a | TIME N/a

MEDICATIONS TAKEN Insulin, Paxil ØDrug allergies

NARRATIVE: (Include chief complaint, history, pt. exam, impression, therapy)

38 y.o. ♂ found lying supine on sofa. Per wife, pt. took his insulin but did not eat. Pt. responsive to painful Stimuli only; Combative when aroused. Per wife, pt. has Hx of IDDM and depression. Ø other PMHx. Initial assessment findings revealed patent airway, tachypnea, and tachycardia Ø gross bleeding or S/s of trauma. Applied O2 @ 15 L/min via NRB Mask. D-Stick: 34 mg/dL. Per protocol, initiated IV NS c̄ 18 ga. cath in Ⓛ hand @ 0827. At 0828, gave 50mL of 50% Dextrose IVP. Reassessment p̄ D50 revealed that pt. was conscious + Alert, asking "what happened." Advised pt. of Situation + of need to go to hospital; he agreed. Baseline Vital Signs taken @ 0830 (see flow chart). ECG reveals Sinus Tach @ 104 BPM s̄ ectopy. Loaded pt. into unit + began transport to hospital. Medical Control notified @ 0834; Ø further orders. Continued O2 and reassessed Blood Sugar (105 mg/dL). Head to toe exam was unremarkable; pt. remained Conscious + alert throughout transport. Vital Signs repeated (see flow chart). ECG revealed NSR. Pupils E/R to light.

Arrived @ receiving facility @ 0855; Pt. Condition remained unchanged. ~~Verbal~~ Verbal report given to ED physician. Cleared receiving facility @ 0908 and returned to service.

Per Medic 52 Badge #1715

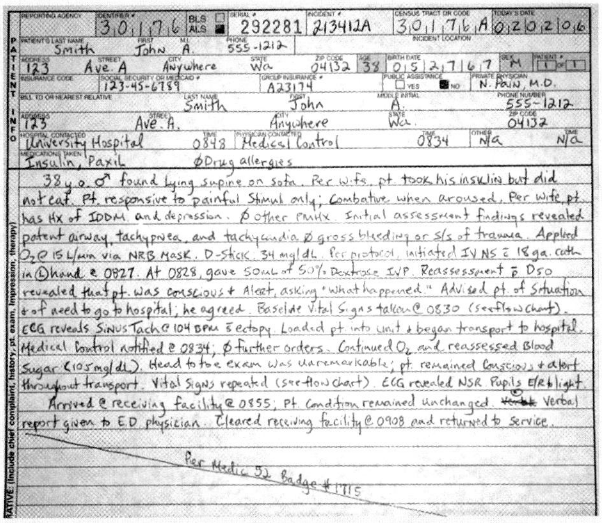

FIGURE 11-6 A complete and well-written report can be the provider's best defense in a legal dispute.

When writing a run report or patient report form, the provider should ask him- or herself the following questions FIGURE 11-6:

- Would I be comfortable defending this report in a court of law several years from now?
- Would someone reading this report have a clear understanding of why an ambulance was called, what the assessment findings were, what treatment was provided, and how the patient responded to any interventions?

A well-written report should be accurate, complete, and legible. Remember the cardinal rule of documentation: *If you didn't write it, you didn't do it*. Pertinent positive findings (patient has pain) as well as pertinent negative (patient has no pain) findings should be documented. In a court of law, the judge may very well apply this rule and not permit a provider to testify regarding any care or treatment that was not documented on the run report. A well-written report may be a provider's best defense in a lawsuit challenging the quality of the care provided. On the other hand, a poorly written report can be devastating and result in a bad outcome in court despite the fact that the quality of care delivered on scene was excellent.

CHAPTER RESOURCES

CASE STUDY ANSWERS

1 This patient told you she did not want your help. Does she have the ability to refuse your care?

This patient lacks the ability to refuse medical care based on her altered level of consciousness, inability to respond to questions appropriately, disorientation, and the apparently overwhelming influence of drugs or alcohol. Other factors that would affect the patient's ability to consent to or refuse care include underlying mental disease, shock or head injury, altered vital signs, or preexisting mental capacity issues.

2 When this patient became unconscious, you began to treat her for possible injury or intoxication. What legal doctrine allowed you to care for her without her verbal permission?

Implied consent (also known as the emergency doctrine) allows the provider to provide immediate emergency care to an individual who lacks the ability to make a rational decision. Implied consent is deemed appropriate to use only in serious cases that require immediate treatment to stabilize an injury or illness. This patient may have a head injury that, if left untreated, could progress to disability or death.

3 This patient stumbled away from you during your attempt to assess her and sustained injury to her hands and knee. What elements would be required to claim malpractice?

Injury sustained by the patient while you are caring for her is a serious event and should be fully documented. To claim malpractice she would have to prove four key things: You had a duty to act, you breached that duty, she was injured, and the injury came from your breach of duty.

4 You have completed your transportation of the patient to the hospital and are returning to your station when the dispatcher asks you to contact the police officer who is completing the report on the patient. He asks for information about the patient to fill in the details on his report. What information can you give to him?

Information regarding a patient is guarded under several laws and often local policies. Although the urge to assist the police may be strong, consider what information is able to be exchanged and under what circumstances in your system.

Trauma in Motion

1. If a patient admits a crime to you during your assessment, can you follow up with the police?
2. A patient has tried to commit suicide by hanging. During your assessment he requests that you leave him alone. If he is awake and alert and understands his medical condition, can you honor his request?
3. A patient admits to having three drinks tonight and then getting in a minor collision with his car, leaving him with a laceration to the head. He does not want to go to the hospital. Does he have the ability to refuse care?
4. What is your agency's protocol for interacting with law enforcement when a patient is in police custody?
5. How can a well-written patient care report keep you from having to testify in court?

References and Resources

Cohn B, Azzara AJ. *Legal Aspects of Emergency Medical Services*. W.B. Saunders: New York; 1998.

Emergency Medical Treatment and Active Labor Act. 42 USC Sect. 1395 dd.

Grubb A, Kennedy I. *Medical Law*, 3rd ed. London: Butterworths; 2000.

Moy MM. *The EMTALA Answer Book*. Aspen Publishing: New York; 2008.

Rozofsky F. *Informed Consent*, 2nd ed. Little, Brown: London; 1994.

Schneid T. *Legal Liabilities in Emergency Medical Services*. Taylor & Francis: London; 2001.

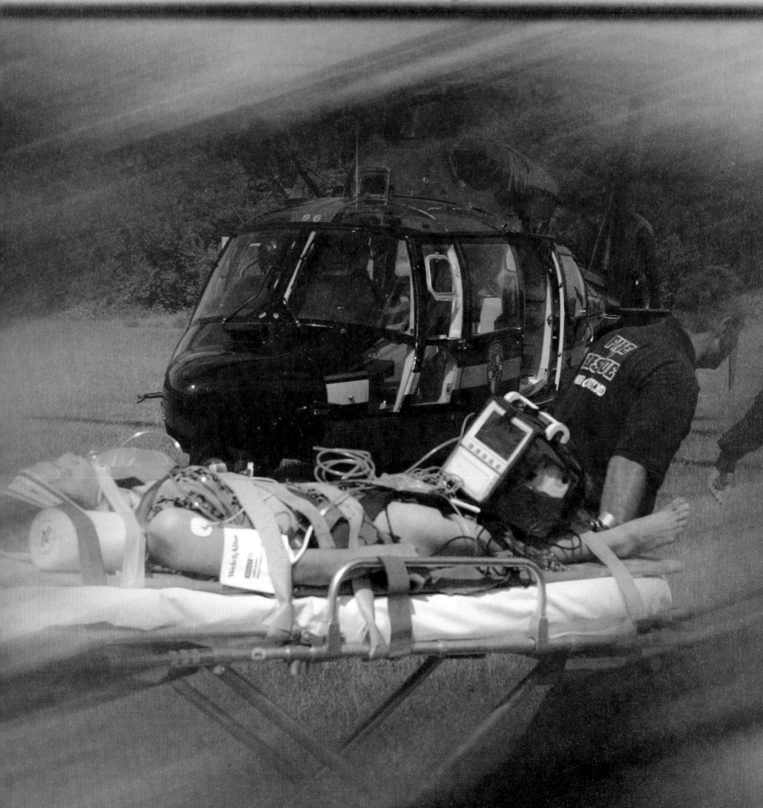

You are dispatched to a motor vehicle collision as the third ambulance for multiple patients. The first arriving units set up a command post and rescue has been working to extricate the passengers from a vehicle that has rolled over an embankment at the edge of a roadway. As you arrive, you are directed to a 20-year-old woman who was an unrestrained rear seat passenger. Because of her position in the vehicle, your patient has been removed directly to a long backboard prior to your arrival. The previous ambulance crews have removed two seriously injured patients and found the driver of the vehicle to be deceased.

Your assessment reveals a young woman secured to a long backboard who complains that she cannot feel her legs. You confirm the loss of motor function and sensation below her lower chest and begin a rapid trauma/secondary assessment. During the assessment you locate deformity and bruising over the thoracic spine at the T-8 level and several abrasions on her head and arms. Vital signs include a pulse of 120 beats/min, blood pressure of 84/40 mm Hg, and respirations of 22 breaths/min and shallow. Her skin is warm and pink. You complete the immobilization of the patient to the long backboard.

The local community hospital is a 40-minute drive and the closest trauma center is over an hour by ground. By air, the transport time is 18 minutes to the trauma center. The weather is clear and there is ample space to land a helicopter.

1 What is the best way to determine which patients should be treated when limited providers are available?

2 What are the resources a trauma center would have available for your patient that a community hospital may not?

3 What are the types of patients best suited to triage to a trauma center?

4 Is there a danger of sending too many patients to one hospital?

5 What are the transport considerations for this patient?

Introduction

Trauma is recognized as a serious health care problem worldwide and it is accepted that trauma should be addressed in a systematic manner. The majority of injuries seen by prehospital providers are of minor or moderate severity, and the number of patients is typically handled by a single ambulance crew. Occasionally, the provider will be faced with making decisions regarding the severely injured patient requiring specialized trauma care. For a trauma system to be optimally effective it is critical to use a method of differentiating those patients who require the specialized expertise and resources of a **trauma center** (hospital that specializes in the care of the severely injured) from those who can be cared for in a community hospital. Rapid field assessment and triage to an appropriate facility are essential in any functioning trauma system.

Triage of Multiple Casualties

A **mass casualty incident (MCI)** is defined as an incident that has more patients than a system can handle using everyday procedures and equipment. (Urban emergency medical service [EMS] systems often have more assets available than smaller rural EMS groups.) It is not uncommon to have more than one patient at a trauma scene, and most operational plans are designed to handle these situations. MCIs often require multiple EMS agencies and may require law enforcement, rescue, fire suppression, hazmat, or other specialized groups. The **incident command system (ICS)** was developed to help manage a situation that has become bigger than a local system can control without help **FIGURE 12-1**.

Because an MCI exceeds the ability of the system to handle either the number of patients or the number of severely injured ones in the early stages, additional resources must be called for using **mutual aid agreements** set up ahead of an event like this. Agreements with neighboring agencies often include how and when the other agency will enter the scene and how they will interact within the ICS. These agreements have very localized information and the local protocols should be reviewed frequently.

Triage is the sorting of patients first based on their need for initial care and then based on an appropriate facility that is able to provide an appropriate level of care. **Mass casualty triage** is the process of determining, in the presence of an overwhelming number of injuries, which patients get treated and/or transported based on the resources available to provide treatment and transportation.

The scope of the incident can be as great as the London underground bombing **FIGURE 12-2** or as small as a motor vehicle crash that exceeds your agency's available units.

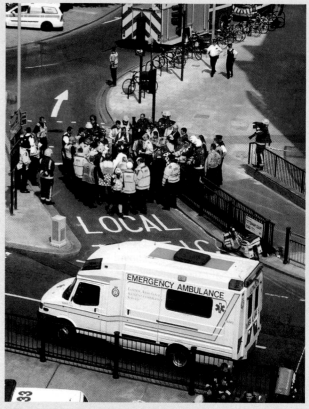

FIGURE 12-1 Many types of agencies can work under the ICS.

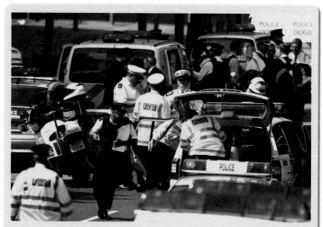

FIGURE 12-2 Emergency responders treated 700 injured and 56 dead at the scene of the London underground bombing.

Triage Systems

Using a system will make it easy for any trained provider to perform the task of field triage. Several different systems are used around the world but most have similar steps and sorting methods. Primary triage is used to sort patients at the scene of an MCI to allow a limited number of responders to provide the most efficient care to the most people affected by the event. Secondary triage includes efforts such as Triage SORT, Secondary Assessment of Victim Endpoint (SAVE), and System of Risk Triage, which usually requires an increase in the number of providers and available resources. Several of the primary methods of triage are discussed here.

Simple triage and rapid treatment (START) is a basic triage system that can be performed by trained first responders in emergencies. It is not intended to supersede medical personnel or techniques. It was developed at Hoag Hospital in Newport, California, and has been used effectively in MCIs throughout the world, including the 1989 Northridge California earthquake, the 1992 and 2001 New York World Trade Center attacks, and the 1995 Oklahoma City bombing. In an effort to maximize the use of limited resources, the triage function at any scene can be performed by the lowest trained provider capable of performing it properly. This keeps the limited advanced resources free to perform the more critical task of treating the injured and allows arriving care providers to be directed to those with the most urgent needs without spending valuable time with patients who are either only mildly injured or are most likely not going to survive.

START triage uses respirations, pulse, and mental status (RPM) to assign priority. Patients with no respirations receive an attempt to open the airway and reevaluation. Respirations are divided at the 30 breaths/min mark; pulse is based on a capillary refill time of 2 seconds; and mental status is assessed by asking the patient to follow a simple command. An alternative to the START triage tool used for pediatric patients is the JumpSTART triage method. In JumpSTART triage, children who are not breathing after having their airway opened are given five rescue breaths and are reevaluated for spontaneous breathing. Respirations must be between 15 and 45 breaths/min, and mental status should be appropriate to age.

The triage sieve is another tool used by providers to provide primary triage at the scene of an MCI. The triage sieve was originally introduced as part of the Major Incident Medical Management and Support (MIMMS) course for health care providers. Documented use of the triage sieve includes a train wreck in Balochistan, Pakistan, where 122 patients were encountered. Used in the UK and parts of Australia, the triage sieve uses the ability to walk, an open airway, respiratory rate (between 10 and 29 breaths/min), and heart rate to assign priority to each patient. Follow-up to the triage sieve is completed using the Triage SORT system.

In the triage sieve, patients are placed into one of four categories based on the assessment findings. Associated with the development of the triage sieve is the **Pediatric**

Triage Tape (PTT). Although the parameters of the PTT are the same as the triage sieve, the values are changed based on patient height measured by the tape. A child's height is related to his or her weight, which is related to their age, thus making the tool age-appropriate.

The **Move, Assess, Sort, and Send (MASS)** triage system, introduced by the Advanced Disaster Life Support (ADLS) course, uses an initial step of asking the casualties who can walk to move to a separate location while the ones who cannot walk are asked to raise their hands to wave. Triage is started on the patients who do not move. These patients either cannot understand the command or are not able to move, making them a higher priority. The patients are then assessed based on the START or any of the sorting methods available and separated into four categories.

The **CareFlight** triage system operates similar to the START system but uses only observations that require no vital sign measurements. Because it does not use measurement of vitals, it is appropriate for pediatric use. Designed and used in Australia and also used in South Africa, its documented usage includes the 2002 Bali nightclub bombing. It has been validated in large-scale studies using patients presenting to an emergency department but, as with the other methods, it has no documented large-scale field validity studies.

The **Sort, Assess, Lifesaving interventions, and Treatment and/or Transport (SALT)** triage system begins by using a global sorting of the mass of casualties similar to the MASS system. This initial step identifies the casualties who are able to understand verbal instructions and are therefore likely to have good perfusion. The casualties are given a collection point to move to for further instructions. This is in an attempt to decrease casualties leaving the scene and overwhelming local hospital resources before EMS can begin to move the highest priority patients. The SALT method differs from others in its lifesaving intervention steps, which include bleeding control, opening the airway, two rescue breaths for children, needle decompression for tension pneumothorax, and auto-injector antidotes. Patients are then sorted into one of five categories.

The **Sacco Triage Method** uses a proprietary computer-based program designed to match victims with available resources. Casualties are assigned a score based on respiratory rate, pulse rate, and motor response. Before scoring a patient, initial care such as opening the airway, chest decompression, and bleeding control should be completed. The score is then put into a computer program along with the available resources on the scene and in the regional hospitals. An algorithm provides a score for each patient that will change with the available resources, maximizing the chances for survival. Patients are scored for transport individually and not sorted into categories.

Triage Categories

A provider assigned to triage will be required to assess all patients at a scene to determine the initial severity of each. This initial assessment can be done in 30 to 60 seconds per patient. Four to five categories are used by most systems to determine patient acuity:

1. **Red tag or flag**: This category is used for patients with critical injuries who are unstable but salvageable. Patients placed in the red category usually fail the ABCs. They require treatment immediately to fix a problem in the ABCs.
2. **Yellow tag or flag**: Yellow category patients are categorized as serious. These patients will pass the ABCs but usually have a significant injury preventing them from walking from the scene of the injury. These injuries are often musculoskeletal in nature.
3. **Green tag or flag**: The color green has a connection with "go" and patients within this category are usually able to ambulate on their own from the scene. It is often helpful to move into a triage situation with a large number of patients and ask the victims who can walk to move themselves to a secure area. This will decrease the number of patients who will have to be initially triaged and open the area for additional personnel to assist in triage or treatment. These patients will need to be triaged later, but the patients who are left will be the ones more desperately needing assistance.

This is where the major systems begin to differ. Many of the systems provide for the categorizing of patients who are dead at the scene of the incident. Some systems also provide for a category of patients who are expected, or who are not expected, to be salvageable using the available resources. This category often assigns specific physiologic parameters to qualify the casualties assigned.

4. **Black (or sometimes white) tag or flag**: Patients who present with no breathing after an attempt to open the airway or who have injuries incompatible with life are placed into this category.
5. **Grey, white, or blue tag or flag**: (The color used for this category is not universal and a blue tag or flag is often used to signify a patient who requires decontamination from a hazardous materials exposure.) Expectant or patients who are expected to die due to an overwhelming injury are placed in this category. A patient who does not breathe after the airway is opened but may have a pulse would be placed in this category, as would a patient with an open head wound with brain matter missing. Depending on the type of incident involved, the number of patients in this category may be few or overwhelming. It should be noted that the patients initially placed into this category should be retriaged as soon as additional resources become available.

Triage is a process that can change with time. After the initial triage is done, a patient will be seen by different providers giving further assessment or treatment. At each step, the triage category of the patient may change. It is possible that a patient who initially is able to walk from the scene presents with a complaint that will move them to a yellow or red category. Retriaging requires tracking the changes to the patient. This can be done by simply tearing off additional segments of some triage tags or adding another triage tag to the patient **FIGURE 12-3**. In large incidents, this triage tag may become the only record required to be completed for each of the patients.

When an additional triage tag is added to a patient during retriaging, the triage officer must remember to change the patient count to track the number of patients seen at the incident. See your local protocols for the accepted way to document retriaging.

Incident Command System

The ICS was initially developed to enable fire fighters on large-scale wildfires to work together under one commander: the **incident commander**. The ICS has since become a more universal way to manage everyday scenes that have several units or agencies working together

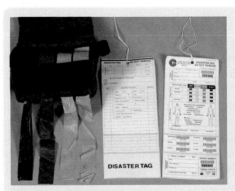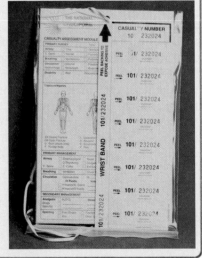

FIGURE 12-3 Triage tags are simple devices used to keep track of patients at a multicasualty incident.

FIGURE 12-4. The command position should be filled by the first unit responding when they realize the scale of the incident will be larger than a single unit can handle. This command position can then be handed off to more qualified personnel as the incident unfolds (which, in some countries, may be the police). The incident commander will often appoint several units to deal with specialized tasks such as medical patient care, law enforcement, fire suppression, or extrication FIGURE 12-5.

With patients requiring medical care, the incident commander will often open the position of medical or EMS unit. This unit will have several tasks that may be handled by one person or may require additional positions depending on the scale of the incident. These positions include the medi-

cal unit chief and triage, treatment, transport, and staging officers. Several of these tasks may be completed by a single person; in larger incidents all providers may be separated by space and function.

The **triage officer** (or the providers assigned by the triage officer in a larger scene) is charged with utilizing the agencies' initial triage system and provides little or no treatment to patients. The triage officer must continue sorting patients into their medical needs and counting the overall number of patients to be treated until all patients have been triaged. An accurate accounting for all patients must be started from the onset of the incident and follow to the completion of the incident. Although most triaging will be done at the scene of the incident, safety issues may require that triaging be completed after rescue or decontamination has been completed.

The **treatment officer or casualty clearing officer** will set up an area suitable for immediate patient care needs. This officer will supervise medical care given to patients at the scene and keep a record of the patients seen. The treatment unit will be the first place most patients will be completely assessed and treatment will begin. This area should be close enough for immediate access to patients, yet far enough away to allow a zone of safety for the providers to care for the injured. The treatment officer has the added responsibility of retriaging all patients to determine if they still meet the original triage decision. Medical personnel with the highest levels of training should be used to provide the care in the treatment area.

Transport officers or ambulance loading officers organize transport of patients from the scene, ensuring patients are distributed to appropriate hospitals and preventing hospital overloading. Part of this organization involves contacting receiving hospitals to advise them of the number and condition of patients. A transportation log must be completed to accurately account for all patients treated at the scene. Most triage tags have options for numbering patients to account for each from the time of triage through arrival at the hospitals.

Staging is used to collect incoming providers, equipment, and ambulances, and move them to where they are needed. The **staging officer or ambulance parking officer** coordinates the physical location and approach of incoming resources, including additional ambulances and requests for aeromedical resources. Additional personnel who wish to help at the scene should be funneled through the staging officer for assignment to an appropriate area.

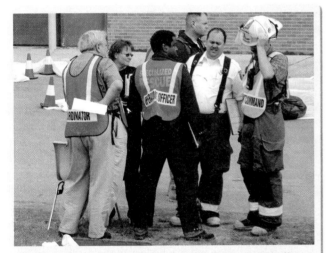

FIGURE 12-4 The incident commander will appoint officers to handle tasks on scenes with large numbers of victims.

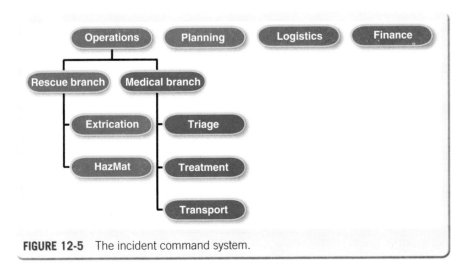

FIGURE 12-5 The incident command system.

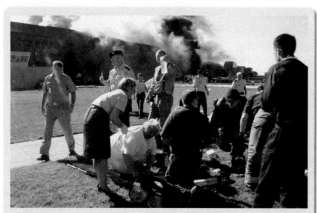

FIGURE 12-6 Providers must be able to assess each patient and move to the next quickly to care for the most people with the limited resources initially available.

Initial Triage Assessment

The initial/primary assessment used in triaging multiple patients focuses on the ABCs, including the level of consciousness (LOC). As you approach a patient, formulate your general impression. Age of the patient, what position they are found in, activity or awareness of their surroundings, work of breathing, and external bleeding are visual cues to the assessment of a patient. In the United Kingdom, this initial triage assessment is referred to as the *triage sieve*.

Airway and Breathing

Quickly assess for breathing. If the patient is breathing, determine whether the ventilations are of an adequate rate (between 12 and 29 breaths/min) and depth (good chest rise). If the patient requires assistance, the patient is tagged with a red tag. If the patient is not breathing, open the airway and check for breathing again. If there is no breathing after opening the airway, the patient is tagged black. Move on to the next patient. The triage officer's job is just to triage, not to treat patients **FIGURE 12-6**.

Circulation

Assess for a pulse. Radial pulses may provide information to help you assess the quality of pulses. If there is no radial pulse, move immediately to a carotid pulse. If no pulse is felt, tag the patient with black. Patients with a weak pulse should be tagged red. Check for external bleeding. Remem-

ber that treatment is left for the next providers. If bleeding is present, however, and the patient is conscious, have the patient hold pressure using a piece of clothing for a bandage until the next provider arrives. Tourniquets should be considered for patients presenting with catastrophic bleeding from an extremity.

Level of Consciousness

To finish the initial triage assessment, check the LOC. Patients who are not awake but respond only to pain, or patients who are unconscious, should be tagged red. If the patient is awake or can be awakened by voice, but is confused and has good ABCs, he or she should be tagged yellow.

Special Considerations

There are several special considerations when treating patients at a large incident. The objective of triaging patients is to provide the most amount of care to the patients who are most likely to survive. This can be difficult to determine in a 60-second assessment, but the factors that influence this decision can include the patient's age. When a young patient and an older patient have the same injuries, the younger patient usually has the better chance of survival. Another factor is the patient's overall health. Patients who are healthier before the incident are more likely to survive than patients who have other medical conditions. Efforts should be made in the treatment area to determine the best use of resources by retriaging patients as they are treated.

When rescuers working at the scene become ill or injured, they should be treated as quickly as possible **FIGURE 12-7**. Providers need to be assured that if they become injured they will not be lost in the mass of patients. Providing immediate care to our colleagues will bring them back to the incident quicker and give peace of mind to the other providers that they will be taken care of in the event of injury. The psychological impact of providers when an injured provider appears stuck sitting at a scene can be devastating and reduce their ability to provide care.

Children may not respond to the same stimuli that adults do when assessing the airway and breathing. If a child does not begin breathing after opening the airway, provide five rescue breaths. If the child begins breathing, tag the patient red and move on; if there is no breathing, tag them black. Respiratory rates for children should be between 15 and 45 breaths/min. Any breathing above or below this should be tagged red. Because pulses are often hard to find in young patients, patients who are breathing but have no pulse should be tagged red until retriaging can occur.

Which system you use to triage patients may be dictated by state, regional, local, or department/service protocols. Whatever system is used, providers within that EMS system should not only be aware of the triage system, but also practice it regularly.

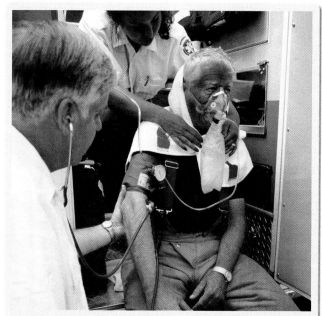

FIGURE 12-7 Injured rescuers should receive immediate care and should not fall into the triage system.

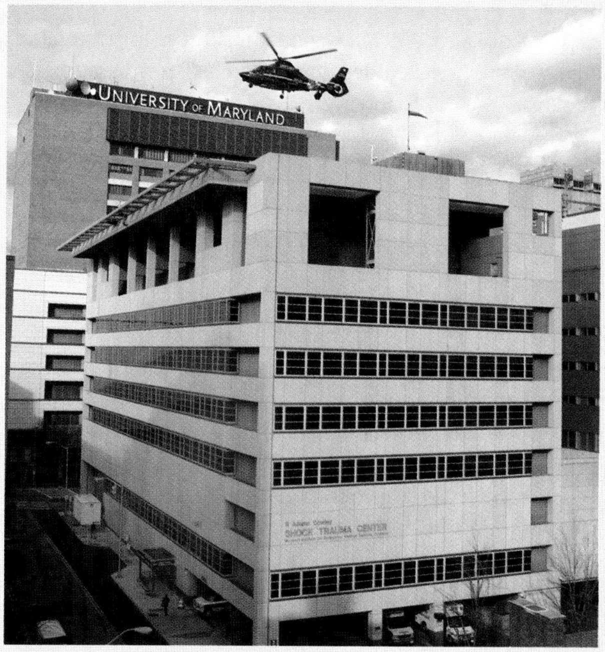

FIGURE 12-8 Designated trauma centers are an important component of any state's overall trauma system.

Trauma Centers

Treatment of the acutely injured has been recognized as significantly different from treatment of the ill since the time of Napoleon when early trauma systems were born in continental Europe. In the United Kingdom, the Birmingham Accident Hospital and Rehabilitation Centre opened in 1941 and was dedicated to the treatment and rehabilitation of the injured by specially trained staff.

In 1966, at the direction of the U.S. Department of Transportation, a study was published that changed the way injuries were dealt with throughout the United States. This paper, *Accidental Death and Disability: The Neglected Disease of Modern Society*, published by the National Academy of Sciences National Research Council, was charged with answering this question: Why are so many people dying on U.S. roadways? As a result of that paper, the U.S. Congress was persuaded to put forth money in the form of block grants to the individual states to develop systems to deal with the cause of the death and disability in the report—trauma.

The recommendations in the report focused mainly on improving emergency medical care, but also recommended completing additional research and injury prevention policy. In 1985, *Injury in America—A Continuing Public Health Problem* reexamined the original 1966 paper and recommended a major national program of research to increase injury prevention and control. The *Report on the Management of Patients with Major Injuries* from the Royal College of Surgeons of England and the British Orthopaedic Association led to the introduction of advanced trauma life support (ATLS) as well as trauma centers in the United Kingdom.

Systems designed to care for acutely injured victims of trauma began to be developed during the 1980s throughout North America, Europe, Asia, Australia, and South Africa.

The formation of trauma systems in the United States initiated many other changes. Organizations that previously had no connection to prehospital care began to influence it and to be influenced by it. One such agency is the American College of Surgeons (ACS). Prior to the development of emergency medical services, its scope of authority reached only to surgeons and hospitals. As a result of the advancement of EMS and the additional trauma patients being brought into hospitals, the ACS began to make recommendations that would affect EMS. One area it influenced was the development of standards for trauma center designation **FIGURE 12-8** .

Trauma centers are hospitals that specialize in the care of the severely injured. The ACS does not *officially* designate hospitals as trauma centers, but describes their categorization as a process by which government entities, or others with the requisite power, are authorized to designate the trauma levels. The self-appointed mission of the ACS is limited to confirming and reporting on the ability of any given hospital to comply with the ACS standard of care known as *Resources for Optimal Care of the Injured Patient*.

Trauma Level Designation

The ACS Committee on Trauma has identified four levels of trauma care: Levels I, II, III, and IV. These designations reflect a health care facility's ability to care for trauma patients.

Level I

Level I trauma centers are regional resources for trauma care delivery systems. Facilities designated as Level I trauma centers must have the following:

- 24-hour in-house coverage by general surgeons
- Availability of care in specialties such as orthopaedic surgery, neurosurgery, anesthesiology, emergency medicine, radiology, internal medicine, and critical care
- Capability of cardiac, hand, pediatric, and microvascular surgery and hemodialysis
- Leadership in prevention, public education, and continuing education of trauma team members
- Commitment to continued improvement through a comprehensive quality assessment program and organized research to help direct new innovations in trauma care

Health care facilities in this category tend to provide residency training and specialized patient care services, for example computed tomography (CT) scanning, magnetic resonance imaging (MRI), and thoracic surgery.

Level II

Level II trauma centers provide initial care to stabilize trauma patients, regardless of the severity of their injuries. If necessary, patients are then transferred to Level I trauma centers. Facilities designated as Level II trauma centers must have the following:

- 24-hour immediate coverage by general surgeons
- Availability of orthopaedic surgery, neurosurgery, anesthesiology, emergency medicine, radiology, and critical care
- Commitment to trauma prevention and continuing education of trauma team members
- Continued improvement in trauma care through a comprehensive quality assessment program

Level II trauma centers often have the same capabilities and resources as Level I trauma centers, but may not have surgical or medical subspecialties for ongoing care of complex injuries. Tertiary care needs such as cardiac surgery, hemodialysis, and microvascular surgery may be referred to a Level I trauma center. General surgeons must be available, though they may be on-call. This level of trauma center often provides residency training as well.

Level III

The primary function of Level III trauma centers is to arrange for rapid transfer of severely injured patients to Level I or II trauma centers. Facilities designated as Level III trauma centers must have the following:

- 24-hour immediate coverage by emergency medicine physicians and prompt availability of general surgeons and anesthesiologists

- Program dedicated to continued improvement in trauma care through a comprehensive quality assessment program
- Transfer agreements for patients requiring more comprehensive care at a Level I or Level II trauma center
- Commitment to continuing education of nursing and allied health personnel or the trauma team
- Involvement with prevention and an active outreach program for their referring communities
- Dedication to improving trauma care through a comprehensive quality assessment program

Level IV

Level IV trauma centers provide advanced trauma life support. Facilities designated as Level IV trauma centers must have the following:

- Basic emergency department facilities to implement trauma life support protocols and 24-hour laboratory coverage
- Formal transfer agreements outlining guidelines for transfer to higher level trauma centers
- Commitment to continued improvement of trauma care activities through a formal quality assessment program
- Involvement in prevention, outreach, and education within their community

Because Level IV trauma centers are typically in remote locations and physicians may not be available, trauma patients will often be transferred to Level I or II trauma centers. The United Kingdom does not have Level IV centers, but instead designates minor injury units for lesser levels of injury. Because these are often in remote locations, many areas of Europe and the United States do not have them.

> **TIP**
>
> ### Specialty Trauma Centers
> Although not a separate designation by the ACS, some regional specialty facilities have expertise in specific disciplines. Examples include pediatric trauma, burns, spinal cord trauma, and replantation specialists.

Criteria for Determining Trauma Center Patients

The criteria for determining which patients should be taken to a trauma center vary by location, as do most medical protocols. The provider must always adhere to his or her local protocol, policies, and guidelines. The criteria for transport to a trauma center as defined by the ACS provide a process

TABLE 12-1	Criteria for Triaging Patients to a Trauma Center
Physiologic	• GCS (Glasgow Coma Scale score) < 14 • SBP (systolic blood pressure) < 90 mm Hg • RR (respiratory rate) < 10 or > 29 breaths/min • RR < 20 for infants younger than 1 year old Some systems also include: • RTS (revised trauma score) < 11 • PTS (pediatric trauma score) < 9
Anatomic	• Flail chest • Two or more proximal long bone fractures • Amputation proximal to the wrist or ankle • Penetrating trauma to the head, neck, torso, or extremities proximal to the elbow or knee • Paralysis • Pelvic fractures • Crushed, degloved, or mangled extremity • Open or depressed skull fractures

Mechanism of Trauma	• High-risk motor vehicle collision
	  • Ejection (partial or complete) from vehicle
	  • Death in same passenger compartment
	  • Intrusion into occupant compartment > 12″ (30 cm) or > 18″ (45 cm) at any site
	  • Vehicle telemetry data consistent with high risk of injury
	• Auto vs. pedestrian/bicyclist thrown or run over or auto-pedestrian injury at > 20 mph (32 km/h)
	• Falls > 20′ (6 m); for children, > 10′ (3 m), or two to three times the child's height
	• Motorcycle collision at > 20 mph (32 km/h)
	Some systems also include:
	• Vehicle rollover with unrestrained passenger
	• Extrication time > 20 minutes

Alternate Rationale	• Patient older than 55 years old
	• Children should be preferentially triaged to pediatric-capable trauma centers
	• Pregnancy > 20 weeks
	• Anticoagulant and bleeding disorders
	• Burns
	  • Without other trauma: triage to burns facility
	  • With trauma mechanisms: triage to trauma center
	• Time-sensitive extremity injury (eg, open fracture, fracture with neurovascular compromise)
	• End-stage renal disease requiring dialysis
	• EMS provider judgment
	Some systems also include:
	• Known cardiac disease or respiratory disease comorbidity
	• Known immunosuppressed patient
	• Type 1 diabetes, cirrhosis, morbid obesity, or coagulopathy

for choosing the most appropriate facility. **TABLE 12-1** lists the order in which criteria should be evaluated. If any of these criteria are met, transfer the patient to a trauma center.

Providers must always have as much of the big picture as possible available to them before making a decision as to what level of trauma care the patient needs and where they will best receive that care. A number of different criteria must be considered to make the decision in the best interest of the patient.

Physiologic Criteria

The **Glasgow Coma Scale (GCS)** is a measure that aims to give a reliable, objective recording of a patient's level of consciousness **TABLE 12-2** **PROCEDURE 3**. It is used for both initial and continuing assessment. A patient is assessed against the criteria of the scale, and point values between 3 (indicating deep unconsciousness) and 15 are assigned based on the patient's best response to the three criteria tested.

TABLE 12-2   Glasgow Coma Scale

	Adult	Child (age 1–5)	Infant (age <1)
Eye opening	4 Spontaneous	4 Spontaneous	4 Spontaneous
	3 Voice	3 To shouting/voice	3 To shouting/voice
	2 Pain stimulation	2 Pain stimulation	2 Pain stimulation
	1 None	1 None	1 None
Verbal	5 Oriented	5 Cry, smile, coo, words correct for age	5 Coos, babbles
	4 Disoriented	4 Cries, inappropriate words for age	4 Irritable cries
	3 Inappropriate words	3 Inappropriate cry or scream	3 Cries to pain
	2 Incomprehensible	2 Grunts	2 Moans, grunts
	1 None	1 None	1 None
Motor	6 Obeys	6 Spontaneous	6 Spontaneous
	5 Localizes pain	5 Localizes pain	5 Localizes pain
	4 Withdraws from pain	4 Withdraws from pain	4 Withdraws from pain
	3 Decorticate	3 Decorticate	3 Flexion
	2 Decerebrate	2 Decerebrate	2 Extension
	1 None	1 None	1 None

Values: A score between 13 and 15 may indicate a mild head injury.
A score between 9 and 12 may indicate a moderate head injury.
A score of 8 or less indicates a severe head injury and endotracheal intubation is usually required (but may not be possible without rapid sequence intubation [RSI]).

TABLE 12-3   Revised Trauma Score

Glasgow Coma Score (GCS)	Systolic Blood Pressure (mm Hg)	Respiratory Rate (breaths/min)
4 = (13–15)	4 = (> 89)	4 = (10–29)
3 = (9–12)	3 = (76–89)	3 = (> 29)
2 = (6–8)	2 = (50–75)	2 = (6–9)
1 = (4–5)	1 = (1–49)	1 = (1–5)
0 = (3)	0 = (0)	0 = (0)

Another criterion for triage to a Level I trauma center is a respiratory rate below 10 breaths/min or over 29 breaths/min. In either case, the provider should be supplementing the patient's respirations with 100% oxygen and using a bag mask while awaiting a successful intubation.

Additionally, a systolic blood pressure of less then 90 mm Hg should trigger a referral to a Level I trauma center. In addition to the provider supporting the blood pressure, he or she should also administer 100% oxygen by partial rebreathing mask (or by bag mask) and large-bore intravenous fluids until blood or blood products can be replaced.

In addition to the GCS, the **revised trauma score (RTS)** is another tool to help providers determine the need to divert to a trauma center. The RTS is scored based on the first assessment of the patient and combines the GCS, systolic blood pressure, and respiratory rate. Each category is given a score of 0–4 and then the three categories are totaled **TABLE 12-3**.

The score range is 0–12. Patients with an RTS of 12 are considered stable. Scores of 11 or less are considered critical and should be triaged to a trauma center.

The **pediatric trauma score (PTS)** is a tool aimed at evaluating the severity of injury for children **TABLE 12-4**.

Anatomic Criteria

There are also several anatomic criteria that could indicate that a patient needs to be transported to a trauma center. These injuries are indicative of higher mortality and indicate a higher level of care is needed:

- Flail chest
- Two or more proximal long bone fractures
- Amputation proximal to the wrist or ankle

TABLE 12-4 Pediatric Trauma Score				
Components	**+2**	**+1**	**−1**	**Score**
Weight	> 20 kg (44 lb)	10–20 kg (22–44 lb)	< 10 kg (22 lb)	
Airway	Patent	Maintainable	Unmaintainable	
Systolic blood pressure pulses	> 90 Radial	50–90 Carotid	< 50 Nonpalpable	
Central nervous system	Awake	+LOC (responsive)	Unresponsive	
Fractures	None	Closed or suspected	Multiple closed or open	
Wounds	None	Minor	Major, penetrating, or burns > 10%	
TOTAL SCORE				
9–12: Minor trauma. Use local guidelines/protocols.				
6–8: Potentially life threatening. Suggests need for trauma center.				
0–5: Life threatening. Need for trauma center.				
< 0: Usually fatal. Transport to nearest facility.				

- Penetrating trauma to the head, neck, torso, or extremities proximal to the elbow or knee
- Paralysis
- Pelvic fractures
- Crushed, degloved, or mangled extremity
- Open or depressed skull fracture

In addition to the guidelines used by the ACS, many local protocols include the following:

- Head injury with altered LOC
- Chest injury with respiratory distress

Mechanism of Trauma

A number of subjective or partially subjective criteria also need to be considered. These all have to do with the **mechanism of trauma**, or how the injuries were sustained. When combined with physiologic changes and anatomic injuries, consideration of the mechanism of trauma can improve the provider's ability to make good judgments.

The provider must take into account not just what he or she can see as far as injuries to the patient, but also what else may have been damaged in the event and to what extent it was involved. These criteria are as follows:

- High-risk motor vehicle collision
  - Ejection (partial or complete) from automobile
  - Death in same passenger compartment
  - Intrusion into occupant compartment > 12″ (30 cm) or > 18″ (45 cm) at any site
  - Vehicle telemetry data consistent with high risk of injury
- Auto vs. pedestrian/bicyclist thrown or run over or auto–pedestrian injury at > 20 mph (32 km/h)
- Falls > 20′ (6 m); for children, > 10′ (3 m), or two to three times the child's height
- Motorcycle collision at > 20 mph (32 km/h)
- Vehicle rollover with unrestrained passenger
- Extrication time > 20 minutes

This list is finite but includes items that call for the prehospital provider to make subjective estimates. As providers we must act as patient advocates and always err on the side of caution for the patient.

Alternate Rationale

Several other situations could cause the prehospital provider to triage a patient to a trauma center even if the patient did not meet the above criteria. Most of these are due to underlying conditions that can lead to a patient being less able to respond to the injured state the way a normal or healthy patient might. The following are some of these conditions:

- Patient older than 55 years old
- Children should be preferentially triaged to pediatric-capable trauma centers
- Pregnancy > 20 weeks
- Anticoagulant and bleeding disorders
- Burns
  - Without other trauma: triage to burns facility
  - With trauma mechanisms: triage to trauma center
- Time-sensitive extremity injury (eg, open fracture, fracture with neurovascular compromise)
- End-stage renal disease requiring dialysis
- EMS provider judgment
- Known immunosuppressed patient (including status postorgan transplant, cancer patients undergoing radiation or chemotherapy, and HIV-positive patients)
- Known cardiac or respiratory comorbidity
- Type 1 diabetes, cirrhosis, morbid obesity, or coagulopathy

It must be stated that not all patients who fit into these classifications will have worse than normal outcomes, but because of the potential for a worse outcome, providers need to be more proactive to benefit the patient's chance of recovery. Patients with burns and trauma for whom the burn injury poses the greatest risk of morbidity or

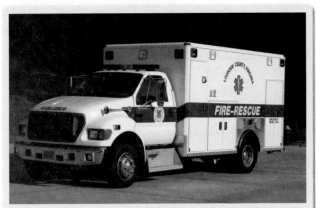

FIGURE 12-9 Ambulances have the advantage of being available in most types of weather.

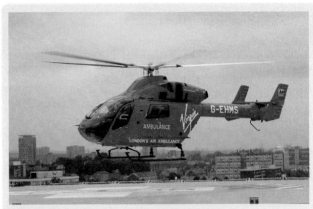

FIGURE 12-10 Helicopters and fixed-wing aircraft can be time-saving transportation considerations when available.

mortality should be transferred to a burn center, while trauma patients with burns whose injury poses the greatest threat should go to the trauma center. The EMS provider should have the ability to triage an injured patient to a trauma center based on scene observations when the patient does not fit the above criteria.

Transport Options
Ground Ambulance

Most systems will use an ambulance to transport patients to a medical facility capable of caring for the injured. Ambulances have advantages and disadvantages. Most are well equipped and have enough room to access a patient easily. Most will operate in a variety of weather conditions but may be hampered by extremes **FIGURE 12-9**. Traffic can be a distinct disadvantage when dealing with a severely injured trauma patient who requires immediate care to survive, and distance becomes another issue when time is of the essence.

Air Ambulance

The use of aeromedical evacuation has been a topic of much concern over the years. After the use of helicopters proved their efficacy in the conflicts in Korea and Vietnam, they began to be adopted for civilian use. Since then, they have

proliferated to become an available resource in most EMS systems **FIGURE 12-10**.

Each jurisdiction has developed its own policies for aeromedical use, including the criteria for the use, established guidelines for landing zones and safety, protocols for ensuring the safety of the aeromedical crew, and minimum crew credentials.

Several factors must be considered when a request is made for aeromedical evacuation of a patient from the trauma scene:

- The time needed to transport a patient by ground to an appropriate facility poses a threat to the patient's survival and recovery.
- Weather, road, and traffic conditions would seriously delay the patient's access to definitive care.
- Critical care personnel and equipment are needed to care for the patient adequately during transport.

Care to the injured can be greatly enhanced through the use of a trauma system. Systematic stabilization and rapid transport to an appropriate hospital capable of caring for the trauma patient makes EMS an integral part of trauma care. The time and preparation every prehospital provider takes to prevent increased levels of shock and injury at every level truly makes a difference.

CHAPTER RESOURCES

CASE STUDY ANSWERS

1 What is the best way to determine which patients should be treated when limited providers are available?

Incidents with multiple patients require a triaging of the patients to best match the needs of the patients with the available resources. Triage can be done using several methods; the START triage method has been used in many large-scale incidents.

2 What are the resources a trauma center would have available for your patient that a community hospital may not?

Trauma centers (or trauma hospitals) specialize in the care of the multiply injured patient. Starting with an expertise in assessment technologies, timely surgical care, and continuing through rehabilitation, the trauma center provides injured patients with the specialized care needed for survival of severe injuries.

3 What are the types of patients best suited to triage to a trauma center?

Triage to a trauma center should be decided based on local protocols; however, there are often three or four categories to help the provider decide if their patient meets the requirements. Looking at the physiologic parameters, anatomic injuries, and mechanism of injury is often required, but age and previous conditions may cause a patient to be better handled in a trauma center for more mild forms of injury.

4 Is there a danger of sending too many patients to one hospital?

Any hospital, even a large one, can be overwhelmed by too many patients at one time. Local protocols often provide for regional differences in care levels, but sending patients to a trauma center when they do not meet the requirements may overburden the hospital, and patients who require higher-level care may be delayed. This is known as overtriage, and although it is built into the system, providers should do their best to assess patients to determine their needs.

5 What are the transport considerations for this patient?

Due to her limb paralysis and decreased blood pressure, this patient should be seen in a trauma center. The extended transport time may make aeromedical transport a viable option. Aeromedical transportation can also be beneficial when several patients have been sent to the closest trauma center available and additional patients need to be sent to a more distant facility.

Trauma in Motion

1. At what number of patients does your system become overwhelmed and require additional resources? How do you request these resources?
2. When was the last time you reviewed the multicasualty triage tags used by your department?
3. Which hospitals in your area have specialty care capabilities such as burn care or spinal trauma care?
4. What aeromedical resources are available in your area and what are their limitations for use?

References and Resources

Albert J, Phillips H. Trauma care systems in the United Kingdom. *Injury Int J Care Injured.* 2003; 34:728–734.

American Academy of Orthopaedic Surgeons. Pollak AN, ed. *Nancy Caroline's Emergency Care in the Streets*, 6th ed. Sudbury, MA: Jones and Bartlett; 2007.

American College of Surgeons. *Resources for Optimal Care of the Injured Patient.* Chicago: American College of Surgeons; 2006.

American College of Surgeons Committee on Trauma. *Advanced Trauma Life Support for Doctors: Student Course Manual.* Chicago: American College of Surgeons; 2004.

Asaeda G. The day that the START triage system came to a STOP: Observations from the World Trade Center disaster. *Acad Emerg Med.* 2002; 9(3):255–256.

Benson M, Koenig KL, Schultz CH. Disaster triage: START, then SAVE—A new method of dynamic triage for victims of a catastrophic earthquake. *Prehospital Disast Med.* 1996; 11(2):117–124.

Centers for Disease Control and Prevention. Injuries and mass casualty events: information for health professionals. Available at: http://emergency.cdc.gov/masscasualties/injuriespro.asp. Accessed June 2, 2009.

Commission on Life Sciences. *Injury in America—A Continuing Public Health Problem.* Washington, DC: National Academies Press; 1985.

Coule P, Dallas C, James J, et al. eds. Basic Disaster Life Support (BDLS) Provider Manual. Chicago: American Medical Association; 2003.

Dai K, Xu Z, Zhu L. Trauma care systems in China. *Injury Int J Care Injured.* 2003; 34:664–668.

Garner A, Lee A, Harrison K, Schultz CH. Comparative analysis of multiple-casualty incident triage algorithms. *Ann Emerg Med.* 2001; 38(5):541–548.

Goosen J, Bowley DM, Degiannis E, Plani F. Trauma care systems in South Africa. *Injury Int J Care Injured.* 2003; 34:704–708.

Hines S, Payne A, Edmondson J, et al. Bombs under London. The EMS response plan that worked. *JEMS.* 2005; 30:58–67.

Hodgetts TJ, Hall J, Maconochie I, Smart C. Pediatric Triage Tape. *Prehospital Immediate Care* 1998; 2:155–159.

Hogan DE, Waeckerle JF, Dire DJ, et al. Emergency department impact of the Oklahoma City terrorist bombing. *Ann Emerg Med.* 1999; 34:160–167.

Institute of Medicine. *Accidental Death and Disability: The Neglected Disease of Modern Society.* Washington, DC: National Academy of Science, National Research Council; 1966.

Jenkins JL, McCarthy ML, Sauer LM, et al. Mass-casualty triage: time for an evidence-based approach. *Prehosp Disast Med.* 2008; 23(1):3–8.

Joshipura MK. Trauma care in India: current scenario. *World J Surg.* 2008; 32:1613–1617.

Joshipura M, Mock C, Goosen J, Peden M. Essential trauma care: strengthening trauma systems round the world. *Injury.* 2004; 34:841–845.

Kortbeek JB, Buckley R. Trauma care systems in Canada. *Injury.* 2003; 34:658–663.

Lee WH, Chiu TF, Ng CJ, et al. Emergency medical preparedness and response to a Singapore airliner crash. *Acad Emerg Med.* 2002; 9:194–198.

Lerner EB, et al. Mass casualty triage: an evaluation of the data and development of a proposed national guideline. *Disaster Med Public Health Preparedness.* 2008; 2(Suppl 1):S25–S34.

Liberman M, Mulder DS, Lavoie A, Sampalis JS. Implementation of a trauma care system: evolution through evaluation. *J Trauma.* 2004; 56:1330–1335.

Malik ZU, Pervez M, Safdar A, Masood T, et al. Triage and management of mass casualties in a train accident. *J Coll Physicians Surg Pak.* 2004; 14(2):108–111.

Nocera A, Garner A. An Australian mass casualty incident triage system for the future based upon triage mistakes of the past: the Homebush triage standard. *Aust NZ J Surg.* 1999; 69:603–608.

Romig LE. Pediatric triage: a system to JumpSTART your triage of young patients at MCIs. *JEMS* 2002; 27(7):52–53.

Royal College of Surgeons of England. *Report of the Working Party on the Management of Patients with Major Injuries.* London: Royal College of Surgeons; 1988.

Royal College of Surgeons of England, British Orthopaedic Association. *Better Care for the Severely Injured.* London: Royal College of Surgeons of England; 2000.

Sacco WJ, Navin M, Fiedler EA. Precise formulation and evidence-based application of resource-constrained triage. *Acad Emerg Med.* 2005; 12(8):759–770.

Tran MD, Garner AA, Morrison I, et al. The Bali bombing: civilian aeromedical evacuation. *Med J Aust.* 2003; 179(7):353–356.

Trauma.org. History of trauma: trauma systems. Available at: www.trauma.org/archive/history/systems.html. Accessed August 7, 2008.

Wallis LA, Carley S. Comparison of paediatric major incident primary triage tools. *Emerg Med J.* 2006; 23(6):475–478.

Wallis LA, Carley S. Validation of the paediatric triage tape. *Emerg Med J.* 2006; 23(1):47–50.

Westhoff J, Hildebrand M, Grotz M, et al. Trauma care in Germany. *Injury Int J Care Injured.* 2003; 34:674–683.

13 Secondary Transport Issues

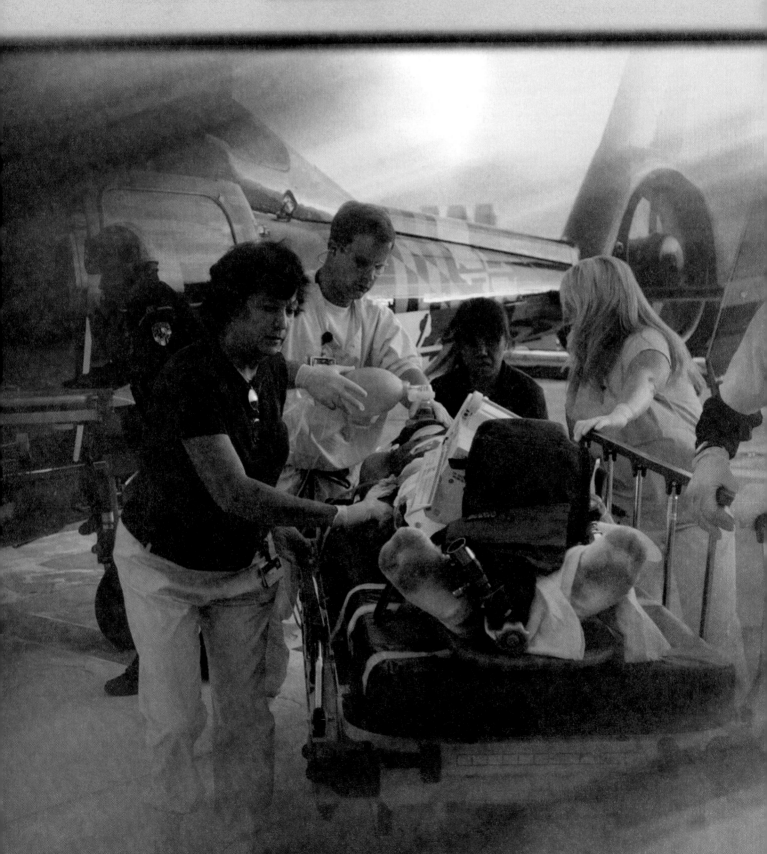

Your crew has been called to transfer a 20-year-old man who was struck by a car and taken to the closest hospital by his friend. The community hospital does not have trauma capabilities and quickly determined that this patient needed transport. At the time of the request for transport, they reported a patient with respiratory failure and hypotension.

You arrive at the small community hospital approximately 2 hours after the injury occurred. The patient has been intubated and is on a ventilator. He is immobilized on a long backboard with a cervical collar and has two IV lines running. He is approximately 68″ (173 cm) tall and weighs about 165 pounds (75 kg). The patient has a current heart rate of 130 beats/min that appears to be sinus tachycardia on the monitor. Blood pressure is 84/66 mm Hg, and Spo_2 is 97%. The ventilator settings are Vt 550, F 14, Fio_2 1.0, I:E 1:2, PIP 22, Pplat 20, and PEEP 5 on SIMV. He also has a urinary catheter inserted.

You begin your physical assessment of the patient and find the patient intubated with a 7.0-cm endotracheal tube (ETT) with a depth of 24 cm at the teeth, equal lung sounds on auscultation, a bruise and abrasion to the left side of the chest, and a fractured left forearm. Pupils are equal and reactive to light (PEARL); however, the patient does not respond to pain. The transferring nurse reports the patient was paralyzed with vecuronium and has received fentanyl and ketamine to sedate him. She also states the patient has received 3 L of normal saline in an attempt to keep his blood pressure up. A type and screening has been sent and two units of whole blood have been ordered but have not yet been started. You note 600 mL of clear yellow urine in the urinary collection bag.

A review of his labs and radiology reports shows an arterial blood gas (ABG; pH 7.01, Pco_2 72, HCO_3 10, Po_2 265, BD −4), hemoglobin 8 g/dL, hematocrit 32%, lactate 4.2 mEq/L, Na+ 185, and K+ 6.7. Urinalysis reveals no hematuria. Chest x-ray shows the ETT placed approximately 1 cm above the carina, and two fractures are noted in ribs 9 and 10 in the left axillary region. The computerized tomographic (CT) report indicates no acute brain trauma, no c-spine abnormalities, and a splenic laceration and left lower lung contusion.

1 How does your assessment differ when the patient is an interhospital transfer compared to a trauma scene response?

2 What are the priorities during the patient's physical exam?

3 What do this patient's laboratory results help to confirm as part of his diagnosis?

4 Is this patient ready for immediate departure?

5 What are the potential problems with care that this patient may present en route?

Introduction

The regionalization of trauma care around the world has resulted in a significant improvement in the quality of care for injured patients over the last 3 decades. Local trauma systems facilitate the direct transport of severely injured patients to hospitals well equipped to care for the overwhelming majority of injuries. Unfortunately, many individuals are injured in areas far from a regional level I or II trauma center (see Chapter 12). As a result, the initial treating facility is unlikely to have the resources necessary to care for the multi-trauma patient. For these patients, interfacility transfer can be lifesaving. Having providers and transportation trained and dedicated for this purpose is crucial.

Secondary transport, or **critical care transport**, can be defined as a provision of en route intensive care–level services during the transport of a critically ill patient between medical treatment facilities (MTFs). It should not be confused with initial advanced life support patient care and transport from the point of injury, as occurs routinely with local fire and emergency medical services (EMS) agencies. Critical care transport patients have been assessed and treated by a provider in a designated hospital, aid station, emergency room, or other place where critical care services can be initiated. An example is the transport of a severely injured patient from a community hospital with limited resources to a regional trauma center. In this scenario, the patient has been evaluated and a determination made that the patient will benefit from treatment not available at the originating facility. These local facilities may initiate advanced critical care therapies while waiting for the transport team to arrive. Interventions may then be monitored by the critical care transport team and the therapies themselves may then be adjusted by these advanced level providers while en route. The ultimate goal of this level of care is to maintain, if not improve, the patient's condition during transport.

Although the providers may be similar or the same in some cases, an essential component to critical care transport is the communication between transferring and receiving providers to ensure that the receiving facility can accommodate the specific needs of the patient. Critical care transport can also involve the transport of patients from places of equivalent capabilities for reasons of patient or family convenience or payment capability. In this case, patient transfer is elective and should be performed only if the patient's condition is likely to be unaffected by the transport. Regardless, the goal of transport is to maintain the patient's condition during transit.

Critical Care Providers

Traditional critical care transport teams are composed of a nurse/nurse or nurse/paramedic combination. These individuals are required to have a higher level of certification than their hospital-based counterparts **TABLE 13-1**. In some cases, physicians and/or other care specialists are required, depending on the patient, travel time, and transport platform. Regardless of the type of provider, all team members should be specifically trained for critical care transport, and in most cases advanced certifications are required **FIGURE 13-1**. At a minimum, all providers should be certified in advanced cardiac life support (ACLS) and pediatric advanced life support (PALS), and neonatal resuscitation as appropriate. It is not uncommon to have a transport vehicle staffed with a neonatal or pediatric intensive care transport team, an aortic balloon pump, or a burn team. On rare occasions, a patient may require **extracorporeal life support/extracorporeal membrane oxygenation (ECLS/ECMO)** and be accompanied by nurses and/or physicians with special training in this treatment modality. For all these reasons, this level of patient transport should be considered a highly specialized field. The transport model is expandable to address individual patient requirements.

TABLE 13-1 Examples of Advanced Certification Requirements	
Provider	**Training Certification**
EMT-Basic	Additional training is often required based on the needs of the transport team.
Paramedic	Flight Paramedic Certification (FP-C) or Critical Care Paramedic Certification (CCP-C)
Nurse	Certified Emergency Nurse (CEN), Critical Care Registered Nurse (CCRN), or Certified Flight Registered Nurse (CFRN)
Physician	Flight medicine, Critical Care Air Transport, En route Care Course

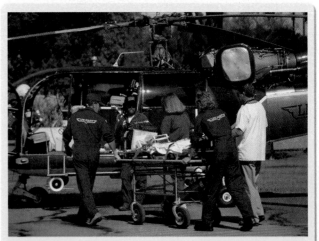

FIGURE 13-1 A critical care transport team often includes different types of providers.

Mode of Transport

Ground Ambulance

The origin of the ambulance can be seen as early as the battles of the Crusades where the men wounded in battle were transported to centralized treatment centers by horse-drawn carts. These carts were primarily used for other tasks, including removing the waste products from the camp-grounds. In the late 1700s, Baron Dominique-Jean Larrey began transporting the injured soldiers of Napoleon's army from the battlefield by horse and carriage or horse-pulled stretcher. The baron would later call this the "flying ambulance." During the late phases of the Civil War in the United States, dedicated ambulances were utilized to transport patients. In 1865, recognizing the usefulness of this patient transport platform, the Cincinnati Commercial Hospital in Ohio became the first civilian hospital-based ambulance service. The first motorized ambulances were used during the Spanish-American War at the urging of then US President William McKinley. Ironically, President McKinley was the first president to be transported by motorized ambulance in 1901 when he was shot in Buffalo, New York. Since that time, ground ambulances have become the mainstay of medical transport around the globe.

Rotary-Wing Aircraft

The first planned helicopter medical missions by the US Army occurred during the Korean War using Stokes-style baskets affixed to the helicopter skids. During this time, the British Royal Air Force (RAF) had become very successful in rescue missions to recover downed pilots; however, although the health of their victims was important, the missions were not geared toward medical treatment. The use of helicopters for medical transport increased after this because it was seen as an efficient way to remove critically wounded soldiers from the battlefield. During the Vietnam War, the number of patients transported via helicopter increased substantially and resulted in a significant decrease in the interval between injury and initial medical care with improved casualty survival.

In 1969, the US government experimented with programs in Mississippi and Texas using helicopters with civilian medical crews to transport trauma patients from the field. The first permanent civilian-based rotor-wing air ambulance began in 1970 in Harlaching, Germany, and was named *Christoph 1* after Saint Christopher. Helicopter transport was later adopted by the civilian community and in 1972 both Loma Linda Hospital in California and Saint Anthony Central Hospital in Denver, Colorado, developed helicopter programs. Today, tens of thousands of critically ill patients are transported via helicopter each year.

Fixed-Wing Aircraft

Although there was planning in the works for medical flight since the early 1900s, the first fixed-wing medical flight occurred in 1915 during World War I. At this time the French and Serbian Air Forces evacuated wounded Serbian soldiers by plane across Albania during the retreat to the Adriatic Sea. Fixed-wing aircraft were mainly utilized as first response vehicles, transporting soldiers from the battlefield to a hospital. In 1928, the first full-time air ambulance service was established in the Australian outback and became known as the *Royal Flying Doctor Service*.

Fixed-wing medical evacuation was embraced slowly over the next 50 years in both military and civilian settings. During the Vietnam conflict, aeromedical evacuation of stable patients became common. The US Air Force further enhanced aeromedical care through the development of Critical Care Air Transport Teams (CCATTs). First utilized in the late 1990s, this asset has now transported thousands of coalition forces patients, as well as civilian casualties, from battlefield hospitals to more definitive facilities throughout the world.

Maritime Vessels

The relatively long transport times associated with transport by ship make this a poor choice for transport of critically ill patients. In most cases of maritime transport, the host country's navy is tasked with providing maritime medical care and transportation of injured mariners. Utilizing these assets brings with them the specialized vessels/vehicles and training required for embarkation over water, generally including hoist capabilities. For the most part, this type of transport more closely approximates first responder care, although in some cases the patients will have been treated and stabilized by advanced providers while aboard the ship.

Choosing the Mode of Transport

Multiple factors should be considered when determining the mode of transport. Patient stability, distance, and geography are all important considerations. Weather is often a limiting factor given the minimum visibility requirements for rotary-wing aircraft. In some cases, delayed transport may be a better option than immediate transport because weather delays en route may put excess stress on the patient and the crew as well as deplete necessary supplies **TABLE 13-2**.

The most common decision requires deciding between transport by ground ambulance or rotary-wing aircraft. Each has advantages and disadvantages; however, the most compelling reason to choose one over the other is often transport time. Local traffic considerations, patient considerations, and aircraft or ambulance accessibility may favor one mode over the other when distances are short.

TIP

A list of trauma centers in the United States can be found at the American Trauma Society's website: www.amtrauma.org.

Decisions on Crew Configuration and Scope of Practice

THE AIR- AND LAND-BASED CRITICAL CARE TRANSPORT INDUSTRY has grown significantly in the past 3 decades. Crew configurations have also evolved due to a growth in provider type and scope of practice. As a result of increased crew depth and breadth, the debate over crew configuration has also grown. This section will review and discuss key considerations when deciding on the optimal crew configuration for an air or land critical care transport program.

Traditional EMS systems respond to emergency and nonemergency calls originating from a public service answering point. Their mandate is to respond rapidly when the public calls for help. Their scope is the traditional basic and advanced life support care, supported by other public service agencies such as fire and police services. In many jurisdictions, the EMS service is integrated with other public service agencies to form a safety net for the community as a whole.

Air- and land-based critical care transport services differ from their EMS counterparts in both mandate and scope. Although they may work in partnership with other public service agencies, their roles extend beyond emergency response. Some function as a backup to the public safety net, providing yet another, more advanced layer of prehospital care. More importantly, critical care transport services provide hospital- and intensive-level care to patients being transferred between health care institutions. In a regional health care system where centers of excellence provide tertiary or quaternary care services, critical care transfers are essential links in the delivery of health care.

The debate continues over what constitutes "critical care" and who is best suited to deliver care in the transport setting. In most parts of Europe, Asia, and Australia, physicians are the principal transport care providers. Their specialties include anesthesia, emergency medicine, critical care, surgery, and internal medicine. In contrast, North American transport services utilize a mix of physicians, nurses, paramedics, and respiratory therapists. Individual services choose a particular configuration and are convinced theirs is the best choice. Instead of basing optimal configurations on individual or expert opinion, a review of the medical literature can help.

Physicians appear to be a sound choice as a crew member. Although this may seem logical and supported to improve outcome for patients with certain injuries or illnesses, the literature does not universally support the presence of a physician in all cases.[1] Some studies compared outcomes for patients based on the presence or absence of physicians as part of the prehospital response.[2–4] The studies determined that physicians do not necessarily improve patient outcome. Studies have also examined the impact of physicians in hospital transfers. Although physicians did decrease the number of adverse events and errors, there was no significant impact on patient outcome.[5] The role of a physician in the transport setting may be limited to patients with specific or multisystem problems that require complex and very specialized care.

What is clear is that scope of practice is a key predictor of patient safety and well-being.[5,6] With that in mind, the best crew configuration should include the ability to manage patients requiring critical care therapies, interventions, and continuation of specialized care while in transport. For example, the crew should be well trained, familiar with, and have skills maintained in advanced airway maneuvers, management of an intubated and mechanically ventilated patient, vasopressor and inotrope therapy, invasive lines and tubes, and interpretation of laboratory and imaging studies. The scope of practice, not the provider title itself (physician, nurse, etc.), is what should define the optimal crew configuration.

The literature is also very clear that scope of practice and skill set are not enough to ensure patient safety and well-being. The other key predictor of patient outcome is the crew's specific training and familiarity in the transport environment.[6–8] Patients transported by crews who are specifically trained and routinely work in the

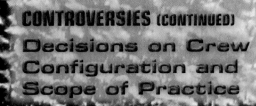

transport setting have fewer adverse events and experience better outcomes compared to similar providers who work predominantly in the hospital setting. Training and experience in the transport setting is a key determinant of patient safety that cannot be overlooked when determining optimal crew configuration. Once again, it is transport-specific training and experience, not the provider title, that determines the best transport crew.

The final debate is what defines terms such as *trained*, *experience*, *skills maintenance*, or for that matter, *critical care*. In some locales, the terms are economically driven as a means to generate revenue. National expert groups have defined clinical practice guidelines that apply in the transport setting.[9] For example, the number of intubations needed to acquire and maintain an appropriate level of practice was derived from large cohorts of paramedics.[10,11] Although controversial, possibly because some services do not meet these levels, the use of evidence-based training goals and objectives is the only way to ensure providers have the skills to ensure the best possible outcomes.

Perhaps the most controversial definition is for critical care. There are few national or international definitions for critical care. One national definition, developed by the Paramedic Association of Canada, defines the knowledge base, training, and skill maintenance requirements for all aspects of professional practice at this level.[12] The definition also serves as the accreditation standard for paramedic training institutions in Canada. Although this occupational competency profile is not entirely based on hard, reproducible evidence, it is a template based on the consensus of national experts on the definition of critical care. This makes a consistent, national definition possible and avoids inconsistencies and potential error when interacting with hospitals and other health care providers.

The optimal crew configuration is based on a mix of providers who meet the patient care needs in a particular transport setting, and who are intimately familiar with the transport setting. The configuration is not specific to provider type. Finally, the term *critical care* is not useful unless it clearly defines a scope of practice that suits the needs of the patient population served by the transport service. Optimal crew configurations may differ between settings, but these principles can help ensure a particular crew meets the needs in that setting.

Russell D. MacDonald, MD, MPH, FCPC, FRCPC
Medical Director, Research Program, Ornge Transport Medicine
Assistant Professor, Division of Emergency Medicine
Faculty of Medicine, University of Toronto
Toronto, Ontario, Canada

References

1. Boktker MT, Bakke SA, Christensen EF. A systematic review of controlled studies: do physicians increase survival with prehospital treatment? *Scan J Trauma Resus Emerg Med.* 2009;17:12(doi:10.1186/1757-78241-17-12).

2. Lirola TT, Laaksonen MI, Vahlberg MJ, Palve HK. Effect of physician-staffed helicopter emergency medical service on blunt trauma patient survival and prehospital care. *Eur J Emerg Med.* 2006;13(6):335–339.

3. Estner HL, Günzel C, Ndrepepa G, et al. Outcome after out-of-hospital cardiac arrest in a physician-staffed emergency medical system according to the Utstein style. *Am Heart J.* 2007;153(5):792–799.

4. Cameron S, Pereira P, Mulcahy R, Seymour J. Helicopter primary retrieval: tasking who should do it? *Emerg Med Austral.* 2005;17:387–391.

5. Edge WE. Reduction of morbidity in interhospital transport by specialized pediatric staff. *Crit Care Med.* 1994;22(7):1186–1191.

6. Hatherill M, Waggie Z, Reynolds L, Argent A. Transport of critically ill children in a resource-limited setting. *Intensive Care Med.* 2003;29(9):1547–1554.

7. Vos GD, Nissen AC, Nieman FH, et al. Comparison of interhospital pediatric intensive care transport accompanied by a referring specialist or a specialist retrieval team. *Intensive Care Med.* 2004;30(2):302–308.

8. Bellingan G, Olivier T, Batson S, Webb A. Comparison of a specialist retrieval team with current United Kingdom practice for the transport of critically ill patients. *Intensive Care Med.* 2000;26(6):740–744.

9. National Association of EMS Physicians. Position statements. Available at: http://www.naemsp.org/position.html. Accessed March 25, 2009.

10. Wang HE, Abo BN, Lave JR, Yealy DM. How would minimum experience standards affect the distribution of out-of-hospital endotracheal intubations? *Ann Emerg Med.* 2007;50(3):246–252.

11. Wang HE, Yealy DM. How many attempts are required to accomplish out-of-hospital endotracheal intubation? *Acad Emerg Med.* 2006;13(4):372–377.

12. Paramedic Association of Canada. National occupational competency profile (NOCP). Available at: http://www.paramedic.ca/Content.aspx?ContentID=4&ContentTypeID=2. Accessed March 25, 2009.

TABLE 13-2   Modes of Transportation

Mode of Transportation	Advantages	Disadvantages
Ground ambulance	• Most common vehicle used in patient transport • Can accommodate a wide variety of patients • Minimal limitations on weight, girth, and length • More readily available because there are statistically more ground assets than air assets • Cheaper to maintain than other vehicles • Can accommodate a larger transport team compared to rotor aircraft • Fuel is much more readily available than for other vehicles • Not affected by weather or flight ceiling restrictions • Does not have to locate a helipad	• Affected by heavy city traffic • Typically limited to legal speed limit • Effective transport range is less than 150 miles (240 km) in most areas • Potentially lengthy transport times to definitive care • Very difficult/uncomfortable on prolonged transports, risking motion sickness, added fatigue, and stress • Use in long transports may put a strain on local resources
Rotor-wing aircraft	• Speed is 100–180 mph (160–290 km/h) • Range is generally 150 miles (240 km) from home station; refueling can extend that range • Capable of bringing certain elements of an emergency room to the scene • Rapid transport to an appropriate level of care • Transport time may effectively be reduced to one fourth the time of ground vehicles • Higher level of care offered • Can overcome obstacles that are either man made (rush hour traffic) or naturally occurring (regional flooding) • If solid standard operating procedures are in place, they can take the place of the need to contact medical control, allowing earlier implementation of care • No runway needed • In a mass casualty incident (MCI), using a helicopter can relieve the load on the local trauma center and deliver patients to trauma centers farther away • Public safety aircraft with a medical component may be utilized in MCIs	• Most expensive cost per mile vehicle in medical transport • Unless EMS system allows for early or simultaneous activation, you may have a delay in aircraft arrival • There is an increased element of danger for all involved: ground crews, patient, and flight crews • When you consider load time on scene and offload time at the hospital, air transport may not be time saving • Highest cost of maintenance • Fewer available vehicles • Need for an available landing zone close to the hospital • Need for support ground resources and ground units • Weather can be a limiting factor, depending on whether the flight crew is certified to fly under instrument flight rules (IFR) and whether they use night vision goggles • Patient size, weight, and girth could be a limiting factor depending on the airframe used
Fixed-wing aircraft	• Speed is 120–450 mph (193–725 km/h) • Range is in excess of 2,000 miles (3,200 km) • Longer range than ground or helicopter transports • Minimal refueling stops required • Multiple patient abilities • Weights and balance less of an issue compared to helicopters • Pressurized cabins may alleviate the effects of altitude on the body	• The need for a runway near the origination and destination locations • The aircraft may have other roles; it may need to be converted for air medical • May not have usable electrical fixtures for your equipment • May not have oxygen on board the airframe

The decision to transport via fixed-wing aircraft is primarily determined by distance. This mode of travel requires special considerations due to gas expansion that can occur when taking the patient up to altitude. This is particularly important in patients with the potential for trapped gas expansion such as pneumothorax, pneumocephalus, or intraocular air. Choosing the appropriate platform is important in ensuring a timely and safe transport.

Assessment of the Patient Prior to Transport

History

A thorough history and physical exam should be obtained with a specific focus on the mechanism of injury, known injuries, treatment provided, and the presence of significant preexisting conditions. Although this may be in progress or incomplete depending on the facility and time from injury, it will provide a starting point from which a more detailed, focused history can be obtained. In some cases, the patient may have been hospitalized for several days prior to transport, so this information can be quite extensive.

Critical information includes:

- **Mechanism of injury:** This provides critical information with respect to the expected types of injuries and the potential for missed injuries. Possible scenarios include a motor vehicle collision involving rollover or occupant ejection, auto versus pedestrian accident, or stab or gunshot wound.
- **Injuries identified during primary and secondary assessments:** These should be communicated clearly from the transferring provider. Any wounds should be inspected and documented, and a plan determined for care during transport.
- **Abnormal vital signs:** Knowing this information can help to anticipate a problem that may occur during transport. For instance, hypotension, severe tachycardia, and tachypnea suggest hemorrhagic or other forms of shock and place the patient at high risk of decomposition and death during transport. Severe hypoxemia should be quickly identified and remedied if possible.
- **Treatments rendered:** Pay specific attention to the administration of sedatives and paralytics and to the method of airway stabilization, like endotracheal tube placement and confirmation. The exam should be as comprehensive as time allows and should include a neurologic assessment. It should document any intravenous lines, what type they are, where they are located, whether all the ports are functional, and when the line was placed. All other tubes, including chest tubes, Jackson-Pratt drains, urinary catheters, colostomy bags, and gastric or jejunostomy-tube drains should be identified and noted. Determine the patient's current mental status so any changes during

transport can easily be identified. Also investigate how the patient initially arrived to the facility so their baseline mental status can be conveyed to the accepting hospital.

Past medical history is important to ascertain conditions that may affect the patient's stability and management during transport. Significant cardiopulmonary or renal disease should be identified, because both may impact drug dosing and/or side effects during transport. Surgical history is important to ascertain prior to flight. Reconsider air transportation of a patient if they have been extubated within the last 12 hours, due to potential decompensation from the stressors of flight. In general, patients with a traumatic eye injury or free air in the globe should not fly. Individuals who have recently had eye surgery should be evaluated for possible complications in flight. Patients who had recent retina surgery, where a gas bubble was placed in the eye, should not fly because of **Boyle's law**, which states that the volume of the gas bubble will expand as the altitude is increased. Flights after radial keratotomy (RK) surgery, because of ocular hypoxia, can cause a distortion in the RK scar. Corneal lens implants, photorefractive keratotomy (PRK), and LASIK surgery do not have the same problem, but should be evaluated before flight if within 1 month from the date of surgery. Often case-by-case evaluations are done by the flight surgeon to determine whether a patient is able to be transported.

Medication allergies as well as a home and hospital medication list should be documented. In particular, the use of anticoagulants, warfarin or heparin, or antiplatelet agents such as aspirin or clopidogrel (Plavix) should be noted given the increased risk of bleeding complications. A brief social history should be obtained, including tobacco, alcohol, or drug use, which may place the patient at greater risk for withdrawal delirium or seizures during long transports, especially when the patient has been hospitalized for more than 24 hours prior to transport.

Predeparture Physical Exam

A focused physical exam provides real-time information concerning the current status of injuries and treatments noted in the history. It begins with a full set of vital signs, including oxygen saturation and current oxygen requirement. Note how many liters of supplemental oxygen the patient is using to maintain their oxygenation level. A head-to-toe evaluation augments the transferring provider's assessment and may result in the finding of additional injuries.

TIP

Similar to the rapid trauma/secondary assessment, the physical exam done prior to transporting the patient will have the benefit of a stable environment and additional diagnostic equipment.

In some cases, these may need to be addressed prior to patient departure. Documentation of motor function and neurologic status via measures like the Glasgow Coma Scale (GCS) are critical during this phase because patients with head or vertebral column fractures may worsen prior to, or during, transport **PROCEDURE 3** . Always log roll the patient and ensure an adequate examination of the back, flank, gluteal, and perineal areas. This can be done during the physical transfer of the patient to the transport stretcher.

Pertinent Laboratory and Radiographic Data

The results of imaging and laboratory studies should be reviewed with an emphasis on values that may lead to significant patient compromise during transport. Examples include hemoglobin, hematocrit, platelet count, coagulation parameters, critical electrolytes, and blood gas analysis. Anticipating the need for transfusion, the treatment of life-threatening hypoglycemia, or an electrolyte abnormality is important. During long transports, some of these values may need to be repeated to monitor progress. Familiarity and access to point-of-care devices such as glucometers and blood gas machines (eg, i-STAT) may be necessary during long fixed-wing transports. Given the impact of air travel on hemoglobin oxygen saturation, some patients will require transfusions when this value falls below 8.0 g/dL to maintain adequate oxygen delivery. It is important to ensure this has been addressed when possible prior to transport to minimize the need for in-flight transfusion and the associated risks **TABLE 13-3** .

Electrolytes

When patients arrive at the hospital, part of the routine work-up involves screening lab work, which includes general chemistry and complete blood count. The general chemistry panel typically includes electrolytes, bicarbonate, glucose, and renal function. In terms of electrolytes, potassium is one of the key components to address **TABLE 13-4** . Hypokalemia or low potassium can be asymptomatic in mild cases but in more severe cases can affect major organ systems. It can also cause nerve and muscle weakness, including respiratory muscles, and cardiovascular dysfunction including irregular heart rhythms like ventricular

arrhythmias, particularly in patients with underlying cardiac conditions. Electrocardiogram (ECG) findings of hypokalemia include flattening or inversion of T waves, increased prominence of U waves, depression of ST segment, and ventricular ectopy **FIGURE 13-2** . Cardiac symptoms are the most worrisome for excess potassium or hyperkalemia. ECG findings for hyperkalemia include peaked T wave,

TABLE 13-3 Blood Values

Complete Blood Count (CBC)	Values	May Indicate
Red blood cells (RBCs)	Males: 4.7–6.1 million cells/μL Females: 4.2–5.4 million cells/μL	High: dehydration Low: bleeding
White blood cells (WBCs)	4,500–10,500 cells/mm³	High: Infection, tissue damage (eg, burns), severe emotional or psychological stress
Hematocrit (varies with altitude)	Males: 40.7–50.3% Females: 36.1–44%	High: Burns, dehydration Low: Anemia, blood loss, destruction of red blood cells associated with blood transfusion
Hemoglobin	Males: 13.8–17.2 g/dL Females: 12.1–15.1 g/dL	High: Chronic low blood oxygen levels Low: Blood loss, destruction of red blood cells associated with blood transfusion
Platelets	140–400 × 10⁹/L	High: Anemia Low: Post-massive blood transfusion, disseminated intravascular coagulation (DIC)

TABLE 13-4 Interpreting Electrolyte Values

Normal Parameters for Electrolytes	Adult Values	May Indicate
Na⁺ (Sodium)	135–145 mEq/L	High: Large normal saline boluses, sweating, burns Low: Dehydration
K⁺ (Potassium)	3.5–5.5 mEq/L	High: Blood transfusion, crushed tissue injury, red blood cell destruction, acidosis Low: Vomiting, prolonged use of NG suctioning
Cl⁻ (Chloride)	95–105 mEq/L	High: Metabolic acidosis, respiratory alkalosis Low: Metabolic alkalosis, overhydration, burns
BUN (Blood urea nitrogen)	6–23 mg/dL	Hypovolemia, shock
Creatinine	0.6–1.4 mg/dL	High: Dehydration, reduced kidney blood flow, kidney failure, rhabdomyolysis
Glucose	70–110 mg/dL	High or low may cause altered mental states
CO₂ (Carbon dioxide)	24–30 mEq/L	Low: Metabolic acidosis, ethelyne glycol poisoning, methanol poisoning, salicylate toxicity High: Excessive vomiting

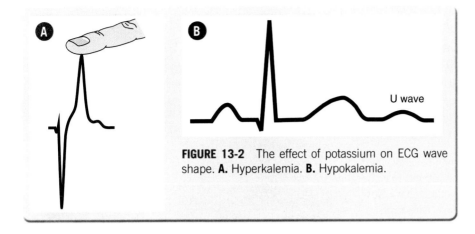

FIGURE 13-2 The effect of potassium on ECG wave shape. **A.** Hyperkalemia. **B.** Hypokalemia.

TABLE 13-5 Acid-Base Status		
Blood Gas (at sea level)	**Normal Parameters (arterial)**	**Normal Parameters (mixed venous)**
pH	7.35–7.45	7.31–7.41
Pa_{O_2}	75–100 mm Hg	35–40 mm Hg
Pa_{CO_2}	35–45 mm Hg	40–50 mm Hg
Sa_{O_2}	94–100%	70–75%
HCO_3 (Bicarbonate)	22–26 mEq/L	22–26 mEq/L
BE (Base excess)	−2 to +2	

flattened P wave, prolonged PR interval, widened QRS complex, ventricular fibrillation, and at the most severe cardiac arrest.

Acid-Base Status

Acid-base status is important for the patient's metabolic and respiratory status. An arterial blood gas is a reliable tool prior to transport that may be used to determine whether the patient is in <u>acidosis</u>, an acid excess state, or in <u>alkalosis</u>, a base excess state. Using the patient's lab information, the provider can determine whether the patient has a metabolic or respiratory acidosis or alkalosis **TABLE 13-5**. The normal serum pH for a human is approximately 7.4.

> **TIP**
>
> When reading blood gasses, a pH that is lower than normal shows acidosis whereas a higher than normal pH is alkalosis.

Respiratory Acidosis

Respiratory acidosis is represented by a decreased pH and an increased Pa_{CO_2}. Common causes for respiratory acidosis include severe pulmonary disease, respiratory muscle fatigue, and respiratory depression from head trauma or drugs like anesthetics or sedatives. Other causes include neuromuscular diseases, like poliomyelitis and myasthenia,

or obesity and alveolar hypoventilation syndromes.

Metabolic Acidosis

A metabolic acidosis presents with a pH of less than 7.4 and decreased serum bicarbonate level (HCO_3). If the patient has a metabolic acidosis, it is important to determine whether it is a non-anion gap or anion gap metabolic acidosis. The anion gap represents unmeasured anions in plasma including proteins, phosphate, sulfate, and organic anions. The equation for determining anion gap is:

$$Na - (Cl + HCO_3)$$

If the anion gap is greater than 12, the patient has a condition consistent with an anion gap metabolic acidosis. Common causes for this include methanol or ethylene glycol ingestion (automobile antifreeze), uremia, diabetic ketoacidosis, paraldehyde ingestion, lactic acidosis, and salicylate (aspirin) ingestion.

> **TIP**
>
> A blood gas showing respiratory acidosis will have a low pH, increased Pa_{CO_2}, and normal HCO_3. A blood gas showing metabolic acidosis will have a low pH, normal to high Pa_{CO_2}, and high HCO_3.

Respiratory Alkalosis

Respiratory alkalosis is noted with an elevated pH and decreased Pa_{CO_2}. Causes of respiratory alkalosis include central nervous system injury like head injury or stroke, salicylate ingestion, pregnancy, liver failure, and an early sign in gram-negative sepsis. Possible pulmonary causes of respiratory alkalosis include hyperventilation, pneumonia, pulmonary embolism, and asthma. The kidneys respond to this at altitude by producing increased amounts of urine, which results in an increase in red blood cells.

Metabolic Alkalosis

Metabolic alkalosis presents with increased pH greater than 7.4, increased serum HCO_3, and decreased Pa_{CO_2}. The differential diagnosis for metabolic alkalosis is dependent on the upright and supine posture, potassium level, and renin-aldosterone system. It also is affected by whether the patient is adequately hydrated. Some causes of metabolic alkalosis include vomiting, gastric aspiration, diuretics, posthypercapnic state, renal artery stenosis, primary aldosteronism, Cushing's syndrome, and potassium depletion and edematous states.

Glucose

Glucose is another important value to monitor. Tight glucose control has become a key factor in good wound healing and improved outcomes after myocardial infarction and

> **TIP**
>
> A blood gas showing respiratory alkalosis will have a high pH, decreased $Paco_2$, and normal HCO_3. A blood gas showing metabolic alkalosis will have a high pH, normal to low $Paco_2$, and high HCO_3.

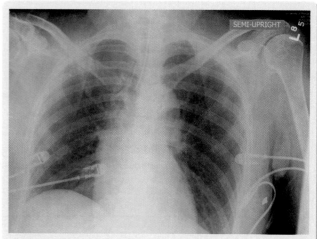

FIGURE 13-3 The provider should be able to interpret simple radiologic findings that would affect the transport of their patient.

cerebrovascular accidents. Many patients may have elevated blood glucose because of a stress response; others may be newly diagnosed patients with diabetes. Facilities have now adopted insulin protocols for their intensive care units to maintain good glycemic control. On the opposite end of the spectrum, it is just as essential to be aware of when a patient develops a low blood glucose. Hypoglycemia can mimic other conditions; patients experiencing this may present to medical personnel with altered mental status, confusion, tremors, or sweats.

Coagulation Studies

Coagulation studies provide information about how well a patient is clotting and are important to review prior to departure **TABLE 13-6**. The prothrombin time (PT) is a measure of the extrinsic and common pathways of clotting activity. Some of the causes for the PT to be elevated include liver disease, warfarin therapy, vitamin K deficiency, lupus anticoagulant, Factor VII deficiency, and Factor VII inhibitor. The partial thromboplastin time (PTT) measures the activity of the intrinsic and common pathways of coagulation. Common causes for a prolonged PTT include heparin therapy, factor inhibitor, Von Willebrand's disease, lupus anticoagulant, and Factor VIII, IX, XI, or XII deficiency. It is important to be familiar with these values because if either the PT or PTT is prolonged it indicates that the patient is at an increased risk for bleeding. Therefore, it will be important to anticipate, when possible, how to stop bleeding during transport with these patients.

Radiographic Data

Just as the history, physical exam, and laboratory data are part of the initial assessment, radiographic data help to provide details to the picture of the patient's clinical status.

Radiographic data should be reviewed with attention to acute injury that may cause problems during transport. A chest radiograph should be done immediately prior to transport to ensure adequate endotracheal tube position and to evaluate for untreated pulmonary pathology such as pneumonia, fluid or blood in the lungs, or pneumothorax and significant lung collapse **FIGURE 13-3**. This may also be used to confirm the placement of a chest tube, central venous catheter, or gastric decompression tube. The results of **computerized tomographic (CT)** studies should be known to identify the presence of significant intra-abdominal, intrathoracic, or intracranial blood that could prompt further treatment at the transferring location or en route. Whenever possible, this data should be transmitted to the accepting physician prior to transport to ensure that the patient is not transferred prematurely and the receiving facility has the necessary resources to care for the patient.

An essential component of the patient's record is copies of all radiographs performed at the transferring institution. Dictated or handwritten interpretations are often contained in the paper packet; however, the actual radiographs or electronic media containing this data are more useful to the receiving facility. Often, the reason for transport is to bring the patient to a specialized center and allow these specialized providers access to the raw data of the CT, magnetic resonance imaging (MRI), or radiograph. This will result in a more thorough evaluation without unnecessarily repeating invasive or expensive tests.

A transport provider should be familiar with basic radiographic interpretation. A systematic approach should be used each time an imaging study is read so as not to miss any possible pathology. Begin by checking the patient's name on the image to make sure that it belongs to the appropriate patient. For a chest radiograph, begin with

TABLE 13-6	Coagulation Studies
Test	**Normal**
PT (Prothrombin time)	10–12 seconds (can vary between labs)
PTT (Partial thromboplastin time)	30–45 seconds (can vary between labs)
INR (International normalized ratio)	1–2 (without anticoagulant therapy)

the airway and determine whether the trachea is midline, whether there is an endotracheal tube, and whether it is at the appropriate level above the <u>carina</u>. Determine whether the trachea and mainstem bronchi are patent. Then check the bones and document any abnormalities or fractures. Next assess the <u>cardiac silhouette</u> for any enlargement or any disruption or obscuring of the silhouette, which could indicate a mass or infiltrate.

The posterior-anterior (PA) view is better for assessing heart size. The anterior-posterior (AP) view magnifies the heart silhouette and blurs the pulmonary vessels. Identify the diaphragm for clear, sharp costophrenic and costocardiac margins; any obscuring of the margins could be a sign of an infiltrate versus fluid accumulation. Also, look for possible air under the diaphragm that would indicate a perforation of either the stomach, small intestine, or large intestine; this is an acute abdominal process and is typically a surgical emergency. Review the lung fields for any possible pathology like increased interstitial markings, air bronchograms, or increased vascularity, which could suggest possible pneumonia, congestive heart failure, or lung injury. Finally, review the radiograph for Swan-Ganz or other lumen-style central venous access catheter placement. Evaluate the quality of the film and determine whether the patient took a good inspiration, typically indicated if 10 ribs can be counted.

Blood and Body Fluid Cultures

Other results of interest include cultures of blood, urine, sputum, and stool. These are often initially obtained if the physician thinks the patient's condition is likely due to infection. Cultures provide information regarding what bacteria, virus, or fungus may be causing the illness. The results of blood and other body fluid cultures are important for secondary transport because of the potential need for isolation or specific contact precautions. Respiratory precautions may be required for certain pulmonary diseases such as tuberculosis, severe acute respiratory syndrome (SARS), and avian influenza. Bacterial infection or colonization with methicillin-resistant staphylococcus aureus (MRSA) or vancomycin-resistant enterococcus (VRE) will require specific contact precautions during transport and specific cleaning procedures after transport.

Packaging the Patient

Securing the patient, with all of the transport equipment, can be challenging. Commercially available devices can help with securing equipment and range in complexity from litter attachments to custom critical care transport modules. Providers must have access to critical patient areas including the airway and invasive monitoring/vascular access ports whenever possible. Specific injury areas that require close monitoring should also be reachable. Care should be taken to pad areas at risk for pressure ulceration, especially during long transports. Pressure sores can develop early and are

difficult and costly to treat, even in tertiary referral hospitals. Every effort should be made to avoid this complication when time and resources permit. Patients who have undergone oral surgery and have their jaw wired should have wire cutters with them during transport. For patients being transported by air, circumferential casts or bandaging should be evaluated and replaced or modified to prevent compartment syndrome.

After packaging, lines and tubes should be rechecked for security and function prior to leaving the transferring facility. When an IV is functioning marginally or does not appear functional, it should be replaced prior to transport. Replacing critical lines such as chest tubes, arterial lines, and central venous line catheters is difficult during transport. A discussion of potential problems should occur prior to transport with the transferring provider including what care should be initiated if a critical tube were to become inadvertently dislodged, especially if replacement is beyond the skill level of the en route care providers. For example, loss of the arterial line is generally well tolerated because cuff pressures can be used during the remaining transport. In contrast, a chest tube during air transport may be critical to prevent the development of a tension pneumothorax. In this situation, the solution may be frequent assessment or, alternatively, immediate needle decompression, depending on the patient's injuries, current clinical stability, and remaining transport time. During transport, consider closing off chest tubes with a Heimlich valve or water seal. These options should be anticipated and discussed with either the transferring or accepting provider prior to transport.

Prior to considering air transport, the patient's physical size should be considered due to transport restrictions. It is important to note that in some smaller versions of rotor and fixed-wing air transport vehicles there are set guidelines regarding the maximum weight, length, and girth of a patient. These guidelines are set up to address the aircraft's weights and balances. These issues also become a concern because the size of the patient may affect safe access to the patient during transport. You should also take into account the size, weight, and girth of your equipment. Equipment such as an infant <u>isolette</u> may add a significant challenge in some aircraft, but it must be considered especially when transporting pregnant patients. Ground ambulances are much less affected by these issues.

Equipment Preparation

Preparation and pre-mission testing are critical to minimize the risk of equipment malfunction during transport. After receiving a transport request and a brief summary of the patient, identify necessary equipment and supplies and include calculations that account for unanticipated delays. This is especially true for aeromedical transport because weather, traffic, and mechanical problems may delay arrival and patient handoff. Even during long ground transport distances, vehicle problems can result in long delays. Poor planning may leave your patient without pain or sedative medication, or in the worst case, without required oxygen. A general rule is to carry backup pieces of critical equipment, including additional batteries and fuses, and enough supplies to account for two to two and a half times the door-to-door travel time. This is in addition to a standard emergency set that your local jurisdiction may require. Oxygen calculations should also be accomplished. Determine your number of patients and account for both their current need and what their oxygen demand may be if they decompensate. Although calculating gaseous oxygen is straightforward, you should know that you may be able to utilize oxygen onboard from airframes that utilize a liquid oxygen system or LOX. In LOX systems, 1 liter of liquid oxygen produces 862 liters of gaseous oxygen.

Perform a complete equipment function check prior to patient loading. Aeromedical transport equipment, in particular, is subjected to harsher than normal conditions. The extremes of temperature and the barometric pressure changes shorten the life span of most devices. Power requirements should be considered and equipment and power source compatibility checked prior to committing to a transport. For devices with a backup or primary battery source, check the charges and ensure spare batteries are available. Remember, battery life can decrease with battery age and intensity of use, including the number of variables monitored, frequency of ventilation, and temperature. In all cases, power cords and charging devices should be available in the event the time spent at the transferring facility is excessive. This allows the transport equipment to run on the facility's AC power during the delay and a maximal charge is available during transport. Flights occurring internationally have the added concern of power conversion. All converters and adapters must be hospital grade.

Finally, ensure compatibility with any needed specialty equipment. Neonatal transport units, **aortic balloon pumps**, or ECLS/ECMO devices may have specific power requirements that are incompatible with the transport vehicle power output. Frequency converters are available if this problem is anticipated. All devices require preapproval for flight due to safety concerns regarding the patient and the flight crew. In emergency cases, waivers can be obtained.

Transport equipment varies based on mission requirements, transport mode, space considerations, cost, availability, and personal preference. Regardless, all critical care patient transports have the basic requirements listed in **TABLE 13-7**.

TABLE 13-7 Basic Critical Care Equipment Requirements

Equipment	Features/Functions	Advantages	Disadvantages
Ventilator	• Adjusts for barometric pressure changes	• Standard ventilator functions including pressure control and pressure support	• Ventilator may shut off during prolonged suctioning. • Blown fuses may occur on aircraft/vehicle power.
Monitor and defibrillator	• Noninvasive blood pressure (NIBP), continuous cardiac monitoring, temperature, pulse oximetry, continuous capnography	• Ability to monitor several patient indicators simultaneously • Most have biphasic defibrillation capabilities	• Leads may not match the originating facility. • Ensure that your setting is age appropriate.
Portable suction	• Continuous and intermittent suctioning	• Quick removal of vomitus and blood via suction • Able to be connected to chest tubes	• Ensure the device is set up prior to accepting patients.
Blood gas analyzer	• Delivers lab-accurate testing for blood gases, electrolytes, chemistries, hematology, and glucose • Some models include coagulation and cardiac markers (troponin)	• Invaluable tool for prolonged transport of critical patients	• Most devices will not operate if the temperature is outside of the machine's posted temperature limits. • Make sure to take extra cartridges from different lot numbers. A bad lot number can keep the machine from working during transport.
Infusion device	• May deliver several simultaneous medications	• Separate delivery channels for separate intravenous infusions	• Tubing must be compatible with the device. • Air in the line from movement is very common and will trigger an alarm.

Emergency Medications

The emergency kit should contain supplies capable of supporting a critically ill patient in the event of an unanticipated delay that exceeds the planned mission supplies **TABLE 13-8**. It is similar to a "crash cart" found in most intensive care units with additional medications for longer term care. Keep in mind that the contents of this kit may differ among jurisdictions.

In-Transit Care

The intensity of critical care while en route depends on many factors that include the patient, transport distance, mode and capabilities during transport, and the skill level of the provider(s). In general, critical care transport should adhere to a similar standard as that of a fixed intensive care unit. In some cases the intensive care physician will be traveling with the patient. More commonly, the physician will be

TABLE 13-8	**Emergency Kit**	
Category	**Type of Emergency**	**Equipment and Medication**
Airway		• Nasopharyngeal airway • Oropharyngeal airway • Supraglottic airway (LMA, King LT) • Intubation set
Breathing	Bronchospasm	• Salbutamol/albuterol MDI • Ipratropium/Atrovent MDI
	Mucous plugging	• Suction catheters • Saline
	Tension pneumothorax	• 14-gauge 3 1/4″ angiocatheter • Pneumothorax kit to include but not limited to: catheter introducer needle, Heimlich valve, syringe, one-way stopcock • Chest tube kit (if applicable)
Circulation	Vascular access	• Intravenous cannulas • Intraosseous access kit • Central venous access kit
	Hypotension/shock	• Intravenous fluids • Vasoactive medications
	Cardiac arrest	• Standard ACLS medications • Defibrillator/pacing pads • Lead pads
	Myocardial infarction	• Aspirin • Nitroglycerin • Morphine • Oxygen • Heparin
Disability	Sedation	• Propofol • Midazolam
	Analgesia	• Fentanyl • Morphine • Hydromorphone • Oral acetaminophen or paracetamol
	Seizures	• Lorazepam IV • Phenytoin IV • Phenobarbital IV
	Agitation	• Halperidol • Midazolam
	Elevated intracranial pressure	• Mannitol • 3% sodium chloride

(continues)

TABLE 13-8	Emergency Kit (Continued)	
Category	**Type of Emergency**	**Equipment and Medication**
Infection		• Ertapenem IV • Moxifloxacin IV • Metronidazole IV
Inflammation	Anaphylaxis	• Hydrocortisone injection • Dexamethasone injection • Diphenhydramine injection • Epinephrine 1:1000
	Fever	• Acetaminophen (paracetamol) (oral and rectal)
Gastrointestinal	Antiemetic	• Odansetron (IV and oral) • Compazine (IV and oral)
	Gastroesophageal reflux disease (GERD)	• Omeprazole IV • Ranitidine
	Antidiarrheal	• Loperamide
Patient safety		• Patient restraints • Wire cutters for mandibular wiring • Cast cutter to remove patient casts
Antisepsis		• Sharps container • Alcohol swabs • Chloraprep swabs • Chlorhexadine • Alcohol-based hand gel
Lines/tubes		• Nasogastric/orogastric tubes (adult/pediatric) • Urinary catheters (adult/pediatric) • Extra primary and accessory IV line tubing
Bandaging/tape		• Gauze rolls • 4″ self-adherent elastic bandage • 4″ × 4″ gauze pads • 2″ × 2″ gauze pads • Armboard splints (securing IVs) • Small and medium occlusive dressings • 1″ and 2″ tape • Tourniquet

available by radio or mobile phone. It should be noted that regardless of the provider's qualifications or the presence of advanced equipment, all patients are at risk during transport and the goal is to minimize the impact of transport on the patient's physiology.

Vital signs and pertinent physical exam findings should be obtained every 5 to 15 minutes depending on the stability of the patient, ongoing interventions, and the duration of transport. This should include recording the cardiac rhythm, heart rate, blood pressure, respiratory rate, oxygen saturation, capnography, urine output, and Glasgow Coma Scale (GCS) score. Lines and tubes should be assessed for function and security before and after patient movement and hourly during transport. In addition, always recheck function during changes in patient status. A dislodged or obstructed endotracheal tube is one of the most common

causes for respiratory decompensation during transport. Pertinent physical exam components should be assessed hourly, including pupillary response, gross motor function, and specific injury assessments such as an abdominal exam or a distal pulse assessment. For longer transports, blood gas monitoring and other specific laboratory values should be checked, depending on the patient. Complications of trauma can include bleeding, coagulopathy, and electrolyte abnormalities, and many of these can be followed using a point-of-care testing device such as the i-STAT blood analyzer.

Routine treatment occurs regularly when caring for patients, and it should be provided during transport. This care includes ventilator care (including suctioning), administration of maintenance or resuscitation fluid, pain control or sedation, and the administration of vasoactive or cardiotonic agents. For longer transports, patients may require scheduled medications such as antibiotics, anticonvulsants, or prophylactic medications for deep venous thrombosis or gastric stress ulceration. En route transfusion deserves special attention given the risk of transfusion reaction.

Blood Transfusion

Blood product transfusion is an essential part of the resuscitation of the severely injured patient. In the setting of severe hemorrhagic shock, transfusion combined with hemorrhage control can be lifesaving. During critical care transport, this is the primary available treatment for hemorrhagic shock, and every effort should be made to anticipate the need for and to carry blood products in transit when possible. Of course, as with any invasive treatment, there are risks. The primary risks involve transfusion reactions that range in severity from a low-grade fever to massive hemolysis and death. Ensuring compatibility is the best way to minimize this risk. Once blood product administration has begun, careful monitoring is necessary to intervene at the first sign of a reaction.

There are multiple blood group antigen systems. The two initial antigen groups used to type and screen blood products are the ABO blood group system and the Rh system. Within the ABO system, there are four main groups: A, B, AB, and O. The O group lacks A or B antigens. The majority of individuals make antibodies to the AB antigen that they lack. For instance, the A blood group has anti-B antibodies called **isoagglutinins**. Type AB patients do not have either isoagglutinin, but type O individuals have both anti-A and anti-B antibodies. Type O individuals are considered universal donors and type AB are universal recipients. The Rh system is based primarily on the presence of the D antigen on a red blood cell (RBC) membrane protein. If the D antigen is present, the patient is Rh positive; if it is not present, the patient is Rh negative. Prior to transfusion, a type and screen is performed on the patient to determine the ABO and Rh phenotype of the recipient for the transfusion. Once it is determined that the patient will need a transfusion, crossmatching is ordered to make sure the blood does not have any antigens for which the patient has clinically significant antibodies.

The primary blood transfusion products are:

- **Packed red blood cells (pRBCs)** increase oxygen-carrying capacity in the anemic patient. A single unit has a volume of approximately 230 mL. Transfused pRBCs should be typed and crossmatched, to be type specific, or type O blood can be used in an emergency.
- **Plasma** contains primarily clotting factors and should be administered in patients who have had significant blood loss (> 30%) or to patients with underlying coagulation dysfunction.
- **Platelets** are used to help reduce the incidence of bleeding in the setting of thrombocytopenia or decreased platelet count. Single platelet concentrates are roughly 50 mL in volume and increase the

recipient's count approximately 10,000 per cubic milliliter. "Pooled" platelets are a collection of single platelet concentrates (50 mL) from a "pool" of five to eight donors; these may raise the recipient's platelet count by up to 50,000 per cubic milliliter, depending on the quantity from each concentrate. Today, the most common form is a platelet apheresis. This is a large number of platelets obtained through continuous inline extraction from a single donor using an apheresis machine. The result is approximately 400 mL in volume, which can raise the recipient's platelet count by approximately 50,000 per cubic milliliter. It has the additional benefit of exposing the patient to only a single donor. Platelets cannot be refrigerated and can be stored for only up to 5 days using a specialized mixing device to prevent aggregation. In addition, platelets cannot be infused in a massive transfusion device due to the risk of platelet destruction.

- **Cryoprecipitate** is a liquid suspension of concentrated clotting factors and has the primary advantage of giving large amounts of clotting proteins in a small volume. Cryoprecipitate is indicated in states of low fibrinogen (less than 100 mg/dL) or factor VIII and von Willebrand factor deficiencies.
- **Fresh whole blood (FWB)** contains all components and provides the oxygen-carrying capacity of packed RBCs and the hemostatic capacity of plasma and platelets in a single 450-mL unit. In addition, the blood is "fresh," which allows maximal function of the components. The major drawbacks include availability and the potential for suboptimal testing. FWB must be type and Rh matched to the patient. Despite the potential benefits and recent enthusiasm for use in combat environments, it is rarely, if ever, used in the civilian sector.

It should be noted that almost all products (except FWB) are refrigerated prior to administration, and an untoward side effect of massive transfusion is hypothermia. This can be avoided by using a blood warmer or rapid transfusion device. Unfortunately, these are generally not available during transport. A second common problem with massive transfusion is hypocalcemia secondary to the sequestration of calcium by citrate, the anticoagulant used in stored pRBCs. Careful monitoring and replacement can prevent this life-threatening complication.

Blood Transfusion Reactions

The most common transfusion reaction, assuming appropriate crossmatching and administration, is a mild reaction consisting of a low-grade fever and chills **TABLE 13-9**. Febrile nonhemolytic transfusion reaction presents with chills and rigors and a temperature change of 1°C (1.8°F) or greater. This is typically a diagnosis or exclusion of other causes for fever. The reaction can be decreased by premedicating with antipyretics like acetaminophen, but this is typically saved for patients with recurrent reactions.

TABLE 13-9   Transfusion Reactions

Reaction	Onset	Signs and Symptoms	Treatment
Febrile	Within 30–90 minutes of starting the infusion	Fever, chills	Stop the infusion
Anaphylactic	Within 30 minutes of starting infusion	Urticaria, wheezing, hypotension	Stop the infusion; provide epinephrine and steroids
Hemolytic	Shortly after beginning transfusion	Fever, chills, dyspnea, back pain	Stop the transfusion, supportive care
Cardiovascular overload	Anytime during or immediately following the infusion	Cough, cyanosis, pulmonary edema	Stop the transfusion; provide oxygen and diuretics

More severe cases can involve anaphylactic reactions consisting of a pruritic rash, bronchospasm, and cardiovascular collapse. Anaphylactic reactions occur in up to 1% of patients receiving transfusions and are often caused by foreign proteins in the plasma. Mild cases of anaphylaxis can be treated with antihistamines and slowing of the transfusion. Cases involving dyspnea, stridor, hypotension, tachycardia, loss of consciousness, cardiac arrhythmia, shock, and cardiac arrest require the infusion to be stopped and are treated with antihistamines, bronchodilators, steroids, and in severe cases, epinephrine.

The most severe transfusion reactions are **immune-mediated hemolytic reactions** due to serum antibodies. Delayed hemolytic transfusion reactions occur in patients who had previous transfusion or crossmatching difficulties. These occur in patients who have prior sensitization to RBC alloantigens. This results in massive red blood cell destruction and profound shock. Fever, chills, hypotension, tachypnea, and tachycardia are often seen immediately during and following transfusion when this occurs. Treatment consists of immediately stopping the transfusion, ensuring adequate intravascular volume and urine output, and providing cardiovascular support when necessary. Inducing diuresis using mannitol may be of some benefit to minimize the potential for heme pigment injury to the kidney. The patient should be monitored for disseminated intravascular coagulation (DIC), which may be a lethal consequence of this type of reaction. Delayed hemolytic reactions can occur but may be less severe.

Patients with underlying cardiac disease are at risk for overload, especially during rapid infusions. Signs and symptoms include tachypnea, cough, pulmonary edema, tachycardia, and signs of congestive heart failure. If the signs are mild, the transfusion can be slowed. Signs of cardiovascular collapse should be managed aggressively by stopping the infusion and increasing the patient's oxygen and use of diuretics.

Transferring Care to the Receiving Facility

Arrival at the destination facility is often a relief for transport providers, especially when the transported patients require a high intensity of care. This period, however, is generally one of the most dangerous times during critical care transport. Crew fatigue compounds the difficulties, and continued vigilance is required until the receiving providers have assumed complete control of the patient. A dislodged endotracheal tube or unrecognized tension pneumothorax that occurs during the last 15 minutes of care can be equally lethal as one that occurs in the first 15 minutes of care, and may be less easily recognized due to fatigue or communication errors between teams. The transport providers should provide a thorough report to the receiving team including any changes in the patient's condition and treatments rendered en route.

Considerations Unique to Aeromedical Transport

In general, the physiologic dysfunction that occurs with critical illness is worsened at significant elevation. The majority of pressurized cabins are calibrated for 5,000 to 8,000 feet (1,524 to 2,438 m) above sea level. Changes in the patient's condition should be anticipated and in some cases treated prior to flight. As discussed earlier in the chapter, a thorough medical history is critical as is an understanding of the patient's affliction (trauma vs medical), the capabilities of the aircraft (ie, ability to adjust cabin pressurization), the duration of flight, and the capabilities of the receiving medical treatment facility.

Stresses of Flight

Dysbarism refers to medical conditions that occur as a result of changes in ambient air pressure. Mechanical problems secondary to closed space gas expansion during takeoff and landing can occur and result in significant pain. Areas at risk in all individuals include the paranasal sinuses, lungs, and gastrointestinal tract. In particular, patients with upper respiratory infections, pneumothorax, or a mechanical bowel obstruction are susceptible to injuries related to dysbarism. Other traumatic injuries including penetrating brain injuries with **pneumocephalus** or globe injuries with intraocular air may significantly worsen when flying at a normal cabin pressure, 5,000 to 8,000 feet (1,524 to 2,438 m) above sea level, due to the consequences of even small amounts of gas expansion in these areas. Fluid-filled compartments may also be at risk for compartment syndrome. **Compartment syndrome** is defined as perfusion pressure lower than tissue pressure in a closed compartment space. This is often identified by a loss of a distal pulse; however, the progressive swelling due to ischemia and reperfusion injury may be a much more significant factor than changes in cabin pressure. Identification and monitoring of high-risk patients during the pretransport preparation is critical to avoid irreversible complications. In the setting of a prolonged fixed-wing flight, typically greater than 2 hours, high-risk patients should be considered for surgical decompression of areas of concern prior to transport, if possible.

In addition, all circumferential dressings should be conforming but not overly tight and casts should be bivalved or cut to allow expansion. Patients should not be flown with air splints, military antishock trousers (MAST), or pneumatic stockings applied. Air in ETT cuffs may be manually adjusted for the changes in gas expansion or may be replaced with saline. Close monitoring during transport is essential to recognize these subtle and unpredictable complications.

Hyper/hypothermia can occur because there is a change of 1°C (33.8°F) for every 330′ (100 m) in altitude. Frequent temperature monitoring and appropriate preventive measures including head covering and insulated blankets are the primary treatment.

Noise and vibration effects during flight may be variable depending on the type of aircraft, the type of injury or illness, and the patient. Transport planes are relatively stable platforms; however, noise and vibration can still have significant consequences including patient fatigue. Providing ear protection and extra padding for immobilized fractures are simple maneuvers to increase the comfort of the patient. In some cases, the effects of vibration can be life threatening. Patients with significant vertebral column fractures can be at serious risk for spinal cord injury if improperly immobilized, especially when transported on a smaller aircraft or helicopter. Additional care may be required to minimize the risk of further injury during transport. Finally, the increased psychological stress of excess noise and vibration results in an increased metabolic rate and oxygen demand. This may be particularly important for small children and neonates.

Anxiety and sleep deprivation are common in critically ill patients. The physical movement, unfamiliar environment, or a preexisting fear of flight all serve to increase anxiety during transport. It is important to remember that despite every effort to ensure patient stability and comfort, patient transport is a significant stress for the patient.

Hypoxia

Hypoxia is an issue in aeromedical evacuation, and its toll on the body increases as the patient is taken to higher altitudes. Patients who are on a ventilator will generally be unaffected because their concentration of oxygen is being manually controlled. However, there may be significant consequences for those who are breathing unassisted, especially if there is a history of acute or chronic cardiopulmonary disease because with these disease processes patients may have lost their body's natural capabilities to deal with low oxygen states. Patients at significant risk include those with chronic obstructive pulmonary disease (COPD) and those with ischemic heart disease.

The brain is extremely sensitive to oxygen deprivation, and hypoxia is common at elevations above 10,000′. At extreme altitudes (greater than 20,000′ [6,096 m]), the partial pressure of oxygen is less than half that at sea level. This can have immediate and profound effects on the cognitive and physical functions of patients and crew members. This can result in loss of consciousness and in severe cases, death.

Cabin Decompression

Loss of cabin pressurization is an in-flight emergency; aeromedical crew members should be able to recognize the symptoms of decompression and be familiar with emergency procedures prior to takeoff. The main consequences are hypoxia and decompression sickness. Signs and symptoms of cabin decompression that crew members or patients may experience are listed in **TABLE 13-10**.

There are two main types of decompression:

- **Slow decompression:** May be insidious and results in gradual hypoxia, the signs of which may go unnoticed. It may not trigger the cabin pressurization alarm so it is imperative that the flight crew is aware of their individual signs of hypoxia.
- **Rapid decompression:** Occurs instantaneously and may be associated with fog and noise occurring as liquid material rapidly vaporizes and gas expands. Hypoxia occurs rapidly in the absence of oxygen administration. In addition, rapid gas expansion in the blood and tissue can result in decompression sickness. In rare cases, gas embolism can occur.

The corrective action in instances of aircraft decompressions is for the pilot, flight crew members, and passengers to immediately go on 100% oxygen and for the aircraft to descend below a flight level of approximately 10,000′ (3,048 m) where ambient oxygen is acceptable to sustain life and cognitive function without the use of supplemental oxygen.

Time of useful consciousness (TUC) is the period during which adequate cognitive function persists in a hypoxic environment. Beyond this, judgment and dexterity are impaired and, ultimately, consciousness is lost.

TABLE 13-10 Decompression Signs and Symptoms	
Signs	**Symptoms**
Rapid breathing	Air hunger
Cyanosis	Dizziness
Poor coordination	Headache
Lethargy	Mental and muscle fatigue
Poor judgment	Nausea
	Hot and cold flashes
	Tingling
	Euphoria
	Visual impairment

The signs of hypoxia may be subtle; ideally all aeromedical providers would undergo specific training in an altitude chamber designed to familiarize them with the sensory and motor changes that can occur during decompression. Currently, only the US Air Force mandates that all aircrew members receive initial and refresher training in an altitude chamber. The time spent in this chamber simulates in-flight aircraft emergencies and allows personnel the opportunity to gain an improved understanding of their individual symptoms. Many international aeromedical agencies do not have this requirement due to the potential of actually inducing decompression sickness (DCS) during the time in the chamber. It is for this reason, as well as because of the high cost of an altitude chamber, that it is not a requirement in many of these agencies.

Decompression Illness

Decompression sickness (DCS), also known as the *bends* or *caisson disease*, is a medical emergency that occurs when there is a supersaturation of dissolved nitrogen in the tissues that expands to form small gaseous bubbles. This occurs most commonly in the joint spaces (elbows, shoulders, hip, wrists, knees, ankles), but a more severe form can occur in the central nervous system and result in paralysis or death. Other symptoms include itching with or without a skin rash and loss of sensation. If caused by altitude, pain can occur immediately or up to many hours later.

Air embolism is a related process caused by sudden expansion of dissolved gas in the bloodstream. This results in embolization and occlusion of blood flow to a vital organ such as the brain, heart, or lungs, and can have many of the same symptoms as DCS. The two conditions are grouped together under the name decompression illness (DCI). Both cases require immediate recompression that often requires decreasing the cabin and/or aircraft altitude to as close to sea level as the airframe can accommodate.

Aircraft Safety

In rotary or fixed-wing transport, it is important to be familiar with aircraft safety procedures as well as how to safely approach the aircraft.

Fixed-wing aircraft should not be approached unless instructed to do so by a crew member; those not instructed to do so should stay outside of the circle of safety. The *circle of safety* is an imaginary circle that encompasses the aircraft, keeping individuals 10′ (3 m) from the wing tip, nose, and tail of the airframe. If approaching while the engines are running, the tail distance may increase to up to 300′ (91 m).

In rotary aircraft, the landing zone (LZ) often is predetermined. Understanding the limitations of rotary-wing aircraft can be useful, particularly in austere or rural settings. Helicopter landing zones (HLZs) have specific space requirements. The minimums vary depending on the airframe; all require a clear approach and departure path with a minimum area of at least 75′ by 75′ (23 m × 23 m) during daylight and 100′ by 100′ (30 m × 30 m) during night/low light landings **FIGURE 13-4**. In addition, hazards should be marked and the locations of power lines, fences, antennae, trees, poles, and buildings should be conveyed to the inbound helicopter. The

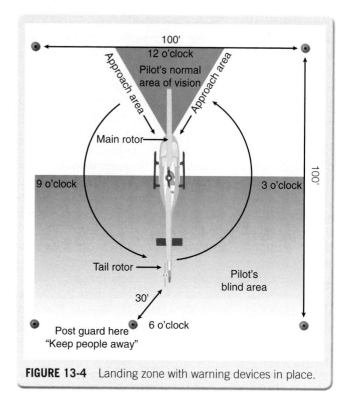

FIGURE 13-4 Landing zone with warning devices in place.

pilot and flight crew will let you know from the air whether a particular location is satisfactory.

Although patient loading is generally performed before aircraft startup, on rare occasions, patients will be loaded onto a running helicopter, also known as a "hot onload." Safety is paramount. Eye and hearing protection should be worn by all individuals operating near the aircraft as well as by the patient being transported. When transporting patients, *do not approach the airframe* unless explicitly instructed to by a crew member. To keep the risks to on-scene personnel to a minimum, only those necessary for patient movement should approach the aircraft. It is important to realize that any location within the rotor area is a danger zone. Always approach the aircraft from the 10 o'clock to 2 o'clock position or within 45 degrees of the nose. This allows for continuous eye contact with the pilot or crew chief. The same route that you used to approach the aircraft should be used when departing the aircraft. Be aware that sudden wind gusts may cause depression of the main rotor blades to as low as 4′ in some cases. In addition, the tail rotor rotates with such velocity that it may be invisible, particularly at night. Finally, never approach or depart the aircraft from the uphill side, given the risk of main rotor injury or death. Diligence and good situational awareness are imperative when dealing with an operational aircraft.

Similar to onloading, "hot offloads" are generally unnecessary, although they should be considered for patients who have a sudden decompensation en route or during a multiple or mass casualty incident that results in the need to rapidly clear the landing zone for additional aircraft. Each facility has its own regulations governing hot offloads; local transport crews should be familiar with the indications and necessary safety procedures.

CHAPTER RESOURCES

CASE STUDY ANSWERS

1 How does your assessment differ when the patient is an interhospital transfer compared to a trauma scene response?

Because initial stabilization of the patient has been started, your exam will require a review of the treatments provided prior to your arrival. Trauma systems, and EMS in particular, have changed the flow of trauma patients toward primary intake at a trauma hospital. This has been shown to reduce morbidity and mortality. However, it has decreased the number of trauma patients seen in community hospitals and therefore the familiarity of the staff at those hospitals to recognize and stabilize these patients. Careful attention must be taken to fully evaluate your patient to prevent less obvious injuries from being overlooked.

2 What are the priorities during the patient's physical exam?

The priorities continue to be based on life threats. The simple ABCs of the initial/primary assessment now contain more points to look at. Is the patient intubated? Is it the right size? How was positioning confirmed? What medications were used to paralyze or sedate him? If he is not intubated, will he need to be intubated to complete your transfer? Many of these same questions are asked in a field situation, but the same technology often is not available to help answer them. Has a chest radiograph been done to confirm ETT placement? What are his ABGs? These additional diagnostic tools allow the provider to complete a much more thorough examination and develop a more defined plan for the transport.

3 What do this patient's laboratory results help to confirm as part of his diagnosis?

His ABG shows a mixed respiratory/metabolic acidosis; combined with the increased lactate level this confirms a diagnosis of shock. Hemoglobin, hematocrit, and Na^+ levels correspond with the large amount of normal saline that has been administered. The radiograph confirms good ETT placement and shows several rib fractures that may complicate continued patient care. Radiology report on the CT confirms bleeding from the spleen is most likely the cause of the shock.

4 Is this patient ready for immediate departure?

This patient has had whole blood ordered; however, it has not been started. Given time constraints it could be started in the stable environment of the facility to assess potential adverse reactions. Also, the patient's ventilator settings are slightly off, and adding tidal volume could help the patient compensate for the acidosis. These can be changed en route if time is critical, but having the ability to make the patient more stable before transport is preferred.

5 What are the potential problems with care that this patient may present en route?

This patient has had his airway secured and is being ventilated. He has or will have blood replacement products being delivered and has been sedated or paralyzed for transport. Potential issues that may present include dislodging the ETT, failure of the ventilator, development of a pneumothorax due to the ventilator, and cardiovascular collapse due to decompensated shock and the added stresses of transportation. Prior to transport the team must make plans to identify and mediate these and other complications.

Trauma in Motion

1. What options are available in your area if the transport of a critical patient is interrupted by mechanical failure or weather-related safety issues?
2. Do you feel the training that you received is appropriate to the level that you operate at? Should it be more intensive, or were you trained for more than you are allowed to do?
3. When a transfer comes in for your crew, do the crew members have the ability to delay or cancel a response due to safety concerns?
4. Does long transport time affect the ability of the crew to provide care?

References and Resources

American Trauma Society. American College of Surgeons Committee on Trauma classification system of trauma center care. 1996. Available at: http://www.amtrauma.org/tiep/reports/ACSClassification.html. Accessed May 7, 2009.

American Trauma Society. Trauma Information Exchange Program (TIEP). 1996. Available at: http://amtrauma.org/tiep/reports/publicreports.html. Accessed April 17, 2009.

Barillo DJ, Renz E. An emergency medical bag set for long-range aeromedical transportation. *Am J Disaster Med.* 2008; 3(2):79–86.

Bartolacci RA, Munford B, Lee A, McDougall P. Air medical scene response to blunt trauma: effect on early survival. *Med J Austral.* 1998; 169:612–616.

Belway D, Dodek PM, Keenan S, Norena M, Wong H. The role of transport intervals in outcomes for critically ill patients who are transferred to referral centers. *J Crit Care.* 2008; 23(3):287–294.

Beninati W, Meyer MT, Carter TE. The critical care air transport program. *Crit Care Med.* 2008; 36(7 Suppl):S370–S376.

Biewener A, Aschenbrenner U, Rammelt S, Grass R, Zwipp H. Impact of helicopter transport and hospital level on mortality in polytrauma patients. *J Trauma.* 2004; 56:94–98.

Brathwaite CEM, Rosko M, McDowell R, et al. A critical analysis of on-scene helicopter transport on survival in a statewide trauma system. *J Trauma Inj Infect Crit Care.* 1998; 45:140–146.

Davis JR, Johnson R, Stepanek J, Fogarty JA. *Fundamentals of Aerospace Medicine,* 4th ed. Philadelphia, PA: Lippincott, Williams and Wilkins; 2008.

Diaz MA, Hendey GW, Bivins HG. When is a helicopter faster? A comparison of helicopter and ground ambulance transport times. *J Trauma.* 2005; 58:148–153.

Dugdale DC III. CBC. 2008. Available at: http://www.nlm.nih.gov/medlineplus/ency/article/003642.htm. Accessed April 15, 2009.

Fan E, MacDonald RD, Adhikari NKJ, et al. Outcomes of interfacility critical care adult patient transport: a systematic review. *Crit Care.* 2006; 10(1):R6.

Ford M, Delaney KA, Ling L, Erickson T. *Clinical Toxicology,* 1st ed. Philadelphia, PA: Saunders; 2000.

Gray A, Bush S, Whitely S. Secondary transport of the critically ill and injured adult. *Emerg Med J.* 2004; 21(3):281–285.

Grissom TE. Critical care air transport: patient flight physiology and organizational considerations. In: Hurd WW, Jernigan JG, eds. *Aeromedical Evacuation: Management of Acute and Stabilized Patients.* New York: Springer; 2002:111–135.

Hoffman R, Benz Jr EJ, Shattil SJ, et al., eds. *Hematology: Basic Principles and Practice,* 4th ed. Philadelphia, PA: Churchill Livingston; 2005:2674.

Holleran RS. *Air and Surface Patient Transport Principles and Practice,* 3rd ed. St. Louis, MO: Mosby; 2003.

Jacobs LM, Bennett B. A critical care helicopter system in trauma. *J Natl Med Assoc.* 1989; 81(11):1157–1167.

Kashani KB, Farmer JC. The support of severe respiratory failure beyond the hospital and during transportation. *Curr Opin Crit Care.* 2006; 12(1):43–49.

Ligtenberg JJ, Arnold LG, Stienstra Y, van der Werf TS, Meertens J, Tulleken JE, et al. Quality of interhospital transport of critically ill patients: a prospective audit. *Crit Care.* 2005; 9(4):R446–R451.

Margolis SA, Carter T, Dunn EV, Reed RL. The health status of community based elderly in the United Arab Emirates. *Arch Gerontol Geriatr.* 2003; 37(1):1–12.

Mason RJ, Broaddus VC, Murray JF, Nadel JA. *Murray and Nadel's Textbook of Respiratory Medicine,* 4th ed. Philadelphia, PA: Saunders; 2005.

McPherson RA, Pincus MR. *Henry's Clinical Diagnosis and Management by Laboratory Methods,* 21st ed. Philadelphia, PA: WB Saunders; 2007:459–460.

Moylan JA. Impact of helicopters on trauma care and clinical results. *Ann Surg.* 1988; 208(6):673–678.

Renz EM, Cancio LC, Barillo DJ, et al. Long range transport of war-related burn casualties. *J Trauma.* 2008; 64(2 Suppl): S136–S144; discussion S144–S145.

Rockwood CA Jr, Mann CM, Farrington JD, et al. History of emergency medical services in the United States. *J Trauma.* 1976; 16(4):299–308.

Schmidt US, Frame SB, Nerlich ML, et al. On-scene helicopter transport of patients with multiple injuries—comparison of a German and an American system. *J Trauma.* 1992; 33:548–553.

Schwartz RB, McManus Jr JG, Swienton RE. *Tactical Emergency Medicine.* Philadelphia, PA: Lippincott, Williams and Wilkins; 2008.

Seymour CW, Kahn JM, Schwab CW, Fuchs BD. Adverse events during rotary-wing transport of mechanically ventilated patients: a retrospective cohort study. *Crit Care.* 2008; 12(3):R71.

Woodward GA. *Guidelines for Air and Ground Transport of Neonatal and Pediatric Patients*, 3rd ed. Elk Grove Village, IL: American Academy of Pediatrics; 2007.

Procedures

PROCEDURE 1
Initial/Primary Assessment

Introduction

Trauma patients can present with a multitude of injuries, all with varying (and sometimes misleading) degrees of severity. The initial/primary assessment is a critical component in the care of these patients; it is imperative that life threats be identified and resolved quickly. The initial/primary assessment provides a systematic approach to find and treat life-threatening conditions. It is important to remember that the quality of the assessment usually determines the quality of the care.

Indications, Contraindications, and Equipment

Indications	Trauma patients
Contraindications	None
Equipment	Exam gloves and goggles Airway supplies Ventilation supplies Oxygen Hemorrhage-control supplies Stethoscope

Rationale

Because trauma patients can have injuries ranging from superficial to life threatening, it is important to have an organized system to prioritize the assessment to locate injuries that will cause death if left untreated. The initial/primary assessment is an effective way to identify "primary" life threats rapidly and to manage them. When treating the critically injured patient, the prehospital care provider may never conduct more than an initial/primary assessment if care is required to support the ABCs. The emphasis is on rapid evaluation, initiation of resuscitation, and transportation to an appropriate medical facility.

Possible Complications

The only complications associated with trauma assessments occur when life-threatening assessment findings are missed. When an orderly and complete process is followed, the findings are less likely to be misinterpreted and interventions can be completed in an efficient manner.

Procedure

Before the patient assessment begins, evaluation of the scene for the safety of EMS providers, other responders, victims, and bystanders must be completed.

1 Quickly assess the mechanism of injury to determine if spinal precautions should be used.

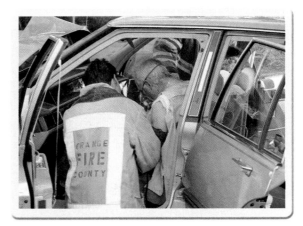

2 Assess the airway and begin steps to open and maintain it.
  a. Stabilize the c-spine if indicated.
  b. Control any gross exsanguinating (catastrophic) hemorrhage.

3 Determine the adequacy of breathing and support it to maintain adequate oxygenation.
  a. Expose the chest and visually assess for symmetry of movement.
  b. Listen to the chest to assess for the presence and equality of lung sounds.
  c. Palpate the chest to check the stability of the rib cage.

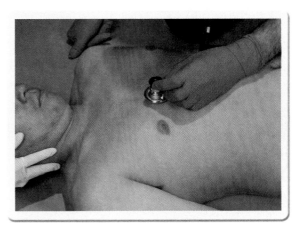

4 Evaluate the quality of pulses and assess for blood losses.
   a. Check distal pulses for presence, rate, and quality.
   b. Control any external bleeding that continues.
   c. Check capillary refill.
   d. Check areas that may hide internal bleeding: the abdomen, the pelvis, and the long bones of the upper arm and leg.

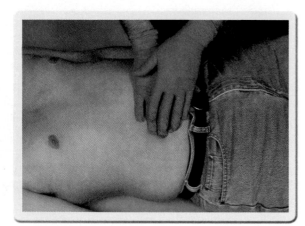

5 Assess gross neurologic function.
   a. AVPU score for brain function.
   b. Have patient move feet or toes to determine spinal cord function.

6 Treat any deficiencies noted in the assessment as they are found.
   a. Open and secure the airway.
   b. Begin ventilations if needed.
   c. Secure chest wall injuries that may impair ventilations.
   d. Control external bleeding and begin rapid transport for signs of internal bleeding.
   e. Complete spinal immobilization where required.

7 Complete initial vital signs and SAMPLE history during preparation for transport.

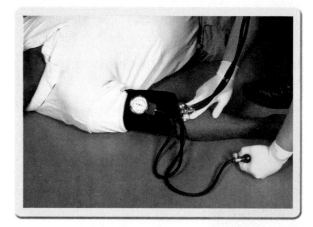

PROCEDURE 2
Rapid Trauma/Secondary Assessment

Introduction

A rapid assessment is required to find additional life-threatening injuries following the initial/primary assessment. When treating injuries associated with the initial/primary assessment, providers should defer the rapid trauma/secondary assessment and detailed exam until transportation has begun. In the unconscious patient or patient with decreased level of consciousness, this systematic approach helps find additional injuries. Patients who are able to communicate their injuries should have their injuries assessed and stabilized.

Indications, Contraindications, and Equipment

Indications	Trauma patients
Contraindications	None
Equipment	Exam gloves and goggles Oxygen Stethoscope

Rationale

Because trauma patients are not always capable of verbalizing their injuries, it is important to have a system to locate injuries that a patient may have incurred. The rapid trauma/secondary assessment is a head-to-toe approach to assess the entire body for injuries.

Possible Complications

The only complications associated with trauma assessments occur when life-threatening assessment findings are missed. When an orderly and complete process is followed, the findings are less likely to be misinterpreted and interventions can be completed in an efficient manner.

Procedure

Head and Neck

1 Start the assessment at the patient's head, inspecting and palpating the skull for any asymmetry (such as knots or depressions) or bleeding.

2 Quickly look in and behind the patient's ears for blood, cerebrospinal fluid (CSF), or bruising. Speak into each ear and ask the patient if the sound is equal.

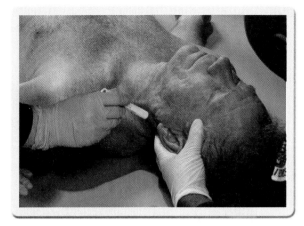

3 Check the pupils for size, equality, and response to light. Palpate the orbits around the eyes, doing both sides in unison. Feel from the nose out to the lateral edge, including upper and lower ridges. If the patient is responsive, assess the eye movements through the visual fields. Have the patient read an eye card or other item and describe any visual changes they may be experiencing.

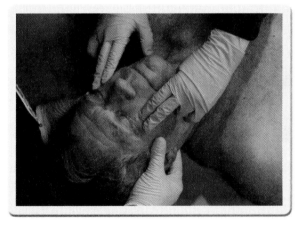

4 Inspect the nose for bleeding and other signs of trauma, such as tenderness or swelling.

5 Assess the mouth for blood or other fluids that may need suctioning. If the patient is unresponsive, open the mouth and look for injury or a need for suctioning. Check for broken or uneven teeth. If the patient is responsive, have them open and close the jaw to assess the mandible and the temporomandibular joint.

6 Palpate down the posterior cervical spine, feeling for any step-offs and looking for any signs of trauma. Be alert for point tenderness on the central cervical spine.

7 Assess the neck for jugular venous distension (JVD), subcutaneous emphysema (a sign of air leaking from the chest), or tracheal shift (a very late sign of a pneumothorax) per local protocols.

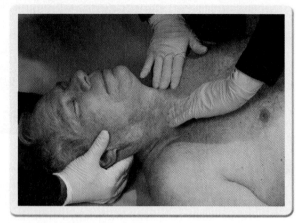

Chest

8 Inspect and palpate the chest. Place your thumbs in the suprasternal notch and follow both clavicles out to the shoulder girdle, keeping the clavicles (commonly fractured bones) between your thumb and finger. At the same time, inspect the chest for symmetric rise and fall and for any signs of retractions or other excessive work of breathing.

9 Gently place your palm on the sternum; press down and then side-to-side to check stability as you assess for a flail chest or fractured sternum.

10 Spread your fingers and surround the rib cage under the armpits and then at the costal margin to assess for fractured ribs or a flail chest. If you find large bruised areas, make special mental note: a flail segment may not show the classic paradoxical ("seesaw") movement because the body is still splinting the segment with muscle spasm.

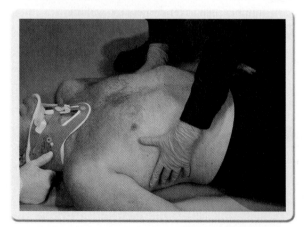

11 Listen to the lung sounds. Evaluate for the presence, depth, and equality of breath sounds.

Abdomen

12 Inspect and palpate the abdomen, being alert for rigidity, guarding, wounds, bruising, and tenderness. While palpating the upper abdomen, have the patient take a deep breath and assess for increasing tenderness. Peritoneal signs can be assessed by checking rebound tenderness. Be quick but thorough with your assessment of the abdomen.

Back

13 When you log roll the patient to move him or her to a backboard, examine and palpate the thoracic and lumbar spine for step-offs and tenderness. Also look for puncture wounds or other signs of trauma along the back.

Note: The back assessment may be completed at any time during the rapid trauma/secondary assessment that the patient needs to be moved for assessment or treatment.

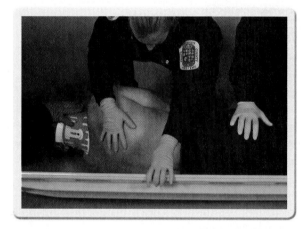

Pelvis

14 Move to the pelvic girdle and gently but firmly assess flexion and compression by pressing downward on the iliac crest and then moving the pressure inward, feeling for any sign (instability or pain) that the pelvic girdle is damaged. (Note that this technique of pressing inward is not used in all areas. Be sure to follow local protocols.)

15 Gently palpate over the bladder. If the groin area is wet or bloody or if the patient complains of pain in the area, expose and examine the groin and the genitalia.

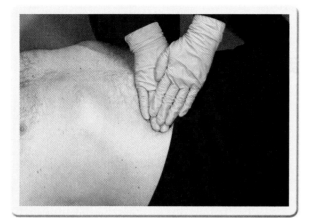

Lower Extremities

16 Inspect and palpate both lower extremities from the hip to the toes, looking for signs of bleeding or swelling. Note whether one extremity is shorter than the other or if either or both are rotated abnormally (signs of fracture or dislocation).

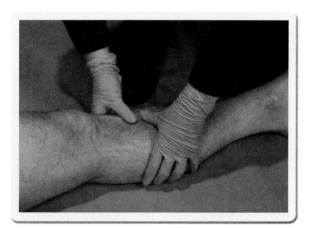

17 Simultaneously assess pedal pulses, noting whether they feel similar. A difference in pulse quality (that is, one weaker than the other) points to a potentially serious vascular disruption.

18 Check capillary refill and skin temperature to assess distal circulation in each extremity.

19 Assess for motor and sensory nerve function if the patient is responsive and cooperative.

Upper Extremities

20 Inspect and palpate both upper extremities from the shoulder to the fingers.

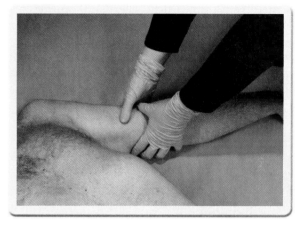

21 Simultaneously assess radial pulses, noting whether they feel similar.

22 Check capillary refill and skin temperature to assess distal circulation in each extremity.

23 Assess for motor and sensory nerve function if the patient is responsive and cooperative.

Treatment and Transport

24 Provide stabilization for all injuries found and begin transport.

25 Reassess the initial/primary assessment frequently because patient condition is prone to change. If the condition deteriorates and requires life-sustaining treatment, discontinue the rapid trauma/secondary assessment and provide immediate care and transportation.

PROCEDURE 3
Glasgow Coma Scale Assessment and Grading

Introduction

It is important to determine the level of consciousness for trauma patients. From levels of disorientation to the severity of a trauma patient's head injury, the ability to qualify and quantify the level can be difficult for the provider to do on scene. The Glasgow Coma Scale (GCS) provides a simple and relatively reproducible assessment of the level of consciousness. Based on an evaluation of the patient's eye opening and verbal and motor responses, the on-scene provider can determine the general severity of the head injury and effectively communicate this to the receiving facility.

Indications, Contraindications, and Equipment

Indications	Altered levels of consciousness Head trauma
Contraindications	None
Equipment	Exam gloves and goggles

Rationale

Patients who have experienced an injury often present with a decreased or decreasing level of consciousness or coma. Prehospital providers must be able to assess the level of responsiveness both to determine the need for treatment and to present a baseline medical exam to the receiving facility to further the patient's care. The GCS is an easily repeated exam tool that enables providers to obtain and relay this information to others quickly and in a useful format.

Possible Complications

Mistaking patient responses while assessing the GCS can lead to incorrect prioritization and/or treatment both prehospitally and during the initial phase of in-hospital care.

Procedure

1 Assess eye opening.
   a. If the patient's eyes are open, the score is 4.
   b. If the eyes are closed, say the patient's name or ask them to open their eyes. If they open, the score is 3.
   c. If the eyes remain closed, apply a painful stimulus such as pressure over a fingernail. If the eyes open, the score is 2.
   d. If the eyes do not open, the score is 1.
   e. Note: If the eyes are swollen and cannot open, the score is omitted for the section and a "C" (for closed) placed in the comments.

2 Assess motor response.
   a. Ask the patient to complete a task ("Lift your arm"). If the patient completes the task with no prompting, the score is 6. Note: Do not ask the patient to squeeze your fingers because this response can be confused with a grasp reflex.
   b. If the patient does not complete the task, apply a painful stimulus to one side of the body. This can be done by putting pressure on a fingernail of one hand, squeezing the trapezius muscle, or applying supraorbital pressure to the rim above the eye. If the patient reaches across the midline in response to the pain (as to push you away), the patient is said to localize pain and the score is 5. Do not use a sternal rub because the result may be confusing to interpret so close to the center.
   c. If the patient responds to the pain by withdrawing from the pain, the score is 4. The trapezius pinch may be better suited to a centralized response and will produce a shrug of the shoulder.

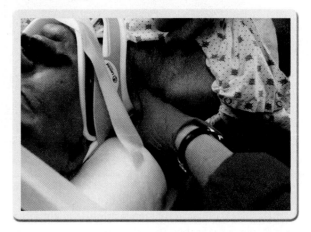

d. If the patient responds to pain by abnormal flexion of the extremity, as seen by wrist flexion, upper arm abduction, or flexion of the fingers over the thumb, the patient is said to be decorticate posturing and receives a score of 3. Also common to the upper arm movements are extension of the head and neck and extension of the lower extremities.

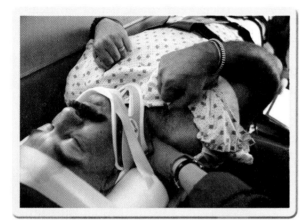

e. If the patient responds to the stimuli with abnormal extension, as seen by internal rotation of the shoulder, pronation of the forearm, and flexion of the wrist, the patient is said to be decerebrate posturing and receives a score of 2. Decerebrate posturing also has extension of the head and neck with extension of the lower extremities. Posturing is a primitive response by the brain to attempt to remove the painful stimuli.

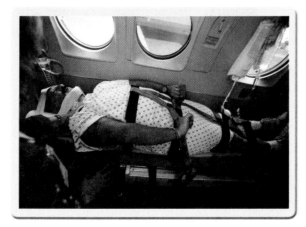

f. If there is no response the score is 1. Note: If the patient is chemically paralyzed or sedated, a "P" or "S" should be inserted into the comments, respectively, and the score omitted for the section.

3 Assess verbal response.

a. Ask the patient questions to determine their orientation to person, place, and time. If the patient is oriented, the score is 5.

b. If the patient forms a complete sentence but the answer is incorrect, the patient is disoriented and the score is a 4.

c. If the patient uses random words that do not fit into a sentence, the score is 3.

d. If the patient cannot make words or just utters moans or incomprehensible sounds, the score is reduced to 2.

e. If the patient does not respond, the score is 1. Note: Patients with a tracheostomy or intubated patients incapable of speaking should have a "T" (for tube) placed in the comments and the score for the section omitted.

4 Calculate the score by adding up the three components (eye opening, motor response, and verbal response). The score will range from 3 to 15 and should be documented with the appropriate letter if a condition produced an abnormally low score (eg, patient with swollen eyes but otherwise normal motor and verbal responses would have a score of "10 C").

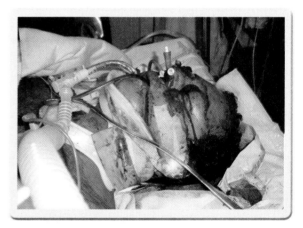

5 Repeat the assessment every 15 minutes to trend changes to the baseline or anytime a significant change is noted.

PROCEDURE 4
Pediatric Glasgow Coma Scale

Introduction

The Pediatric Glasgow Coma Scale (PGCS) can be effective in the assessment of pediatric trauma patients. Much like the adult model, it is based on evaluating the patient's eye opening and verbal and physical responses, but with a special focus on some very age-specific abilities. Perfect scores on the PGCS vary according to age.

Indications, Contraindications, and Equipment

Indications	Altered level of consciousness Head trauma
Contraindications	None
Equipment	Exam gloves and goggles

Rationale

Altered levels of consciousness can be caused by shock, hypoxia, head injury, or other medical conditions in pediatric trauma patients. The PGCS not only allows determination of the patient's level of consciousness, but also gives the provider the ability to relay that information to others quickly.

Possible Complications

Mistaking the patient's age or response while assessing the PGCS can lead to incorrect prioritization and/or treatment.

Procedure

The PGCS is completed the same way the adult GCS is; however, the scoring has to be adjusted to the child's developmental age.

Age 0 to 6 Months

- The best verbal response is normally a cry, though some infants grunt during this period as a response. Normal verbal score is 2.
- The best motor response is usually flexion. Normal motor score is 3.

Age 6 to 12 Months

- The normal infant makes noises. Normal verbal score is 3.
- The infant will usually locate pain but not obey commands. Normal motor score is 4.

Age 12 Months to 2 Years

- Recognizable words are expected. Normal verbal score is 4.
- The toddler will usually locate pain but not obey commands. Normal motor score is 4.

Age 2 Years to 5 Years

- Recognizable words are expected. Normal verbal score is 4.
- The child will usually obey commands. Normal motor score is 5.

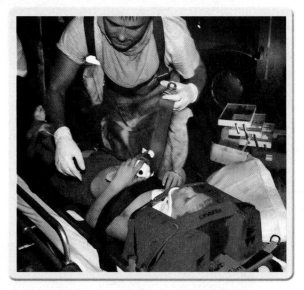

Age 5 Years and Older

- Orientation is defined as awareness of location. Normal verbal score is 5.

PROCEDURE 5
Extremity Assessment

Introduction

The purpose of assessing the extremities of a trauma patient is to find and evaluate injuries and to assess for conditions that could complicate those injuries.

Indications, Contraindications, and Equipment

Indications	Trauma patients
Contraindications	None
Equipment	Exam gloves and goggles
	Trauma shears

Rationale

In addition to looking and palpating for injuries, assessing the trauma patient's extremities for distal pulses and neurodeficits can provide valuable diagnostic clues to the patient's condition. This information can influence the provider's decisions and better guide the care of the patient.

Possible Complications

The complications usually associated with extremity assessments are caused by provider error. When injuries or indicators are missed or findings are misinterpreted, interventions can be either neglected or incorrect.

Procedure

Upper Extremities

1 Perform a distal motor function exam by having the patient shrug their shoulders and then bend the elbow and flex and extend the wrist. Perform the exam with and without resistance. Distal motor functioning can be assessed using an old child's game of "rock, paper, scissors."

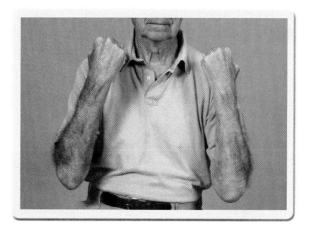

2 Perform a distal sensory exam by assessing sensation to the dorsal side of the thumb and first finger, the palm side of the middle fingers, and the dorsal side of the pinky and ring fingers. Have the patient compare the sensation bilaterally.

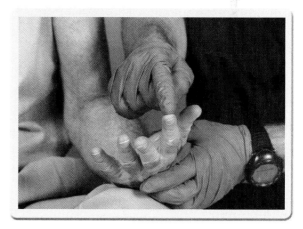

3 Assess the range of motion (ROM) passively in each arm, stopping immediately if pain is elicited. Compare the ROM from side to side to determine equality of movement.

Lower Extremities

1 Perform a distal motor function exam by having the patient lift their legs off the ground, then bend at the knee and flex and extend the foot. Perform the exam with and without resistance. Bilateral loss of motor function suggests a spinal cord injury, whereas unilateral loss of function is most likely musculoskeletal in origin.

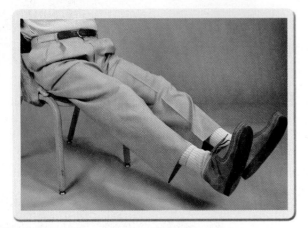

2 Perform a distal sensory exam by assessing sensation to the top and bottom of the foot on each side. Have the patient compare the sensation bilaterally.

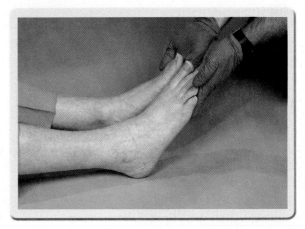

3 Assess the range of motion (ROM) passively in each leg, stopping immediately if pain is elicited. Compare the ROM from side to side to determine equality of movement.

PROCEDURE 6
Jaw-Thrust Maneuver

Introduction

When assessing for airway patency in a trauma patient, it is critical to maintain neutral immobilization of the patient's cervical spine. Because the jaw-thrust maneuver requires no additional equipment, every provider level should utilize it when an initial airway is needed during assessment. The jaw-thrust maneuver, when performed correctly, allows the tongue to be moved from the airway without compromising the alignment of the cervical spine.

Indications, Contraindications, and Equipment

Indications	Unresponsive trauma patients with suspected spinal injury who are unable to maintain a patent airway
Contraindications	Responsive trauma patients whose mouth cannot be opened
Equipment	Exam gloves and goggles

Rationale

Tongue occlusion of the upper airway can be a problem with altered and unresponsive trauma patients. The jaw-thrust maneuver moves the lower jaw anteriorly, thus separating the tongue from the soft tissue of the posterior airway while protecting the neutral positioning of the cervical spine.

Possible Complications

This airway technique cannot be maintained if the patient becomes responsive or combative, and it makes it difficult to use bag-mask ventilation devices with a single rescuer.

Procedure

1. Place the thumbs of both hands on the zygomatic arches of the patient's face.
2. Position fingers under the mandible near the temporomandibular joint.
3. Displace the mandible anteriorly while holding the head stable to avoid c-spine movement.

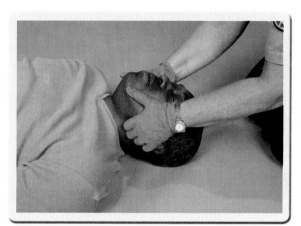

PROCEDURE 7
Trauma Chin Lift

Introduction

When assessing for airway patency in a trauma patient, it is critical to maintain neutral immobilization of the patient's cervical spine. The trauma chin lift is often used in conjunction with the jaw-thrust maneuver to maintain a patent airway until an adjunct can be placed. When performed correctly, the trauma chin lift allows the tongue to be moved from the airway without compromising the alignment of the cervical spine.

Indications, Contraindications, and Equipment

Indications	Unresponsive trauma patients with suspected spinal injury who are unable to maintain a patent airway
Contraindications	Responsive trauma patients whose mouths cannot be opened
Equipment	Exam gloves and goggles

Rationale

Tongue occlusion of the upper airway can be a problem with altered and unresponsive trauma patients. The trauma chin lift moves the lower jaw anteriorly, thus separating the tongue from the soft tissue of the airway while protecting the neutral positioning of the cervical spine.

Possible Complications

This airway technique cannot be maintained if the patient becomes responsive or combative, and it makes it difficult to use bag-mask ventilation devices.

Procedure

1. Place the fingers of one hand under the mandible while the thumb is inserted into the mouth, grasping the lower incisors.

2. Gently lift the mandible anteriorly.

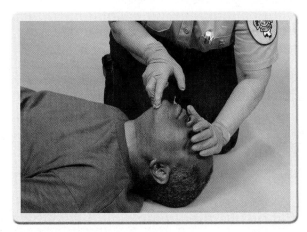

PROCEDURE 8
Intubation With C-Spine Stabilization

Introduction

The need to take c-spine precautions is common when caring for trauma patients, but this can cause challenges when intubation is necessary. Although laryngoscopy and intubation can be performed very carefully in this situation, extensive manipulation of the head and neck is sometimes required to visualize the cords.

Indications, Contraindications, and Equipment

Indications	Patients with suspected cervical spine injuries who require airway or breathing control
Contraindications	Responsive patients or patients with an intact gag reflex
Equipment	Exam gloves and goggles Intubation equipment Tape or tube-securing device Capnometry or placement confirmation device Bag-mask device Oxygen

Rationale

Manipulating the head and neck of a patient with possible cervical spine injuries can worsen the damage or create new injuries. Because standard intubation technique sometimes requires the patient's neck to be hyperextended, other options should be considered when laryngoscopy would require too much movement. One of the most common alternatives in these situations is digital intubation, where the provider feels for the glottic opening with the index and middle fingers and slides the tube in place by palpation.

Possible Complications

With standard methods of intubation, excessive movement of the patient's head and neck can cause further injury. Also, as with any attempt at laryngoscopy, damage to the teeth and airway tissue is a possibility.

Procedure

1. If a cervical spine fracture is suspected, maintain stabilization of the neck.

2. Ensure that adequate ventilations are provided and preoxygenate the patient.

3. Assemble the equipment.

4. Have an assistant maintain manual immobilization of the head and neck while the cervical collar (if present) is loosened. The assistant should position him- or herself alongside the patient in a face-to-face direction. Stabilization should support the head but leave the mandible free for movement to facilitate intubation.

5. Insert the laryngoscope and visualize the vocal cords. Pass the endotracheal tube (ET) through the vocal cords.

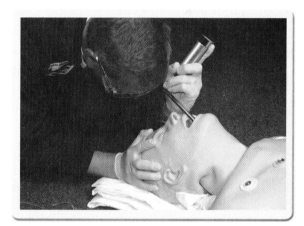

6. Inflate the cuff of the ET tube with enough air to provide an adequate seal.

7 Check the placement of the tube by ventilating with a bag-mask device and auscultating the lung fields.

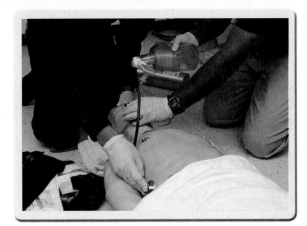

8 Confirm placement of the ET tube with a secondary method such as capnometry or an esophageal detection device.

9 Secure the tube.

10 Reattach the cervical collar or place a cervical collar if one has not been applied.

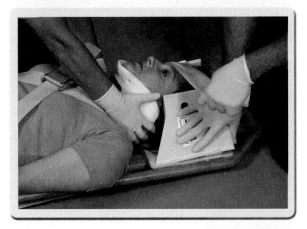

11 Move the patient to a long backboard and secure the patient.

12 Repeat confirmation of ET tube placement following the move.

PROCEDURE 9
Face-to-Face Intubation

Introduction

In traumatic injury, one of the highest priorities for pre-hospital providers is airway management. Often patients are entrapped by materials, requiring the provider to care for the patient in an austere environment. When a patient who requires intubation cannot be moved into a position normally used to intubate, an alternative is the face-to-face method. This method has been referred to in the literature as inverse intubation, the tomahawk method, or the ice pick method.

Indications, Contraindications, and Equipment

Indications	A patient who requires intubation but has limited access or is unable to be moved into a neutral position normally associated with intubation
Contraindications	The provider must be familiar with the technique and be skilled in intubation before attempting.
	Should be used only when intubation is immediately required
Equipment	Exam gloves and goggles Intubation equipment A Macintosh (curved) blade is preferred for the technique. Tape or tube-securing device Capnometry or placement confirmation device Bag-mask device Oxygen

Rationale

Effective management of the airway of a patient who is entrapped or otherwise obstructed may require an alternative approach. Proficiency in multiple airway techniques is essential. When intubation is required in a patient who presents in an awkward position or suboptimal conditions exist for intubation, an alternative technique can be used. The face-to-face method of intubation allows access to the airway when another position may not be available.

Possible Complications

Intubation is a skill that requires a high degree of proficiency. Contributing to the difficulty is that the anatomy of the airway will be upside down when compared to a standard intubation. Because this technique is often used under austere conditions, the provider must be the most skilled available. Esophageal intubation, mainstem intubation, airway trauma, bleeding, airway occlusion, cervical spine injury, and death are all possible complications.

Procedure

1 If a cervical spine fracture is suspected, maintain stabilization of the neck.

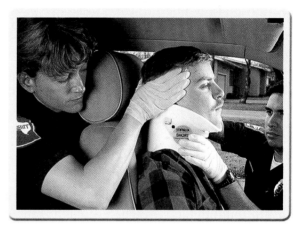

2 Ensure that adequate ventilations are provided and preoxygenate the patient.

3 Assemble the equipment. A curved laryngoscope blade is preferred for this technique.

4 Have an assistant maintain manual immobilization of the head.

5 Hold the laryngoscope in the right hand and advance into the mouth toward the uvula, then pull downward along the tongue. Pull the scope anteriorly to open the airway.

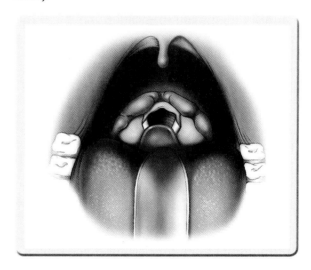

6 Visualize the vocal cords. Remember that the anatomy will be reversed compared to a standard intubation. Pass the endotracheal tube (ET) through the vocal cords.

7 Inflate the cuff of the ET tube with enough air to provide an adequate seal.

8 Check the placement of the ET tube by ventilating with a bag-mask device and auscultating the lung fields.

9 Confirm placement of the ET tube with a secondary method.

10 Secure the tube.

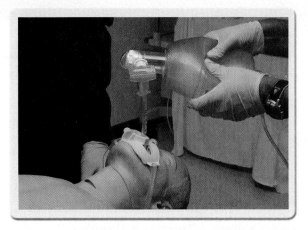

11 Reconfirm ET tube placement throughout the extrication and transport process.

PROCEDURE 10
Nasal Intubation

Introduction

Some trauma patients with mandibular fractures or injuries that prevent mouth opening may require advanced airway control while they are still breathing spontaneously or even conscious. Nasal intubation, sometimes called blind nasotracheal intubation, is a very effective technique in those situations but may not be allowed in your jurisdiction. Follow local protocols.

Indications, Contraindications, and Equipment

Indications	Spontaneously breathing trauma patients who require advanced airway control where orotracheal intubation is not possible
Contraindications	Apnea Head trauma with suspected basal skull fracture Midface fractures Deviated septum
Equipment	Exam gloves and goggles Standard orotracheal intubation equipment minus the laryngoscope and stylet Anesthetic and vasoconstrictor sprays

Rationale

Occasionally, trauma patients who are conscious and breathing require advanced airway control, and due to jaw injuries, trismus, or a gag reflex, other airway techniques are not possible. With these patients, being able to insert an ET tube nasally into the trachea will ensure airway control and provide an adequate ventilatory channel if needed.

Possible Complications

Bleeding, due to airway trauma from the procedure, is the most common complication of nasal intubation. Unrecognized esophageal intubation, unrecognized mainstem bronchus intubation, or the inability to intubate can lead to hypoxia and death. Conversion of a cervical vertebral injury without neurologic deficit to a cervical cord injury with neurologic deficit is possible.

Procedure

1. If a cervical spine fracture is suspected, leave the cervical collar in place to assist in maintaining immobilization of the neck.
2. Ensure that adequate ventilations are present and preoxygenate the patient.
3. Assemble the equipment.
4. Preform the ET tube by bending it in a circle.

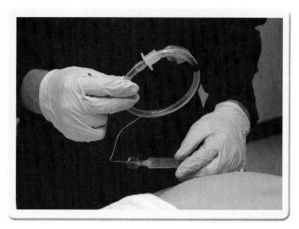

5. If the patient is conscious, spray the nasal passage with an anesthetic and vasoconstrictor to anesthetize and constrict the mucosa. If the patient is unconscious, it is adequate to spray the nasal passage with only a vasoconstrictor.
6. Have an assistant maintain manual immobilization of the head and neck.
7. Lubricate the nasotracheal tube with a water-soluble gel.
8. Insert the tube into the most compliant nostril with the bevel facing the septum.

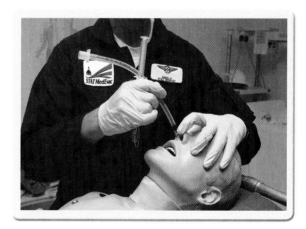

9 Guide the tube slowly but firmly along the nasal floor. The curve of the tube should be aligned to facilitate passage along this curved course.

10 Once the tube has entered the pharynx, listen to the airflow through the ET tube. Advance the tube until the sound of moving air is maximal. While listening to air movement, determine the point of inhalation and advance the tube quickly. If the tube placement is unsuccessful, repeat the procedure.

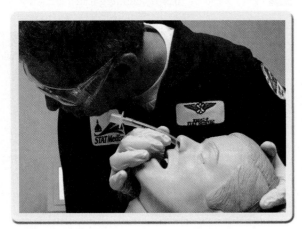

11 Inflate the cuff of the ET tube with enough air to provide an adequate seal.

12 Check the placement of the ET tube by ventilating with a bag-mask device and auscultating the lung fields.

13 Confirm placement of the ET tube with a secondary method.

14 Secure the tube.

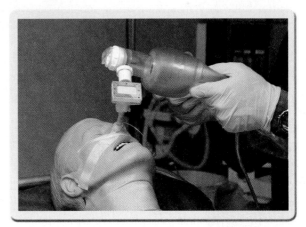

PROCEDURE 11
Needle Cricothyroidotomy

Introduction

When a trauma patient has suffered head, face, or airway injuries that prevent traditional airway controls, a surgical airway must be considered. During preparations for an open cricothyroidotomy, or if transport time to an appropriate care facility is very short, needle cricothyroidotomy may be an effective option.

Indications, Contraindications, and Equipment

Indications	Failure to control airway by any other means Standard airway methods are not possible or contraindicated
Contraindications	None when performed as a lifesaving measure
Equipment	Exam gloves and goggles Antiseptic preps Transtracheal needle and cannula Jet ventilator with valve, tubing, and luer lock Oxygen

Rationale

Head, facial, and upper airway trauma can destroy the patient's airway while making traditional, less-invasive airway techniques impossible or dangerous. In these cases, needle cricothyroidotomy may quickly establish an effective *but temporary* means of ventilation by introducing a catheter into the trachea through which 100% oxygen is forced in 1- to 2-second bursts.

Possible Complications

Inadequate ventilations may lead to hypoxia and death. Esophageal laceration, posterior tracheal wall perforation, or thyroid perforation are possible due to improper placement of the needle. Hematoma in the tissue surrounding the airway or subcutaneous and/or mediastinal emphysema can complicate the airway. If passive exhalation does not occur because of injury or device error and it is not assessed correctly, needle cricothyroidotomy can lead to tension pneumothorax. Also, because this procedure does not provide adequate ventilatory volume, extended use can lead to hypoxia and hypercarbia.

Procedure

1 Assemble and prepare oxygen tubing or a commercial ventilation device.

2 Assemble a 14- or 16-gauge over-the-needle IV catheter to a 10-mL syringe with 3 mL of saline.

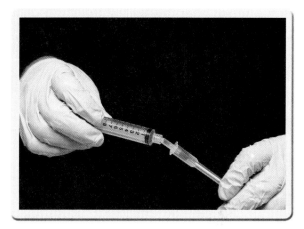

3 Place the patient supine in a neutral position.

4 Prepare the neck using antiseptic swabs.

5 Palpate the cricothyroid membrane. Stabilize the trachea with the thumb and forefinger of one hand to prevent lateral movement of the trachea during the procedure.

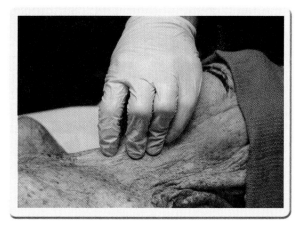

6 Puncture the skin in the midline with the syringe and needle directly over the cricothyroid membrane.

7 Direct the needle at a 45° angle toward the feet (caudally) while applying negative pressure to the syringe.

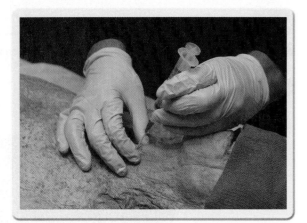

8 Carefully insert the needle through the cricothyroid membrane, aspirating as the needle is advanced.

9 Aspiration of air (seen by bubbles in the saline) signifies entry into the trachea.

10 Remove the syringe and withdraw the needle while gently advancing the catheter downward into position, being careful not to perforate the posterior wall of the trachea.

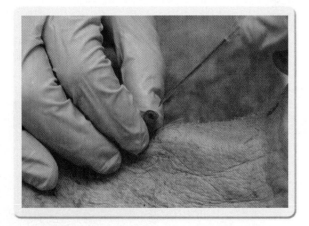

11 Attach the jet ventilator oxygen tubing to the catheter needle hub and secure the catheter to the patient's neck.

12 Ventilation can be achieved by opening the valve on the ventilator or occluding the open hole cut into the oxygen tubing with your thumb for 1 second and releasing it for 4 seconds. After releasing, the patient passively exhales.

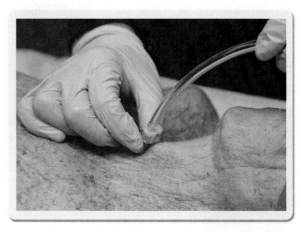

13 Observe for chest inflation and auscultate the chest for adequate ventilation.

Note: Adequate Pao_2 can be maintained for only 30 to 45 minutes, and CO_2 accumulation may occur more rapidly.

PROCEDURE 12
Surgical Cricothyroidotomy

Introduction

Patients who have suffered catastrophic trauma or burns to the face and/or upper airway may be nearly impossible to ventilate with a bag-mask device or to intubate. In these extreme cases, an open (or surgical) cricothyroidotomy may be the only way to establish an airway.

Indications, Contraindications, and Equipment

Indications	Severe burns of upper airway Massive maxillofacial trauma Head injuries resulting in trismus
Contraindications	Inability to locate correct anatomic landmarks Crushing larynx injuries Tracheal transection
Equipment (Minimum)	Scalpel ET or tracheostomy tube Securing device Curved hemostats Suction apparatus Sterile gauze pads Bag-mask device Oxygen Note: Commercially prepared kits may be available

Rationale

Head, facial, and upper airway traumas can destroy the patient's airway while making traditional, less-invasive airway techniques impossible or dangerous. In these cases, a surgical cricothyroidotomy can quickly reestablish an effective airway by introducing a large-bore tube directly into the airway without requiring the manipulation of the trauma patient's cervical spine.

Possible Complications

Hemorrhage or hematoma formation in or around the airway, laceration of the esophagus or the trachea, and aspiration of blood are among the complications associated with a surgical airway procedure. Creation of false passage in the tissues can occur if the tube does not enter the trachea, and mediastinal or subcutaneous emphysema will occur if ventilations are initiated. Vocal cord paralysis and subglottic or laryngeal stenosis (narrowing) are among the complications of the procedure. Using too much force when inserting the tube can perforate the esophagus and damage the laryngeal nerves.

Procedure

1 Check, assemble, and prepare the equipment.

2 Place the patient in a neutral position. Palpate the thyroid notch, the cricothyroid interval, and the sternal notch for orientation.

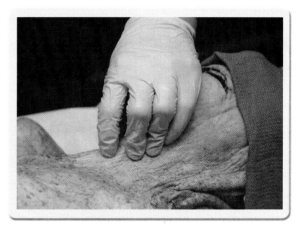

3 Prepare the neck using antiseptic swabs.

4 Stabilize the thyroid cartilage with the left hand and maintain stabilization until the trachea is intubated.

5 Make a 1- to 2-cm vertical incision over the cricothyroid membrane.

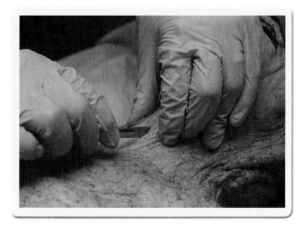

6 Puncture the cricothyroid membrane and make a horizontal cut 1 cm in each direction from the midline.

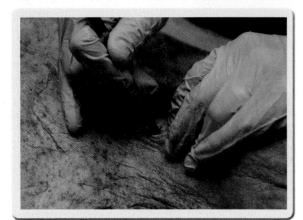

7 Spread the incision with a curved hemostat or tracheal spreader.

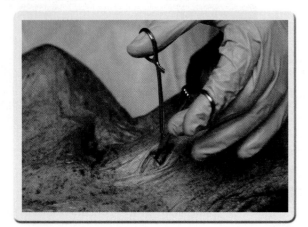

8 Insert an appropriately sized, cuffed ET tube or tracheostomy tube (usually #5 or #6) into the incision, directing the tube distally into the trachea.

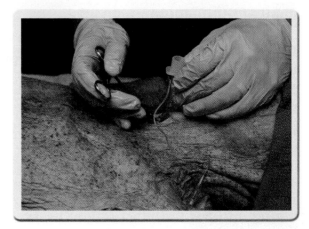

9 Inflate the cuff and ventilate the patient.

10 Observe chest inflation and auscultate the chest for adequate ventilation.

11 Confirm placement of the tube with a secondary method as used in endotracheal intubation.

12 Secure the tube to the patient to prevent dislodging.

Caution: Do not remove any part of the cricoid and/or thyroid cartilages during the procedure.

PROCEDURE 13
Needle Chest Decompression (Needle Thoracentesis)

Introduction

It is not uncommon to encounter tension pneumothoraces when caring for trauma patients who have significant thoracic injuries or mechanisms indicative of them (vehicle collisions, blunt traumas, falls, etc). A tension pneumothorax can occur quickly or be a slowly developing complication that may not always be obvious initially, but if missed it can have serious consequences. In the prehospital environment, a needle chest decompression is the most effective and widely accepted method of treatment.

Indications, Contraindications, and Equipment

Indications	Mechanism suggesting thoracic injury accompanied by: • Difficult ventilation despite open airway • Jugular venous distension • Absent or decreased breath sounds on the affected side • Decreasing cardiac output • Hyperresonance to percussion on the affected side • Tracheal deviation away from the affected side
Contraindications	None in a case of tension pneumothorax
Equipment	Exam gloves and goggles Nonrebreather mask and high-flow oxygen source or bag mask Large-bore IV catheter (18 gauge or larger and 2″ or larger) Alcohol or povidone-iodine (Betadine) preps One-way or flutter valve (commercially prepared device or finger from exam glove) 4″ × 4″ gauze pads Adhesive tape

Rationale

As air escapes from an injured lung and fills the pleural space, pressure builds and can compress the affected lung, heart, and great vessels. The needle chest decompression will release that pressure, allowing the lungs and heart to resume normal function.

Possible Complications

Improper placement of the needle can easily cause injury to the intercostal blood vessels and nerves, resulting in bleeding or prolonged pain. Excessive force during insertion can also injure the lung parenchyma, causing a pneumothorax in an uninjured lung or subcutaneous emphysema from air leaking under the skin. Clotting can occur, causing the tension pneumothorax to return. An additional thoracentesis may be required to redecompress the chest. If the provider is unable to treat the tension pneumothorax, pulselessness (PEA) and death will follow.

Procedure

1 Locate the appropriate site. Find the second or third rib, because you will need to insert the needle just above the third rib into the intercostal space at the midclavicular line on the affected side. If there is significant trauma to the anterior portion of the chest, use the intercostal space between the fourth and fifth ribs at the midaxillary line on the affected side (if allowed by local protocol). The midclavicular approach is preferred, however, because it is usually easier to access with less chance of dislodging the needle.

2 Cleanse the appropriate area using aseptic technique.

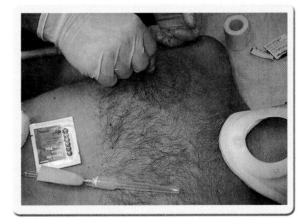

3 Insert the needle at a 90° angle, and listen for the release of air or visualize bubbles through saline in a syringe. If air does not return, make sure the length of the needle is appropriate for the size of the patient, then check the placement and reinsert the needle. Insert the needle just superior to the third rib, midclavicular, or just above the sixth rib, midaxillary. (The nerves, arteries, and veins run along the inferior borders of each rib.)

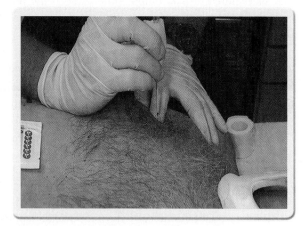

4 Advance the catheter over the needle and place the needle in the sharps container.

5 Some protocols may require placement of a one-way valve to decrease the chance of an open pneumothorax. The size of the catheter and the length prohibit large amounts of air, and an increased risk of pneumothorax is unlikely.

6 Secure the catheter in place in the same manner you would use to secure an impaled object.

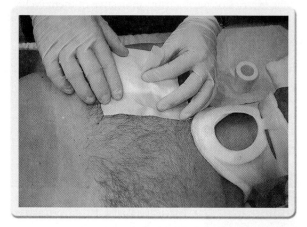

7 Monitor the patient closely for recurrence of the tension pneumothorax. This procedure may need to be repeated several times before arrival at the emergency department.

PROCEDURE 14
Pericardiocentesis

Introduction

Acute cardiac tamponade can be caused by severe thoracic injuries (blunt or penetrating) or any other mechanism that directly injures the heart. If not treated rapidly, it could result in death. Where allowed, a pericardiocentesis is usually the first attempted and least invasive method of cardiac tamponade treatment.

Indications, Contraindications, and Equipment

Indications	Acute pericardial tamponade
Contraindications	None in cases of pericardial tamponade with severe decompensated shock
Equipment	Exam gloves and goggles IV setup and fluid Local anesthetic Intracardiac needle and catheter

Rationale

Trauma to the cardiac muscle causes bleeding into the pericardial sac, which begins to fill and tighten around the heart. This causes a decrease in the ability of the ventricles to effectively pump blood. With pericardiocentesis, the provider introduces a long needle and catheter through the chest wall and into the pericardial membrane. The needle is then withdrawn, leaving the catheter in place and allowing the blood to drain away from the pericardium.

Possible Complications

Aspiration of ventricular blood instead of pericardial blood can occur if the needle is misplaced. A misplaced needle can also lacerate the ventricular epicardium or myocardium, or a coronary artery or vein, leading to new or additional bleeding in the pericardial sac. Pneumothorax can be caused by puncture of the lung, and worsening of pericardial tamponade may develop if puncture of the great vessels occurs. Puncture of the esophagus may cause mediastinitis, and puncture of the peritoneum may present with subsequent peritonitis or a false positive aspirate during the procedure. Finally, ventricular fibrillation can be caused by irritation of the myocardium during the procedure.

Procedure

1 Continually monitor the patient's vital signs and ECG before, during, and after the procedure.

2 Prepare the xiphoid and subxiphoid areas using antiseptic swabs.

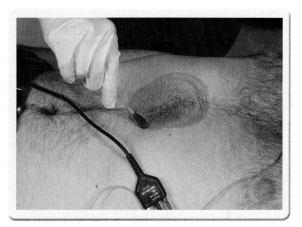

3 Use a 16- to 18-gauge, 6″ (15 cm) or longer over-the-needle catheter, and attach a large, empty syringe with a three-way stopcock.

4 Assess the patient for any mediastinal shift (seen by tracheal deviation or shift in heart tones) that may have caused the heart to shift position significantly.

5 Puncture the skin 1 to 2 cm below and to the left of the xiphoid process, at a 45° angle upward (toward the head) and to the left, aiming toward the tip of the left scapula.

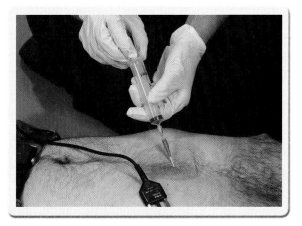

6 If the needle is advanced too far into the ventricular muscle, an injury pattern known as the "current of injury" will appear on the EKG monitor (eg, extreme ST-T wave changes or widened and enlarged QRS complex). If seen, withdraw the needle until the baseline EKG tracing returns. Premature ventricular contractions can also occur secondarily to irritation of the ventricular myocardium.

7 When the needle tip enters the blood-filled pericardial sac, withdraw as much nonclotted blood as possible.

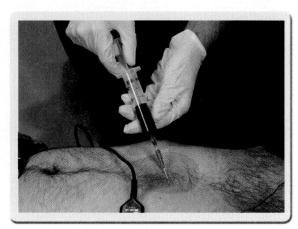

8 During aspiration, the pericardial sac collapses toward the surface of the heart, as does the needle tip. Subsequently, a current of injury pattern appears. This indicates that the needle should be withdrawn slightly. Should this injury pattern persist, withdraw the needle completely.

9 After aspiration is completed, remove the syringe and attach a three-way stopcock, leaving the stopcock closed. Secure the catheter in place.

10 If the cardiac tamponade symptoms persist, the stopcock may be opened and the pericardial sac reaspirated.

PROCEDURE 15
Spinal Assessment for Immobilization

Introduction

Although cervical spine stabilization is a standard priority on approach, not all trauma patients require spinal immobilization. There are certain indicators that allow a provider to decide against initiating or maintaining spinal stabilization, but this decision should not be made lightly because a mistake could have serious consequences for the patient. Many EMS organizations have local protocols about spinal clearance, and those protocols should be followed.

Indications, Contraindications, and Equipment

Indications	Patient is alert and oriented and is not intoxicated No signs or symptoms of spinal injury No neck or back pain or discomfort No neurodeficits
Contraindications	Any signs, symptoms, or suspicion of spinal injury
Equipment	Exam gloves and goggles

Rationale

Studies indicate that fewer than 10% of patients suffering from major trauma or serious head injuries also have spinal injuries, yet it is common for all trauma patients to be placed in full spinal immobilization prior to transport. Although it is better to err on the side of comprehensive spinal care, there are competent trauma patients who present with no pain, no injury, and no neurologic indicators of spinal trauma who do not need to be immobilized.

Possible Complications

Deciding against taking spinal precautions with a trauma patient who actually does have a spinal injury can lead to serious consequences such as chronic pain or weakness, or even quadriplegia. It is also important not to decide against spinal precautions with a patient who is still experiencing the effects of adrenaline, because it may mask pain and some neurodeficits.

Procedure

1 Determine the level of consciousness. If decreased, immobilize the trauma patient's spine (any GCS less than 15, including young children whose PGCS may not equal 15).

2 Determine the mechanism of injury.

Blunt Trauma

1 Palpate for tenderness or deformity along the center of the spine.

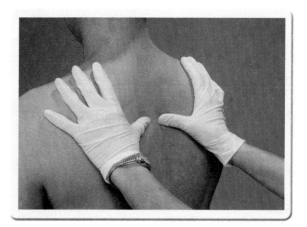

2 Assess the extremities for neurodeficits or complaints.

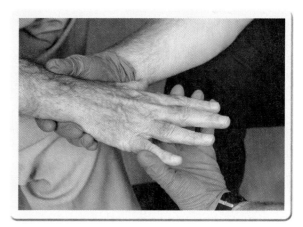

3 Consider the mechanism of injury. Is the mechanism suggestive of spinal injury?
  a. Mechanisms that produce a violent impact to the head, neck, torso, or pelvis
  b. Mechanisms that produce a sudden acceleration or deceleration of the spine or bending motion to the spine
  c. Ejection or fall from a moving vehicle including nonmotorized devices such as a bicycle or skateboard
  d. Diving accident where the head or neck was struck
  e. All persons over the age of 65 with a mechanism suggesting neck or back injury

4 If the patient is alert, has no spine pain or tenderness, no neurologic deficit, and the mechanism is not concerning, no immobilization may be needed.

5 Is there a presence or suspicion of alcohol or drugs involved that would alter the senses?

6 Is there a distracting injury? Distracting injury may include:
   a. Long bone fractures
   b. Abdominal injury with tenderness or pain
   c. Large lacerations, crush injury, or degloving injury
   d. Large burns
   e. Any other injuries that can cause functional disability

7 Can the patient and provider communicate? The patient must be able to participate in their assessment. (Participation difficulties can include speech and hearing disabilities and foreign languages without a reliable translator.)

8 If the patient is positive for any of the assessment points above, immobilize the spine.

9 If not, immobilization may not be needed.

Penetrating Trauma

1 Assess for penetrating trauma to the head, neck, or torso.

2 Palpate the spine and assess the neurologic status in the extremities.

3 If the GCS is less than 15, there is evidence of external injury to the spine, or there is neurologic impairment, immobilize the spine.

4 If there is no external injury to the spine and there are no neurologic impairments, spinal immobilization is not indicated.

Note: When in doubt, use clinical judgment and immobilize the spine.

PROCEDURE 16
Cervical Collar Sizing and Placement

Introduction

For trauma patients with suspected spinal injuries, or mechanisms indicative of them, manual immobilization followed by mechanical cervical immobilization can help to prevent further injury during transport. A properly sized and placed cervical collar is an important component of full immobilization.

Indications, Contraindications, and Equipment

Indications	Penetrating wounds near the spine
	Falls
	Severe blunt injuries above the chest
	Diving injuries
	High-speed motor vehicle collisions
Contraindications	Injury preventing neutral head alignment
	Inadequate size of collar to match the patient
Equipment	Exam gloves and goggles
	Cervical collars in multiple sizes to fit the patient

Rationale

Neck and back injuries can result in problems with stability of the spinal column. Damage to the spinal cord can occur when the unstable spine is moved. A cervical collar, as part of full spinal immobilization, can help to prevent additional trauma to the spinal column or cord caused by head and neck movement. When measured and correctly placed, the collar will fit snugly under the chin and be supported on the chest, minimizing flexion and extension of the cervical spine.

Possible Complications

Improperly sized cervical collars can cause excessive head movement, hyperextension of the neck, or pressure on the trachea, jugular veins, or carotid arteries. If the collar is too tall for the patient, it can also prevent jaw movement, which could compromise the airway in some situations.

Procedure

1 Begin manual in-line stabilization by holding the head firmly with both hands.

2 Support the lower jaw with your index and middle fingers and support the head with your palms. If the patient's head is not facing forward, gently move it until the patient's eyes are looking straight ahead and the head and torso are in line. Never twist, flex, or extend the head or neck excessively. Do not remove your hands from the patient's head until the patient is properly secured to a backboard and the head is immobilized.

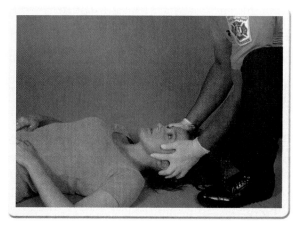

3 Assess distal pulses and neurologic function in each extremity.

4 Measure the patient for correct collar size based on the manufacturer's specifications.

5 Place the chin support snugly underneath the chin. While maintaining manual in-line stabilization, wrap the collar around the neck and secure the collar to the far side of the chin support. A cervical collar is used in addition to—not instead of—manual in-line cervical spine immobilization. Recheck that the patient is in a neutral in-line position.

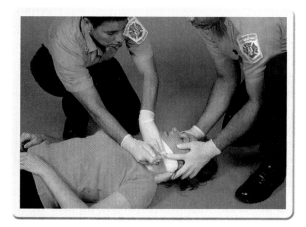

6 Secure the patient with a spinal immobilization device capable of immobilizing the entire spine.

PROCEDURE 17
Long Backboard With a Supine Patient

Introduction

When responding to trauma patients, the need for spinal immobilization should always be evaluated. Not only is the long backboard the most commonly used device for full spinal immobilization, it is also effective when rapid stabilization of the multiple trauma patient is indicated.

Indications, Contraindications, and Equipment

Indications	Mechanism indicating possible spinal injury Spinal injury as assessed by neurologic symptoms, pain, or tenderness to the spine Multisystem trauma including extremity fractures
Contraindications	Patients who cannot be placed into a supine position because it would compromise the ABCs Patients who cannot be moved to a neutral in-line position due to injury (eg, impaled object, movement is restricted)
Equipment	Exam gloves and goggles Cervical collar Long backboard with straps Head-securing device Extra padding

Rationale

Back and neck injuries can cause damage to the spinal cord in numerous ways, from twisting and hyperextension to crushing and severing traumas. Properly securing the patient to a long backboard can help to prevent injury or additional spinal damage caused by excessive movement during transport.

Possible Complications

Most of the complications associated with long backboards are related to improper application. Not securing a patient sufficiently can cause excessive movement and subsequent spinal damage. Securing a patient too tightly can cause circulatory complications and unnecessary pain. Patients who are left secured to a long backboard for prolonged periods are prone to increased pain and pressure sores. These patients often remain on the board following transport to the hospital.

Procedure

1. Begin by providing manual in-line stabilization to the head and neck.

2. If the patient's head is not facing forward, gently move it until the patient's eyes are looking straight ahead and the head and torso are in line. Never twist, flex, or extend the head or neck excessively. Do not discontinue stabilization until the patient is properly secured to a backboard and the head is immobilized.

3. Assess distal pulses and neurologic function in each extremity.

4. Apply an appropriately sized cervical collar.

5. Another provider should position the immobilization device (backboard) alongside the patient.

6. On command, the rescuers should roll the patient toward themselves. Slide the board under the patient. The team should then roll the patient back onto the board, avoiding rotation of the head, shoulders, and pelvis.

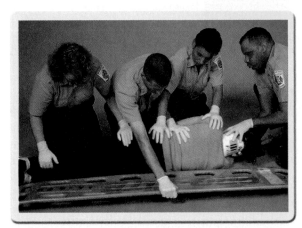

7. Make sure the patient is centered on the board. This should be accomplished by moving the patient as a unit.

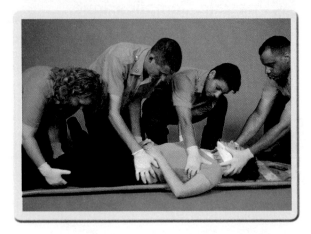

8 Secure the upper torso to the board once the patient is centered on the backboard.

9 Secure the pelvis and upper legs, using padding as needed. For the pelvis, use straps over the iliac crests and/or groin loops (leg straps).

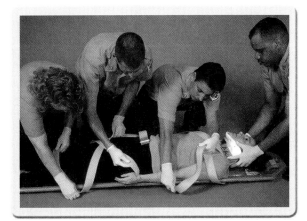

10 Immobilize the head to the board by positioning a commercial immobilization device or using towel rolls. Secure the head to the board only after straps have secured the torso. If the head is secured first and the body shifts, the spine may be compromised. Securing the majority of the body weight first provides better protection.

11 Secure the head by strapping or taping the head immobilization device across the forehead. To prevent airway problems and maintain access to the airway, do not tape over the throat or chin. Instead, tape across the cervical collar just under the chin without covering the opening.

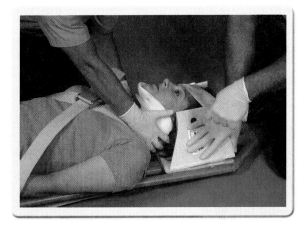

12 Check and readjust straps as needed to ensure that the entire body is snugly secured and will not slide during movement of the board or patient transport.

13 Reassess distal function in each extremity and continue to do so periodically.

PROCEDURE 18
Short Backboard/Vest-Type Device

Introduction

When responding to trauma patients, the need for spinal immobilization should always be evaluated. For those patients who are found in a seated position, a short backboard or vest-type extrication device will often be the most effective means of spinal immobilization.

Indications, Contraindications, and Equipment

Indications	Seated patient with: • Mechanism indicating possible spinal injury • Spinal injury as assessed by neurologic symptoms, pain, or tenderness to the spine
Contraindications	A vest-type device could cause hypoventilation in a patient experiencing difficulty breathing.
Equipment	Exam gloves and goggles Cervical collar Short backboard or vest-type device Head-securing device Extra padding

Rationale

Back and neck injuries can damage the spinal cord in numerous ways, from twisting and hyperextension to crushing and severing traumas. Properly securing the patient to an appropriate spinal immobilization device can help to prevent injury or additional spinal damage caused by excessive movement during extrication and transport.

Possible Complications

Most of the complications associated with spinal immobilization devices are actually related to improper application. Not securing a patient sufficiently can cause excessive movement and subsequent spinal damage, and securing a patient too tightly can cause respiratory complaints and unnecessary pain.

Procedure

1 Stabilize the head and maintain manual in-line stabilization until the patient is secured to the long backboard.

2 Assess distal pulses and neurologic function in each extremity.

3 Apply the rigid cervical collar.

4 Insert a short spine immobilization device between the patient's upper back and the seat back.

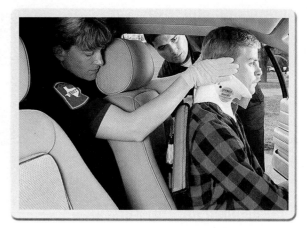

5 Open the board's side flaps (if present) and position them around the patient's torso, snug to the armpits.

6 Once the device is properly positioned, secure the upper torso straps.

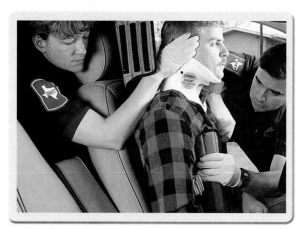

7 Position and fasten both groin loops (leg straps). Pad the groin as needed. Check all torso straps and make sure they are secure. Make any adjustments necessary without excessive movement of the patient.

8 Pad any space between the patient's head and the device.

9 Secure the forehead strap or tape the head securely, then fasten the lower head strap around the rigid cervical collar.

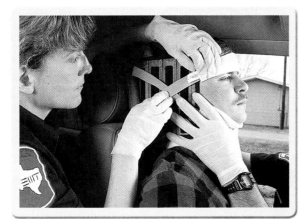

10 Place the long backboard next to the patient's buttocks, perpendicular to the trunk.

11 Turn the patient parallel to the long backboard.

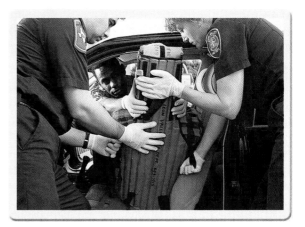

12 Lift the patient and the vest-type device together as a unit (without rotating the patient), and slip the long backboard under the patient and device.

13 Release the leg straps and loosen the chest strap to allow the legs to straighten and give the chest room to expand fully.

14 Secure the short device and long backboard together. Do not remove the vest-type device from the patient.

15 Reassess distal function in all four extremities.

PROCEDURE 19
Vacuum Mattress

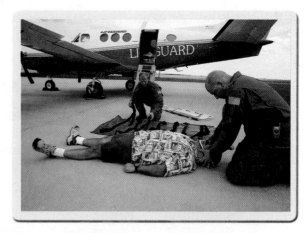

Introduction

The vacuum mattress provides immobilization by molding to the specific contours of the patient's body, reducing pressure point tenderness. The mattress also provides thermal insulation, decreasing the potential for hypothermia, and is the standard equipment used to transport patients with spinal injuries in the United Kingdom. A drawback to the device is its thickness, requiring careful patient movement to maintain spinal stabilization during the application procedure.

Indications, Contraindications, and Equipment

Indications	Mechanism indicating possible spinal injury Spinal injury as assessed by neurologic symptoms, pain, or tenderness to the spine
Contraindications	Limited to patients weighing less than 350 lb (160 kg)
Equipment	Exam gloves and goggles Cervical collar Vacuum mattress

Rationale

Properly securing potential spinal injury patients can help prevent additional injury caused by excessive spinal movement. The vacuum mattress can provide an alternative to a long backboard for spinal immobilization with more patient comfort and a greater degree of immobilization.

Possible Complications

Complications associated with vacuum mattress use are related to not securing the patient sufficiently, which can cause excessive movement and subsequent spinal damage, paralysis, pain, and death.

Procedure

1 If spinal injury is suspected, establish manual, in-line stabilization, apply a properly sized cervical collar, and instruct the patient to remain still.

2 Prepare and position the vacuum mattress appropriately next to the patient.

3 Remove any sharp or bulky items that may damage the vacuum splint.

4 Move the patient onto the vacuum mattress using another immobilization device such as a scoop stretcher, maintaining spinal alignment.

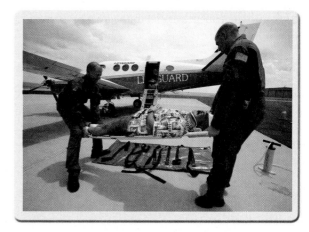

5 Locate the patient in the center of the vacuum mattress, moving the patient as a unit.

6 Lift the edges of the mattress to conform around the contour of the patient, starting at the head.

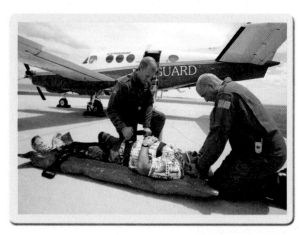

7 Secure the patient to the vacuum mattress with straps securing the chest, hips, and legs.

8 Evacuate the air from the vacuum mattress until it becomes rigid.

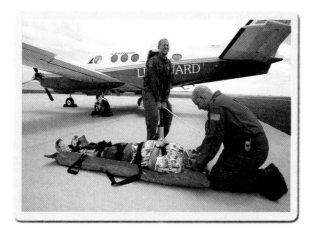

9 Disconnect the vacuum pump and ensure that the valve is closed or secured.

10 Reassess and adjust the straps around the chest, hips, and legs.

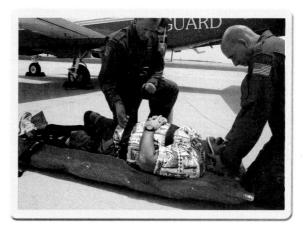

11 Stabilize the head in a neutral position and secure it to the vacuum mattress last.

12 Reassess the patient's circulatory, motor, and sensory function.

PROCEDURE 20
Scoop (Orthopaedic) Stretcher

Introduction

Trauma patients can be found in numerous challenging locations, some of which do not lend themselves to standard patient movement techniques and equipment. To help responders overcome these challenges, there are several different types of patient movement devices, each suited to specific needs. A scoop stretcher can be a very effective option for patient movement.

Indications, Contraindications, and Equipment

Indications	Supine patient in close quarters Suspected fractured hip
Contraindications	Obesity
Equipment	Exam gloves and goggles Scoop stretcher Long backboard or wheeled gurney

Rationale

With some trauma patients, log rolling, carrying, or dragging is difficult or impossible due to space restrictions or type of injury. A scoop stretcher is the solution in some of these cases because it can be broken apart, moved into confined spaces, and reassembled under the patient. This device is also preferred for patients with certain musculoskeletal injuries who would not tolerate being log rolled or moved using an extremity lift.

Possible Complications

The most common complication encountered when using a scoop stretcher is that the device can pinch the patient, the patient's clothing, or even flooring material when reassembled. Inadequate stabilization during transfer can cause excessive movement and subsequent spinal damage, paralysis, pain, and death.

Procedure

1 If spinal injury is suspected, establish manual in-line stabilization, apply a properly sized cervical collar, and instruct the patient to remain still.

2 Adjust the stretcher to the length of the patient.

3 Separate the stretcher into right and left halves.

4 Position the stretcher halves on opposite sides of the patient.

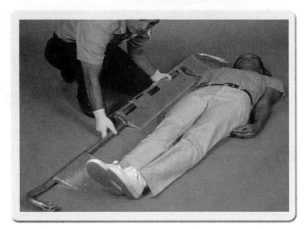

5 Slightly log roll the patient away from you and slide the stretcher half under the patient.

6 Assemble the head end of the stretcher.

7 Log roll the patient toward you while the other rescuer brings the foot ends of the stretcher together and latches them in place.

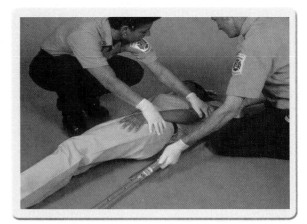

8 Pad the patient's head.

9 Secure the patient's trunk and lower extremities with three straps positioned at the patient's chest, pelvis, and knees.

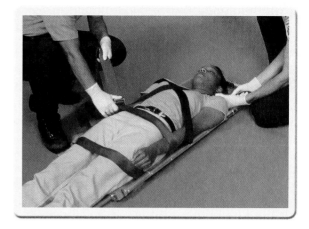

10 Immobilize the patient's head with a forehead strap.

PROCEDURE 21
Helmet Removal

Introduction

Many people wear helmets to protect the head from injury during high risk activities such as motorcycle riding or contact sports. When these helmets fit snugly to the head, the head can be stabilized by securing the outside of the helmet. Control of a patient's airway may require removal of the helmet. Even in the best of circumstances, spinal movement will take place. Trained personnel can minimize the movement of the spine while removing the helmet.

Indications, Contraindications, and Equipment

Indications	The helmet and chin strap fail to hold the head securely, as with a loose-fitting helmet. The helmet and chin strap design prevent adequate airway control, even after the removal of the face mask. A helmet with a face mask that cannot be removed after a reasonable amount of time. The helmet prevents proper immobilization for transport.
Contraindications	Untrained personnel should not attempt helmet removal on a patient with suspected spinal injury unless an obvious airway obstruction is evident and failure to remove the helmet would compromise the patient.
Equipment	Exam gloves and goggles Cervical collar Long backboard with straps Head-securing device Extra padding

Rationale

Patients wearing a helmet who have sustained traumatic injury and require airway management should have the helmet removed. Some sports helmets will allow airway management after removal of the face shield component of the helmet. Removal of the helmet may compromise c-spine stability and should be done with a two-person technique to minimize spinal impact.

Possible Complications

Various countries and jurisdictions have differing views on whether a helmet should be left on a patient. For example, in the United Kingdom, standard practice dictates that a helmet should always be removed, regardless of the situation.

Some local protocols dictate that when a patient with a helmet is able to maintain their own airway and the helmet is secure to the head, the patient should be immobilized with the helmet in place because doing so could limit the risk of pain or paralysis. The helmet can be removed in the emergency department by cutting the helmet from ear to ear with a cast saw.

Procedure

Only providers who are familiar with the procedure should attempt helmet removal. A single rescuer should not attempt helmet removal because the maneuver requires two providers.

1 Have your partner kneel at the patient's head. Leave enough room to remove the helmet. Kneel on one side of the patient, at the shoulder area.

2 Have your partner stabilize the helmet to prevent movement of the head. The face strap can then be loosened.

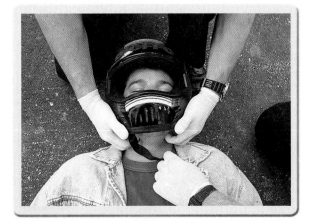

3 Open the face shield, if there is one, and assess the patient's airway and breathing.

4 Place one hand on the patient's lower jaw at the angle of the jaw and the other behind the head in the back of the helmet. Have your partner reach into the sides of the helmet near the ears and pull the sides of the helmet away from the patient's head.

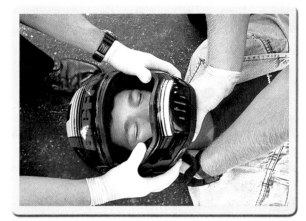

5 Gently slip the helmet partly off the patient's head, stopping when the helmet reaches the halfway point.

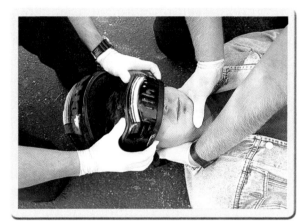

6 Reposition the hand under the head to support the weight while maintaining stabilization and preventing the head from falling back once the helmet is completely removed.

7 Remove the helmet and provide manual in-line cervical spine stabilization.

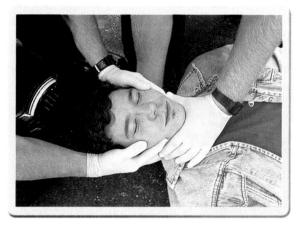

8 Apply a rigid cervical collar and secure the patient to a long backboard.

Note: Padding may be needed under the shoulders to prevent flexion of the neck if the helmet is left in place.

PROCEDURE 22
Rapid Extrication From a Motor Vehicle

Introduction

Rapid extrication from a motor vehicle is needed to care for life-threatening conditions where providers must minimize movement of the spine. This choreographed movement tries to decrease the chance of a spinal injury worsening with movement; however, it does not stabilize the spine like other methods and should be used with caution.

Indications, Contraindications, and Equipment

Indications	Patients seated in a vehicle:
	• With immediate threats to airway, breathing, or circulation that require immediate treatment
	• With a life threat due to a safety hazard (eg, fire, submersion in water, hazardous materials)
	• Who are blocking access to a patient with life threats, although they do not have life-threatening injury themselves
Contraindications	Patients who do not meet the indications above
Equipment	Exam gloves and goggles
	Cervical collar
	Long backboard with straps
	Head-securing device
	Extra padding

Rationale

Rapid extrication should be used to move a patient from a motor vehicle to a long backboard quickly to treat life threats. These injuries may include care required to manage an airway, support breathing, or care for bleeding or shock. They also include conditions that could threaten the safety or life of the patient or provider, such as fire, hazardous materials, or rising water levels. The third and final reason for rapid extrication is to provide life-supporting care to a patient who is blocked by the first patient. An example would be a passenger trapped in a vehicle with a wall blocking access to their side and the driver seated in the access from the other side. The driver should be rapidly extricated to provide care to the passenger.

Possible Complications

Because rapid extrication is a method to move the patient quickly but does not immobilize the spine prior to moving, the risks include pain, paralysis, and death.

Procedure

The rapid extrication technique requires a team of three providers who are knowledgeable and practiced in the procedure. Follow these steps:

1 The first rescuer provides manual in-line stabilization of the patient's head and cervical spine from behind. Support may be applied from the side, if necessary, by reaching through the door.

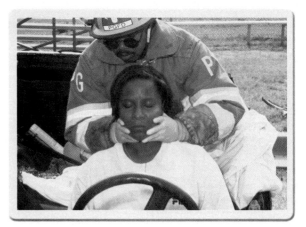

2 The second rescuer serves as a team leader and gives the commands to coordinate the team's moves until the patient is supine on the backboard. Because the second rescuer lifts and turns the patient's torso, he or she must be physically capable of moving the patient. The second rescuer works from the victim's doorway. If the first rescuer is also working from that doorway, the second rescuer should stand closer to the door hinges toward the front of the vehicle. The second rescuer applies a rigid cervical collar and performs the initial/primary assessment.

3 The second rescuer provides continuous support of the patient's torso until the patient is supine on the backboard. Once the second rescuer takes control of the torso, usually in the form of a body hug, he or she should not let go of the patient for any reason. Some type of cross-chest shoulder hug usually works well, but you must decide which method will work best for any given patient. You cannot simply reach into the car and grab the patient, because this will twist the patient's torso. You must rotate the patient as a unit.

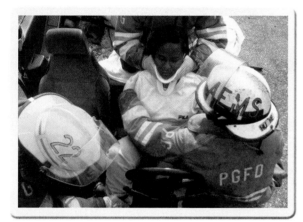

4 The third rescuer works from the other side of the car (if possible) and rotates the patient's legs and feet as the torso is turned, ensuring that they are free of the pedals and any other obstruction. The third rescuer should first carefully move the patient's nearer leg laterally, without rotating the patient's pelvis and lower spine. The pelvis and lower spine rotate only as the third rescuer moves the second leg during the next step. Moving the nearer leg first makes it much easier to move the second leg in concert with the rest of the body. Once the third rescuer moves the legs together, the legs should be moved as a unit.

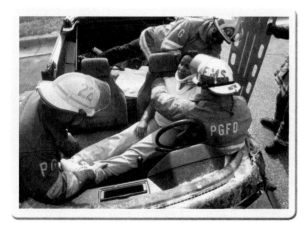

5 Rotate the patient 90° so the back faces out the victim's door and the feet are on the seat next to the victim. This coordinated movement is done in three or four short, quick, one-eighth turns. The second rescuer coordinates the sequence of moves and the first rescuer directs each quick turn by saying, "Ready, turn" or "Ready, move." Hand position changes should be made between moves.

6 In most cases, the first rescuer will be working from behind. At some point, either because the doorpost is in the way or because he or she cannot reach further from their location, the first rescuer will be unable to follow the torso rotation. At that time, the third rescuer should assume temporary manual in-line stabilization of the head and neck until the first rescuer can regain control of the head from outside the vehicle. If a fourth rescuer is present, the fourth rescuer stands next to the second rescuer. The fourth rescuer takes control of the head and neck from outside the vehicle without involving the third rescuer. As soon as the change has been made, the rotation can continue.

7 Once the patient has been fully rotated, the backboard is placed against the patient's buttocks on the seat. Do not try to wedge the backboard under the patient. If only three rescuers are present, place the backboard within arm's reach of the victim's door before the move so that the board can be pulled into place when needed; the far end of the board can be left on the ground. When a fourth rescuer is available, the first rescuer exits the car, places the backboard against the patient's buttocks, and maintains pressure in toward the vehicle from the far end of the board. When the door opening allows, some rescuers prefer to insert the backboard onto the car seat before the patient is rotated.

8 As soon as the patient has been rotated and the backboard is in place, the second and third rescuers lower the patient onto the board while supporting the head and torso so that neutral alignment is maintained. The first rescuer holds the backboard until the patient is secured.

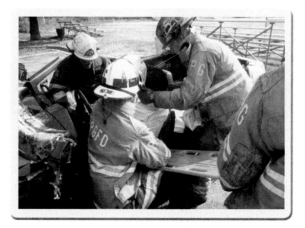

9 The third rescuer moves across the seat to be in position at the patient's hips. If the third rescuer stays at the patient's knees or feet, he or she will be ineffective in helping to move the body's weight. The knees and feet follow the hips.

10 The fourth rescuer maintains in-line support of the head and takes over giving the commands. If a fourth rescuer is not present, you can direct a volunteer to assist you. The second rescuer maintains direction of the extrication; this rescuer stands with his or her back to the door, facing the rear of the vehicle. The backboard should be immediately in front of the third rescuer. The second rescuer grasps the patient's shoulders or armpits. On command, the second and third rescuers slide the patient 8″ to 12″ (20 to 30 cm) along the backboard, repeating this slide until the patient's hips are firmly on the backboard.

11 The third rescuer gets out of the vehicle and moves to the opposite side of the backboard, across from the second rescuer. The third rescuer takes control at the shoulders and the second rescuer moves back to take control of the hips. On command, these two rescuers move the patient along the board in 8″- to 12″- (20- to 30-cm) slides until the patient is completely on the board.

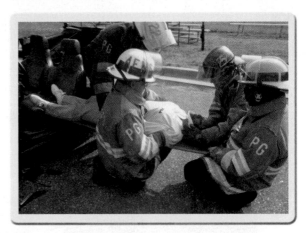

12 The first (or fourth) rescuer continues to maintain manual in-line support of the head. The second and third rescuers grasp their side of the board, and then carry it and the patient away from the vehicle onto the prepared cot nearby.

PROCEDURE 23
Standing Backboard

Introduction

Occasionally patients requiring spinal immobilization will be found in an upright or semi-upright position. To minimize spinal movement of these patients, a technique of moving them directly to a long backboard is required. Patients who are walking at the scene should be evaluated for the need for spinal immobilization.

Indications, Contraindications, and Equipment

Indications	For patients who are found in an upright (standing) or semi-upright position at the trauma scene and require spinal immobilization
Contraindications	Having a patient stand to place the long backboard Having the patient ambulate to the long backboard Lack of properly sized crew configuration to complete the procedure safely
Equipment	Exam gloves and goggles Cervical collar Long backboard with straps Head-securing device Extra padding

Rationale

Because trauma victims are found in different body positions following injury, alternate methods of immobilization may be required. One such position is the upright or semi-upright (standing) position. To minimize movement and safely move the patient to a neutral (supine) position, the long backboard can be used.

Possible Complications

Movement of a patient found standing on a scene with a spinal injury could cause an unstable injury to worsen or a stable injury to become unstable. Permanent paralysis, persistent pain, or death can result.

Procedure

1 Establish manual in-line stabilization, apply a properly sized cervical collar, and instruct the patient to remain still. Explain the procedure to the patient.

2 Position the board upright, directly behind the patient.

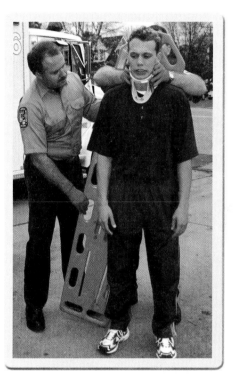

3 Two rescuers stand on either side of the patient; the third is directly behind the patient, maintaining immobilization.

4 The two rescuers grasp the handholds at shoulder level or slightly above by reaching under the patient's arms while standing at either side.

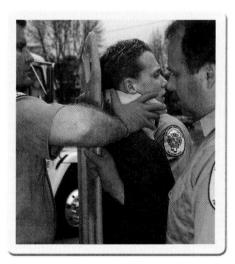

5 The two rescuers support the patient with the other hand and prepare to lower the patient to the ground.

6 The two rescuers place the foot closest to the board against the base at the ground and step forward on the second foot to keep the board from sliding.

7 Carefully lower the patient as a unit under the direction of the rescuer at the head. The rescuer at the head must make sure the head stays against the board and must carefully rotate his or her hands while the patient is being lowered to maintain in-line stabilization.

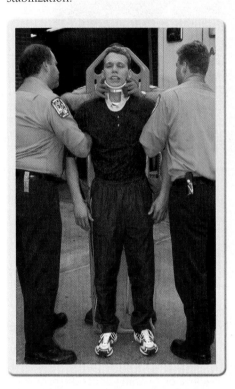

8 Move the patient to the proper positioning on the long backboard with in-line stabilization. Secure the patient to the long backboard with straps.

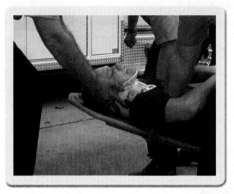

9 Reassess distal function in all four extremities.

PROCEDURE 24
Pediatric Spinal Immobilization

Introduction

Just as with adults, pediatric trauma patients often require spinal immobilization. Because of children's unique anatomic features, adult spinal immobilization equipment must be adapted to fit. Commercially made pediatric boards or vacuum mattresses offer unique features, making spinal immobilization of small children and infants easier.

Indications, Contraindications, and Equipment

Indications	Mechanism indicating possible spinal injury Spinal injury as assessed by neurologic symptoms, pain, or tenderness to the spine
Contraindications	Patient size is over the height and weight specifications of the device
Equipment	Exam gloves and goggles Cervical collar (if correct size is available) Long backboard with extra padding or pediatric board with straps or child vacuum mattress

Rationale

Due to pediatric anatomy, specifically the larger occipital region of the skull, traditional spinal immobilization on a standard backboard is discouraged for small children. Pediatric boards traditionally have a head segment slightly lower than the body segment to keep patients in a neutral, in-line position while not compromising the airway. Many boards also have additional straps to keep uncooperative pediatric patients from moving and compromising immobilization. These modifications can be made to standard adult long backboards using extra padding when pediatric-specific equipment is unavailable. Child-sized vacuum mattresses can provide more support and proper positioning of the spine than a traditional long backboard.

Possible Complications

If the pediatric patient is secured to the pediatric board with an improperly sized cervical collar or movement occurs from inadequately securing the child, additional spinal injury and/or respiratory difficulty can result.

Procedure

1 Begin by providing manual in-line stabilization to the head and neck.

2 If the patient's head is not facing forward, gently move it until the patient's eyes are looking straight ahead and the head and torso are in line. Never twist, flex, or extend the head or neck excessively. Do not stop stabilization until the patient is properly secured to a backboard and the head is immobilized.

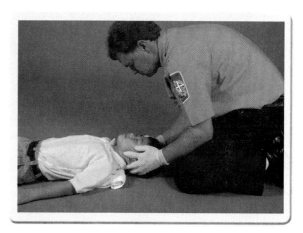

3 Assess distal pulses and neurologic function in each extremity.

4 Apply an appropriately sized cervical collar. If a collar will not fit correctly, omit this step and move on.

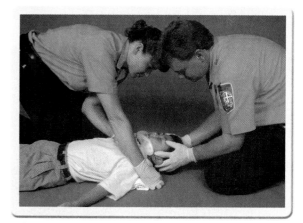

5 Another provider should position the immobilization device or backboard alongside the patient. If a long backboard is used, 1″ (2.5 cm) of padding should be placed on the board in the area that will support the child's torso.

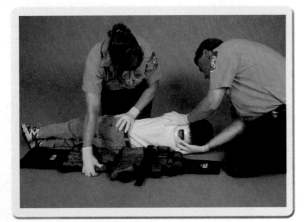

6 On command, two or three rescuers should roll the patient toward themselves. With small children, the child may be lifted straight up and moved as a unit onto the board. Slide the board under the patient.

7 Make sure the patient is centered on the board. This should be accomplished by moving the patient as a unit.

8 Secure the upper torso to the board once the patient is centered on the backboard. For children placed on adult backboards, padding must be added along the lateral aspects to pad the voids left under the straps.

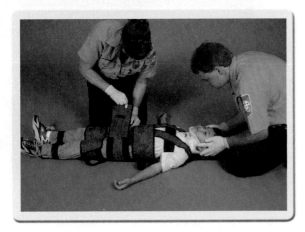

9 Secure the pelvis and upper legs, using padding as needed. For the pelvis, use straps over the iliac crests and/or groin loops (leg straps).

10 Immobilize the head to the board by positioning towel rolls or blocks next to the head. If a properly sized cervical collar is unavailable, secure towels or blankets along the lateral sides of the head and neck. Secure the head to the board only after straps have secured the torso.

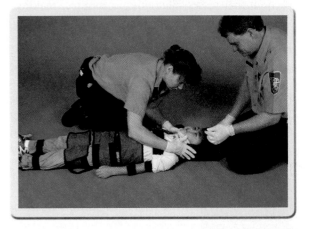

11 Secure the head by taping across the forehead. To prevent airway problems and maintain access to the airway, do not tape over the throat or chin.

12 Check and readjust straps as needed to ensure that the entire body is snugly secured and will not slide during movement of the board or patient transport.

13 Reassess distal function in each extremity and continue to do so periodically.

PROCEDURE 25
Bandaging of Bleeding Wounds

Introduction

Immobilizing injuries and controlling blood loss are two of the most common responsibilities in the care of trauma patients. Proper bandaging can effectively immobilize most injuries, and after direct pressure, it is the best method to control blood loss and keep wounds clean.

Indications, Contraindications, and Equipment

Indications	Painful, swollen, or deformed injuries Open injuries Impaled objects Amputations
Contraindications	None
Equipment	Exam gloves and goggles Dressing material (gauze pads, trauma dressing, etc) Bandaging material (eg, roller gauze, triangle bandages)

Rationale

Whether initially open or closed, injuries that are not immobilized can cause more damage and quickly become more serious. Also, bleeding that is not significantly slowed or stopped using pressure, clotting agents, and bandaging can lead to hypoperfusion and death.

Possible Complications

Poorly sized dressings may either be ineffective or prevent adequate inspection of the injury site. Circumferential bandaging may be applied too tightly or become too tight when the injured area swells, causing possible distal ischemia. Bandages left soaked with blood or other body fluids for too long may invite infection.

Procedure

1 Apply a sterile dressing over the entire wound. Apply pressure to the dressing with a gloved hand. Pressure should be applied for at least 5 minutes to allow sufficient time for the wound to develop a clot.

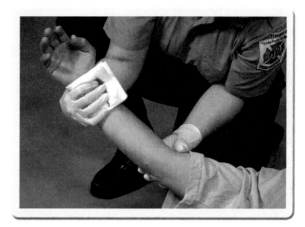

2 Maintain the pressure while securing the dressing with a roller bandage.

3 If bleeding continues or recurs, leave the original dressing in place. Apply a tourniquet to the arm proximal to the zone or injury and just below the axilla. Be sure to advise hospital personnel that tourniquet application was necessary in order to control hemorrhage.

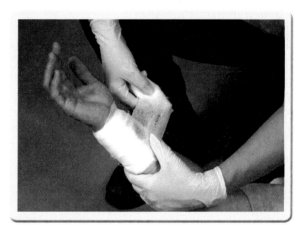

4 Special considerations:
  a. Wounds to the neck that may involve the large blood vessels should have an occlusive dressing to protect against air entering the bloodstream.
  b. Wounds inside the oral cavity may require airway control before bleeding can be stopped.
  c. Bleeding from the vagina or rectum following sexual trauma should have direct pressure applied only if the trauma is external. Bleeding leaking from the orifice should have an external pad applied.

PROCEDURE 26
Sealing Open Chest Wounds

Introduction

Penetrating chest injuries create a unique problem for pre-hospital care providers because with each inhalation the pressure in the chest decreases, pulling outside air into the chest cavity through the wound. This eventually creates a pneumothorax with potentially deadly consequences. Bandaging open chest wounds properly is critical to the patient's survival.

Indications, Contraindications, and Equipment

Indications	Penetrating (sucking) chest injury
Contraindications	None
Equipment	Exam gloves and goggles Sterile occlusive dressing or commercial device Tape

Rationale

To prevent a buildup of air in the chest cavity following an open chest injury, air must be prevented from entering through the wound. This can be accomplished with a secure occlusive dressing, which stops air from moving in either direction through the wound. If too much pressure has already built up in the chest cavity, creating a tension pneumothorax, the occlusive dressing should be opened to allow excess air to escape from it and then resealed (sometimes called burping a wound).

Possible Complications

Improperly bandaging or fully occluding an open chest injury can sometimes lead to a tension pneumothorax and death.

Procedure

1 Immediately upon locating an open wound to the chest that presents with air movement through the wound, the opening should be covered with a gloved hand, preventing outside air from entering the chest.

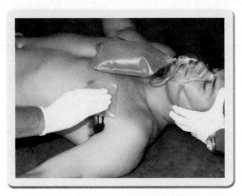

2 An occlusive dressing or commercial device should be placed over the entire wound. If an occlusive dressing is unavailable, a plastic wrapper from a bandage can be substituted.

3 Secure the dressing by taping the edges of the bandage to the chest wall. Some protocols require only three sides of the dressing to be taped so air trapped inside the chest can leak past the dressing. When negative pressure is being exerted, however, the bandage is pulled tight to the wound, preventing air movement.

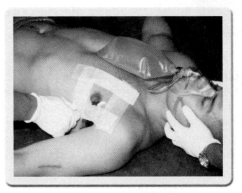

4 Assess the patient for signs of a pneumothorax. If signs of a tension pneumothorax develop, open the dressing and allow air to exit through the wound.

PROCEDURE 27
Tourniquet Application

Introduction

Occasionally, trauma patients will suffer from seemingly unstoppable external bleeding secondary to massive extremity injuries. Direct pressure may fail to stop the blood loss, leaving the application of a tourniquet to save the patient's life.

Indications, Contraindications, and Equipment

Indications	External extremity bleeding that is uncontrollable by direct pressure application
Contraindications	None when used as a lifesaving technique
Equipment	Exam gloves and goggles Commercially available tourniquet kit

Rationale

If vessels are damaged in ways that prevent them from constricting (usually following a crush, open fracture, or amputation injury) and the provider has tried and failed to control blood loss using direct pressure, a tourniquet should be applied to compress the injured vessels and stop the bleeding.

Possible Complications

Improper placement or technique can result in failure to control bleeding.

Procedure

1 Hold direct pressure over the bleeding site.

2 Place the tourniquet around the extremity in the proximal arm or proximal thigh as near the axilla or groin as possible.

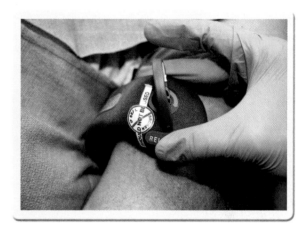

3 Click the buckle into place and pull the strap tight.

4 Turn the tightening dial clockwise until pulses are no longer palpable distal to the tourniquet or until bleeding has been controlled.

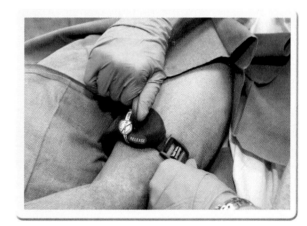

5 To release the tourniquet at the hospital, or if otherwise instructed by medical control, push the release button and pull the strap back. Be aware that bleeding may rapidly return upon tourniquet release and that you should be prepared to reapply it immediately if necessary.

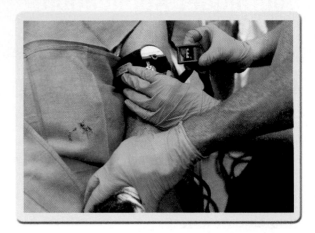

PROCEDURE 28
Bandaging Burns

Introduction

Burn dressings and bandages serve three purposes: protect against infection, decrease heat loss, and provide comfort. Functionally, bandages serve to isolate the wound from the environment and absorb drainage from wounds. Cover the burns with sterile, dry gauze bandage and wrap loosely to avoid putting pressure on the burned skin. Bandaging keeps air off the burn, reduces pain, and protects blisters that may have formed.

Indications, Contraindications, and Equipment

Indications	Partial- or full-thickness burns where the skin has blistered or is not intact
Contraindications	Burns from hazardous materials that have not been decontaminated in the field
Equipment	Exam gloves and goggles Sterile gauze pads Sterile field/drape Roller gauze

Rationale

Burn victims require an immediate evaluation of the basic ABCs prior to treating the burn itself. After the ABCs, burns should be treated with loose, dry sterile gauze to help prevent infection and to provide comfort.

Possible Complications

Possible complications of burn care include treating the burn prior to treating the ABCs. Burn victims who suffer from an inhalation burn require airway management prior to wrapping individual burns on the extremities. Applying bandages too tight can cause additional pain and compromise blood flow to an area that is already compromised.

Procedure

1 After the ABCs have been managed and the burn process has been stopped, prepare the patient by administering pain medication.

2 Expose only the area on the patient that is needed for wound care. Unnecessary exposure can cause additional heat loss and increase patient anxiety.

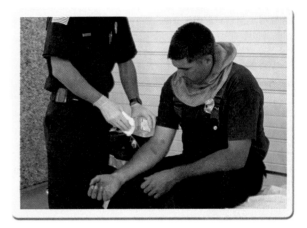

3 Open the sterile dressing using a clean technique and place the field/towel next to the wound.

4 Put on sterile gloves.

5 Apply the sterile gauze dressing over the affected area.

6 Apply the roller gauze loosely around the sterile gauze.

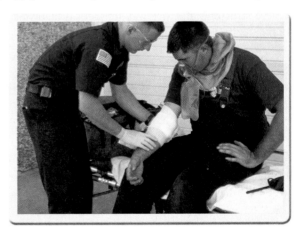

7 Apply tape to secure the gauze in place.

PROCEDURE 29
Bandaging Eyes

Introduction

Injury to the eye can be both physically and emotionally painful. Proper care of an injury can reduce the chance of further injury. Covering eye injuries decreases movement of the eye and will decrease the pain felt by the patient. Additionally, covering the uninjured eye will decrease the movement caused by accommodation of the eyes.

Indications, Contraindications, and Equipment

Indications	Penetrating eye trauma Foreign body/substance in the eye Laceration to the eye or eyelid
Contraindications	If further damage would be caused with the implementation of bandaging
Equipment	Exam gloves and goggles Tape Gauze Eye shield/paper or plastic cup

Rationale

Bandaging or covering the eye prevents further damage to the eye structures and vision of the person following acute injury.

Possible Complications

Direct pressure to the eye injury can cause additional pain and damage to the patient's eye, its structures, or vision.

Procedure

1 Place the patient in a semi-Fowler's position on the stretcher.

2 Gently and without touching the eye itself, apply a piece of gauze that covers the entire eye.

3 Again gently, and without applying pressure to the eye, apply the eye shield to the affected eye.

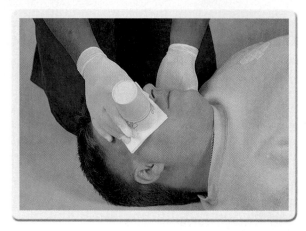

4 Tape the eye shield in place without applying direct pressure to the eye.

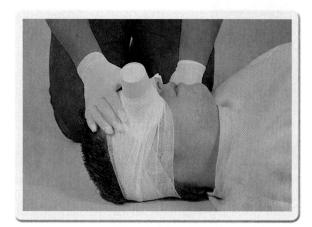

PROCEDURE 30
Irrigating Eyes

Introduction

Foreign substances in the eye cause pain and damage if not removed. Chemical exposures and loose debris can be removed by irrigating the eye. Copious amounts of water or saline are often required to clear chemical exposures while debris may be cleared quicker. Eye irrigation is used to flush any foreign substance from the eye with the intent to prevent further damage to the eye.

Indications, Contraindications, and Equipment

Indications	Foreign body or substance in the eye
Contraindications	Laceration to the eye causing exposure of the contents of the globe or avulsion of the lens
Equipment	Exam gloves Basin 1,000 mL normal saline for each eye Tubing or syringe/Morgan lens/IV tubing/eye wash station

Rationale

Irrigating an eye clears the eye of a chemical or foreign body that is causing (or may cause) pain, visual disturbances, or blindness. Clearing of foreign materials requires flushing for at least 5 minutes, while chemical exposures will require continuous flushing for 20 to 30 minutes with at least 1,000 mL of fluid.

Possible Complications

Possible complications include irrigating the eyes incorrectly, causing recontamination of the eyes. Using an irrigation solution that would cause a reaction is contraindicated with the substance in the eye. And irrigating an eye wound that has an open injury to the globe or laceration or detachment of the lens may cause additional damage and should not be attempted.

Procedure

1 Place patient on their back with a towel around their neck. Place the basin next to the patient's ear on the affected side to help collect the irrigation fluids. If only one eye is affected, the patient can be turned slightly to the affected side.

2 Prepare the equipment to flush, including the fluid and tubing or syringe.

3 Begin flushing at the bridge of the nose, allowing the excess to flow toward the affected side. This will keep the run-off from contaminating the unaffected eye.

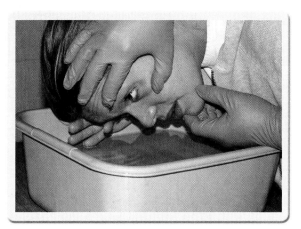

4 Infuse the 1,000 mL of normal saline.

5 Place a dry gauze pad lightly over the eye. Do not allow patient to rub the eyes.

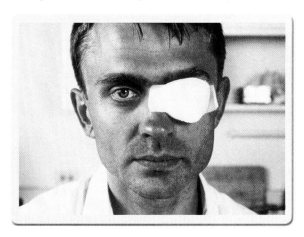

6 If both eyes need irrigation, start the procedure over with an entirely new setup or irrigate both eyes simultaneously.

7 Be careful not to recontaminate the eye that was previously irrigated.

PROCEDURE 31
Splinting (Board, Fitted, and Formable)

Introduction

The need to splint injured extremities is common while caring for trauma patients; board splints, fitted splints, and formable splints are three often used splint types.

Indications, Contraindications, and Equipment

Indications	Painful, swollen, and deformed extremities
Contraindications	Critical trauma necessitating immediate transport
Equipment	Exam gloves and goggles Commercially available splints Improvised splinting materials Triangle bandages Roller gauze

Rationale

Injured extremities can cause severe pain and additional damage if not immobilized properly. Board, fitted, or formable splints can be used to secure limbs and joints in place quickly and effectively, thus reducing pain and preventing further injury.

Possible Complications

If the splint is applied too tightly, or subsequent swelling makes it too tight, poor circulation and associated complications may occur in the distal extremity.

Procedure

There are many types of splints available to the provider. It is the provider's responsibility to understand the mechanism of the splints available to them. The following is a generalized approach to splinting:

1 Support and stabilize the injured limb, applying traction if needed to bring the limb into anatomic position.

2 Gently place the injured limb onto or into the splint according to the manufacturer's instructions.

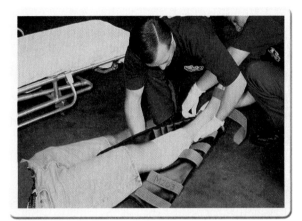

3 Pad any voids to avoid movement.

4 Secure the splint to the limb.

5 Check distal pulses, motor function, and sensation and monitor them en route.

PROCEDURE 32
Traction Splints

Introduction

Traumatic femur fractures can cause tremendous pain as well as damage to muscles, blood vessels, and nerves. Traction splinting is the most common method of caring for isolated femur fractures in the prehospital setting, but is not used in all countries. Please follow local protocols.

Indications, Contraindications, and Equipment

Indications	Isolated femur fracture
Contraindications	Lower leg, knee, or hip injuries
Equipment	Exam gloves and goggles Unipolar traction device (Sager style) Bipolar traction device (Hare or Donway style) Long backboard

Rationale

Because the muscles surrounding the femur are large and powerful, instability of the bone can easily cause the muscles to contract and spasm, pulling the fractured bone ends past each other and causing severe damage to the surrounding tissues. The traction splint will forcibly extend the muscle and realign the bone ends.

Possible Complications

Inconsistent or unstable traction can worsen tissue and vascular injuries as well as create more pain for the patient. Also, taking the time to apply traction devices to a multisystem trauma patient could risk patient deterioration and delay definitive care.

Procedure

There are several types of splints available to the provider. It is the provider's responsibility to understand the mechanism of the splints available to them. The following is a generalized approach to traction splinting:

1 Cut open the patient's pant (trouser) leg or otherwise expose the injured lower extremity. Be sure to assess the pulse, motor function, and sensation distal to the injury.

2 Place the splint beside the patient's uninjured leg, and adjust it to the proper length.

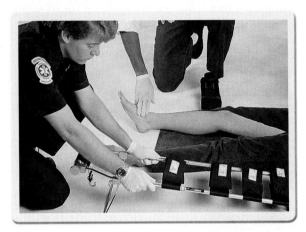

3 Manually support and stabilize the injured limb so that no motion occurs at the fracture site while a second provider fastens the appropriate-sized ankle strap around the patient's ankle and foot.

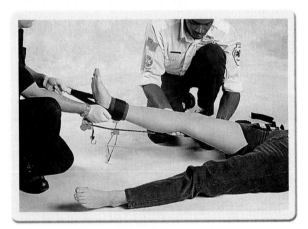

4 Support the leg at the site of the suspected injury while the second provider manually applies gentle longitudinal traction to the ankle strap and foot. Use only enough force to align (reposition) the limb so that it will fit into the splint. Do not attempt to align the fracture fragments anatomically.

5 Slide the splint into position, making certain that it is seated well.

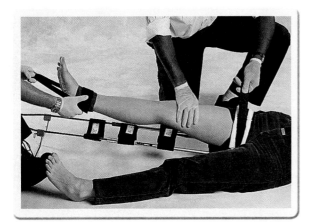

6 Pad the groin area and gently apply the ischial or thigh strap.

7 Connect the loops of the ankle strap to the end of the splint. Then apply gentle traction to the connecting strap between the ankle strap and the splint, just strong enough to maintain limb alignment. Adequate traction has been applied when the leg is the same length as the other leg or the patient feels relief.

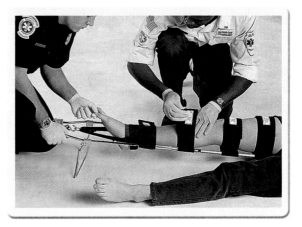

8 Once proper traction has been applied, fasten the support straps so that the limb is securely held in the splint. Check all proximal and distal support straps to make sure they are secure.

9 Reassess distal pulses, motor function, and sensation.

10 Place the patient on a long backboard or vacuum mattress for transport.

PROCEDURE 33
Air Splint

Introduction

Air splints are soft, formed cylinders that use air pressure to immobilize fractures of the lower leg or forearm and to control bleeding. Air splints are not used in all areas; refer to your local protocols.

Indications, Contraindications, and Equipment

Indications	Fractures of the lower leg or forearm Nonarterial bleeding from severe soft-tissue injuries of the lower leg or forearm
Contraindications	Long bone injuries at or higher than the elbow or knee Arterial hemorrhaging of the lower leg or forearm Angulated fractures Open fractures with exposed bone ends
Equipment	Exam gloves and goggles Air splint Inflation system

Rationale

The cylindrical shape of an air splint helps keep extremities aligned, and the even air pressure can assist with the control of internal and external bleeding.

Possible Complications

Changes in atmospheric pressure or ambient temperatures can increase or decrease the air pressure in the splint, causing it to become either too soft or too tight.

Procedure

1 Support the patient's injured limb until splinting is accomplished.

2 Place your arm through the splint. Extend your hand beyond the splint and grasp the hand or foot of the injured limb.

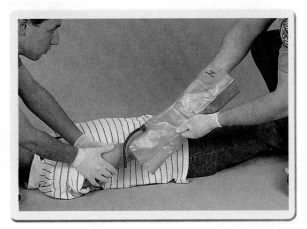

3 Apply gentle traction to the hand or foot while sliding the splint onto the injured limb. The hand or foot of the injured limb should always be included in the splint.

4 Inflate the splint by pump or by mouth.

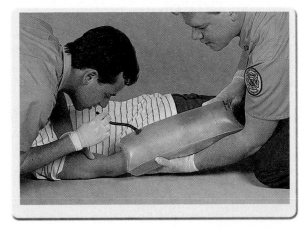

5 Test the pressure in the splint.

6 Check and record pulse, motor, and sensory functions, and monitor them en route.

PROCEDURE 34
Vacuum Splint

Introduction

A vacuum splint is a formable plastic device that is wrapped around an injured limb. When the air is drawn out, the splint hardens and secures the limb in position.

Indications, Contraindications, and Equipment

Indications	Swollen, painful, or deformed extremity Long bone fracture
Contraindications	Uncontrolled bleeding Protruding bone ends
Equipment	Exam gloves and goggles Vacuum splint device Air evacuation device

Rationale

The malleability of the vacuum splint makes it very useful for extremity splinting in most trauma situations.

Possible Complications

When air is evacuated from the splint, the splint can shrink and become too tight.

Procedure

1 Support and stabilize the injured limb, applying traction if needed.

2 Gently place the injured limb onto the vacuum splint and wrap the splint around the limb.

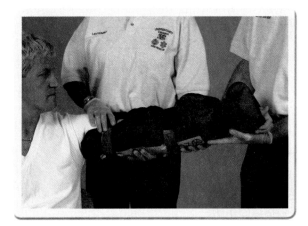

3 Draw the air out of the splint through the suction valve, then seal the valve. Once the valve is sealed, the vacuum splint becomes rigid, conforming to the shape of the deformed limb and stabilizing it.

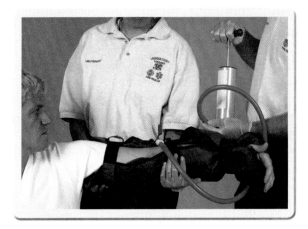

4 Check distal pulses, motor function, and sensation and monitor them en route.

PROCEDURE 35
Splinting the Pelvis

Introduction

The bones of the pelvis form a generally rounded shape. When the pelvis is fractured and deformed, the loss of structure will allow excessive bleeding to occur. Bringing the shape back to the pelvis is the best way to control bleeding.

Indications, Contraindications, and Equipment

Indications	A pelvic fracture that presents with deformity of the pelvis
Contraindications	None in the emergent setting
Equipment	Exam gloves Blanket, sheet, or commercial pelvic sling

Rationale

The bones of the pelvis are very vascular and bleed when fractured. When the fracture becomes displaced, the shape of the pelvis becomes deformed. To slow the bleeding, the shape of the pelvis must be restored.

Possible Complications

Excessive manipulation of the fractured pelvis can allow additional bleeding to occur and delay definitive care. Shock, long-term disability, and death are all possible.

Procedure

1 Assess the pelvis for signs of potential fracture.

2 Slide the sheet or pelvic sling under the patient at the level of the greater trochanters.

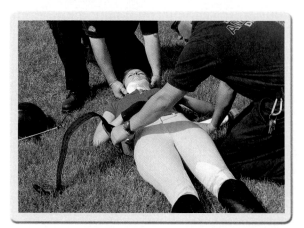

3 Draw the ends of the sheet or sling together, creating circumferential tension.

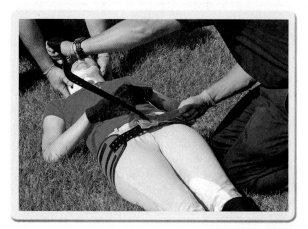

4 Secure the sheet or commercial sling to keep tension on the pelvis.

5 Reassess the patient for distal pulses and neurologic status.

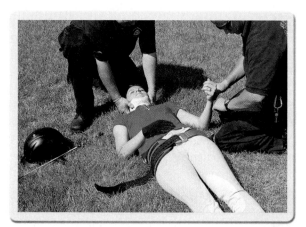

6 Move the patient to a spinal immobilization device and secure for transport.

PROCEDURE 36
PASG/MAST

Introduction

The pneumatic antishock garment (PASG) (also known as a military antishock trouser [MAST]) is an inflatable device that applies circumferential pressure to a patient's legs and abdomen. It is most commonly used with trauma patients to help control severe bleeding and counteract hypotension. In some countries, the PASG/MAST is not used outside of the military. Be sure to follow local protocols.

Indications, Contraindications, and Equipment

Indications	Suspected pelvic fracture with hypotension Severe hypotension Suspected intraperitoneal or retroperitoneal bleeding with hypotension
Contraindications	Penetrating thoracic trauma Lower extremity injuries without hypotension Evisceration of abdominal organs Objects impaled in the abdomen Pregnancy Acute pulmonary edema Traumatic cardiac arrest Severe head injuries
Equipment	Exam gloves and goggles PASG/MAST Stethoscope Blood pressure cuff

Rationale

The even, circumferential pressure applied by the garment can help control blood loss, increase a patient's blood pressure, splint pelvis fractures, and sometimes splint lower extremity injuries (although the device usually offers only marginal effectiveness when used to splint the lower extremities).

Possible Complications

Increasing the patient's blood pressure prior to controlling bleeding may cause increased blood loss, and compartment syndrome of the lower leg is possible if extremity fractures are present. Also, puncture of the PASG can result in loss of pressure if exposed bone ends are not properly padded.

Procedure

1 Rapidly expose and examine the areas to be covered by the PASG/MAST. Pad any exposed bone ends to prevent puncture of the garment as it is inflated.

2 Apply the garment. Position the top of the PASG/MAST below the lowest rib to ensure that it does not compromise chest expansion.

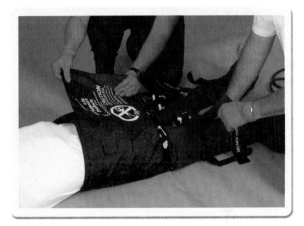

3 Close and fasten both leg compartments and the abdominal compartment.

4 Open the stopcocks (valves) to the compartments you are preparing to inflate, ensuring that the other compartments are closed off.

5 Auscultate for breath sounds, looking for signs of pulmonary edema.

6 Inflate the compartments with the foot pump until the Velcro crackles. Turn off compartment valves after inflation to maintain pressure in the garment. When using the device to stabilize pelvic fractures, apply pressure only until the garment is firm to the touch. Overinflation may cause the bones to shift, causing further injury.

7 Assess the patient's blood pressure and monitor frequently.

Note: Use of PASG/MAST has become controversial in recent years. Know your local protocol regarding this device. In severely injured patients, deflating the device can take between 20 and 60 minutes, causing a delay in treatment.

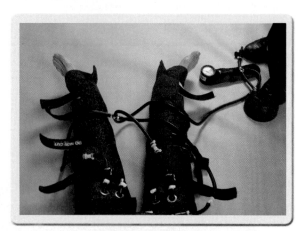

Glossary

abandonment The termination of the provider-patient relationship without providing for the appropriate continuation of care.

acceleration (a) The rate of change of velocity that an object is subjected to, whether speeding up or slowing down.

Achilles tendon The strong, fibrous cord that attaches the muscles in the back of the leg to the heel.

acidosis An excess of hydrogen ions in the body, which causes the pH to drop below 7.35.

acromioclavicular joint The shoulder.

active external rewarming Applying heat directly to the skin to rewarm the body.

active internal rewarming Directing the heat into the core and essentially warming the body from the inside.

adventitious Abnormal.

afterdrop Situation in which cold blood sequestered in the peripheral areas of the body is moved into the core.

afterload The pressure against which the heart must pump.

agnosia The inability to comprehend auditory, visual, or sensational stimuli, even though the eyes, ears, and other sensory organs are intact.

air embolism A process caused by sudden expansion of dissolved gas in the bloodstream. This results in embolization and occlusion of blood flow to a vital organ such as the brain, heart, or lungs.

alkalosis A decrease in the number of hydrogen ions in the body, causing the pH to increase above 7.45.

alveoli Small air sacs in the lungs.

amputation The complete separation or loss of a body part, usually a finger, toe, arm, or leg.

angiotensin II Hormone that helps reduce urine production.

anterior-posterior compression fracture (straddle fracture) Fracture associated with a slight widening of the pubic symphysis along with a fracture at the sacroiliac joint, whereby the pelvis is separated both front and back.

anterograde (posttraumatic) amnesia A loss of memory relating to events that occurred after an injury.

antidiuretic hormone (ADH) Hormone released from the pituitary gland to stimulate the kidneys to retain water and sodium; also called vasopressin.

aorta The large blood vessel near the heart.

aortic balloon pump A mechanical device used to decrease oxygen demand while increasing cardiac output. The device uses a balloon inserted in the aorta to inflate and deflate timed with the cardiac cycle.

aphasia The inability to communicate through speech, writing, or signs because of brain dysfunction.

apraxia The inability to perform purposeful movements when the motor and sensory organs are not directly impaired.

aqueous humor Clear watery fluid that fills the anterior chamber of the globe of the eye.

arachnoid mater The second meningeal layer, a delicate, transparent membrane.

arterial pressure points Locations on extremities where large arteries from the trunk of the body pass near bones as they enter the extremity.

arteriosclerosis The stiffening of vessel walls.

ataxia Lack of muscular coordination.

autonomic nervous system System that controls the cardiovascular system and is composed of two competing subsystems.

avulsion A three-sided cut that leaves a flap of skin and soft tissue attached to the body on the fourth side.

avulsion fracture An injury to the bone where a tendon or ligament attaches to the bone.

axon A long, slender extension of a neuron that conducts electrical impulses away from the neuronal soma in the brain.

bariatrics The branch of medicine that deals with obesity and related health issues.

barometric energy Energy resulting from sudden and radical changes in pressure, often during diving or flying.

basal metabolic rate (BMR) The number of kilocalories created by the body per hour.

Bennett's fracture Fracture of the base of the thumb.

biomechanics The study of the physiology and mechanics of a living organism using the tools of mechanical engineering.

blast front The leading edge of a shock wave.

blunt trauma Injuries in which the tissues are not penetrated by an external object.

boxer's fracture Metacarpal neck fracture of the little finger.

Boyle's law A gas law that states that pressure and volume of gas are directly proportional. Important because the volume of air will increase if the patient is moved to a higher altitude, as occurs during flight transfers.

bradypnea Slow respiratory rate.

brain stem Structure located at the base of the brain that connects the spinal cord to the remainder of the brain. It houses many structures that are critical to the maintenance of vital functions.

breach of duty When the provider deviates from what would be considered good and accepted practice.

bronchi The two main branches of the trachea.

bronchiole Small tube that branches from the bronchi to the alveoli in the lungs.

bronchorrhea Excessive mucus production by the bronchial mucus membrane.

burn Diffuse soft tissue injury created by destructive energy transfer via radiation, thermal energy, or electrical energy.

burn shock Shock that occurs because of fluid loss across the damaged skin and because of a series of volume shifts within the body itself.

bursa A synovial-like membrane around the joint to protect it and to decrease the friction of rubbing tendons over their boney prominences.

calcaneus The bone in the back of the foot, commonly referred to as the *heel*.

cancellous bone The inner spongy bone.

capnography The monitoring of the rise and fall of $ETCO_2$ levels over time.

carbon monoxide (CO) Odorless, colorless, and tasteless gas produced by incomplete combustion of fuels.

carboxyhemoglobin (COHb) Hemoglobin loaded with carbon monoxide.

cardiac contusion Bruise on the heart.

cardiac output A measurement of the amount of blood that the heart moves over time.

cardiac silhouette The shadow produced by the heart on a radiograph.

cardiogenic shock Shock that results from a weakening pumping action of the heart.

cardiovascular system System that consists of the heart, blood vessels, and circulating blood.

CareFlight A basic triage system that can be performed by trained first responders in emergencies.

carina The ridge at the base of the trachea that separates the right and left main stem bronchi.

catecholamines Chemicals that stimulate an immediate increase in the heart rate and contractile force.

cavitation Cavity formation.

cerebellum Part of the brain responsible for the maintenance of posture and equilibrium and the coordination of skilled movements.

cerebral contusion Brain tissue bruised and damaged in a local area.

cerebral perfusion pressure (CPP) The pressure required to make blood flow through the brain.

cerebrum The largest portion of the brain, which is responsible for higher functions, such as reasoning.

cervical collar Soft or rigid device used to aid in the immobilization of the cervical spine.

cervical spine Includes the first seven bones of the vertebral column and its supporting structures.

chemical energy Energy found in an explosive or an acid, or even from a reaction to an ingested or medically delivered agent or drug.

choroid The vascular membrane that nourishes the retina.

classic heat stroke Condition in which core temperature rises due to exhaustion of the compensatory mechanisms.

closed fracture Any fracture that does not penetrate overlying skin or mucous membrane to the outer air.

coagulation Blood clotting.

coagulative necrosis Where tissue burned by an acid forms a tough layer of scar tissue.

coagulopathies Blood clotting disorders.

collagen Fibrous protein with a very high tensile strength that gives the skin a high resistance to breakage under mechanical stress.

Colles fracture Fracture in which the distal radius fragment is tilted upward or dorsal.

combined mechanical A combination of pelvic fractures due to high-energy impact.

comminuted fracture Fracture in which the bone is crushed, splintered, or broken into multiple fragments.

compartment syndrome The increased tissue pressure from edema and/or hemorrhage within a muscle compartment that gradually compromises vascular perfusion, escalating to ischemia of the tissues and nerves.

complete spinal cord injury Complete disruption of all tracts of the spinal cord, with permanent loss of all cord-mediated functions below the level transaction.

compressive asphyxia The mechanical limitation of the expansion of the chest.

computerized tomography (CT) A radiograph scan that uses a 360° beam to produce cross-sectional images of the body.

conduction The transfer of heat from a source of relatively high heat to one of lower heat through physical contact.

condyloid joints Joints of the jaw and fingers that allow for movement but not rotation.

conjunctiva A delicate mucous membrane that covers the sclera and internal surfaces of the eyelids (except the iris).

consent Permission from a patient to provide treatment. Consent can be considered a function of three significant factors: legal status, decision-making capacity, and information.

contact burns Burns that result from the heating of metal objects on a person or on a person's clothing.

convection Heat transfer through movement of a liquid or air over a surface.

cornea The transparent anterior portion of the eye that overlies the iris and pupil.

cortical bone The hard outer shell, or cortex, of the bone.

cranium Eight bones that encase and protect the brain.

crepitus Crunching of the bone or cartilage.

critical care transport A provision of en-route intensive care–level services during the transport of a critically ill patient between medical treatment facilities.

crush syndrome The result of a severe crushing injury, this condition is characterized by extensive soft tissue damage with excessive blood and fluid loss.

cryoprecipitate A liquid suspension of concentrated clotting factors that has the primary advantage of giving large amounts of clotting proteins in a small volume.

Cullen's sign A bruise-type marking around the umbilicus.

current The flow of power over time.

cyanosis When the skin turns a dusky gray or blue color.

decerebrate (extensor) posturing Rigid extension of the arms and legs, usually accompanied with downward pointing of the toes and arching of the neck.

decision-making capacity The mental capacity to make a rational decision.

decompression sickness A medical emergency that occurs when there is a supersaturation of dissolved nitrogen in the tissues that expands to form small gaseous bubbles. It is also known as the *bends* or *caisson disease*.

decorticate (flexor) posturing Rigidity and flexion of the arms toward the chest as well as extension of the legs.

defasciculating dose Generally 10% of the paralyzing agent that is given to reduce the amount of increased ICP produced by myoclonal fasciculations.

demand pacemakers Pacemakers that sense the natural heart rate and begin pacing only when the natural heart rate drops below the set level.

dermatomes Areas of the skin supplied by particular nerves.

dermis Highly elastic layer of connective tissues composed chiefly of collagen fibers, elastin, and a mucopolysaccharide gel.

diaphragm The thin muscle that is responsible for respirations and serves as a partition between the chest and the abdominal cavities.

diaphysis The long shaft of a long bone.

diastasis A separation or dislocation between two bones that are attached but have no true joint.

diffusion The process in which a gas moves from an area of higher concentration to an area of lower concentration.

digital arteries The arteries of each finger.

diplopia Double vision.

dislocation A complete disruption of a joint with total loss of contact between the joint's articular surfaces.

disseminated intravascular coagulopathy (DIC) A problem with the coagulation system in which more clots are needed than can be created, leading to clots being formed incorrectly, inappropriately, or not at all.

distributive shock Shock caused by an insufficient volume of blood in the vascular space due to an increase in the vascular space (vasodilation).

dura mater A strong, fibrous wrapping and the outermost layer of the meninges.

duty to act An understanding in the relationship that exists between parties that requires the emergency medical service or other provider to respond to a request for assistance. This may arise out of a contract, a statute, a mutual aid agreement, or some other legal relationship.

dysbarism Medical condition that occurs as a result of changes in ambient air pressure.

dysconjugate gaze Condition in which both eyes are not fixated on the same point.

elastin Material that imparts elasticity to the skin, allowing the skin to return to its usual contours.

electrical energy Energy in the form of high-voltage electrocution or a lightning strike.

endocardium The innermost layer of the heart muscle lining the ventricles.

end-tidal carbon dioxide (ETCO$_2$) monitor Equipment that measures the partial pressure of carbon dioxide gas in a sample.

energy dissipation The process by which kinetic energy is transformed into thermal, electrical, chemical, radiant, or mechanical energy.

epidermis Outermost layer of the skin.

epidural (extradural) hematoma An accumulation of blood between the skull and dura mater.

escharotomy An incision into burned tissue that helps decrease pressure on neurovascular structures

evaporation Loss of heat through the transition of water from a liquid state to a gas.

evisceration Wound through which the internal organs are exposed to the outside of the body.

exertional heat stroke Condition in which compensatory cooling mechanisms in the body are overwhelmed by more heat than they can manage.

exothermic reaction Reaction that produces heat.

extracorporeal life support/extracorporeal membrane oxygenation (ECLS/ECMO) A procedure in which a machine continuously pumps blood from the patient through a membrane designed to exchange oxygen and carbon dioxide in the blood. The machine connects through cannulae placed in the large blood vessels.

extracorporeal rewarming Removing the patient's blood from the body, heating it, and then returning it.

fasciculations Uncontrolled quivering of the skeletal muscles.

femoral neck fracture Fracture in which the femoral head is broken at its neck from the femoral shaft.

flail segment Injury in which more than two consecutive ribs are fractured in two or more areas.

flash burn Burn caused by the excessive heat of flashover, resulting in a brownish, discolored partial-thickness burn.

foramen magnum Allows the brain to connect to the spinal cord.

fracture A break in the bone.

fresh whole blood (FWB) Blood that contains all components and provides the oxygen-carrying capacity of packed RBCs and the hemostatic capacity of plasma and platelets in a single 450-mL unit. In addition, the blood is "fresh," which allows maximal function of the components.

frostbite Condition in which the body tissue freezes.

frostnip Condition of superficial and reversible partial freezing of tissues within the body.

full-thickness burn Burn involving destruction of both layers of the skin, including the basement membrane of dermis, which produces new skin cells.

fundus The top portion of the uterus, opposite the cervix.

Glasgow Coma Scale (GCS) A widely accepted method of assessing level of consciousness. It is based on three independent measurements: eye opening, verbal response, and motor response.

gliding joints Joints such as those in the wrists, ankles, and spine that allow bones to glide past each other.

globe Eyeball.

glomerulus The main filter in the nephron of a kidney.

gravid Total pregnancies, but not necessarily carried to term.

gravity (g) The downward acceleration imparted to any object on earth by the effect of the earth's mass.

greenstick fracture A partial break in which the bone does not completely break through the skin.

Grey Turner's sign A delayed sign of internal bleeding that presents as a dark discoloration along the flanks.

gross negligence Conduct that is reckless and bears no relationship to the accepted standard of care.

hair follicles Structures that produce hair and enclose the hair roots.

hairline fracture A small crack in the bone with no displacement of the ends.

hard palate The bony anterior part of the palate, or roof of the mouth.

heat cramps Cramping that can occur in patients who try to replace lost volume with free water.

heat edema Condition in which vasodilation and pooling of fluids in the interstitial space cause swelling in the hands and feet.

heat exchange The movement of heat from one source to another.

heat exhaustion Condition in which water and salt levels within the body have been depleted.

heat production The speed at which the body is burning fuels.

heat syncope Transient syncopal event brought on by heat.

hematocrit Volume of red blood cells per given volume of blood.

hemorrhagic shock Shock from blood loss.

hemothorax Condition in which blood collects between the lung and chest wall.

hinge joints Joints like the knee and elbow that allow movement much like that of a door hinge.

homeostasis Balance.

hyoid bone Bone that supports the tongue and serves as a point of attachment for many important neck and tongue muscles.

hyperpyrexia Very high body temperature.

hypertrophies Enlarges.

hyphema Bleeding into the anterior chamber of the eye that partially or completely obscures vision.

hyponatremia Low sodium levels.

hypoperfusion Another term for shock.

hypothermia Condition in which the body loses more heat than it produces or gains.

hypovolemic shock Shock that reduces the total fluid in the body.

icterus Jaundice.

immune-mediated hemolytic reaction Also known as a hemolytic transfusion reaction, this is a rapid destruction of red blood cells in the transfused blood by the patient's antibodies.

implied consent A legal doctrine that permits a health care provider to render emergency treatment under circumstances in which the patient is incapable of making a rational decision either to consent to or to refuse treatment.

incident command system (ICS) Organizational system developed to help manage a situation that has become bigger than a local system can control without help.

incident commander The one commander at the top of the incident command system.

incision A clean, possibly surgical-type laceration with smooth, straight edges that can be stitched back together easily.

incomplete spinal cord injury Classification of patients who retain some degree of a cord-mediated function 24 hours following an injury.

induction agent Medication used to produce a rapid loss of consciousness to assist in intubation.

integument Skin.

intertrochanter fracture Fracture that occurs just below the neck of the femur.

intracerebral hematoma Bleeding within the brain tissue (parenchyma).

intracranial pressure (ICP) Pressure within the cranial vault.

intramedulary canal The innermost space in long bones, also called the *marrow cavity*.

inverse square law Law of physics that states the strength of the radiation is inversely proportional to the square of the distance from the object. (The further away, the weaker the radiation.)

involuntary muscles Smooth muscles found in the digestive system, blood vessels, bladder, and airway. These muscles have the ability to stretch and hold tension for long periods of time and are controlled by the autonomic or involuntary nervous system.

iris The pigmented part of the eye that surrounds and protects the pupil.

ischemia Inadequate blood flow to the cells.

isoagglutinins An antibody produced by one individual that causes agglutination of red blood cells in another individual.

isolette A clear plastic–enclosed crib that maintains a warm environment for new babies.

joints Articulating bones.

keraunographic marks Fern-like patterns appearing on the skin after a lightning strike. They are also called feathering, lightning prints, or Lichtenberg's figures or flowers.

kinetic energy Energy from motion.

kinetics The study of the relationships among speed, mass, direction of the force, and, for emergency medical providers, the physical injury caused by speed, mass, and force.

Kussmaul's sign Increased jugular filling pressure with inspiration.

kyphosis Misshaping of the bones in the back and neck caused by weakening of neck and upper body muscles. Commonly referred to as humpback or hunchback.

laceration An injury to the skin and its underlying soft tissue.

laryngeal mask airway (LMA) Airway that consists of a tube connected to a pointed oval-shaped inflatable cuff with an opening in the center.

laryngeal tube airway (LTA) Airway with similar form and function to the dual lumen airways, though it is reported to have less resistance on insertion.

lateral compression fracture Fracture involving the transverse fractures of the pubis bone, along with associated sacral compression on the side of impact, or iliac wing fracture on the side of impact.

law of conservation of energy Law that states that energy can be neither created nor destroyed; it can only change form.

Le Fort I fracture A horizontal fracture of the maxilla that involves the hard palate and inferior maxilla.

Le Fort II fracture A pyramidal fracture involving the nasal bone and inferior maxilla.

Le Fort III fracture A fracture of all midfacial bones, separating the entire midface from the cranium.

lens Transparent structure behind the pupil that can alter its thickness to focus light on the retina at the back of the eye.

ligament Fibrous, somewhat stretchy tissue that holds one bone to another, forming the joint.

ligamentum flavum A long elastic band that connects to the anterior surface of the lamina bones.

lightning position Seated, cross-legged position or kneeling position.

liquefactive necrosis When tissue has been burned by an alkali and liquefies and becomes "soapy," allowing the base to burn deeper.

lordosis Forward curvature of the lumbar spine.

mallet finger An injury that occurs when the most distal joint of the finger is forcefully hyperflexed, resulting in a flexion deformity of the distal phalanx, which the patient cannot actively extend.

mandible The large movable bone forming the lower jaw and containing the lower teeth.

mass casualty incident An incident that has more patients than a system can handle using everyday procedures and equipment.

mass casualty triage The process of determining, in the presence of an overwhelming number of injuries, which patients get treated and/or transported based on the resources available to provide treatment and transportation.

mastication Chewing of food by the teeth.

mean arterial pressure (MAP) The average (or mean) blood pressure against the arterial wall during a cardiac cycle.

mechanical energy Energy from motion or energy stored in an object.

mechanism of injury (MOI) The forces that act on the body to cause damage.

mechanism of trauma How injuries were sustained.

mediastinum The center of the chest.

medulla The inferior portion of the midbrain.

meninges Protective layers that surround and enfold the entire central nervous system.

meniscus Shock-absorbing cartilage between the femur and tibia that protects the bone ends from rubbing together.

mesentery Tissue that connects the small intestine to the posterior abdominal wall.

metabolic rate The speed at which your cells are burning fuel.

methemoglobin (MetHb) Compound formed by oxidation of the iron on the hemoglobin.

move, assess, sort, send (MASS) A basic triage system that can be performed by trained first responders in emergencies.

mucopolysaccharide gel Substance that gives the skin resistance to compression.

musculoskeletal system The bones, tendons, ligaments, and voluntary muscles that give the body its form and movement.

mutual aid agreements Agreements with neighboring agencies that often include how and when the other agency will enter the scene and how they will interact within the incident command system.

myocardium The heart muscle.

myoglobin The oxygen-transporting protein found in muscle cells.

nasal septum The separation between the nostrils, located in the midline.

negative wave pulse The phase in which pressure is less than atmospheric; it may last 10 times as long as the positive wave pulse.

neurogenic shock Shock resulting from blood vessel dilation caused by a brain or spinal/nerve injury.

neuron Nerve cell.

neuronal soma Cell body.

Newton's first law of motion Law stating that a body at rest will remain at rest (and a body in motion tends to remain in motion at a constant velocity, traveling in a straight line) unless acted on by an outside force.

Newton's second law of motion Law stating that the force an object can exert is the product of its mass times its acceleration.

Newton's third law of motion Law stating that for every action there is an equal and opposite reaction.

nocioceptors Peripheral pain receptors.

oblique fracture Fracture in which the ends of the bone compact at an oblique angle to the long bone itself.

obstructive shock Shock that obstructs the flow of oxygen into the bloodstream and into the starving tissue.

occipital condyles The points of articulation between the skull and the vertebral column that lie on either side of the foramen magnum.

oculomotor nerve The third cranial nerve, which innervates the muscles that cause motion of the eyeballs and upper eyelids.

olecranon The rounded posterior projection commonly called the *elbow*.

open fracture When bone at the fracture site penetrates through soft tissue and skin to become exposed to the outside environment.

open pneumothorax Pneumothorax associated with an open chest wall injury so that air can enter and exit the chest through the exterior wound opening.

optic nerve The second cranial nerve, which transmits nerve impulses necessary for the sense of vision.

orbit Eye socket.

ordinary negligence Errors in judgment, mistakes in treatment, and faulty handling of a patient.

osseous tissue Three-dimensional honeycomb-like structure that gives the bone rigidity and shape.

osteomyelitis Bone infection.

osteoporosis Widespread decrease in bone mass brought on by aging.

oxyhemoglobin (HbO$_2$) Oxygen-rich hemoglobin.

packed red blood cells (pRBCs) A preparation of red blood cells used to correct low blood levels in anemic patients.

palatine bone The irregularly shaped bone in the posterior nasal cavity.

para/parity Pregnancies carried to more than 28 weeks' gestation, regardless of whether delivered dead or alive.

parasympathetic nervous system System primarily responsible for rest and regeneration.

paresthesia Temporary or permanent loss of sensation to an area, often associated with a pins-and-needles feeling.

parietal peritoneum Covering on the abdominal wall that also serves as connective tissue.

parietal pleura A sticky membrane lining the inside of the chest wall.

partial-thickness burn Burn involving the epidermis and varying degrees of the dermis.

passive external rewarming Using the patient's own body heat to rewarm the body.

patella fracture Knee fracture caused by direct trauma to the kneecap.

pathologic fracture Fracture that occurs at a point where the bone is weakened from another disease process.

pathway expansion The tissue displacement that occurs as the result of low-displacement shock waves that travel at the speed of sound in tissue.

pediatric trauma score (PTS) Tool aimed at evaluating the severity of injury for children.

pediatric triage tape Triage system similar to the trauma sieve, but with the values based on the patient's height measured by the tape.

pelvic fracture The disruption of the bony structure of the pelvis.

pelvic girdle Commercial device that provides pelvic immobilization.

penetrating trauma Injuries when tissues are penetrated by single or multiple objects.

perfusion Process that involves moving oxygen and nutrients from outside the body to the tissues and removing the waste products from the tissues.

pericardiocentesis Process that involves penetrating the pericardium with a needle and withdrawing the accumulated blood.

pericardium A very strong fibrous sac that surrounds the heart.

periorbital ecchymosis Raccoon eyes.

peripheral nervous system (PNS) The complex system of nerves that arise from the spinal nerve roots.

petechiae Pinpoint hemorrhages that show up on the skin.

pia mater The third meningeal layer, a thin, translucent, highly vascular membrane that firmly adheres directly to the surface of the brain.

pivot joints Joints of the neck that allow bones to pivot or twist around one another.

plasma The liquid component of blood that contains the coagulation factors and proteins.

platelets Small irregularly shaped cells within the blood whose primary job is to stop bleeding.

plexus Cluster of nerve roots.

pneumocephalus The presence of air or gas in the cranial cavity.

pneumothorax The presence of air in the pleural cavity between the parietal and visceral pleura, which creates a void between the normally contacted pleural surfaces.

polyuria Excessive passage of urine.

pons Structure that lies below the midbrain and above the medulla and contains numerous important nerve fibers.

positive wave pulse The phase of an explosion in which there is a pressure front higher than atmospheric pressure.

postfall syndrome An increased likelihood of a fall based on a previous fall; the patient's resultant lack of confidence with movement and anxiety about potential falls leads to muscle wasting that leaves the patient at a higher risk of future falls.

postpartum After birth.

posturing An abnormal flexion of the arms and extension of the legs associated with increases in intracranial pressure.

potential energy Energy stored in an object.

preload Blood return to the heart.

premedication agents Medications that may be helpful in intubating a patient.

progesterone Hormone produced early in pregnancy by the corpus luteum and later by the placenta. It decreases the threshold of the medullary respiratory center to carbon dioxide.

pronation Rotation of the arm with the palm downward.

pulmonary contusion A bruise of the lung tissue.

pulsus paradoxus Weakening pulse with inspiration.

punctuated burns Small, circular burn marks over dry skin, resembling cigarette burns.

pupil Circular, adjustable opening within the iris through which light passes to the lens.

radial head The proximal articulating end of the radius.

radial head subluxation The most common injury to the upper extremity in infants and children; also known as *nursemaid's elbow*.

radiation The transfer of heat through electromagnetic waves.

rebound tenderness Pain when you release your hand after pressing deeply on a patient.

recruitment A process in which more neurons need to signal more muscle cells to contract to generate a more forceful contraction.

reduced hemoglobin (RHB) Hemoglobin after the oxygen has been released to the cells.

renin-angiotensin-aldosterone system (RAAS) A system that increases systemic vascular resistance and works to increase fluid retention by the kidneys by increasing sodium reabsorption and stimulating the release of antidiuretic hormone (ADH).

residual volume The amount of air left in the lungs at the end of a maximal exhalation.

retina Structure that lies in the posterior aspect of the internal globe and receives light impulses and converts them to nerve signals that are conducted to the brain by the optic nerve and interpreted as vision.

retinal detachment Separation of the inner layers of the retina from the underlying choroid.

retroauricular ecchymosis Battle's sign; bruising behind the ear over the mastoid process.

retrograde amnesia A loss of memory relating to events that occurred before the injury.

retrograde endotracheal intubation (REI) Intubation technique in which a flexible wire is inserted through the cricothyroid membrane to guide the tracheal tube through the mouth into position.

retroperitoneal space The space behind the abdomen.

reverse triage Triage approach based on the concept that patients may be dead simply because of a disconnection between the nervous and cardiovascular systems.

revised trauma score (RTS) Score based on the first assessment of the patient that combines the GCS, systolic blood pressure, and respiratory rate.

rhabdomyolysis Condition in which the breakdown of muscle fibers releases their contents into the bloodstream.

Sacco Triage Method (STM) A triage system that utilizes computer models to sort casualties based on severity and available resources.

saddle joint Joint that allows movement back and forth and side to side but very little rotation. Found in the thumb.

scapula A large, triangular, flat bone on the back side of the rib cage, commonly called the *shoulder blade*.

sclera White of the eye.

sebaceous gland Gland at the neck of each hair follicle that produces an oily substance called sebum.

septic shock Shock resulting from fluid shifts associated with massive infections and poisons.

shivering The rhythmic, involuntary movement of muscles.

shock Condition that results from inadequate flow of oxygen and nutrients to the cells of the body.

simple pneumothorax Condition in which there is air in the pleural space but that air does not build up pressure and is contained to 10%–30% collapse of the lung.

simple triage and rapid treatment (START) A basic triage system that can be performed by trained first responders in emergencies.

Smith fracture Fracture in which the distal fragment is tilted downward or volar.

somatic motor neurons Neurons that transmit electrical stimuli to a muscle, causing it to contract.

sort, assess, lifesaving interventions, and treatment and/or transport (SALT) A triage system that can be performed by trained providers in emergencies.

spiral fracture Fracture that occurs when the bone is twisted apart by a torsional force.

spondylosis Degenerative changes in the spine.

sprain A stretching or partial tearing of a ligament.

stable ankle fractures One-sided fractures of the medial or lateral malleolus.

staging officer or ambulance parking officer Officer who coordinates the physical location and approach of incoming resources, including additional ambulances and aeromedical resources.

strain A stretching or partial tearing of a muscle or musculo-tendinous unit.

stroke volume The volume of blood the heart pumps with each contraction.

subarachnoid Beneath the arachnoid layer covering the brain.

subarachnoid hemorrhage Bleeding into the subarachnoid space, where the CSF circulates.

subcutaneous air Crackling of air under the skin.

subdural Beneath the outermost covering of the brain.

subdural hematoma An accumulation of blood beneath the dura mater but outside the brain.

subluxation A joint malalignment where some part of the opposing joint surfaces remains in contact.

sucking chest wound Open wound of the chest that has air movement through it.

superficial burn Burn that involves the epidermis only.

supination Rotation of the arm with the palm upward.

supraglottic Upper airway.

sympathetic eye movement The movement of both eyes in unison.

sympathetic nervous system System that prepares the body for physical activity during a stressful situation for the body; sometimes known as the "fight or flight" system.

sympathomimetics Medications that increase a patient's basal metabolic rate.

tachypnea Fast respiratory rate.

tendon A very tough, yet flexible band of fibrous tissue that connects the muscle to the bone and is necessary for the muscle to provide movement of a joint.

tension pneumothorax Pneumothorax in which an oblique opening into the pleura occludes and acts as a one-way valve.

tentorium A structure that separates the cerebral hemispheres from the cerebellum and brain stem.

thermal energy Energy stored in objects that is seen as a change in temperature, like the friction in braking on a car or burning of materials.

thromboembolism A blood clot that has broken off and lodged itself elsewhere in the vein, blocking blood flow.

thrombus Blood clot.

tibial plateau fracture Knee fracture that occurs when a victim lands on their feet and the distal femur crushes the tibial head.

tidal volume The amount inspired with each breath.

time of useful consciousness (TUC) The period during which adequate cognitive function persists in a hypoxic environment.

torus fracture An incomplete fracture that is the result of compression force, which leads to a buckling of the pliable cortex. Commonly found in pediatric patients.

transport officer or ambulance clearing officer Officer who organizes transport of patients from the scene, and ensures patients are distributed to appropriate hospitals to prevent hospital overloading.

transverse fracture Fracture that forms a line or break at a right angle to the axis of the bone.

trauma The acute physiologic and structural change (injury) that occurs in a patient's body when an external source of energy dissipates faster than the body's ability to sustain and dissipate it.

trauma center Hospital or other facility that specializes in the care of the severely injured.

traumatic asphyxia Compressive asphyxia resulting from being crushed or pinned under a large weight or force.

treatment officer or casualty clearing officer Officer who supervises medical care given to patients at the scene and keeps a record of the patients seen.

trench foot Condition in which the feet are exposed to long-term and/or repeated insults of hypothermia.

triage The sorting of patients first for their need for initial care and then to an appropriate facility that is able to provide an appropriate level of care.

triage officer Officer charged with utilizing the agencies' initial triage system and providing no treatment to patients.

triage sieve A basic triage system that can be performed by trained first responders in emergencies.

tunica adventitia The external layer of an artery, which is made of connective and elastic tissue, protects the patient from stretch-type injuries and minor puncture wounds, and can limit the chance of hemorrhage.

tunica intima The innermost layer of an artery.

tunica media The smooth, muscular middle layer of an artery.

vagus nerve The 10th cranial nerve, and a bundle of nerves that primarily innervates the parasympathetic nervous system.

vasoconstriction Constriction of the blood vessels.

vasodilation Enlarging of the blood vessels.

velocity (V) The distance an object travels per unit of time.

vena cava A thin-walled vessel that lies along the right side of the spine.

vertebral body The anterior weight-bearing structure, made of bone that provides support and stability.

vertebral column The major structural component of the axial skeleton.

vertical shear Displacement of both the anterior and posterior pelvic ring due to a high-energy impact.

visceral peritoneum A thin visceral covering that covers all the abdominal organs.

visceral pleura A sticky membrane that allows the lungs to stay connected to the rib cage but also move with it.

vital capacity The amount of air that can be exhaled following a maximal inhalation.

vitreous humor Jellylike substance that maintains the shape of the globe.

voltage Amount of power.

voluntary muscles Muscles that we think about moving, then the nervous system tells them to move.

Waddell's triad The pattern of automobile pedestrian injuries in children and people of short stature.

whiplash injury An injury to the cervical vertebrae or their supporting ligaments and muscles, usually resulting from sudden acceleration or deceleration.

work of breathing The effort a person uses to breathe.

zone of coagulation The central area of the skin that suffers the most damage from a burn.

zone of hyperemia The area of a burn that is least affected by the thermal injury.

zone of stasis Burned area that undergoes necrosis.

zygomatic arch The bone that extends along the front of the skull below the orbit(s).

Note: page numbers with italicized *f* or *t* indicate figures or tables respectively.

Airway status. *See also* Airway
    initial assessment of, 30–31, 31*f*, 31*t*
    reassessment of, 40
Alcohol use
    cervical spine injuries and, 126
    traumatic brain injuries and, 114–115
Alert and oriented (A × O) evaluation, 36
Alkali burns
    to eyes, 100, 101*f*, 191
    liquefactive necrosis and, 198, 198*t*
    management of, 213
    treatment in eyes, 103
Alkalosis, 307
Alveoli, 133
Ambulance loading officers, 287
Ambulance parking officers, 287
Ambulances. *See also* Secondary transport; Transport
    ground or air, 294, 294*f*
    sonogram utilization in, 140–141
American College of Surgeons (ACS), 289
Amnesia, 110, 112*t*, 241–242, 241*t*
Amputations
    of ear, 104
    of extremities, 166, 166*f*
    of male genitalia, 155, 156
    proximal to wrist or ankle, 291*t*, 292
Anatomic criteria for triaging patients to trauma center, 291*t*, 292–293
Anemia, oxyhemoglobin saturation and, 59
Aneurysm
    aortic tears and, 148, 148*f*
    subarachnoid hematoma and, 112
Angiotensin II, shock effects on, 78
Angular motorcycle collisions, 15*f*, 16
Animal bites, 166, 279
Ankle injuries, 167, 185
Anterior cruciate ligament (ACL), 162*f*, 167, 183
Anterior-posterior compression fractures of pelvis, 182
Anterograde amnesia, 110, 112*t*
Anticonvulsants, for traumatic brain injuries, 117
Antidiuretic hormone (ADH), shock effects on, 78
Antidotes, radiation burns and, 215, 215*t*

Aorta
    anatomy and physiology, 133, 134*f*
    deceleration injuries to, 7
    layers of, 148*f*
    in pelvic girdle, 135*f*, 136
    shearing forces and, 136
    tears or transection of, 147–148
Aortic balloon pumps, 310
Aphasia, 241
Appearance. *See also* Inspection
    in pediatric assessment, 253, 253*f*, 253*t*
Apraxia, 241
Aqueous humor, 92, 93*f*
Arachnoid mater, 95, 96*f*
Area of impact, in falls, 17*f*, 18
Arm slings, 176*f*, 177. *See also* Upper extremities
Arrhythmias. *See also* Pulse
    age and, 258
    blunt injuries and, 8
    cardiac contusion and, 146
    cold emergencies and, 231
    electrical burns and, 214
    lightning and, 239, 243
Arteries
    air embolism in, pulmonary blast injuries and, 22, 23*f*
    of anterior neck, 91, 91*f*, 92*f*
    bleeding from, 70–71, 70*f*, 166
    bleeding from, epidural hematoma and, 111
    major, anterior neck injuries and, 117
    major, pelvic fractures and, 154
    pressure point for, 71
    pulmonary, 133
    role in cardiovascular system, 68
    of upper and lower extremities, 162–163
Arteriosclerosis, 258
Arteriovenous malformation, subarachnoid hematoma and, 112
Asphyxia
    electricity and, 200
    traumatic, 150–151, 150*f*
Asymmetric pupils, 114, 114*f*, 115
Ataxia, 231

Blunt trauma
    to anterior neck, 117
    aortic tears or transection and, 147
    bladder injuries and, 153
    cardiac tamponade and, 146
    cerebral contusion and, 110
    in children, 251
    closed head injuries due to, 106
    defined, 6, 7, 7f
    depressed skull fractures and, 106–107
    diaphragm injuries and, 149
    evisceration and, 151
    to eyes, 100, 100f
    gastrointestinal tract injury and, 152, 153f
    liver injuries and, 151
    to male genitals, 155
    mandibular fractures due to, 96–97
    maxillary-facial, ventilating patients with, 62
    myocardial rupture and, 147
    pancreatic injuries and, 152
    pelvic fractures and, 154
    to torso, 136
    tracheobronchial injury and, 150
Body armor, blast injuries and, 23, 23f
Body fluid cultures, 309
Body position, falls and, 17f, 18
Body substance isolation, 28, 28, 102, 202, 209t
Body temperature. See also Cold emergencies; Heat
        emergencies
    burns and, 210
    head injuries and, 116
    in injured elderly, 262
    regulation of, 222, 222f, 223f
Bones, 160–161, 161f. See also Carpal bones; Long bones
Bougie stylet, 52, 53f
Bowel, large or small
    deceleration injuries to, 7
    sounds, assessment of, 139, 149, 152
Boxer's fracture, 181, 181f
Boyle's law, 305
Brachial plexus, 91, 163
Bradycardia, 112, 112t, 231, 237. See also Arrhythmias

Bradypnea, 232
Brain. See also Traumatic brain injuries
    aging and, 258–259, 259f
    anatomy and physiology, 93–96
    deceleration injuries to, 7, 7f
    lightning strikes and, 239
    perfusion, general assessment of, 77
Brain stem, 94, 94f
Breach of duty, 277, 278
Breathing. See also Breath sounds; Respiratory patterns;
        Respiratory rate; Work of breathing
    burns and, 203
    cervical spine injuries and, 123
    difficulties, patient priority and, 37
    ear injuries and, 104
    in elderly, 261
    esophageal rupture and, 150
    initial assessment of, 31, 34–35, 34t
    initial triage assessment, 288
    mechanics of, 45f
    in obese patients, 266–267, 266f
    reassessment of, 40
Breath sounds. See also Lung sounds
    auscultation of, confirming tube placement, 51
    hemothorax and, 145
    pulmonary contusion and, 143
    tension pneumothorax and, 145
    types of, 30–31, 31t, 46–47, 46t
Bronchi, 133, 150
Bronchioles, 133
Bronchorrhea, 236
Buckle fracture, 166
Buddy splinting, 176f, 177
Bullard laryngoscope, 52
Bullet impact. See also Gunshot wounds
    injuries due to, 6
Bull's eye lesions, electrical burns and, 199, 200f
Burns
    bandaging, 371
    chemical, 100, 101f, 191, 198, 198f, 198t
    consequences of, 216

Ground ambulance, 294, 294f, 301, 304t

Gum elastic bougie (GEB) stylet, 52, 53f

Gunshot wounds
 characteristics, 19–21, 20f
 to head, 106
 hemostatic agents and hemorrhage control for, 82–83
 to male genitals, 155, 155f
 mandatory reporting of, 279
 maxillary-facial, ventilating patients with, 62
 to musculoskeletal system, 164
 myocardial rupture and, 147
 to torso, 136–137

Gurgling respirations, 30–31, 31t, 46, 46t

H

Hair follicles, 191

Hairline fractures, 165, 165f

Handguns, 19

Hand injuries, 181, 181f, 204

Hard palate, 88, 88f

Hazardous materials scenes, 29, 29f

Head. *See also* Brain; Traumatic brain injuries
 anatomy and physiology, 88–91, 88–91f
 blast injuries to, 22–23
 child vs. adult size of, 248, 248f
 deceleration injuries to, 7, 7f
 injuries in elderly to, 260
 injury with altered LOC, 293
 signs and symptoms of injuries to, 112t
 skull fractures, 107–108, 107–108f
 soft-tissue injuries to, 106, 106f
 up-and-over pathway, motor vehicle injuries and, 11

Headache, 112, 112t

Head and neck trauma
 anatomy and physiology, 88–96
 anterior neck, 117–119
 cervical spine, 119–128
 ear injuries, 104–105
 eye injuries, 99–104
 face injuries, 96–99
 head injuries, 106–108
 oral and dental injuries, 105–106
 traumatic brain injuries, 108–117

Head-on motorcycle collisions, 15–16

Head-on motor vehicle collisions, 6f, 10t

Head tiltňchin lift maneuver, 98, 123

Hearing. *See also* Ears
 ruptured eardrum and, 104

Heart. *See also* Pulse
 anatomy and physiology, 133
 hypertrophies, in elderly, 258
 perfusion, general assessment of, 78
 role in cardiovascular system, 68

Heat. *See also* Heat emergencies
 body temperature regulation and, 222, 223f
 eye burns and, 100, 101f, 191
 pain control and, 175

Heat cramps, 226–227, 227f, 230t

Heat edema, 226, 230t

Heat emergencies
 characteristics, 224
 general management, 225–226
 heat cramps, 226–227, 227f
 heat edema, 226
 heat exhaustion, 228
 heat stroke, 228–230, 229t
 heat syncope, 227–228, 227f
 incidence, 224
 pathophysiology, 225
 signs, symptoms, and treatment, 230t

Heat exchange, 220–222

Heat exhaustion, 228, 230t

Heat production, 220, 222

Heat stroke, 228–230, 229t, 230t

Heat syncope, 227–228, 227f, 230t

Height, of falls, 17–18, 17f

Helicopters, 294, 294f, 301, 304t, 316. *See also* Air ambulances

Helmets, sports
 cervical spine immobilization and, 126, 127f
 removal procedures, 358–359

M

Macintosh laryngoscope blades, 51
Major vessels. *See* Arteries, major; Veins, major
Male genital injuries, 155, 155*f*, 156
Mallet finger, 181, 181*f*
Malpractice claims, 277–278
Mandatory reporting, 279, 279*f*
Mandible
    fractures, 96–97, 97*f*, 98*t*
    stabilization, 99
    structure, 89
MASS (Move, Assess, Sort, and Send) triage
    system, 285
Mass, in physics of injury, 5
Mass casualty incidents (MCIs), 284
Mass casualty triage, 284, 284*f*
Mastication, 93
Maxillary-facial trauma
    fractures, 97, 97*f*, 98*t*
    ventilating patients with, 61–62, 62*f*
Mean arterial pressure (MAP), 109
Mechanical energy, 4, 5
Mechanism of injury (MOI)
    assessment of, 6, 30
    for bladder injuries, 153
    for cervical spine injuries, 125–126
    in elderly, 261
    for eye injuries, 101
    life-threatening, 38–39
    for motor vehicle collisions, 10*t*
    for musculoskeletal injuries, 160, 163–164, 164*f*
    for oral injuries, 105
    for torso injuries, 136–137
Mechanism of trauma for triaging patients to trauma
    center, 291*t*, 293
Medial collateral ligament (MCL), 183
Mediastinitis, 118
Mediastinum, 133
    tension pneumothorax and, 76*f*, 144

Medical history. *See also* Focused history and physical
    exam; History of present injury; SAMPLE history
    burns and, 207
    for elderly patients, 261
    focused, cervical spine injuries and, 124
    musculoskeletal injuries and, 171
    previous, head injuries and, 115
Medications. *See also specific conditions*
    body temperature regulation and, 222, 223*t*
    cold emergencies and, 237
    elderly patients and, 261
    in obese patients, 268
    online medical control vs. standing orders for, 32
    for pain control, 175
    shock assessment and, 80
Medulla, 94
Memory loss, 241–242. *See also* Amnesia
Meninges, 95–96, 96*f*
Meniscus, 183
Mental Capacity Act, U.K., 273
Mental status. *See also* Level of consciousness
    altered, patient priority and, 37
    altered, shock and, 71
    body temperature regulation and, 224
    burns and, 203
    cervical spine injuries and, 123, 126
    generalized hypothermia and, 236
    initial assessment of, 36–37, 36*t*
    reassessment of, 40
Mesentery, 135, 136
Metabolic acidosis, 307
Metabolic alkalosis, 307
Metabolic rate, 222
Metacarpal bones, 161, 180–181, 180*f*
Methemoglobin (metHb), 58
Midbrain, 94, 94*f*
Mild diffuse axonal injuries, 110, 110*t*
Miller laryngoscope blades, 51
Minimal or no response to fluid therapy, 81

Minors
consent to treatment issues for, 272
unaccompanied by parents, treatment of, 274–275
Minute volume. *See also* Ventilation
high respiratory rate vs. low respiratory rate, 58, 58*t*
as measure of breathing adequacy, 31, 34, 34*t*
Miscellaneous blast injuries, 21, 21*f*
Mnemonics
AVPU, of level of consciousness, 36
CHILD ABUSE, 251, 252*t*
LOAD, for premedication agents, 53, 54*t*
OLDEST, for burn assessment, 207
OPQRST, for pain assessment, 171
TICLS, of appearance in children, 253, 253*t*
Moderate diffuse axonal injuries, 110, 110*t*
Monro-Kellie doctrine, 109
Morgan Lens, 214, 214*f*
Motorcycle collisions
characteristics and types, 15–16, 15*f*, 16*f*
triaging patients taken to trauma center and, 293
Motor function exam, musculoskeletal injuries and, 172–173, 173*f*
Motor vehicle collisions. *See also* Blunt trauma; Child safety seats
air bag abrasions in, 14*f*
cerebral concussion and, 110
children and, 251
describing damaged area of vehicle, 9*f*
diffuse axonal injuries and, 110
elderly and, 259, 260, 260*f*
frontal impact, 6*f*, 10–11, 10–12*f*
high-risk, triaging patients taken to trauma center and, 293
lateral impact, 12, 13*f*
as leading cause of death from trauma, 4
mechanism of injury in, 9, 10*t*
patient assessment, 39–40
phases of, 8–9, 9*f*
physics of injury due to, 5
predicting types of injury in, 9*f*, 10

primary traumatic brain injuries and, 108, 108*f*
rapid extrication from, procedure for, 360–362
rear impact, 6*f*, 13, 13*f*
restrained vs. unrestrained occupants in, 11*f*, 14
rollover, 14, 14*f*
rotational impact, 13, 13*f*
side impact, 6*f*
statistics, 9
unique patient populations, 14–15
Mouth
anatomy and physiology, 93
soft-tissue injuries to, 105, 105*f*
Move, Assess, Sort, and Send (MASS) triage system, 285
Mucopolysaccharide gel, 191
Multiple injuries. *See also* Mass casualty triage
patient priority and, 37
Multisystem injuries. *See also* Life-threatening injuries
burns and, 202, 202*f*, 208
heat syncope and, 227
lightning strikes and, 242
maxillary-facial, ventilating patients with, 62
musculoskeletal, 171
pelvic fractures and, 154
single system trauma vs., 38–39, 38*f*
Muscles
electricity and injuries to, 200
injuries to, 167, 170
intercostal, dorsal nerves and, 135
intercostal, flail segments and, 142
lightning strikes and, 240
neck, 91–92, 92*f*
skeletal, 162
Musculoskeletal injuries. *See also* Extremities
assessment and management, 171–177
in elderly, 261
fractures and, 166, 166*f*
ligament injuries and dislocations, 167
mechanism of, 163–164, 164*f*
muscle and tendon, 167, 170, 170*f*
vascular, 170, 170*f*

procedure, 323–325

of torso, 137

Rear impact motor vehicle collisions

direction of force and injuries in, 6*f*

mechanism of injury in, 10*t*, 13

Reassessment, 40

Rebound tenderness, 138–139

Recruitment, 163

Red flag or tag, for triage, 286, 286*f*

Reduced hemoglobin (RHb), 58

Referrals, to burn specialty centers, 216

Referred pain, 136

Refusal of treatment or transport, 273, 276

Renal system. *See also* Kidneys

in elderly, 259

Renin-angiotensinaldosterone system (RAAS), 225

Residual volume, 258

Respiration, 45–46, 46*f*

Respiratory acidosis, 307

Respiratory alkalosis, 307

Respiratory arrest, lightning strikes and, 242

Respiratory patterns

cold emergencies and, 232

generalized hypothermia and, 236

head injuries and, 112, 112*t*, 113, 113*f*

lightning strikes and assessment of, 242*t*

Respiratory rate

acid-base balance in shock and, 78, 78*f*

initial assessment of, 31, 34–35, 34*t*

in pregnant women, 265

in trauma airway assessment, 47

Respiratory system. *See also* Airway

in elderly, 258

in obese patients, 266–267

in pregnant women, 262–263

Restraint asphyxia, 151

Retina, 92, 93*f*

detachment of, 100

Retroauricular ecchymosis, 107, 108*f*

Retrograde amnesia, 110, 112*t*. *See also* Amnesia

Retrograde endotracheal intubation (REI), 53

Retroperitoneal space or area

anatomy and physiology, 135

initial assessment of bleeding in, 36

Reverse triage, 242

Revised trauma score (RTS), triaging patients taken to

trauma center and, 292, 292*t*

Rhabdomyolysis, 54, 228–229

Rib fractures and flail segment, 136, 137*f*, 142

Rifles, 19

Rigid splints, 176, 176*f*

Rocking motion, of laryngoscope, 51, 51*f*

Rollovers, motor vehicle, 14

Rotary-wing aircraft, 294, 294*f*, 301, 304*t*

Rotational impact motor vehicle collisions, 13, 13*f*

Rotation with flexion, of cervical spine, 119

Rule of Nines, 205, 206*f*

Rule of Palms, 205

S

Sacco Triage Method, 285

Sacrum, 135–136, 135*f*

Saddle injuries, 154

Saddle joint, 161

Safety. *See also* Scene safety

aircraft, 316, 316*f*

SALT (Sort, Assess, Lifesaving interventions, and

Treatment and/or Transport) triage system, 285

SAMPLE history. *See also* Focused history and physical

exam; History of present injury; Medical history

for elderly patients, 261

in initial assessment, 39

medications and facial injury, 99

musculoskeletal injuries and, 171

SAM sling, 155

San Diego RSI Trial, 56

Scald burns, 192–193, 192*f*, 193*t*

Scalp, 89*f*

soft-tissue injuries to, 106, 106*f*, 112*t*

Scapula, 160

fractures, 178–179

Credits

Chapter 1

1-1 © Rob Vomund/Dreamstime.com; 1-2 © Craig McAteer/Dreamstime.com; 1-3A © Mrreporter/Dreamstime.com; 1-3B Courtesy of Mark Woolcock; 1-3C © Crystalcraig/Dreamstime.com; 1-4B © Custom Medical Stock Photo; 1-10 © Bsauter/Dreamstime.com; 1-11 © Dan Myers; 1-12 Courtesy of Captain David Jackson, Saginaw Township Fire Department; 1-16 © Lisa F. Young/ShutterStock, Inc; 1-17 © Dennis Wetherhold, Jr; 1-20 © Péter Gudella/Dreamstime.com; 1-22 © Robert Convery/Alamy Images; 1-27 © D. Willoughby/Custom Medical Stock Photo; 1-29A © Chuck Stewart, MD; 1-29B © D. Willoughby/Custom Medical Stock Photography; 1-31 Courtesy of the National Nuclear Security Administration/Nevada Site Office; 1-33 Courtesy of Sgt. Ezekiel R. Kitandwe/U.S. Navy.

Chapter 2

Opener © Stringer Thailand/Reuters; 2-3 © Adam Alberti/NJFirePictures.com; 2-4 © Glen E. Ellman; 2-5 Courtesy of PA3 Brent Erb/U.S. Coast Guard; 2-7 © Scott Downs/Dreamstime.com; 2-8 © Michael Donne/Photo Researchers, Inc; 2-12 Courtesy of ED, Royal North Shore Hospital/NSW Institute of Trauma & Injury; 2-13 © Carolina K. Smith, MD/ShutterStock, Inc.

Chapter 3

Opener © Mark C. Ide; 3-10B, 3-10C © LMA North America, Inc; 3-12 © King Systems; 3-13 Courtesy of Dr. David Alfery/Pulmodyne, Inc.

Chapter 4

Opener © Mark C. Ide.

Chapter 5

5-15 Courtesy of Rhonda Beck; 5-16 Courtesy of Joseph Shiber, MD; 5-31A&B Courtesy of www.DrMomOtoscope.com; 5-32 © E.M. Singletary, MD. Used with permission; 5-46 Courtesy of ED, Royal North Shore Hospital/NSW Institute of Trauma and Injury Management; 5-47 © M. English, MD/Custom Medical Stock Photo; 5-48 © E.M. Singletary, MD. Used with permission; 5-55 © Doug Steley B/Alamy Images.

Chapter 6

Opener © M. English, MD/Custom Medical Stock Photo; 6-13 © Custom Medical Stock Photo; 6-21 © SIU Bio Med Comm./Custom Medical Stock Photo; 6-23 © Chuck Stewart, MD; 6-28A&B Courtesy of ED, Royal North Shore Hospital/NSW Institute of Trauma and Injury Management; 6-29 © Sam Medical Products®; 6-30 © Chuck Stewart, MD.

Chapter 7

Opener © Mark C. Ide; 7-15 Courtesy of London Ambulance Service; 7-16 © Chuck Stewart, MD; 7-26A Courtesy of Heidi Gable (http://www.imageinterpretation.co.uk) and the Norfolk and Norwich University Hospital NHS Foundation Trust; 7-26B Courtesy of Eugene Ko; 7-27 © Custom Medical Stock Photo.

Chapter 8

Opener © Siphiwe Sibeko/Reuters/Landov; 8-3 © J.Yakwichuk/Custom Medical Stock Photo; 8-4 Courtesy of Health Resources and Services Administration, Maternal and Child Health Bureau, Emergency Services for Children Program; 8-5A Courtesy of Lynn Douglas Mouden, DDS, MPH, FIDC, FACD; 8-5B © Shout Pictures/Custom Medical Stock Photo; 8-5C © Chuck Stewart, MD; 8-5D © Bubbles Photolibrary/Alamy Images; 8-5E Courtesy of Ronald L. Deickmann, MD; 8-6 © Kevin Frayer/AP Photos; 8-8 Courtesy of Captain David Jackson, Saginaw Township Fire Department; 8-9 Image of Masimo® Rad-57™ Pulse CO-Oximeter™ is © 2008 Masimo Corporation. All rights reserved. Masimo, Rad-57, and Pulse CO-Oximeter are trademarks of Masimo Corporation; 8-11 © Lisa F. Young/ShutterStock, Inc; 8-12 © Chuck Stewart, MD; 8-13A © E.M. Singletary, MD. Used with permission; 8-13B Courtesy of ED, Royal North Shore Hospital/NSW Institute of Trauma and Injury Management; 8-13C © E.M. Singletary, MD. Used with permission; 8-14A&B © Chuck Stewart, MD; 8-16 © Glen E. Ellman; 8-17 Courtesy of Captain David Jackson, Saginaw Township Fire Department; 8-19B © Amy Walters/ShutterStock, Inc; 8-19C © E.M. Singletary, MD. Used with permission; 8-22 © Guy Croft/Alamy Images; 8-24 © Photofusion Picture Library/Alamy Images; 8-26 © avatra images/Alamy Images; 8-28 Courtesy of MorTan, Inc.

Chapter 9

Opener © Becky Burch, Bartlesville Examiner-Enterprise/AP Photos; 9-2 Courtesy of NWS/NOAA; 9-3 © Jim Cole/AP Photos; 9-4 © Jawwa/Dreamstime.com; 9-9 © Glen E. Ellman; 9-10 © Mark C. Ide; 9-11 From 12-Lead ECG: The Art of Interpretation, courtesy of Tomas B. Garcia, MD; 9-13 Courtesy of Megan T. Guffey; 9-16A Courtesy of Neil Malcom Winkelmann; 9-16B, C&D Courtesy of Dr. Jack Poland/CDC; 9-17 © Andy Barrand, The Herald Republican/AP Photos; 9-19 © AbleStock; 9-20 © Chuck Stewart, MD; 9-21 © E.M. Singletary, MD. Used with permission.

Chapter 10

Opener © Mark C. Ide; 10-1 © Glen E. Ellman; 10-2 Courtesy of Marianne Gausche-Hill, MD, FACEP, FAAP; 10-4 © Sean Clarkson/Alamy Images; 10-5 Courtesy of Ronald A. Dieckmann, MD; 10-6 © John Curtis/age fotostock; 10-7 © Juilya W. Shumskaya/ShutterStock, Inc; 10-8 © Suzanne Tucker/ShutterStock, Inc; 10-10 © Mark C. Ide; 10-14 © Bengt-Goran Carlsson/age foto-stock; 10-15 © 2007 Dan Koester; 10-20 Courtesy of Dr. George Russell; 10-21, 10-22 © Mark C. Ide.

Chapter 11

Opener © Mark C. Ide; 11-1 © Mark C. Ide; 11-3 © Brand X Pictures/Creatas; 11-5 Courtesy of Ronald A. Dieckmann, MD.

Chapter 12

Opener © Mark C. Ide; 12-1 © Robert Robertsson/Reuters/Landov; 12-2 © Andrew Stuart/AP Photos; 12-4 Courtesy of Captain David Jackson, Saginaw Township Fire Department; 12-6 Courtesy of Journalist 1st Class Mark D. Faram/U.S. Navy; 12-7 © Photodisc; 12-8 © MIEMSS. Used with permission.

Chapter 13

Opener © Mark C. Ide; 13-1 © Index Stock Images, Inc/Alamy Images; 13-2A&B From 12-Lead ECG: The Art of Interpretation, courtesy of Tomas B. Garcia, MD.

Procedures

Page 321 (top) © Robert Brenner/PhotoEdit, Inc; Page 327 (bottom right) Courtesy of Dr. Ken Harrison, Careflight/NSW Institute of Trauma & Injury Management; Page 328 © Glen E. Ellman; Page 380 EMS facility courtesy of St. Charles County Ambulance District, Missouri, © Ray Kemp/911 Imaging.

Unless otherwise indicated, all photographs and illustrations are under copyright of Jones and Bartlett Publishers, LLC, courtesy of Maryland Institute for Emergency Medical Services Systems, the American Academy of Orthopaedic Surgeons, or have been provided by the authors.